Community Mental Health

A General Introduction

Second Edition

Community Mental Health

A General Introduction

Second Edition

Bernard L. Bloom
University of Colorado

Brooks/Cole Publishing Company
Monterey, California

Brooks/Cole Publishing Company
A Division of Wadsworth, Inc.

Printed in the United States of America

10 9 8 7 6 5 4 3

Library of Congress Cataloging in Publication Data

Bloom, Bernard L., [date]
Community mental health.

Bibliography: p.
Includes indexes.
1. Community mental health services—United States.
I. Title. [DNLM: 1. Community mental health services—
United States. 2. Crisis intervention. WM 30 B655ca]
RA790.6.B62 1983   362.2'0425   83-2841
ISBN 0-534-01408-9

Subject Editor: *Claire Verduin*
Production Editor: *Richard Mason*
Manuscript Editor: *Rephah Berg*
Permissions Editor: *Carline Haga*
Art Coordinator: *Judy Macdonald*
Interior and Cover Design: *Vernon T. Boes*
Cover Illustration: *Lee Phillips*
Typesetting: *Graphic Typesetting Service, Los Angeles, California*

We are each embedded in a community. If we are fortunate, that community provides us with excitement, joy, support, comfort, and strength. I am grateful beyond measure to my first community, my late parents, Lucy and Morris Bloom. As young people, they each left their homes in Poland and found a new life in America. They infused in me an enormous respect, and yet a kind of permanent sadness, for the courage they showed in leaving their families behind, nearly all of whom later perished in the Holocaust.

I want also to acknowledge my wonderful community of today and to thank its most important members—my wife, Joan, and our children, Claire, Paula and Tom, Jaye and John, Deeda, Tracy and Dan, Peter, and Missi. They fill my life to overflowing.

PREFACE

This volume is designed to provide a comprehensive overview of the rapidly expanding field of community mental health. I believe that upper-division and graduate students in social work, psychology, psychiatry, psychiatric nursing, and public health can profit from this treatment of a subject that concerns both clinically and socially oriented professionals.

In the six years since the first edition of this book, the field of community mental health has coalesced around three important themes: community mental health as a set of innovative alternatives to traditional mental health services; community mental health as those activities involved in the prevention of mental disorders; and community mental health as a field concerned with community change.

This second edition reflects that thematic coherence. After an initial part dealing with the development of community mental health as social policy, the following parts deal with the three aforementioned themes. In addition, three new chapters appear in this edition. A chapter on planned short-term therapy (Chapter 2) will be found in the section on alternatives to traditional mental health services. A chapter on stressful life-event theory (Chapter 6) and one on mental health education (Chapter 7) will be found in the section on prevention. In addition, other chapters have been revised and brought up to date.

The field of community mental health is incomparably richer, both in its conceptualizations and in its empirical base, than five years ago. At the same time, there is far less ideological evangelism and far less exhortation. The field is now reasonably well established. Research and practice are developing, sometimes synergistically, sometimes unevenly and independently, but unquestionably developing. I hope this new edition captures that growth.

I want to express my appreciation to those publishers who allowed me to draw on material that previously appeared in their pages—the American Psychological Association, the *Community Mental Health Journal*, Human Sciences Press, the *Annual Review of Psychology*, Guilford Press, and *Multivariate Behavioral Research*. I also want to thank Debbie Casselman, Lisa Frey, Stephen Goldston, Konnie Kindle, Wil Miles, and Jim Wanstrath for their critical reviews of portions of the manuscript, and Dr. William B. Davidson, University of South Carolina, Aiken; Professor Rose C. Dilday, Emory University; Dr. M. Virginia Frazier, California State University, Chico; Dr. Charles J. Holahan, University of Texas; and Dr. Connie Cole Savage, Cheyney State College, for their very useful critical reading of the entire manuscript.

Finally, I want to express special gratitude to Lisa De Hope, who managed, with unfailing good humor, to do the hundreds of things that needed doing during the final preparation of this manuscript. She found books and journal articles in libraries all over this part of the country, helped with proofreading and with putting the references together, and gave up countless hours to make sure that this project came to a successful conclusion.

Bernard L. Bloom

CONTENTS

Community Mental Health

A General Introduction

Second Edition

1

Development of the Community Mental Health Movement

The chapter that follows presents an overview of the origins, social context, and legislative and political history of the field of community mental health. In addition, because the community mental health movement developed out of a conscious social policy, the chapter outlines that policy and discusses some of the major questions that have been raised regarding its validity.

1

Community
Mental Health:
Domain, History,
and Critique

So much has happened since the inauguration of the community mental health movement in the United States that it is hard to believe that it took place as recently as 1963: one can date the inception of the movement to the enactment of Public Law 88–164 (the Mental Retardation Facilities and Community Mental Health Centers Construction Act of 1963) by the United States Congress on October 31, 1963. Actually, however, the community mental health movement has a much longer history. Before outlining the historical antecedents of that movement and showing how it is woven into a broad social fabric, I will introduce the concept of community mental health.

THE CONCEPT OF COMMUNITY MENTAL HEALTH

As the term suggests, *community mental health* refers to all activities undertaken in the community in the name of mental health. Thus, the first characteristic that distinguishes community mental health from more traditional mental-health-related activities is its emphasis on practice in the community, as opposed to practice in institutional settings.

A second characteristic of this orientation is its emphasis on a total community or population rather than on individuals. The term *catchment area* or, more recently, *mental health service area* is used to describe the population of concern to a particular community mental health program. A third dimension is its emphasis on disease-preventive and health-promotive services, as distinguished from therapeutic services. These second and third distinguishing features of the community mental health orientation together represent the application of public health concepts to the field of psychopathology.

A fourth characteristic of the community mental health approach is its emphasis on continuity and comprehensiveness of services. A community mental health program should be a *system* of services with easy flow of patients among its component parts. In addition, a program should meet the full spectrum of mental health needs in the community.

A fifth characteristic is its emphasis on indirect rather than direct services. One indirect service is consultation, in which a mental health professional attempts to make a significant intervention in the lives of a group of people by working with persons who have access to that group, such as teachers, religious leaders, or public health nurses, rather than directly with the group's members. Another indirect service is mental health education, in which mental health professionals, often using the mass media, reach large numbers of people, without seeing them face to face, in order to improve their psychological well-being.

A sixth characteristic is the movement's emphasis on innovative clinical strategies designed to meet the mental health needs of larger numbers of people more promptly, more effectively, and more efficiently than has previously been possible. Of all the approaches used in meeting these objectives, the most effective have been planned short-term therapy and crisis intervention.

A seventh characteristic of the community mental health orientation is its emphasis on a process of thoughtful and realistic planning of mental health programs. Such planning often includes doing demographic analyses of the community being served, specifying unmet mental health needs, identifying populations within the community that run a particularly high risk of developing mental illnesses, coordinating mental health services in a community, and setting priorities for dealing with problems directly or indirectly related to emotional disturbances.

An eighth characteristic is the tapping of new sources of personnel. Rather than viewing the traditional professions of psychiatry, social work, psychiatric nursing, and clinical psychology as the only legitimate sources of mental health center staff, the community mental health orientation seeks to create new types of staff. Such terms as *paraprofessional* and *indigenous mental health worker* have been coined to describe these new colleagues in the community mental health center. These new staff members have less formal training than the traditional mental health professionals but are able to draw on their own skills and life experiences to play useful therapeutic roles in the mental health center.

A ninth characteristic of the community mental health movement is its commitment to what is usually called *community control* or *community involvement*. These terms signify that the mental health professional is not considered the sole source of information about the mental health needs of the community uı the best ways to meet these needs. Rather, the staff of a community mental health center is expected to join with the community to identify needs, propose and evaluate programs to meet these needs, and plan for future program developments. The concept of community control suggests that a community mental health center operates *with* the community and *on behalf of* the community.

A final characteristic of the community mental health orientation is its interest in identifying sources of stress within the community, rather than continuing the traditional assumption that psychopathology originates within the person, lodges within the person, and can be reduced only by effecting changes in the person.

Each of these attributes of the community mental health approach is a response to dissatisfaction with some feature of traditional mental health activities. In the view of many mental health professionals, traditional mental health services—

- have erred in being divorced from the communities where their clients live;
- have been concerned too much with those individuals who find their way to the clinician and too little with the population as a whole—the community's poor as well as its more affluent, its old as well as its young, and its full spectrum of races and ethnic groups;
- have focused almost exclusively on the *treatment* of psychopathology and so have failed to devote adequate resources to activities that might *prevent* certain forms of psychopathology or promote mental health;
- have failed to provide an organized and coordinated *system* of services that meet the community's mental health needs;
- in their almost exclusive emphasis on direct services, have neglected to develop programs for helping other agencies and persons, such as schools, the clergy, public health nurses, or social welfare organizations, to work more effectively with their clients;
- have emphasized long-term therapy to the exclusion of briefer therapeutic strategies that might help greater numbers of clients;
- have not made adequate use of nontraditional sources of personnel;
- have neglected to assess the community's needs in developing mental health services; and
- have failed to identify those community characteristics that enhance or inhibit growth and development and to seek to change stress-producing aspects of the community. (The newly emerging field of community psychology is concerned mainly with strategies of community change. The last chapter provides an introductory view of this field.)

Thus, in an overall sense, community mental health is a point of view. It asserts that mental health services should be available when and where needed, that such services will be more effective if integrated with other human services, and that it would be well to allocate resources to enhance the positive as well as to reduce the negative effects of life experiences. Gonzales, Hays, Bond, and Kelly (in press), reviewing the early conceptions and goals of the community mental health movement, note that

> personal distress was explicitly recognized as a transaction between intrapsychic and interpersonal conditions of the individual *and* qualities of the social environment. By explicitly expressing a public health focus, a new thesis was proclaimed, presenting an alternative approach to understanding and alleviating personal distress, e.g., mental illness could be treated by community services serving populations as well as individuals. Attention to environmental factors [was] included within the definition of mental health care along with individual and small group treatment approaches.

HISTORICAL ANTECEDENTS OF THE
COMMUNITY MENTAL HEALTH MOVEMENT

Two separate historical traditions—one based in mental institutions and the other based in the community—came together shortly after World War II to provide early direction to the community mental health movement.

Throughout history, each major theory of psychopathology has been accompanied by at least one proposal for treatment. The oldest view of psychopathology—that psychiatric disorders arise from the supernatural and that psychiatric patients have been invaded by evil spirits and thus have become evil themselves—brought with it such "treatments" as trephining (cutting a section out of the skull to let the evil spirits escape), beating, burning, or other forms of punishment to drive out the spirits, and exorcism or prayer involving pleading with the spirits to leave the patient. Counteracting this early view, called *demonology,* were the views of Hippocrates and other Greek physicians of the pre-Christian era, who held that mental disorder is a disease process no different from any other disease process, that its origin is thus natural rather than supernatural, and that its treatment should therefore be in the hands of physicians rather than priests. Although the Hippocratic view was an advance over earlier views of the origin of psychopathology, treatments were not necessarily any more humane, and for a thousand years or more the treatments of choice for psychiatric disorders were often just as depletive in character as the treatments for other diseases—purging, bleeding, blistering, and giving drugs to make the patient vomit. The debate raged then, as it continues to do, over whether the psychiatric patient is sick or evil and whether psychopathology is fundamentally a disorder of the body or a disorder of the spirit.

In contrast to those who favored depletive, weakening treatments for diseases, both mental and physical, was a movement whose proponents advocated restorative or strengthening treatments such as bed rest, a cheerful environment, and good nutrition. This new outlook on psychiatric disorders was endorsed by both clergymen and physicians—by persons who believed psychiatric disorders were diseases of the spirit and by those who believed they were diseases of the body. Thus the notion of the *retreat*—a place where troubled persons could go to escape the psychological rigors of their world—was developed by the clergy, while the hospital came to serve the same function in the hands of physicians, particularly during the brief period that came to be known as the era of *moral treatment* (Bockoven, 1963; Dain, 1964).

Development of psychiatric hospitals

Until perhaps 100 years ago, patients who could afford the best medical care available were treated in their homes, while the poor were treated in hospitals, which were originally run by religious orders. This practice was true of psychiatric patients as well. The oldest mental hospital functioning today was started in Valencia, Spain, in 1409 (Andriola & Cata, 1969). The hospital staff held many of the values held by mental hospital workers today. Voluntary admissions were encouraged, and patients were discharged as soon as they were well enough to function in society. Efforts were made to protect as well as treat hospitalized patients and to avoid isolating them from their communities. Between the 15th and 19th centuries, many more hospitals were built in Europe, but the tradition begun in Spain of linking psychiatric hospitals to the community was interrupted.

During the first half of the 19th century, few facilities existed in the United States for the humane treatment of the mentally ill. Those that did exist were privately operated and tended to serve psychiatric patients who were able to pay. The vast majority of psychiatric patients, unable to afford private care, were "treated" in their home communities, together with the physically sick, the poor, the aged, the mentally retarded, and the neglected (see Deutsch, 1949). Some of these "patients" were cared for in their homes. In some communities they were auctioned off; in other communities a contract was made with a single person who, for a fixed fee, agreed to provide care. Finally, some were lodged in prisons or poorhouses, which were usually supported by the local community.

The state-hospital movement began as a protest against these scandalously poor community programs, and the name of Dorothea Dix is permanently identified with this movement (see, for example, Goshen, 1967, pp. 501–504). Going to teach Sunday school in a Massachusetts jail one Sunday in 1841, she was shocked at the conditions and at the fact that there were many obviously mentally disturbed patients among the inmates. She began a long crusade that led to the development of mental hospitals supported by state funds. Before her career ended, 32 state mental hospitals had been built in the United States, care of the mentally ill had been removed from the local community, and the professional orientation toward the insane had been changed from seeing them as no different from paupers or criminals to seeing them as sick people in need of hospital care.

During the early days of state mental hospitals, efforts were made to pattern their programs after the few privately operated psychiatric hospitals then in existence in the United States. In 1842 Charles Dickens visited what is now the Boston State Hospital and reported on his experiences.

> The State Hospital for the insane [is] admirably conducted on those enlightened principles of conciliation and kindness which twenty years ago would have been worse than heretical. . . . The patients . . . work, read, play at skittles, and other games; and when the weather does not admit of their taking exercises out of doors, pass the day together. . . . Every patient in this asylum sits down to dinner every day with a knife and fork; and in the midst of them sits [the superintendent]. . . . At every meal, moral influence alone restrains the more violent among them from cutting the throats of the rest; but the effect of that influence is reduced to an absolute certainty, and is found, even as a means of restraint, to say nothing of it as a means of cure, a hundred times more efficacious than all the strait-waistcoats, fetters, and handcuffs, that ignorance, prejudice, and cruelty have manufactured since the creation of the world. . . . In the labour department, every patient is as freely trusted with the tools of his trade as if he were a sane man. In the garden, and on the farm, they work with spades, rakes, and hoes. For amuse-ment, they walk, run, fish, paint, read, and ride out to take the air in carriages provided for the purpose. They have among themselves a sewing society to make clothes for the poor, which holds meetings, passes resolutions, never comes to fisticuffs or bowie-knives as sane assemblies have been known to do elsewhere; and conducts all its proceedings with the greatest decorum. . . . They are cheerful, tranquil, and healthy. . . . Once a week they have a ball, in which the Doctor and his family, with all the nurses and attendants, take an active part. . . . Immense politeness and good-breeding are observed throughout. . . . one great feature of this system is the inculcation and encouragement, even among such unhappy persons, of a decent self-respect [1842, pp. 105–111].

Rise and fall of moral treatment

The private hospitals founded in the United States in the late 18th and early 19th centuries were influenced in large measure by European experiences that had shown that humane treatment was not only more satisfying to admin-ister but more effective than the chains, purging, and bloodletting of earlier years. The most influential European was the French psychiatrist Philippe Pinel, superintendent of two Parisian psychiatric hospitals. Serving as what is now called a role model, he set an example of how patients should behave. He was inspired to do this by a mental hospital director who taught him about the curability of insanity. In 1806 Pinel wrote:

> Forgetting the empty honours of my titular distinction as a physician, I viewed the scene that was opened to me with the eyes of common sense and unprejudiced observation. I saw a great number of maniacs assembled together, and submitted to a regular system of discipline. Their disorders presented an endless variety of character: but their discordant movements were regulated . . . by the greatest possible skill, and even extravagance and disorder were marshalled into order

and harmony. I then discovered, that insanity was curable in many instances, by mildness of treatment and attention to the state of the mind exclusively, and when coercion was indispensable, that it might be very effectually applied without corporal indignity. . . . I saw, with wonder, the resources of nature when left to herself, or skilfully assisted in her efforts. . . . Attention to these principles alone will, frequently, not only lay the foundation of, but complete a cure: while neglect of them may exasperate each succeeding paroxysm, till, at length, the disease becomes established, continued in its form, and incurable. The successful application of moral regimen exclusively, gives great weight to the supposition, that, in a majority of instances, there is no organic lesion of the brain [Pinel, 1962, pp. 5, 108–109; see also Joint Commission on Mental Illness and Health, 1961, pp. 28–32, and Ewalt & Ewalt, 1969].

In 1813 Samuel Tuke, the British physician who directed the York Retreat, founded by his grandfather some years earlier, described the rationale of moral treatment by noting that "most insane persons, have a considerable degree of self command; and . . . the employment and cultivation of this remaining power, is found to be attended with the most salutary effects" (Goshen, 1967, p. 494). Writing in 1866, Seguin noted that

long before physicians had conceived the plan of correcting the false ideas and feelings of a lunatic by purgatives, or the cranial depressions of an idiot by bleeding, Spain had produced several generations of monks who treated with the greatest success all kinds of mental diseases without drugs, by moral training alone. Certain regular labors, the performance of simple and assiduous duties, an enlightened and sovereign volition, watching constantly over the patients, such were the only remedies employed [Goshen, 1967, pp. 165–166].

Reform in the care of the mentally ill, which started a century ago, was part of a larger movement in the United States whose objectives included prison reform, abolition of slavery, and women's suffrage and which reflected a growing optimism—a belief in human perfectibility rather than predestination.

Unfortunately, a series of events resulted in the virtual destruction of the moral-treatment movement during the next several decades. By the late 19th century, state mental hospitals had grown in size and number, but the quality of the treatment had so deteriorated that they were hardly better than the community programs they had been built to replace. Too little money was allocated by states for the care of the mentally ill in the new state hospitals, and not enough training programs existed to produce the number of skilled employees needed, even where money was available to hire them. In addition, a growing antagonism toward foreign-born people was developing as a consequence of the waves of immigration into the United States, and both the poor and the mentally disordered were heavily overrepresented among the foreign-born. At Worcester State Hospital in Massachusetts, the proportion of foreign-born among all admissions climbed from 10% in 1844 to 47% in 1863. Nearly half of all first admissions into Worcester State Hospital between 1893 and 1933 were foreign-born, and most of these foreign-born patients were destitute (Bockoven, 1963, p. 24). Thus, hospitals for the mentally ill became overcrowded with people for whom many Americans had little sympathy, and adequate treatment became an impossibility. At Worcester State Hospital, for example, between the 1830s and the 1870s, the average daily population was about 400, and the average length of hospitalization was about one year. By 1950 there were 2500 patients in the hospital, and the average length of hospitalization had increased to nearly five years (Bockoven, 1963, p. 23; see also Grob, 1966).

Meanwhile, the profession of psychiatry was developing as a specialty of medicine, and humane, "moral" treatment could hardly be thought of as medical in character. For psychiatrists to develop and maintain some respectability among their medical colleagues, they had to find organic causes and organic treatments. As medical schools became the loci of medical training, the psychiatrists who were interested in moral treatment found no one to replace themselves.

As a consequence of all these events, state psychiatric hospitals were not able to deliver on their promises. Recovery rates decreased and hospitals gradually filled up with chronic, virtually untreatable patients. What had started as an era of optimism regressed to belief in the notions of heredity, predisposition, organic pathology, and incurability.

The deterioration of state mental hospitals continued until after World War II. A few hospitals were unusually well staffed, but on the whole, hospitals functioned with appropriations averaging two or three dollars per patient per day. Staffs were overworked, frequently untrained, and ill paid, and little that could reasonably be called "treatment" took place. Between 1845 and 1945, the United States saw the establishment of almost 300 state mental hospitals, nearly all of which—after an initial flurry of enthusiasm and hope—quickly lapsed into vast storehouses for some of the most disabled and miserable people in the country. By 1955, on an average day, nearly 600,000 persons occupied beds in mental hospitals supported by state or county funds. Both the importance and the plight of state mental hospitals can be seen in the following figures. Of the 1,241,000 people who were patients at any time in psychiatric hospitals in the United States in 1957, including public, private, and Veterans Administration hospitals, nearly 840,000 (approximately two-thirds) were in state mental institutions. In 1960, while general medical hospitals had a daily patient cost of more than $27 and private psychiatric hospitals and psychiatric units in general hospitals expended about $17 per patient per day, daily costs in state mental institutions averaged less than $4.50 per patient. By 1976 the average daily expenditures per patient in state mental institutions had increased to $43.55 (Witkin, 1979), but general-hospital expenses per patient per day averaged $173.68 (U.S. Department of Health, Education and Welfare, 1978b). In 1971 court action had to be brought against one state before it provided proper treatment to the patients in its state hospital. The Department of Justice, in this suit, noted that placement in this state mental hospital "means not only the absence of treatment but indeed is probably and therapeutic and harmful to those unfortunate victims. . . . Treatment is still an elusive concept and is far from reality . . . and has retrogressed since the 19th century when the institution was founded. It simply does not exist for those who are unfortunate enough to be old, mentally ill, or unwanted . . . and placed by the State in its human warehouse" ("Federal Court Upholds Right to Treatment," 1972, p. 1).

Alarm at the growing failure of psychiatric institutions to provide effective care was not only based on humanitarian grounds. New symptoms that developed after hospital admission began to appear in patients with increasing frequency—symptoms that were thought to be brought about by the deficiencies in psychiatric care just described. These symptoms, grouped together under the term *social breakdown syndrome* (American Public Health Association, 1962; Gruenberg, 1980), included severe withdrawal, loss of interest in social functioning and in personal appearance, anger, assaultiveness, and personal dilapidation. The social breakdown syndrome was thought to be socially determined, a consequence of hospitalization almost regardless of initial diagnosis, and responsible for the growing chronic character of psychopathology. Because the social breakdown syndrome was thought to be the result of deficiencies in psychiatric care, changes in the organization of that care would be required before the syndrome could be controlled.

Changes in institutional psychiatric care

In the most forward-looking state mental hospitals, starting in about 1950, three developments took place that set the stage for a major shift in the orientation of mental health professionals toward institutional psychiatric care. First, the field of psychopharmacology began its current period of rapid growth with the development of new tranquilizing drugs. These drugs reduced anxiety, discomfort, and bizarre behavior in many patients, thus speeding discharge from psychiatric hospitals. Because these drugs modified the emotional components of psychiatric disorders without impairing intellectual capacities, they were far superior to the sedating drugs that had been in use until that time. Not only was recovery accelerated, but many patients were able to function in the community by continuing use of these drugs at home (see Cole & Gerard, 1959; Kolb, 1968b, pp. 574ff.; Pasamanick, Scarpitti, & Dinitz, 1967).

The second factor was the development of the philosophy of the *therapeutic community*. This orientation to psychiatric treatment grew out of the axiom that therapeutic potential resides in patients as well as staff. According to this philosophy, a democratic community composed of patients and staff working together could take advantage of this therapeutic potential and thereby increase the effectiveness of psychological treatment. The name of Maxwell Jones is most prominently associated with this movement, which began in England and Scotland under his leadership and spread rapidly to many U.S.

psychiatric hospitals (Jones, 1968). When psychiatric inpatient wards were converted into therapeutic communities, patients and staff began to share responsibility for assessing patient behavior and making recommendations for treatment planning. Patients had to justify their requests for discharge or for changes in treatment status not only to the professional staff but to their fellow patients, and with this orientation to treatment, clinical improvement appeared to be faster and longer-lasting.

The third development was geographic decentralization in large state mental hospitals; patients were placed in wards according to their place of residence before hospitalization. What started out simply as an administrative reorganization rapidly developed into the vehicle for the establishment of working relationships between the hospitals and the communities they served. Before geographic decentralization, state mental hospitals were just as functionally isolated from their communities as they were geographically isolated.

You can best appreciate the significance of geographic decentralization if you understand what it replaced. As state mental hospitals increased in size, the general pattern of administrative organization came to involve an admitting service for newly arriving patients, several acute treatment services to which most patients were transferred after initial diagnostic studies had been completed, and several chronic treatment services to which patients who had not recovered sufficiently to be discharged were transferred. Both acute and chronic treatment services were frequently organized around treatment modalities, so that there were electrical shock treatment wards, insulin treatment wards, wards for patients who had special dietary restrictions or certain physical diseases, wards for elderly patients, wards for alcoholics, and so on. The most highly trained staff members as well as the greatest number of staff members tended to work in admission and acute treatment services, while on chronic wards there were fewer personnel, particularly fewer well-trained personnel, as well as fewer amenities. An aura of hopelessness pervaded these chronic "back wards"; neither patients nor staff aspired to very much in the way of therapeutic progress, and these wards became custodial in the worst sense of the term. In most state mental hospitals, a majority of patients were lodged in these chronic treatment wards. That is, few patients recovered quickly after admission and were discharged; many were transferred to chronic treatment wards, where they remained for years, often for decades, or even for life.

The concept of geographic decentralization, or regionalization, was an attempt to break out of this administrative pattern. Patients of all degrees and types of psychopathology began to be housed according to their home communities, so that on one ward might be placed all patients from a particular city. Admission services were abolished. Newly admitted patients were sent directly to their geographic units. Hospital staff was equitably distributed across geographic units. The only exceptions to geographic decentralization were made for those patients who required such specialized services that it would be impossible to duplicate them in each geographic unit. Thus, most geographically decentralized hospitals maintained a centralized medical facility for the treatment of patients with physical diseases, and most decentralized hospitals were required to maintain separate facilities for those convicted of criminal acts. Many decentralized hospitals continued to have special treatment facilities for psychiatrically disturbed children. But in all hospitals that underwent geographic decentralization, the vast majority of patients lived in wards with their neighbors, as it were. The strong could help the weak. The community had a particular section of the hospital with which it could identify. Hospital personnel had a rationale for spending part of their time in the community from which their patients came, first in providing aftercare services and later in providing alternatives to hospitalization in collaboration with community-based agencies. And finally, decision making was decentralized; decisions about patient care came to be made at ward level rather than at higher administrative levels.

These three developments—tranquilizing drugs, the therapeutic community, and geographic decentralization—worked together to democratize the clinical decision-making process, establish closer working relationships between the hospital and the community, and lower the hospital census. The price paid for these developments, however, was a growing tendency for mental health professionals to see all psychiatric hospitalizations as undesirable. The National Institute of Mental Health funded studies to examine how hospitalization could be prevented (see Pasamanick et al., 1967, for example). State hospitals were envisioned as being converted into community mental health centers (Levy, 1965) or vocational training schools (Stewart, Lafave, Grunberg, & Herjanic, 1968). If they were to remain open to receive psychiatric patients, it was thought, they would have to be much smaller and would need to become far more integrated into the community they served than was typical (Baker, Schulberg, & O'Brien, 1969; Ozarin & Levinson, 1969).

A few authors cautioned against excessively rapid abandonment of the psychiatric hospital. Mendel (1967) noted that hospitalization may be the treatment of choice for (1) persons who are so disturbed that they cannot maintain useful relationships with therapists as outpatients, (2) persons whose impulse control is so poor that they frighten those members of their families who must care for them, (3) individuals whose psychopathology has alienated them from family and friends, who now refuse to care for them, (4) persons who are malnourished or who make excessive use of drugs, (5) persons who need to be protected against self-destructive impulses, (6) persons from whom regularly available supportive resources in the community need a brief vacation, and (7) individuals who must be removed from a pathological environment. The Committee on Therapeutic Care of the Group for the Advancement of Psychiatry, in its report *Crisis in Psychiatric Hospitalization* (Group for the Advancement of Psychiatry, 1969), emphasized the vital role of the psychiatric hospital as one point on a comprehensive continuum of psychiatric treatment and provided its own list of indications for hospitalization. More recently, Gruenberg (1974) and Rabiner and Lurie (1974) have also outlined what they believe to be the circumstances under which hospitalization may be the treatment of choice.

Thus, the complex developments that were dramatically changing the public psychiatric hospital were at the same time generating debate over how best to utilize the mental institution in a system of mental health services. Meanwhile, changes were taking place in attitudes toward community-based care.

History of community-based programs

Perhaps the earliest, and certainly the best-known, alternative to institutional care has been provided in the village of Geel, Belgium, since the 13th century (Aring, 1974). Roosens (1979, pp. 27–28) has described the historical origins of this program:

> The Geel care system originated from the cult of Saint Dympna that was celebrated in Geel. . . . as early as 1250, mentally ill people were brought to Geel to seek cures from St. Dympna. According to the legend . . . St. Dympna was the daughter of an Irish king who, after the death of his beautiful wife, fell in love with his own daughter and attempted to marry her. . . . the girl supposedly fled to Flanders in order to escape her father's incestuous passion. She was . . . caught in the Geel region. . . . she let herself be decapitated by her father . . . rather than submit to his dishonorable and repulsive demands. . . . St. Dympna became the patron of the mentally ill and their cure because, by her heroic death, she defeated the evil spirit that had entered into her father to drive him into a rage and madness. As madness was attributed to possession by some evil spirit, the cult of St. Dympna becomes clear.

Until 1800 the therapy for the mentally ill arriving in Geel was under the control of the church and consisted primarily of religious rites and exorcisms. Because of the large numbers of pilgrims to Geel, the church appealed to the community to house them. The boarding system began when these pilgrims were taken into host families and chose to remain there. Perhaps 200 such mentally ill persons were housed in Geel in 1800. Their number increased to over 900 by 1850, about 2000 in 1900, and a peak of 3736 in 1938. Since that time, it has steadily decreased. As of January 1, 1975, 1256 persons lived with about 1000 host families among the 30,000 inhabitants of Geel. The program was no longer the responsibility of the church, however, having become part of the Department of Hospitals of the Belgian Ministry of Public Health and the Family. An additional 259 persons were hospitalized in the state psychiatric hospital in Geel.

Close and interdependent relationships exist between the inpatient psychiatric hospital and the family care program. On an average day, two or three persons are transferred between these two care systems. All new people are admitted to the state psychiatric hospital, and those transferred to the family care program must first spend a period of observation in the hospital. A hospital brochure describes as follows the life of the person in the family care program:

> The patient stays with the foster family. He has his own room and lives his daily life in the family environment. As much as possible he is involved in all the family activities, meals, work, recreation, social relations. In other words he is truly integrated in the new family environment. According to his capabilities and the situation of the foster family he is included in the business of the foster family (farming or commerce) or in the household activities. Some patients fix a few things for neighbors, family or friends of the foster family, others do odd jobs, errands etc. Patients in family care enjoy a great degree of independence and freedom and can enjoy whatever Geel has to offer in the area of recreation and cultural activities [Department of Hospitals, n.d.].

Not all the people in the Geel program are psychiatrically disturbed; about two-thirds are mentally retarded rather than mentally ill. About two-thirds are men. Geel becomes a virtually permanent home for many—the average length of residence in the community is 15–20 years.

Although the Geel program is thoroughly remarkable in its innovativeness and continuity, it is not without problems. According to Roosens, "the medical staff . . . is underpaid, and thus it is difficult to attract candidates for vacant positions. This obviously reduces the capacity of the medical services. Nor are the benefits paid to the host families very attractive, so that here too the care level remains well below what could be attained. All this does not help the institution's reputation in professional circles" (1979, pp. 31–32). Thus, the community-based program in Geel is undergoing many problems faced by similar programs in the United States, and it would be well to keep track of the ways that program goes about dealing with its problems in providing high-quality community-based care. One can even imagine that the family care program in Geel might one day be terminated.

Community-based care developed in the United States in the late 1890s. The view that people are products of their environments as well as of their heredities reemerged, and a new type of institution for care of the mentally ill was advocated. Called a *psychopathic hospital*, it was to be located in the community and was to provide treatment rather than custodial care. The rationale for the psychopathic hospital was based on what were then quite radical ideas. First, it was believed that patients should be identified and treated soon after the onset of their disorder. Second, it was believed that patients should not be isolated from their families, friends, and other sources of support. Third, it was believed that patients' families could provide very useful information to those persons responsible for the patients' treatment and that such information would be far easier to obtain if the treatment facility were in the community. Finally, the psychopathic hospital was designed to stimulate in local physicians an increased interest in the problem of mental illness.

Such hospitals were established in Albany, New York, in 1902, at the University of Michigan in 1906, and, somewhat later, in Boston, Baltimore, Denver, and other cities. Around the same time, community aftercare services for former psychiatric patients began to be offered, psychiatric diagnostic clinics were established as part of some general hospitals, and psychiatric outpatient clinics began to be developed. The first of these clinics opened in 1896 at the University of Pennsylvania, and the community-clinic movement (designed to provide mental health services primarily for children) grew rapidly. By 1925 nearly 400 such clinics were in existence, and by 1932 nearly 700 were listed in a directory of United States psychiatric clinics (Rossi, 1962).

Changes in community attitudes toward the mentally ill were reflected in the development of a citizens' mental hygiene movement. Volunteer organizations raised money to support expanded psychiatric services for children and worked to increase public awareness of the magnitude and severity of the national problem of mental illness. These educational efforts were designed to underline the facts that mental illness and mental health are on a single continuum, that social factors play a role in the development of psychiatric disorders, and that one way to reduce the magnitude of the problem is to identify cases early and treat them promptly. The mental hygiene movement attracted many influential mental health professionals. For example, in 1915, Adolf Meyer, one of the most influential forerunners of the current community mental health movement, proposed the development of community mental hygiene districts; in each of these districts, mental health practitioners would coordinate the services of schools, recreational facilities, churches, law enforcement agencies, and other social service agencies to prevent mental disorders and to foster sound mental health (Rossi, 1962, pp. 87–88).

Maintenance of mental health became a particularly important problem during World War I. The psychiatric casualty rate among soldiers was very high, and efforts at early detection and prompt treatment were highly successful. When the war ended, mental health professionals interested in applying the skills they had learned in the military to the civilian population found much support and good will in the community.

These developments in communities continued until World War II, supported at first by private foundations and individual contributions and later by increasing amounts of public money. Shortly after World War II, the institutional and community developments I've described merged, and efforts to increase federal support for the fight against mental illness began in earnest. The reduction in the size of the state-hospital population and the apparent successes in the development of community services attracted the attention of the federal government, as if at last there were some hope that improvements could be made in what was generally agreed to be a most unsatisfactory state of affairs in the field of psychiatric care.

The federal role in mental health

The developments in institutions and in the community just described helped set the stage for increased federal involvement in the planning and funding of mental health services throughout the country. The continuing failure of most states to appropriate enough funds to support high-quality institutional mental health care suggested that the state-run system needed to be supplemented, and the increasing involvement of institutional programs with the community suggested that community care of the mentally ill might be a feasible alternative. Federal funds and federal consultation were going to be needed. The ever-present danger, however, was that community programs would do no better than the state hospitals had done or than communities had done before the advent of the state hospital.

Before World War II, the federal government had played a very small role in the support of mental health services in the United States (Levine, 1981). In 1929 a narcotics division had been established within the U.S. Public Health Service. A year later, that division was reorganized into the Division of Mental Hygiene and given more responsibility and authority. Several Veterans Administration psychiatric hospitals were operating, the U.S. Public Health Service operated several hospitals for psychiatric patients, and two federally supported hospitals for drug addicts were in existence.

The first piece of federal legislation of significance enacted after World War II was the National Mental Health Act (Public Law 79-487), in July 1946. Its purpose was the

> improvement of the mental health of the people of the United States through the conducting of researches, investigations, experiments, and demonstrations relating to the cause, diagnosis, and treatment of psychiatric disorders; assisting and fostering such research activity by public and private agencies, and promoting the coordination of all such researches and activities and the useful application of their result; training personnel in matters relating to mental health; and developing, and assisting States in the use of, the most effective methods of prevention, diagnosis and treatment of psychotic disorders [U.S. Congress, 1946, p. 1].

The act created the National Institute of Mental Health (NIMH), which was to be advised by a newly established National Advisory Mental Health Council. During its first ten years, NIMH became both the intellectual and the financial source for much that was innovative in American mental health training, research, and practice. Least affected by the existence of NIMH were the state hospitals, all of which continued to function almost exclusively on the basis of state appropriations.

In addition, the National Mental Health Act encouraged each state or territory to designate one agency to serve as the mental health authority of that state and inaugurated a state grant-in-aid program to assist these mental health authorities in improving the quality of community-based mental health services. The act provided that staff members of NIMH be deployed throughout the country as regional consultants to these mental health authorities. Finally, the act established both research-grant and training-grant programs.

Because certain ideological and practical considerations help to shape all American social policy, most pieces of social legislation have a number of characteristics in common (Freedman, 1967; Ryan, 1969). First, American social policy is characterized by pluralism—"a multitude of governmental structures and private groups, each with its own power and strength, sometimes acting cooperatively, often competitively" (Freedman, 1967, p. 488). Second, social policy is characterized by pragmatism—"Americans focus always on that which works, and policy, political or otherwise, is acceptable which produces desired results" (Freedman, pp. 488–489). Third, there is (or has been until quite recently) an emphasis on short-term goals, at the expense of long-term planning, particularly in matters of health, education, and welfare. Fourth, changes are made by the addition of new structures and agencies. Fifth, change is venerated. Finally, social policy has to deal with the fact that development of social services throughout the United States is very uneven, so that different amounts and types of assistance must be provided to different regions of the country.

Many of these characteristics can be seen in the National Mental Health Act. A new administrative structure (NIMH) was created. That structure's relationship to other, already established agencies with similar missions was not made clear. The act, rather than extolling any particular ideology, encouraged mental health practitioners to do whatever seemed effective. Its modes of functioning put a premium on short-term strategies and short-term goals.

In 1955 three developments took place that were to have enormous impact on continued federal participation in mental health care. First, that year was the turning point in the population of state mental hospitals. Whether because of tranquilizers, because of the therapeutic community, because of changes in the nature and prevalence of serious mental disorder, or because of the slowly increasing availability of mental health facilities in the community, the resident patient population in state mental hospitals began to decline. At first, the decline was slow, averaging about 1 to 2% per year. From a high of nearly 600,000 in 1955, the number of patients in residence declined to 500,000 by 1963. Since 1964 this decrease has accelerated. Resident patient population had declined to 171,000 by the end of 1976 (Bethel & Redick, 1972; Bethel, 1973, 1974; Meyer, 1975; Witkin, 1979). This astonishing drop in patient population, amounting to more than 70% in 21 years, has occurred in spite of a generally increasing number of admissions during the same period.

In 1955 about 170,000 people were admitted to state mental hospitals. By 1967 the number had virtually doubled. Between 1967 and 1971 admissions rose by nearly 5% each year, to more than 402,000 in 1971. Not until 1972 did admissions to state mental hospitals begin to stabilize at about 400,000 per year. Clearly, with decreasing numbers of patients in residence at the same time that increasing numbers were being admitted, the average length of hospitalization was decreasing significantly. Each year, patients were being discharged into the community more and more rapidly.

The second development was that the U.S. Congress enacted legislation enabling NIMH to provide demonstration-grant support to help mental hospitals upgrade their therapeutic programs. And third, Congress, responding to the growing pressure for a general reassessment of the mental health program in the United States, enacted the Mental Health Study Act (Public Law 84-182) to provide for "an objective, thorough, and nationwide analysis and reevaluation of the human and economic problems of mental illness" (Joint Commission on Mental Illness and Health, 1961, p. 301). Within five years more than a million dollars had been appropriated for this study, and another $140,000 had been donated by a variety of professional and philanthropic organizations, including the Rockefeller Brothers Fund, the Smith, Kline, and French Foundation, the Benjamin Rosenthal Foundation, the American Legion, and the National Association for Mental Health, to name just a few. The final report of the Joint Commission on Mental Illness and Health, which had been formed to carry out this congressional mandate, was delivered in 1961 to Congress along with a set of supporting monographs. It was entitled *Action for Mental Health*. The supporting documents dealt with such diverse topics as current concepts of positive mental health, the economics of mental illness, mental health staffing trends, how Americans view their mental health, epidemiology and mental illness, and religion and mental health.

While the joint commission was carrying out its task, the surgeon general appointed two committees with overlapping responsibilities—one to consider the planning of facilities for mental health services (see U.S. Department of Health, Education and Welfare, 1961) and one to consider mental health activities in the context of comprehensive health programs in the community (see U.S. Department of Health, Education and Welfare, 1963).

Thus, beginning after World War II and accelerating in the late 1950s, various developments took place both in the federal government and in mental health institutions that culminated in an increased role for the federal government in the planning and support of mental health services. The exact character of that role has varied tremendously as a function of the social philosophy of each government administration, however, and as we will see, progress in improving the nature and quality of American mental health services has been very uneven.

Recommendations of the Joint Commission on Mental Illness and Health

After documenting the urgent need for improved mental health services, the joint commission recommended that more funds be allocated for basic and applied research, for training, and for expanded services to the mentally ill. With regard to these expanded services, the commission suggested (1) immediate and intensive care for acutely disturbed mental patients in outpatient community mental health clinics created at the rate of one clinic per 50,000 population, inpatient psychiatric units located in every general hospital with 100 or more beds, and intensive psychiatric treatment centers of no more than 1000 beds each (to be developed by converting existing state mental hospitals), (2) improved care of chronic mental patients in other converted state mental hospitals, again involving no more than 1000 beds, (3) improved and expanded aftercare, partial hospitalization (hospitalization for less than 24 hours a day), and rehabilitation services, and (4) expanded mental health education to inform the public about psychological disorders and to reduce the public's tendency to reject the mentally ill. To meet the cost of improved mental health services, the commission recommended, public expenditures (state and federal) should be doubled in five years and tripled in ten, with the bulk of the expense of the expanded services to be borne by the federal government.

When the joint commission's final report reached the desk of President Kennedy, it found a very receptive audience. In order to convert the reports into a coherent, politically persuasive recommendation for a national mental health program, the president asked the secretary of labor, the secretary of health, education and welfare, and the administrator of veterans affairs to join representatives of the Bureau of the Budget and the Council of Economic Advisers and staff members of the National Institute of Mental Health in studying the documents and preparing a set of recommendations. Developing these recommendations required a good deal of careful negotiating, since these people had somewhat differing ideas about what the best kind of mental health program would be (see Connery et al., 1968, Chapter 3, and Duhl & Leopold, 1968, pp. 10–11). These recommendations were submitted to the president in December 1962, and after careful consideration the president, on February 5, 1963, transmitted to Congress a special message on mental health and mental retardation. In his message, he proposed a national mental health program that would require new legislation for its implementation. This special message was of historic importance because it was the first time in American history that a message on the topic of mental health and illness was delivered by a president. It is important to examine this message, because it set the stage for the introduction of special legislation into the Congress that was enacted into law nine months later. The message dealt with both mental illness and mental retardation; the sections dealing with mental illness will be examined in special detail.

The president's message on mental illness

The president asserted that "mental illness and mental retardation are among our most critical health problems. They occur more frequently, affect more people, require more prolonged treatment, cause more suffering by the families of the afflicted, waste more of our human resources, and constitute more financial drain upon both the Public Treasury and the personal finances of the individual families than any other single condition" (pp. 1–2).[1] After reviewing the critical conditions of state mental hospitals, he suggested that

---

[1]This and the following five quotations are from *Message from the President of the United States Relative to Mental Illness and Mental Retardation*, by J. F. Kennedy. 88th Congress, First Session, U.S. House of Representatives Document No. 58. Washington, D.C.: U.S. Government Printing Office, 1963.

the time had come for a "bold new approach." This approach would involve working toward three objectives. First, he said,

> we must seek out the causes of mental illness and of mental retardation and eradicate them. . . . For prevention is far more desirable for all concerned. It is far more economical and it is far more likely to be successful. Prevention will require both selected specific programs directed especially at known causes, and the general strengthening of our fundamental community, social welfare, and educational programs which can do much to eliminate or correct the harsh environmental conditions which often are associated with mental retardation and mental illness [p. 2].

Second, "we must strengthen the underlying resources of knowledge and, above all, of skilled manpower which are necessary to mount and sustain our attack on mental disability for many years to come" (pp. 2–3). And, third, "we must strengthen and improve the programs and facilities serving the mentally ill" (p. 3). As to the specifics of the "bold new approach," the president proposed

> a national mental health program to assist in the inauguration of a wholly new emphasis and approach to care for the mentally ill. . . . Central to a new mental health program is comprehensive community care. . . . We need a new type of health facility, one which will return mental health care to the main stream of American medicine, and at the same time upgrade mental health services. I recommend, therefore, that the Congress (1) authorize grants to the States for the construction of comprehensive community mental health centers . . . (2) authorize short-term project grants for the initial staffing costs of comprehensive community mental health centers . . . and (3) to facilitate the preparation of community plans for these new facilities as a necessary preliminary to any construction or staffing assistance, appropriate $4.2 million for planning grants under the National Institute of Mental Health [pp. 3–5].

In addition to this major proposal for the establishment of comprehensive community mental health centers, the president also proposed grants to improve care in state mental hospitals and increased appropriations for research and training. With respect to improved patient care in state mental hospitals, the president suggested that "until the community mental health program develops fully, it is imperative that the quality of care in existing State mental institutions be improved. . . . If we launch a broad new mental health program now, it will be possible within a decade or two to reduce the number of patients now under custodial care by 50 percent or more" (pp. 4–6).

The community mental health center concept combined the most forward-looking aspects of the joint commission's report into a single, comprehensive program. Unwritten in the president's message was his view that state mental hospitals as they existed in 1963 were to be virtually phased out and replaced by the new community mental health centers. Thus, in 1963, as in 1946, a sharp demarcation was drawn between state mental hospitals and community-based programs, and once again, those mental health professionals whose

primary identification was with high-quality mental hospital care found themselves on the defensive. The president's message touched on most of the
distinguishing features of the community mental health orientation mentioned
earlier: the emphasis on community rather than institutional care, the focus
on total community and on prevention, the emphasis on rational planning as
the basis for center construction and staffing, and a strong interest in identifying stress-inducing aspects of the community.

In some ways, the most innovative characteristic of the proposed community mental health center was to be its emphasis on comprehensiveness.
Most existing mental (and general) health services were scattered, poorly coordinated, and differentially available to various segments of the population. In
contrast, it was hoped, the new facilities would not only restore and maintain
health but also prevent disorder; in addition, the centers were to provide
continuity of care and to offer high-quality care promptly to the total population. The concept of comprehensiveness meant that

> all mental health services are to be available to all the people of a community—
> the rich and the poor, the young and the old, the resident and the transient, the
> healthy who are merely curious or in need of education, and the ill who are mildly
> neurotic or severely psychotic, and the chronic cases of illness as well as the acute.
> They all comprise a community, and a comprehensive community mental health
> center, to deserve the name, must serve them all [Brown & Cain, 1964, pp.
> 834–835].

Community mental health centers were not designed to replace existing
mental health services. Rather, they were envisioned as agencies that would
maintain an overview of a community's mental health needs while providing
preventive and therapeutic programs so that, in collaboration with other existing mental health services, those needs could be met. Private-sector services
were expected to continue, along with publicly funded mental health agencies
that did not aspire to become mental health centers. The community mental
health center, however, would be charged with an entirely novel responsibility—namely, ensuring that the comprehensive mental health needs of a community would be identified and met.

Passage of the Community Mental Health Centers Act

Hearings began shortly after the president's 1963 message to Congress,
and a variety of proposals designed to implement the president's ideas were
introduced into both the Senate and the House. As the hearings progressed,
it became clear that there was substantial support for federal funding of construction of new facilities but opposition to federal subsidies of staff salaries.
The greatest opposition to subsidy by the federal government of the initial
costs of staffing community mental health centers came from the American
Medical Association. In their testimony in the House and Senate, AMA representatives indicated that "once reliance is placed on Federal subsidy for

staffing, the role of the Federal Government, as a provider of funds, will not easily be terminated" (Bartemeier, 1963, p. 88). The AMA, representing primarily the interests of physicians in solo, fee-for-service practice, had a long history of opposition to any other form of practice or payment. Since 1920, it had been consistently opposed to Medicare. In the interest of maintaining the economic viability of the medical profession, it had favored restricting the numbers of students admitted to medical school and had opposed any subsidy program to assist students with the costs of medical education. Since the early 1930s, the AMA had been opposed to prepaid group health plans, group medical practice, or such voluntary insurance programs as Blue Cross or Blue Shield. Only in 1949, when it became clear that legislation supporting some form of compulsory medical insurance might be enacted, did the AMA go on record as favoring voluntary medical insurance programs (Harris, 1969; Tunley, 1966).

But it was not the AMA alone that questioned the staffing legislation. Many members of Congress felt reluctant to have the federal government get into what they felt was primarily a state or local matter. If, as promised by the proponents of the staffing legislation, the states or local communities would assume all staffing costs in four years, why not insist that they absorb those costs from the very beginning? And if, as the proponents argued, the states needed help with some proportion of the initial costs of staffing the community mental health center, why 75%, as the proponents suggested? Why not 50% or 25%?

As a consequence of these and other objections to the staffing component of the community mental health legislative proposals, while the Senate passed the bill including staffing provisions in May 1963, the House approved the legislation without staffing provisions. In its committee report, the House noted that "it is the strong belief of the committee that Federal support is necessary to assist in the creation of community mental health services, but such Federal support should be so tailored as not to result in the Federal Government assuming the traditional responsibility of the States, localities, and the medical profession for the care and treatment of the mentally ill" (Committee on Interstate and Foreign Commerce, 1963, p. 13). In the conference of the House and Senate in late October, the staffing provision was finally deleted, but the construction program was extended from two years to three. Final passage by both houses of Congress took place quickly, and the Community Mental Health Centers Act was signed into law by President Kennedy on October 31, 1963—less than a month before his death.

The staffing provisions were reintroduced into Congress in the next session, which was under President Johnson's leadership, and these provisions were speedily approved in August 1965 as amendments to the construction legislation in virtually the same form as proposed by President Kennedy two and a half years before. The disappearance of opposition to the federal staffing assistance seemed to be due to two factors. First, there was strong sentiment

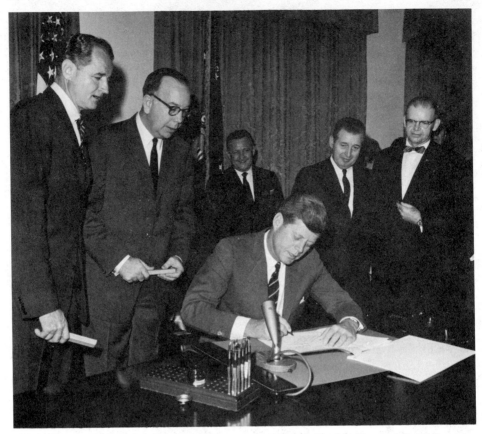

President Kennedy signs the Community Mental Health Centers Act into law, October 31, 1963. *(Photo courtesy of the John F. Kennedy Library.)*

in Congress in favor of completing the work started by President Kennedy and interrupted by his death; second, the AMA had no longer been able to oppose effectively the passage of Medicare legislation, and Medicare had been signed into law the month before. The AMA had been defeated after more than 40 years of opposition to Medicare, and in the groundswell of public calls for improved medical care, particularly for those who could not afford fee-for-service medicine, it prudently decided not to oppose the staffing proposal. Both the construction and staffing components of the community mental health center legislation have since been extended, although, as will be seen later, the road toward the goal of comprehensive community mental health centers for the entire population of the United States has been far from smooth.

As a consequence of the planning grants awarded to each state and territory in the United States before the enactment of the community mental health center legislation, mental health needs and resources had been inventoried. Each state had been divided into catchment areas, each with a population limit of 75,000 to 200,000; the catchment areas of each state were ranked by need for improved mental health services. The community mental health center construction and staffing legislation appropriated funds that could be combined with nonfederal funds for construction and staffing of the mental health center to be built in each catchment area. The federal share of construction costs ranged from one-third to two-thirds of the total cost (depending on the affluence of each state); as for staffing costs, the federal share was to start at 75% and decrease by 15% each year until it reached 30%, after which time nonfederal funds entirely were to be used. Some 1500 catchment areas were created in the United States, and the hope was that in the coming decade each such area would be served by one of these centers.

The act required that the centers provide five essential services: inpatient care, outpatient care, emergency services, partial hospitalization, and consultation and education. Eventually, five additional services were also to be provided: diagnostic services, rehabilitation services, precare and aftercare services, training, and research and evaluation. The services provided in each mental health center were to be available to all residents of the catchment area, including those unable to pay, and were to be readily accessible to the community being served. Further, the centers were to meet a number of regulatory requirements that would help ensure continuity of care. These requirements included (1) that a person eligible for treatment in one element of a community mental health center be eligible in all elements, (2) that patients be readily transferable from one element to another, (3) that clinical information about patients be shared by all elements of the mental health center, (4) that staff members be able to move among treatment elements in order to follow their patients, and (5) that no minimum period of residence in the catchment area be imposed as a requirement for treatment (see U.S. Department of Health, Education and Welfare, 1964).

Years of planning thus culminated in strikingly innovative federal legislation. The legislation was designed to make mental health services available in communities throughout the United States and to put into practice newly emerging mental health techniques such as consultation and crisis intervention—techniques that seemed to offer means of preventing and treating mental disorders more quickly and more successfully than had ever been possible.

Changes in the Community Mental Health Centers Act

In the years since the passage of the Community Mental Health Centers Act in 1963, the U.S. Congress has on numerous occasions extended or amended the act. The first of these amendments (Public Law 89-105), which added the staffing provisions to the original construction act, has already been discussed. Between 1967 and 1975, Congress enacted further legislation that revised and extended the community mental health movement. In 1967 P.L. 90-31 authorized funds for additional construction and staffing of community mental health centers. In 1968 P.L. 90-574 authorized appropriations of funds for construction and staffing of facilities for the prevention and treatment of alcoholism and narcotics addiction. In 1970 P.L. 91-211 made some modifications in the basic concepts of funding for community mental health centers and also added services for children to the growing list of responsibilities of community mental health centers (Joint Commission on Mental Health of Children, 1969; Ozarin & Feldman, 1971). In 1970 P.L. 91-513 added services for persons with drug-abuse and drug-dependence problems to the list of community mental health responsibilities.

The U.S. political and social climate was undergoing a dramatic change during the early 1970s. The high level of federal support for innovative social programs suffered a sharp setback as a conservative presidential administration became preoccupied with the war in Vietnam and with the current inflation and recession. In 1973 P.L. 93-45 extended the community mental health centers program for only one year, in the face of growing opposition to this

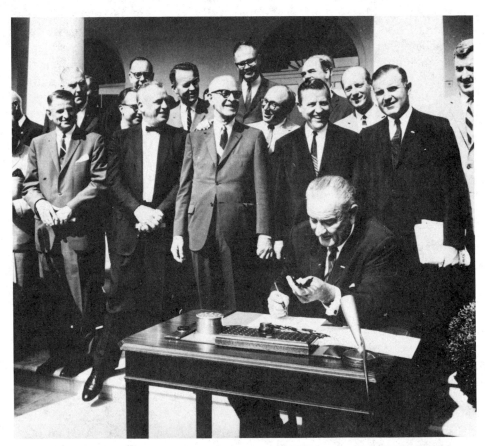

President Johnson signing P.L. 89-105, August 4, 1965. (*Courtesy of The National Park Service.*)

and many other social programs by the Nixon and Ford administrations. In 1974 the president successfully vetoed efforts to extend the legislation, but in 1975 Congress was able to enact an extension of the community mental health centers program (P.L. 94-63) over a presidential veto.

1977: The President's Commission on Mental Health.   Jimmy Carter, elected to the presidency in 1976, brought with him a long-standing family interest in mental health. Both he and his wife, Rosalynn, had been actively involved in improving the quality of mental health services in Georgia while he was governor, and they attempted to apply at the national level a procedure that had been very effective in Georgia at the state level. Mrs. Carter described that process in the following words:

> I became interested in mental health while campaigning . . . for Jimmy when he ran for Governor. I had so many people ask me then, "What will you do for my retarded child? I have a son who is in the 7th grade who is emotionally disturbed. . . . What will your husband do to help him if he is elected Governor?" . . . One night I had decided that I wanted to work with the mental health program when Jimmy was Governor. . . . I was campaigning in a little community in Georgia. . . . and I found out that Jimmy was going to be in that same town that night— which was great. I never saw him in the campaign. So I stayed and got in the back of the auditorium while he spoke. After his speech was over, I got in line, went down with everybody else, shook hands with him. He shook my hand before he saw who I was, and then he said, "What are you doing here?" And I said, "I came to see what you are going to do about the mental health program in Georgia." He said, "We are going to have the best one in the United States, and I am going to put you in charge of it." Well, he didn't put me in charge of it, of course. But he did appoint me to the Governor's Commission to improve services to the mentally and emotionally handicapped. I worked with that commission and we were very pleased with what we were able to do. . . . We submitted a report. We inventoried the needs in the State and gave a report to Jimmy. He implemented almost all of it in his reorganization of State government [Office of the White House Press Secretary, 1977b].

On February 17, 1977, less than one month after President Carter was inaugurated, he signed an executive order creating the President's Commission on Mental Health. The commission was charged with the responsibility to conduct hearings and undertake comprehensive inquiries and studies to identify the mental health needs of the nation and to make recommendations to the president on how the United States might best meet these needs. The commission was to complete its final report within 15 months. Specifically, the commission was asked to identify

> (1) How the mentally ill, emotionally disturbed, and mentally retarded are being served, to what extent they are being underserved, and who is affected by such underservice; (2) The projected needs for dealing with emotional stress during the next twenty-five years; (3) The various ways the President, the Congress, and the Federal Government may most efficiently support the treatment of the under-

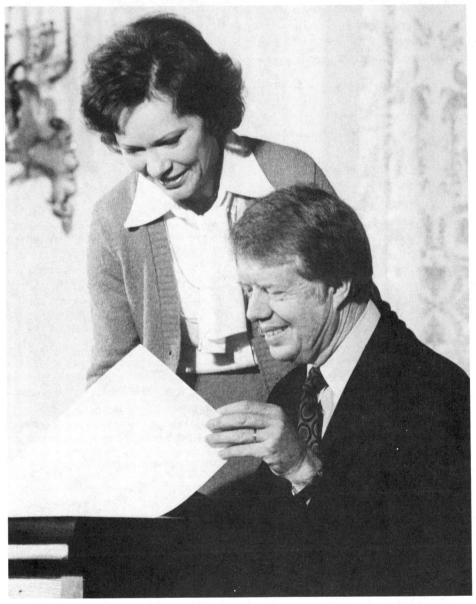

President and Mrs. Carter signing the order creating the President's Commission on Mental Health, February 17, 1977. (*Courtesy of the White House.*)

served mentally ill, emotionally disturbed, and mentally retarded; (4) Various methods for coordinating a unified approach to all mental health and people-helping services; (5) The types of research the Federal Government should support to further the prevention and treatment of mental illness and mental retardation; (6) What role the various educational systems, volunteer agencies and other people-helping institutions can perform to minimize emotional disturbance in our country; and (7) As nearly as possible, what programs will cost, when the money should be spent, and how the financing should be divided among Federal, State and local governments, and the private sector [Office of the White House Press Secretary, 1977a].

The commission went about its task by creating a number of topical areas, such as nature and scope of the problems; access and barriers to care; deinstitutionalization, rehabilitation, and long-term care; cost and financing; prevention; public attitudes and the use of media for promotion of mental health; and mental health of minority populations. The commission identified more than 450 national experts, who served on task panels in each of these areas. The task panels met during 1977 and submitted their reports to the commission, which, in turn, prepared its final report for the president, which was delivered in April 1978. In many ways, its report, along with the set of task-panel reports, represented a major updating of the documents prepared 16 years earlier by the Joint Commission on Mental Illness and Health.

The report of the President's Commission on Mental Health included more than 100 specific recommendations for meeting the country's mental health needs. The general goal of a national mental health program that was articulated by the commission was that high-quality mental health care should be available to all who need it and at reasonable cost.

To achieve that goal, the commission proposed that, during the next decade, the country must take steps to

Develop networks of high quality, comprehensive mental health services throughout the country which are sufficiently flexible to respond to changing circumstances and to the diverse racial and cultural backgrounds of individuals. . . . ; Adequately finance mental health services with public and private funds; Assure that appropriately trained mental health personnel will be available where they are needed; Make available where and when they are needed services and personnel for populations with special needs, such as children, adolescents, and the elderly; Establish a national priority to meet the needs of people with chronic mental illness; Coordinate mental health services more closely with each other, with general health and other human services, and with those personal and social support systems that strengthen our neighborhoods and communities; Broaden the base of knowledge about the nature and treatment of mental disabilities; Undertake a concerted national effort to prevent mental disabilities; Assure that mental health services and programs operate within basic principles protecting human rights and guaranteeing freedom of choice [President's Commission on Mental Health, 1978, pp. 9–10].

The specific recommendations dealt with community supports, a responsive service system, insurance for the future, new directions for personnel, protecting basic rights, expanding the knowledge base, a strategy for prevention, and improving public understanding.

With regard to establishing new services within the public sector, the commission recommended a new, more flexible federal grant program for community mental health services, with priority going to unserved and underserved areas; services for children, adolescents, and the elderly; specialized services for racial and ethnic minority populations; and services for people with chronic mental illness. With regard to strengthening existing services, the commission recommended greater flexibility in delineating catchment-area boundaries and encouragement of cross-catchment-area program development.

As for meeting the needs of the chronically mentally ill, the commission recommended the development of a national plan for the continued phasing down and, where appropriate, closing of large state mental hospitals; upgrading service quality in the remaining state hospitals; and allocating increased resources for the development of comprehensive, integrated systems of care that would include community-based services and the remaining smaller state hospitals.

Regarding the need to expand the knowledge base, the commission recommended that priority be given to rebuilding the mental health research capacity over the next ten years and to investing an amount of money commensurate with the level of the problems associated with mental health, alcoholism, and drug abuse. It recommended a review of how the federal government currently supported and trained research personnel and a sensible increase over the next decade in that support to enhance our ability to train needed research personnel. In addition, it recommended immediate efforts to gather reliable data on the incidence of mental health problems and the use of mental health services, expanded research on the ways mental health services were being delivered and the policies affecting these services, and research directed toward understanding major mental illnesses and mental retardation, as well as the basic psychological, sociological, biological, and developmental processes associated with these disorders.

As for the prevention of mental disorders, the commission recommended that a center for prevention be established in the National Institute of Mental Health with primary prevention as its first priority.

1980: The Mental Health Systems Act. Existing authority for most programs supported under the Community Mental Health Centers Act had been continued by the previous Congress by the enactment of P.L. 95-622, which was to expire in September 1980. With this fact in mind, Congress began hearings in early 1979 to examine the recommendations of the President's Commission on Mental Health and to enact legislation implementing them. The community mental health centers program had passed the halfway mark in providing total national coverage of comprehensive community-based mental health services. This had been achieved with a federal expenditure of $2.29 billion over 13 years. This federal investment had generated well over double that amount in state and local funds and receipts for community mental health services. More important, as a result of this legislation and other federal and state initiatives, there had been a dramatic shift from inpatient to outpatient mental health care. Over the previous ten years, utilization rates for outpatient care had increased fourfold, while the number of psychiatric hospital beds in the United States had decreased by 36%. Since the inception of the community mental health centers program, federal funds had assisted in the initiation of 763 community mental health centers, putting clinical care, preventive services, and social services within reach of over 110 million people, or 50% of the population.

By the summer of 1980, the House and the Senate had each passed their versions of an act to continue the community mental health centers program. In September 1980 the two branches of Congress agreed on a single act, and President Carter signed P.L. 96-398 (the Mental Health Systems Act) into law on October 7, 1980, one month before the presidential election.

The Mental Health Systems Act authorized funds to continue many of the provisions of the original community mental health centers program and to implement other provisions that were instituted to reflect the changing nature of mental health needs and mental health services. These new provisions included grants specifically for the treatment of the chronically mentally ill, for severely disturbed children and adolescents, and for unserved or underserved populations as locally determined. The coordinating role of the state mental health authority was expanded by requiring its prior approval of grant applications.

Furthermore, the National Institute of Mental Health was directed to establish an administrative unit that would "(1) design national goals and establish national priorities for (A) the prevention of mental illness, and (B) the promotion of mental health, (2) encourage and assist local entities and state agencies to achieve the goals and priorities described in paragraph (1), and (3) develop and coordinate Federal prevention policies and programs and to assure increased focus on the prevention of mental illness and the promotion of mental health" (U.S. Congress, 1980, p. 1596).

1981: The election of Ronald Reagan.   As President Carter's term came to an end, the National Institute of Mental Health had begun the planning for implementing the newly enacted program. But the 1980 election campaign was waged largely in the economic sector. Ronald Reagan proposed a series of measures to reduce the inflation that had gripped the United States for more than a decade, including a sharp reduction in federal participation in social programs and an increase in the freedom of each state to deal in its own way with social problems. President Reagan proposed providing relatively unencumbered sums of federal money to each state in the form of block grants. It had historically been customary for Congress to distribute most of its appropriations to states in the form of earmarked categorical grants—that is, specified sums of money for dealing with specific problems. This block-grant proposal would save money because the total amount distributed to states would be far less than the sum of all of the categorical funds allocated for the same purposes in previous years.

Following Reagan's victory in November 1980, as part of the enactment of the budget, all the budgetary authorizations of the Mental Health Systems Act were repealed. By 1981, individual states were preparing to support part of the cost of social programs by using the block grants. Mental health services are included in a block grant called the "health services block." But a specific sum of money has been earmarked for mental health, alcohol, and drug-abuse programs, and some restrictions are imposed on the states' freedom to transfer funds from one program to another. In addition, states are required to fund existing community mental health centers for the duration of their federal funding commitments.

It is not at all clear how each state will choose to deal with its social needs and social programs, given that it will have far less federal money available for that purpose, or how it will choose to allocate that money among competing needs. What does seem clear is that if services are not to decrease, states and local governments will have to provide funds previously provided by the federal government.

But what may turn out to be the most important aspect of the block-grant strategy, from the point of view of social policy, is one of its side effects. States and local communities will now have to consider resource-allocation issues that formerly were the responsibility of the federal government. In that process, they may find themselves asking for information about community needs and community resources—requests that are far more in keeping with a community mental health orientation than ever before.

COMMUNITY MENTAL HEALTH AS SOCIAL POLICY

In addition to a set of specified rules and regulations, the Community Mental Health Centers Act, like many other pieces of federal legislation, carried with it a belief system—that is, an ideology (see Levine, 1981; Mechanic, 1969). In some legislation, this ideology is made explicit, but more often it is implicit and has to be found between the lines or identified inductively. A set of social values guides legislation in the field of human services, and an informed public should be aware of these values in order to be able to react constructively to such legislation.

Social policies need not be permanent and, indeed, rarely are. As we have seen, it is not uncommon for newly elected officials to institute major changes in such policies. These policies guide a broad spectrum of legislative activity, and federal social policies provide direction to the legislative and executive acts of state and municipal governments.

In place of the carefully orchestrated roles for the federal government, states, and local communities that had been built into the original community mental health legislation, the election of Ronald Reagan brought a dramatic change in the political philosophy governing federal/state relations. The Reagan administration supported the concept of strong state government and a relatively weak federal government, a position often called *states' rights*. With this change in social policy, there is far less interdependence between the federal government and the states. Furthermore, the federal government plays a far less active role in helping the states to develop or evaluate their social programs or in maintaining parallel progress in social programs among the states.

In addition, community mental health centers legislation, like virtually all federal legislation in which funds are made available to states for some purpose, is based on the social policy of distributing funds in proportion to need— that is, giving more money to poorer states than to more affluent ones. A third social policy explicit in all the community mental health centers legislation is the concept of the geographically defined mental health service area—that is, a definition of community based exclusively on geographic and topographic characteristics. A fourth social policy is the effort to integrate mental health and general health services.

In associating the community mental health center with physicians and hospitals, the policy seems to assert that emotional disorders are primarily biological and require, among other responses, medical treatment, often including hospitalization. This assertion would seem inconsistent with the bulk of the evidence. At the same time, however, the policy recognizes the special role of the general hospital as the locus of what is ordinarily the highest-quality community health care and serves to induce the general hospital to concern itself more with the treatment of emotionally disordered persons, even when such treatment is not medical in nature. In other words, the policy encourages the general hospital to broaden its view of its role in the community.

One can argue that the fundamental objective of this policy is to involve the family physician, or, in more modern terms, the *primary care physician*, in the internal workings of the community mental health center—that is, to encourage the integration of medical with psychological or psychiatric care. Allowing local primary care physicians to assist in the care of their patients within the community mental health center must also be seen as part of the federal social policy of encouraging the closer collaboration of primary care physicians with psychiatrists and other mental health professionals.

Not far beneath the surface of the Community Mental Health Centers Act, then, is a view of a single integrated and comprehensive community-based health delivery system attending equally to the biological and psychological problems of the individual—a view, interestingly enough, that is inconsistent with the concept of the community mental health center. Yet, that view appears to be consistent with a good deal of contemporary research that links biological, psychological, and sociocultural factors together in understanding health and disease.

Two other social policies embedded within the funding of the community mental health centers program by the U.S. Congress were that federal funds should be used to expand locally supported programs rather than substitute for local sources of support and, perhaps most controversial of all, that federal funds should be used only to start programs rather than to support local programs in perpetuity (Bloom, 1977a).

None of these social policies is without controversy. The struggle for supremacy between cities and states and between states and the federal government has existed for some time, as has the tendency for cities and the federal government to bypass states in their dealings with each other. Much bitterness surrounds the issue of resource redistribution. States that pay more into the federal government want more in return. More affluent states provide more social services for their citizens and often resent the ease with which citizens from less affluent sections of the country move into their areas in order to take advantage of these benefits. To many people, defining the community solely on the basis of geography is too limiting. For these critics, interdependence is the true test of community—a test that may link coal miners or professors to one another across great distances but may fail to link next-door neighbors who are strangers to each other. There is a strong conviction among the public, probably stronger than many realize, that people who have more ought to be able to buy higher-quality medical and psychiatric care (see Whittington, 1965, for example) and that the civil-rights movement is all too often an excuse for giving someone something for nothing.

THE RIGHTS OF PSYCHIATRIC PATIENTS

The Community Mental Health Centers Act broke fresh ground with regard to a number of patient-rights issues and thus can be seen as part of the broader civil-rights movement (Bloom & Asher, 1982a, 1982b). Although courts have long been involved in general issues of civil rights, for the first 175 years of this country's history, courts maintained a hands-off policy regarding the role of social institutions in protecting those rights. On the rare occasions when grievances were brought to a court's attention, whether concerning prisons, schools, hospitals, or other caregiving settings, courts almost invariably deferred to the presumed expertise of the professionals who operated those institutions. The court was unwilling to substitute its judgment for that of the staff in such settings, and it lacked the confidence and competence to review or to fashion remedies affecting the quality of life, programming, or treatment within these human service delivery settings.

Starting about 1955, this state of affairs began a process of dramatic and accelerating change, and the courts are now increasingly involved in the day-to-day operations of a wide variety of human service delivery settings. The reasons for this profound change in the role of the court in the evaluation of human services are multiple and interactive. First, a series of prison atrocities was brought to the attention of the public and the court. Graves of decapitated prisoners were dug up in the pasturelands of prison farms in Arkansas. California prison strip cells were exposed to the public eye, and numerous torture devices used on prisoners were discovered. Factual accounts of such blatant cruelty served to outrage the public, and it became impossible for the courts to continue deferring to the expertise of institutional staff. Courts could continue to assert that they were not expert in identifying high-quality care, but they now felt no hesitancy in making assertions about unacceptably low-quality care.

Second, the activist posture of the Warren Court permitted cases to be argued that the Supreme Court had previously refused to consider. Out of these arguments came the initial decisions on school desegregation and decisions protecting the civil rights of members of the Armed Forces, rights of the poor and of welfare recipients, rights of draftees and draft evaders, tenants and landlords, parolees, debtors, and, more recently, environmentalists. The general impact of these decisions was to establish the principle that constitutional liberties and legislated services were not privileges—they were rights.

Third, changes were beginning in the practice of law and in the character of new lawyers. Federal funds became available for the practice of public-interest law and for the provision of legal services to the poor, a group historically denied adequate legal representation. Well-trained young attorneys became attracted to this new arena of legal practice. State and national bar associations, along with a number of private foundations, became interested in and supportive of the practice of public-interest law.

Finally, long-standing practices of authority figures were challenged. The general erosion of the status of authority figures—including directors of human service delivery systems, teachers, physicians, husbands, and parents—along with the reaction against paternalism, altruism, and benevolence that had begun in the 1960s, constituted another aspect of the historical context of the civil-rights movement.

Interest in protecting the civil rights of psychiatric patients developed rather late in this sequence of events. Because psychiatric patients are in a treatment setting (often under involuntary civil commitment), issues related to the protection of their civil rights are unusually complex. And because psychiatric patients are sometimes not fully rational, protection of their civil rights is doubly complex.

Among the patient-rights issues addressed in the original community mental health centers legislation were the interrelated issues of "right to treatment" and "the least restrictive alternative." In the Mental Health Systems Act, a special section was enacted specifically concerning mental health rights and advocacy.

In the original mental health centers legislation, community services were to be provided without regard to race, creed, or color and without regard to length of residence in the community or to ability to pay. This last requirement had an escape clause, however. The act specified that a state must obtain assurance from a local applicant for a community mental health center grant that a reasonable volume of services would be provided to persons unable to pay for them, but at the same time the state could recommend exempting an applicant from this requirement if it was judged financially unfeasible. Implicit in these regulations was the social policy that, ultimately, every catchment area must be able to provide as much mental health service as is needed in the community—this a far less restrictive setting than the often geographically remote state mental hospital—and that under no circumstances will a person in need of services be denied them. This is a long-term objective, and it was tempered by realistic short-term considerations. For instance, if inpatient services in a particular catchment area are to be provided on the psychiatric ward of a community general hospital, it will not take many nonpaying patients to bankrupt the hospital. The long-term policy takes into consideration the often precarious financial conditions of general hospitals and encourages communities to look toward expanded third-party comprehensive insurance coverage or other prepaid systems for psychiatric as well as medical treatment.

The ill-fated Mental Health Systems Act continued this concern about right to treatment in the least restrictive setting but extended its concerns into other areas of patient rights as well. In addition to requiring that patients have the right to treatment in a setting that restricts their liberty only to the extent necessary to carry out that treatment, the law required an individualized, written treatment plan that was subject to periodic review and revision, ongoing participation by the patient in the development and review of that treatment plan, the right to refuse treatment, the right to freedom from restraint or seclusion other than in an emergency, the right to a humane treatment environment, the right to confidentiality of clinical records, access to such records, private access to the telephone, the mail, and to visitors, and the right to assert that such rights were being abridged. In addition, the Mental Health Systems Act authorized funds to support the development of patient advocacy programs.

CRITICISMS OF THE COMMUNITY
MENTAL HEALTH CENTER MOVEMENT

Few innovative social programs are free from criticism, and often the criticism is not only justified but also persuasive. There has been no shortage of criticism of the community mental health center concept. Such criticism first appeared in published literature in 1965, accelerated rapidly during the next three or four years, tapered off for a number of years, and more recently began to appear as new issues were identified. Perhaps the most influential initial critique of the community mental health center concept was prepared on behalf of the American Psychological Association (Smith & Hobbs, 1966).

The medical model

Initially, criticisms were raised regarding the medical model implicit in the thinking of the original framers of the community mental health center concept (Albee, 1968; Deibert, 1971; Glidewell, 1971; Reiff, 1968; Schwebel, 1972; Shatan, 1969; Smith, 1968). Critics of the medical model have proposed two alternative views of psychopathology—an *educational* model and a *psychosocial* model. The educational model asserts that deviant behavior is learned and, with proper education, can be unlearned and replaced by nondeviant behavior. According to the psychosocial model, emotional disorder emerges from a psychological and a social context, and only attention to these two contexts can reduce the incidence of the kinds of behavior that currently come to the attention of mental health professionals. In his critique of the medical model, Engel has said:

> The dominant model of disease today is biomedical, with molecular biology its basic scientific discipline. . . . It leaves no room within its framework for the social, psychological, and behavioral dimensions of illness. The biomedical model not only requires that disease be dealt with as an entity independent of social behavior, it also demands that behavioral aberrations be explained on the basis of disordered somatic (biochemical or neurophysiological) processes. Thus the biomedical model embraces both reductionism, the philosophic view that complex phenomena are ultimately derived from a single primary principle, and mind-body dualism, the doctrine that separated the mental from the somatic [1977, p. 130].[2]

In contrast to this narrow view of illness and health, Engel has suggested a biopsychosocial model. Such a model

> would acknowledge the fundamental fact that the patient comes to the physician because either he does not know what is wrong, or, if he does, he feels incapable of helping himself. . . . Hence the physician's basic professional knowledge and skills must span the social, psychological, and biological, for his decisions and actions on the patient's behalf involve all three. . . . The development of a biopsychosocial medical model is posed as a challenge for both medicine and psychiatry. For despite the enormous gains which have accrued from biomedical research, there is a growing uneasiness among the public as well as among physicians . . . that health needs are not being met and that biomedical research is not having a sufficient impact in human terms [pp. 133–134].

Financing and personnel

A second criticism concerns issues of financing and personnel. The typical community mental health center has always been far from self-supporting, and as federal funds were to decrease, great concern was raised about where the funds would come from to continue to support the costs of community

[2]From "The Need for a New Medical Model: A Challenge for Biomedicine," by G. L. Engel. In *Science*, April, 1977, Vol. 196, 129–136. Copyright 1977 by the American Association for the Advancement of Science. Reprinted by permission.

mental health programs (Albee, 1968; Bindman, 1966; Jones, 1963; Kubie, 1968; Marvald, 1971; Whittington, 1965; Zusman, 1970).

In addition, there was concern about shortages of professional staff and their maldistribution in the country (Albee, 1968; Feldman, 1971; Glass, 1965; Hersch, 1968; Jones, 1963; Kolb, 1968a; Kubie, 1968; Smith, 1968; Whittington, 1965; Zusman, 1970). A movement toward the development of paraprofessionals had been inaugurated, but questions were raised about the suitability of providing mental health services by persons who did not have traditional mental health professional training (Feldman, 1971; Hallowitz & Riessman, 1967; Halpern, 1969; National Institute of Mental Health, 1974; Shachnow & Matorin, 1969).

Paraprofessionals are now at work throughout the human service delivery system (Robin & Wagenfeld, 1981). They can be found not only in mental health facilities but also in general health care delivery systems, in schools, in the criminal justice system, and serving as alcoholism and drug-abuse counselors. In addition, people in other professional roles often function as caregivers, although their caregiving role is not always acknowledged.

One such group is hairdressers. The interpersonal caregiving behaviors of a group of 90 hairdressers were recently analyzed by Cowen, Gesten, Boike, Norton, Wilson, and DeStefano (1979; see also Cowen, Gesten, Davidson, & Wilson, 1981). An average hairdresser saw more than 50 people each week and spent about 25 minutes talking with each. About one-third of talking time concerned clients' personal problems, many of which were quite serious. Four clusters were identified among these problems: (1) personal problems, such as emotional health, physical health, depression, and anxiety, (2) marital problems, (3) financial problems, and (4) alcohol-related difficulties.

Hairdressers generally felt that listening to customers' interpersonal problems constituted an important part of their functioning. Their techniques for dealing with these problems included friendly denial and support; efforts to help with problem solution; avoidance moves, such as changing the subject; and passive engagement, such as just listening or suggesting that the client should talk to someone else.

There have been a number of evaluations of the functioning of the mental health worker. Durlak (1979; see also Durlak, 1981; Nietzel & Fisher, 1981) examined 42 studies comparing the effectiveness of professional and paraprofessional helpers and concluded that paraprofessionals achieved clinical outcomes equal to or better than those obtained by professionals. Durlak concluded that "professionals do not necessarily possess demonstrably superior clinical skills, in terms of measurable outcome, when compared with paraprofessionals. Moreover, professional mental health education, training, and experience are not necessary prerequisites for an effective helping person" (1979, p. 89).

Strupp and Hadley (1979) contrasted the effectiveness of a group of experienced psychotherapists and a group of college professors who were not mental health professionals but who were known for their abilities to form understanding relationships with students. Each group of therapists saw about 15 student-clients at Vanderbilt University. Strupp and Hadley concluded that "patients undergoing psychotherapy with college professors showed, on the average, quantitatively as much improvement as patients treated by experienced professional psychotherapists. . . . Although some form of treatment appeared to be superior to no treatment, the study, on the whole, lent no support to the major hypothesis that, given a benign human relationship, the technical skills of professional psychotherapists produce measurably greater therapeutic change" (1979, pp. 1134–1135).

Professional competence

Another criticism was directed at the issue of competence and skill. Many critics became alarmed by the apparent tendency to substitute community skills for clinical skills, or what they saw as an escape by mental health professionals away from patients into the community (Bindman, 1966; Bloom, 1977a, 1977b; Bloom & Parad, 1977; Glidewell, 1971; Jones, 1963; Kelly, 1970; Kubie, 1968; Norris, Larsen, Arutunian, Kroll, & Murphy, 1975).

Kubie (1968), for example, warned that mental health professionals have been trained to understand individual behavior in the context of the clinical interview. To the extent that they abandon intensive clinical intervention, they may be giving up their own area of competence for the great unknown of community psychiatry. Kubie wrote:

> Without mature psychiatrists there can be no psychiatry for anyone to know about. Yet learning *about* psychiatry is not the same as becoming a psychiatrist. The latter is more than an indoctrination; it is a continuously evolving life-long therapeutic experience for the psychiatrist which gradually releases him from bondage to his own childhood, thus making possible a process of cognitive, purposive, and emotional maturation. Today the scientific growth of psychiatry is seriously hampered by the fact that so many more people know *about* psychiatry than have gone through this searching, humbling, maturing process of *becoming* [1968, p. 260].

These remarks have general applicability to all mental health professions. Community mental health concepts and techniques should be included in the curriculum throughout the formal training period (Kelly, 1970), and expanded in-service and continuing education programs in the field of community mental health (Bindman, 1966; Bloom, 1977b; Glidewell, 1971) are needed after the completion of formal training.

The Nader report

In 1974 the Center for Study of Responsive Law, headed by Ralph Nader, prepared a general critique of the community mental health center movement (Chu, 1974; Chu & Trotter, 1974). This report was particularly critical of the mental health center concept. It was subsequently characterized by others as grossly distorted, exaggerated, destructive, dogmatic, one-sided, and simplistic, and its authors as impatient, uncharitable, immodest, naive, muckraking, and biased (Cole, 1974; Farnsworth, 1974; Marmor, 1974; see also Bloom, 1977a).

The approach used by the Nader group was what they called *investigative journalism*—the analysis and presentation of selected facts, theories, and policies from the point of view of educated laypersons. This method does not have the virtue of a true program evaluation, although its findings may be equally valid and persuasive. The authors examined the congressional intent of the legislation creating community mental health centers, talked with numerous NIMH officials, legislators, and others, and visited five representative mental health centers in Washington, D.C.; Bakersfield, California; Atlanta, Georgia; New York City; and Pontiac, Michigan.

The report criticized the requirement that each center provide five essential services, holding that it would have been far more appropriate for the legislation to have permitted each community to decide its own most appropriate alternatives to traditional mental health services. The report criticized the disease-oriented medical model, insisting that the largest category of psychiatric patients do not appear to have any disease. It criticized the tendency of some applicants for construction grants to take federal money on any pretense and then to use it to meet the needs of their own agencies—a practice the authors called *benevolent profiteering*. It criticized the fact that highly trained and paid psychiatrists often ended up spending much of their time in administrative activities for which they had never been trained and very little time doing the work they were trained for.

The report also criticized the lack of emphasis on preventive intervention, the NIMH insistence on using a geographic definition of community (see also Zusman, 1969), the failure of mental health centers to publicize the fact of their existence and the nature of their services, the failure of NIMH to require coordination and collaboration among services within service areas, and the failure of most centers to involve representative citizen groups in a meaningful policy-making role. Perhaps most important, the report criticized the failure of NIMH to require some form of evaluation and accountability from mental health centers receiving federal funds.

This critique was prepared nearly a decade ago, and in retrospect there is reason to conclude that most of what it identified so early as deficiencies in the implementation of the community mental health centers movement have been shown to be genuine deficiencies.

DEINSTITUTIONALIZATION
AND THE CONCEPT OF COMMUNITY CARE

From what this chapter has said thus far about the development of the community mental health movement, it might appear that there is universal agreement that treatment in the community is to be preferred over treatment in the geographically remote mental hospital. But a high level of agreement has never existed, and considerable doubt has been expressed about the basic concept of community care. The earliest, and in many ways the most eloquent, defense of the state mental hospital was delivered by Albert J. Glass in 1964, when he was director of the Oklahoma Department of Mental Health. Basing his comments on the fact that the quality of care in many state mental hospitals had been improving rapidly, Glass (1965) made a number of cogent assertions: (1) the stigma of psychiatric hospitalization is just as great regardless of where the patient is hospitalized; (2) the patient is just as removed from his or her community by being hospitalized in the psychiatric unit of a local general hospital as by being hospitalized in a more remote mental hospital; (3) treatment can begin just as early in a state mental hospital as in a general hospital; (4) community aftercare services are equally available to patients discharged from state mental hospitals and patients discharged from general hospitals; and (5) general-hospital psychiatric care is considerably more expensive than care of similar quality in a state-operated facility. Thus, Glass was not persuaded that there was a need for inpatient facilities in local communities.

But perhaps even more important were his other observations. First, he asserted, as have Titmuss (1965), Kolb (1968a), and Kubie (1968), that in many cases treatment may be more effective if the patient is removed from his or her home community and from the sources of stress that were at least partly responsible for his or her condition. Kubie asked "Would it be wise to launch the treatment of a malarial patient in the very malarial swamp in which he had contracted his illness?" (p. 262).[3] Second, Glass asserted that treatment facilities (including staff and programs) may be substantially better in many state mental hospitals than in the typical psychiatric unit in a general hospital and that long hospitalization (which local general hospitals are usually unable to provide) is sometimes necessary. He, along with Kubie, was critical of the typical psychiatric unit in a general hospital because it has few full-time, well-trained staff members and often no supportive services and programs, such as occupational or recreational therapy. Thus, the position of these critics is that state-hospital care is certainly no worse, and often substantially better, than local general-hospital psychiatric care (see also Arnhoff, 1975; Cumming & Cumming, 1965; Dunham, 1965; Glasscote & Gudeman, 1969, especially pp. 158–169; Shatan, 1969).

Enough time has passed to allow evaluation of this group of criticisms in the light of events that have taken place since these early warnings. As already pointed out, since 1955 there has been an accelerating decrease in the number of patients in public mental hospitals in the United States on any given day (Greenblatt, 1974). In reviewing the consequences of this policy of transferring

---

[3]From "Pitfalls of Community Psychiatry," by L. S. Kubie, *Archives of General Psychiatry*, 1968, *18*, 257–266. Copyright 1968 by the American Medical Association. This and all other quotations from this source are reprinted by permission.

care of the mentally ill from the hospital to the community, Kirk and Therrien (1975) have reminded us that "one thrust of the community-mental-health movement has been unmistakably clear: the de-emphasis of the state hospital and long-term custodial care, and the support given to a more decentralized, short-term treatment-oriented system of mental health services available in the local community" (p. 209).

Evaluating the consequences of this thrust is a complex task. In evaluating the assertion that the decrease in hospital population was related to the increase in the availability of community-based mental health services, one is hard put to account for the substantial mismatch in the ages of the patients in question. Of the total decrease in inpatient residents of state and county mental hospitals, almost 60% was among persons aged 55 and above. In contrast, fewer than 5% of the patients seen in community mental health centers are in this age range (Chu & Trotter, 1974, p. 41). Furthermore, research studies to determine whether expanded community services result in decreased state-hospital admissions have yielded inconsistent findings. In a 3-county area in Kansas that began to be served by a community mental health program, state-hospital admissions decreased (Kentsmith, Menninger, & Coyne, 1975). In contrast, in a 17-county area in Minnesota, part of which began to be served by a new community mental health facility, state-hospital admission rate also declined, but the decline was no greater in the area served by the new community facility than in the area not served by it (Aanes, Klaessy, & Wills, 1975; Bockoven & Solomon, 1975).

Beliefs underlying deinstitutionalization

Kirk and Therrien (1975) argue that although community mental health centers were established partly to supplement traditional public mental hospitals, the belief system that underlies community mental health leads the centers to focus on normal populations who are at risk, persons with mild, acute, treatable disorders, and severely disordered persons experiencing their first major psychiatric crisis. What happens to the severely disordered patient who in the past would have been a prime candidate for long-term custodial care? Basing their analysis on an intensive study of one state and on personal observations and experiences in six other states, Kirk and Therrien argue that four myths are developing in community mental health: the myth of *rehabilitation*, the myth of *reintegration*, the myth of *monetary savings*, and the myth of *continuity of care*.

The community mental health movement grew out of the conviction that mental hospitals were as much a cause of chronic mental disorder as a cure and that hospitalization was probably as often harmful as it was helpful. Accordingly, the goal of getting patients out of psychiatric hospitals was the most unequivocal of the early community mental health program objectives. Kirk and Therrien have identified three reasons that achieving this goal may not in fact help the patient: lack of decent community living facilities; attitudes of community-based mental health personnel that make it difficult for them to work effectively or even willingly with discharged hospital patients and attitudes of hospital staff members that make it difficult for them to work in the community; and lack of effective treatment programs in the community for discharged long-term hospital patients. As a result, many discharged psychiatric inpatients are now warehoused in the community under treatment regimens far more custodial than those they experienced in the psychiatric hospital—a fact that has received considerable attention in the press (see Rieder, 1974). The belief that discharging psychiatric patients into the community will hasten their rehabilitation seems to have little basis in fact.

Similarly, it was believed that the return of psychiatric patients to the community would hasten their reintegration into the life of the community. Although public attitudes toward the mentally ill are becoming more favorable, ex-psychiatric patients continue to be rejected by the community, and they are often more isolated after discharge than they were in the public psychiatric hospital.

Further, there is no persuasive evidence that community-based psychiatric care is less expensive than institution-based care, even though it was sometimes argued that treating patients in the community would result in substantial savings. Calculating the true cost of psychiatric care is a very complex task, but Kirk and Therrien make a strong case for their argument that community care is far more expensive than hospital care (see also Cochrane, 1972, pp. 57–58; Robbins, 1982). They cite figures (1975, p. 214), for example, showing that a day of care in the community in California is three times as expensive as a day of care in the public psychiatric hospital. Similar figures have been reported elsewhere. In northwestern Illinois, for example, costs for psychiatric patients treated in regional mental health centers averaged $1000 more per year than for patients treated in the traditional state hospital (Smith & Hart, 1975). The extra cost of community-based care can be acceptable, of course, if the economic benefits of that care (in the form of increased tax revenues or reduced welfare support, for example) exceed the costs. In one of the first attempts to develop a cost analysis of community versus institutional living, Murphy and Datel (1976) projected costs and economic benefits to the community over a ten-year period for a sample of 52 mentally ill or retarded patients, from four institutions in Virginia, who had been in the community an average of 8.5 months. Although the authors caution that the estimates are rough, their results, in contrast to Kirk and Therrien's, suggest that benefits would exceed costs over the ten-year period by more than $20,000 per patient if the patients were to remain in the community.

Finally, largely because of the lack of patient advocacy—the lack of an agency responsible for seeing that the theoretical advantages of continuity of care are attained—this benefit too is more a myth than a reality.

Thus, with respect to the most seriously and most chronically ill psychiatric patients, Kirk and Therrien argue that the early promise of the community mental health philosophy has not been realized. Given the current realities of community-based care, it might be more therapeutic to retain severely ill patients in the hospital until the local community accepts its responsibility to them and acts on it—that is, until the community does what needs to be done to ensure that community-based programs achieve their announced goals.

Difficulties in deinstitutionalization

In a significant number of instances, resources have been taken away from public psychiatric hospitals, in many cases from facilities that rightfully took pride in the high quality of their services, and have been redistributed to community-based programs. The consequence has often been alarming—an obvious reduction in the quality of public psychiatric hospital care without a corresponding increase in the quality of community care.

Lawton, Lipton, Fulcomer, and Kleban (1977) examined the feasibility of deinstitutionalizing the patients in a 550-bed state psychiatric hospital in Pennsylvania. The difficulties in discharging these patients can be seen in their conclusions:

> (1) The great majority of patients . . . were highly dependent, long-term, chronic, and elderly; (2) a minority (18%) were judged capable of living in a location other than a state mental hospital within a period of 1 year; (3) the population actually discharged was primarily an acutely ill, relatively recently admitted group, and (4) existing community facilities would be hard put to accommodate even the small number of patients with the best prognoses. The deficits among the large majority of patients would almost certainly preclude their acceptance by any community facility [p. 1389; see also Kaswan, 1982].

Goplerud (1979) has identified one problem associated with deinstitutionalization—a high mortality rate among patients who are transferred to community facilities, particularly among elderly patients. According to Goplerud, a large proportion of deinstitutionalized elderly psychiatric patients are transferred to community-based nursing homes. Goplerud has noted that if deinstitutionalization is to be considered a therapeutic strategy, one must show "(a) that those persons who go through the process do not experience a greater risk for psychological or physical deterioration than those persons who are not transferred, and (b) that the quality of life and level of functioning of transferred patients are at least equal to or better than that produced by the best treatment available in the state hospital" (1979, p. 318). There is, Goplerud points out, "strong evidence that for at least specific subgroups of the elderly, deinstitutionalization is not only harmful, but often fatal" (p. 318). He specifically identifies the high-risk groups as those elderly patients who are physically frail, nonambulatory, severely cognitively disturbed, and male. He notes that, in one California study, four months after deinstitutionalization five times as many patients who were transferred to another state mental hospital had died as compared with those patients not transferred, and nine times as many had died of those transferred to nursing homes. Goplerud concludes: "The evidence suggests that while relocation may serve the needs of the mental health system, it does not always prove to be beneficial to the patients" (1979, p. 326; see also Craig & Lin, 1981; DeLeon, 1982).

Analyzing the effectiveness of aftercare programs in reducing readmission rates into mental hospitals, McNees, Hannah, Schnelle, and Bratton (1977) found no decrease in recidivism rates in the three counties they studied; however, discharged patients had made little use of community services. Recidivism rates were substantially lower for those former patients who contacted the aftercare program than for those who did not. McNees and colleagues suggested that failure of some community programs might result from a failure to contact newly discharged patients and to involve them in the available community service programs (see also Brown, 1980).

In a similar study, Byers, Cohen, and Harshbarger (1978) examined recidivism rates in three West Virginia counties and concluded that the amount of aftercare received was an important factor in predicting recidivism. In addition, however, current situational factors, such as former patients' living arrangements, appeared even more important in determining the success of the community placement.

Issues in community care

One particularly interesting approach to community care has been practiced at the Southwest Denver Community Mental Health Center for some time. This approach makes use of the homes of carefully screened families in the catchment area who agree to accept up to two patients at a time and receive minimal payment to cover room, board, and care (Polak & Kirby, 1975). Polak, Deever, and Kirby (1977) contrast their program with the mental hospital as described by Rosenhan (1973). Rosenhan noted that psychiatric diagnosis locates the sources of aberration within the individual, rarely within the complex of stimuli that surround him or her. Polak and colleagues diagnose the complex of stimuli in which the client's problems originated in addition to diagnosing the client, and they carry out the diagnostic procedure in the client's home, not in the hospital. Rosenhan noted that it was nearly impossible to distinguish the sane from the insane in psychiatric hospitals. Polak and colleagues assume that no person, sane or insane, needs admission to a psychiatric hospital unless it is proved otherwise; they deemphasize the importance of the diagnosis of illness as a determinant of admission.

Rosenhan noted that staff members spend virtually all their time glassed in and rarely make contact with patients. Polak and colleagues have eliminated staff offices. Rosenhan noted that the hierarchical structure of psychiatric hospitals often facilitates impersonal relationships between staff and patients. Polak and colleagues have replaced the psychiatric hospital with a community alternative that does not encourage impersonality. Finally, Rosenhan noted that whereas patients could diagnose mental illness in the hospital, staff members could not. Polak and colleagues have enlisted the natural skills of patients and community members in the process of diagnosis and treatment and have developed a system for hiring and promotion that is based on practical clinical skills rather than on amount of formal education.

The importance of community support can be seen in the evaluation of a discharge program conducted by Bene-Kociemba, Cotton, and Frank (1979) in an aftercare service associated with a Massachusetts community mental health program. The Ambulatory Community Service dealt with six potential problem areas that discharged patients might have to face—housing, employment, finances, treatment, medication, and leisure—and began working in these areas with patients before discharge. In the sample of 160 patients, the average length of time in the community was 5.1 months at the time of the 6-month follow-up interview and 9.2 months at the 12-month follow-up interview. Achieving this high level of success was not simple, however. The authors comment:

> Most of the discharged state hospital patients we studied were single, unemployed, had major psychiatric illnesses, and had been hospitalized an average of three times. Aftercare assistance during the transition from the hospital to the community was crucial to increased community tenure for this population. Of the specific life management needs of these patients, intervention in the areas of housing, finances, and medication was singularly important in prolonging their stay in the community. Continued community treatment was effective in influencing the community tenure . . . during the first 6 months after discharge.
>
> If the objective of the community mental health movement is to maximize the community care for the state hospital patient, the needs of this patient population demand the provision of concrete, comprehensive community services by the aftercare agencies that subscribe to this objective. Quality patient care for former state hospital patients requires attention to their needs as inpatients while developing their potential for self-care [1979, p. 1560].[4]

Test and Stein (1978) reviewed the research literature contrasting community and institutional treatment of chronic psychiatric patients. They concluded that, with the possible exception of patients with organic brain syndromes, who might be unusually infirm, treatment in some kind of community setting is feasible for most of those patients usually admitted into state mental hospitals. In particular, they noted that community treatment results in less time spent in the hospital, that the symptoms of hospitalized patients do not decrease any more quickly than those of patients treated in the community, that the level of psychosocial functioning is no higher among hospitalized patients than among those treated in the community, and that client satisfaction was uniformly higher among community-based patients than among institutionalized patients. In addition, Test and Stein found that, in studies of

---

[4]From "Predictors of Community Tenure of Discharged State Hospital Patients," by A. Bene-Kociemba, P. G. Cotton, and A. Frank. In *The American Journal of Psychiatry*, Vol. 136, p. 1560. Copyright 1979 by the American Psychiatric Association. Reprinted by permission.

patients discharged into the community before they were judged ready, community placement was successful if there was an active community treatment and support program. Test and Stein conclude that "it is possible to avoid almost completely the hospitalization of most nonorganic chronically disabled patients through the use of community treatment programs . . . as long as the special community treatment program is in effect" (1978, p. 359).

Bachrach (1976) has identified the major issues that must be resolved if the movement toward community care is to succeed. She has grouped these issues into eight categories: (1) issues related to the selection of patients for community care, (2) issues related to the treatment course of patients in the community, including such topics as range of treatment services, level of coordination among community services, and quality and accessibility of services, (3) issues related to the quality of life of patients in the community, (4) issues related to the greater community, such as the effects of the patients on the community, community attitudes toward psychopathology and psychiatric patients, and the effects of discharging psychiatric patients on their families, (5) financial issues, (6) legal and patient-rights issues, (7) informational issues and accountability, such as the need to follow up discharged patients in order to evaluate their progress, and (8) issues arising from the process of deinstitutionalization itself, such as timing, attention to patients' wishes, liaison between hospitals and community agencies, and problems in providing adequate services in hospitals. Bachrach concludes her analysis by noting:

> The deinstitutionalization movement—a movement intended to counteract the effects of dehumanization in mental health care—can best fulfill its promise if certain conditions are met. Individual mental hospitals are most effectively superseded, in accord with the aims of the deinstitutionalization movement, when: (1) there is a thorough understanding of the functions which they serve in American life; (2) consensus is reached as to which of these functions should be continued or discontinued, or which new functions should be added; (3) effective alternatives are established in community settings for the accepted functions; and (4) sufficient time is allowed for the systematic and orderly implementation of new programs and transfer of functions [1976, p. 24].

Bassuk and Gerson have reviewed the major issues in the deinstitutionalization debate in light of their question "how such a well-intentioned reform as deinstitutionalization could have created so many problems" (1978, p. 46). The discharged patient was to be supported by a full spectrum of aftercare services. But communities rarely fulfilled their intended functions in these patients' behalf. Patients' living arrangements were often very poor, especially if they were living on their own. Many drifted to substandard inner-city housing that was unsafe, dirty, and overcrowded. In addition, there were too few rehabilitation programs, vocational training programs, sheltered workshops, job referrals, transportation facilities, and recreational opportunities. These problems, in turn, generally arose out of chronic lack of sufficient personnel and sufficient funds in the agencies responsible for developing expanded community services. Bassuk and Gerson suggest that the first task should be to provide decent places of habitation for discharged psychiatric patients. Indeed, newspaper stories of the plight of the chronic, indigent psychiatric patient now living in the community have little difficulty displaying examples of the generally miserable life such people often must endure. The situation in downtown Denver, Colorado, has been well illustrated by the photographs that accompanied a series of stories on the deinstitutionalized psychiatric patient.

Finally, in a thoughtful defense of the deinstitutionalization movement, Clarke (1979) notes that the initial political motivations for deinstitutionalization stemmed from criticisms of the quality of state-hospital care. Clarke observes: "It is difficult to overstate the brutality of the conditions these reformers were trying to end. The mental health system, from the commitment process to the state hospitals themselves, led to almost unspeakable indignities, privations, and denials of civil rights" (p. 466). In addition, Clarke notes that the courts have reaffirmed that mentally ill patients cannot be denied basic civil rights, that is to say they "cannot be locked away if they have committed no crime, can survive safely in the community, and are not dangerous to themselves or others—even if they are 'crazy' " (p. 475). Moreover, since mental health professionals are such unreliable prognosticators of mentally ill patients' 'dangerousness,' Clarke believes that these patients should be treated in settings no more restrictive than is absolutely necessary (see also Bloom, 1980, pp. 128–134; Bloom & Asher, 1982a.)

In conclusion, Clarke suggests:

> From an analytical viewpoint, deinstitutionalization seems beset by a misperception of its origins, a misreading of its economic history, and a misunderstanding

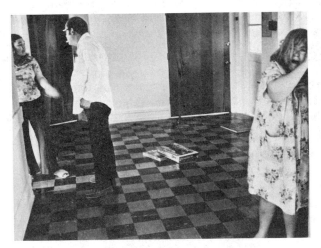 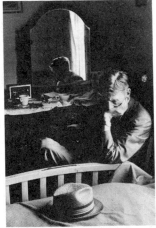

Single room occupancy dwellings for deinstitutionalized psychiatric patients, Denver, Colorado. (*Courtesy of Ernie Leyba.*)

of the nature of chronic mental illness. From a practical viewpoint, deinstitution-alization seems beset by inexorable legal demands for less restrictive care, as well as by a lack of funding. But neither state nor federal policy makers seem likely to commit massive new amounts of money to deinstitutionalization. Thus, the near future will probably witness a slower rate of exodus from state hospitals, better coordination of existing programs, adaptation of already successful models of community care, and innovation only at the fringes of public policy. Given the problems of the past ten years, this may be the best medicine that could be pre-scribed [p. 476].

As is easy to see, the more recent literature on the deinstitutionalization movement is voluminous. I cannot summarize all of it; other analyses of the problems and potentials of the movement that should be read include those by Braun, Kochansky, Shapiro, Greenberg, Gudeman, Johnson, and Shore (1981), Bennett (1979), Carpenter (1978), Fenton, Tessier, and Struening (1979), Klerman (1977), Ozarin and Sharfstein (1978), Rose (1979), Shore and Shapiro (1979), Talbott (1979), and Wolpert and Wolpert (1976).

CONCLUSIONS AND OVERVIEW

President Kennedy's message to Congress in 1963 brought both compas-sion and intellect to bear on what remains one of the most vexing social prob-lems of the 20th century. In that message, the president spelled out the con-ceptual basis for a genuinely revolutionary approach to the philosophy and organization of mental health services. It was not the concept of the com-munity mental health center that was revolutionary. Rather, it was two ideas borrowed, in part, from the field of public health that made it seem as if the golden age of mental health had at last arrived. First, the president proposed that the mental health system think of itself as responsible for everyone's mental health. Second, the president's ways of viewing prevention were unu-sually sophisticated. They recognized that there was no single cause of mental illness. They accepted the belief that, in some not yet well understood manner, harsh environmental conditions can become internalized and can then man-ifest themselves as emotional disorder.

The last 20 years, however, have been frustrating. First, in the little over a year between that presidential message and the enactment and implemen-tation of the community mental health centers legislation, most of what was truly revolutionary in the president's message disappeared. True, a new men-tal health center was not forbidden to involve itself in preventive services or to care about promoting the psychological well-being of the entire community it served, but neither was it required to do so. The Kennedy administration was concerned about much more than mental health, of course, and left the details of planning community mental health centers up to mental health professionals. The word *community* in the phrase *community mental health center* was virtually lost. What remained was not qualitatively different from what had gone on before, and the first mental health center cliché was born—the community mental health center was called "old wine in new bottles."

Second, Congress nearly killed the community mental health movement with kindness. In 1968, and again in 1970 and 1975, an enthusiastic Congress, impressed by the concept of comprehensive community-based mental health services and centers, began adding new responsibilities to these centers— treatment and rehabilitation of alcoholics and narcotics addicts, child mental health services, services for persons with drug dependencies and for the elderly, and rape prevention, among others.

Third, the executive branch, under the Nixon and Ford administrations, nearly starved the community mental health center movement to death. Starting in 1965, by the process of impoundment later determined to be unconstitutional, the executive branch began to withhold an increasing proportion of the funds authorized by Congress. Between 1969 and 1973, the executive branch permitted the expenditure of only 15% of the $340 million authorized by Congress for community mental health programs.

Finally, mental health professionals both in the community and at NIMH played their own part in the unfolding drama. Outside government, some mental health professionals viewed the new funds as a windfall; others viewed them as a virtual birthright. Construction and staffing funds were sometimes used irresponsibly. Community mental health center programs were insufficiently monitored. According to a report by the American Psychiatric Association, for example, the National Council of Community Mental Health Centers and the Mental Health Association tried to contact the 24-hour emergency services of 99 randomly selected federally funded community mental health centers in 43 states. As you will remember, such 24-hour emergency services are required by law. One-third of the 99 centers failed to answer the phone at all, even after the callers verified the correct numbers with local telephone operators. The failure to have a functioning emergency service, what one NIMH official calls "the most important service a community mental health center can provide to the public at large" (*Psychiatric News*, 1977, p. 17), was not only irresponsible but in direct violation of the law. In addition, 1963–1965 saw the beginning of an exodus of many of NIMH's most competent, experienced, and influential staff members at the very time when the field most desperately needed the intellectual and ideological leadership that they had been providing.

The accomplishments of the nearly two decades of the community mental health center movement have fallen far short of the original hopes of its most vocal proponents. The reasons, as we have seen, are complex. Far fewer than the 1500 community mental health centers originally envisioned have been established, and it now seems likely that they may never be established, at least with federal assistance.

The community mental health program seems to have been most successful in achieving three objectives—returning mental health services to the community, providing indirect services to caretaking agencies and their staffs, and providing short-term services. Far less success has been attained in three other objectives—the building of a community-based, coordinated system capable of meeting all the mental health needs of the community, optimal use of nontraditional sources of personnel, and involvement of the community in developing and evaluating the community mental health program. In three other areas, the community mental health center program has done most poorly—development of a concern for a total population, development of preventive services, and reduction of community stresses and enhancement of community strengths.

It seems clear that the community mental health center program has done best in those endeavors most similar to traditional clinical service activities. The areas of greatest failure have been those most removed from traditional training and practice—the areas in which mental health professionals generally have the least competence and experience. It has recently been conservatively estimated that the cost of mental illness in the United States was nearly $37 billion in 1974, up from $25 billion in 1971 (Levine & Willner, 1976). Of this amount, $14.5 billion was expended to provide direct patient services. In the long run, provision of effective preventive services may be the only feasible way of halting the year-by-year rise in these expenditures; yet, prevention is the very activity in which the community mental health program has done most poorly.

But when the community mental health center movement is viewed as part of a larger social revolution, it can be argued that much of its ideology is having an impact on our society. First, the movement is part of the revolution of social responsibility that includes the civil-rights movement, the efforts to provide equality of public education, and the extension of voting rights to the young and to those citizens who until recently have been effectively disenfranchised. The community mental health movement has called attention to the inequalities in our mental health service delivery system, which has denied adequate services to large numbers of Americans, and there is a growing movement to assure civil and constitutional rights to psychiatric patients. Second, it is part of a geopolitical revolution that has resulted in the establishment of the local community as a unit important enough to receive the direct attention of the federal government. Third, it is part of a planning revolution that now includes highway planning, general hospital construction planning, urban redevelopment, and other projects. Fourth, it is part of a revolution in participation in which growing numbers of citizens in all walks of life are beginning to insist on the right to have a voice in determining how and under what conditions they live and work. And, finally, it is part of a revolution in prevention that is manifested in a growing interest in the prevention of poverty, unnecessary physical disability, malnutrition, and undereducation.

There is considerable evidence that throughout the country public funds are being shifted from hospital to community settings. Public outpatient facilities, including community mental health centers, are competing with state hospitals for scarce resources, and the astonishing ability of outpatient facilities to maintain patients in the community without the need for large inpatient facilities has not gone unnoticed. Publicly supported inpatient facilities are consolidating their services and beginning to recentralize as funds traditionally appropriated to them are diverted into community facilities.

But, at the same time, the justification for the community mental health center is being challenged. Federal support is being sharply reduced. Issues having to do with the treatment of psychiatric patients are being overshadowed by concerns about modifying the organization and financing of general medical care. Psychiatric services, historically more in the public domain than other medical services, are likely to be significantly affected by the public-sector/private-sector debate—that is, the debate over whether medical care should be provided primarily by private, fee-for-service practitioners or by salaried practitioners employed by government agencies—and by proposals for the establishment of better-organized health service programs. There is some interest, at the same time, on the part of the federal government and many state governments, in moving away from direct provision of medical care and toward public support for cost- and quality-conscious private-sector services. Thus, it seems somewhat likely that psychiatric services will gradually be integrated into a system of general, comprehensive health care and that agencies whose exclusive purpose is the provision of psychiatric care may find themselves increasingly unable to justify separate status.

We are living in an era of cost accountability. The community mental health center is being called on to defend its budgetary requests and expenditures as never before. As part of this process, it is being asked to document its effectiveness, and statistics on the provision of direct services may no longer serve as acceptable documentation. Questions being asked by many funding sources are now far more sophisticated. How does a community mental health center know that its services are effective? Can it show that its treated patients are able to contribute in increasing amounts to tax revenues? Can it show a decrease in school-dropout rate, in crimes against persons and property, in drug abuse? Could it provide equally effective services at lower cost? Interest by funding agencies in mental health program evaluation has grown rapidly in the past decade. Unfortunately, fiscal resources to address this interest are now in far shorter supply than was the case when the community mental health movement began.

Most important is the danger that the concern with costs may limit our understanding of mental health to its current inadequate level. As public funds are tied more and more directly to the provision of services, less money will be available for extending our knowledge. To answer every question that has been raised about the organization and effectiveness of mental health services requires resources, and there is a staggering gap between what is known and what needs to be known about the provision of effective psychiatric care and the prevention of mental disorders. The potential of the community mental health movement has not yet been realized, and there is some chance that the mental health center will be supplanted before its potential is ascertained. But to the extent that the emphasis on getting the most for our money requires mental health centers to document the consequences of their efforts, mental health programs may be put on much stronger empirical foundations. And as centers begin to identify the outcomes of their programs, gaps in knowledge will become increasingly apparent. With these gaps revealed, it may become easier to defend the need for resources for the continuation of both basic and applied research on mental health and mental illness.

Alternatives to Traditional Mental Health Services

These three chapters deal with community mental health approaches to the delivery of services to people. Three innovative service approaches are associated with the community mental health movement—planned short-term therapy, crisis intervention, and mental health consultation. Each of these approaches represents an effort to meet the mental-health-related needs of the community. Each approach is a potential solution to the problem posed by the chronic mismatch between the demand for mental health services and their availability. Each is a way of providing help for more people than is possible by traditional long-term psychotherapy. Taken together, these approaches constitute an important and enduring contribution of the community mental health movement to human welfare.

CHAPTER

2

Planned Short-Term Therapy

From the point of view of the ideological foundation of community mental health, the responsibility of providing significant help for all who seek it is a challenge of the first magnitude. In the public sector, at least, planned short-term therapy must be one of the treatments of choice. As we will see, interest in brief therapy has been accelerating in the past 15 years, until now it constitutes a virtual revolution.

The growing interest in short-term therapy—that is, psychotherapy that has a planned duration of between 6 and 12 interviews (Castelnuovo-Tedesco, 1971)—can be seen as part of the constantly developing history of psychotherapy. This interest is, in part, a response to growing dissatisfaction with the gradual lengthening of traditional psychodynamic treatment. Most clinicians who write about brief psychotherapy come out of a psychoanalytic, or psychodynamic, orientation. Psychoanalytic therapy started out as relatively short-term but is now the longest of the psychotherapies. Marmor (1979) has noted that Freud's initial therapy cases were often very short. Bruno Walter, the conductor, was successfully treated by Freud in six sessions. The composer Gustav Mahler was successfully treated in a single four-hour session while strolling through the town of Leyden, Holland (Jones, 1955, Vol. 2, p. 80).

A similar development is currently in an earlier phase in the case of the behavior therapies. These therapies were once thought of as quite brief, but they are now increasing in length. The average length of treatment at the New York City Institute of Behavior Therapy is 50 weekly one-hour sessions (Wilson, 1981). We may find a growing interest in planned short-term therapy among behavior therapists if this increase in duration of treatment continues (see also Butcher & Koss, 1978, pp. 726–727).

Starting in 1963, coincident with the formal beginning of the community mental health movement, a series of major volumes began appearing that described and evaluated some particular form of planned short-term therapy (for example, Bellak & Small, 1965; Haley, 1973; Lewin, 1970; Malan, 1963, 1976; Mann, 1973; Phillips & Wiener, 1966; Sifneos, 1972; Wolberg, 1965b). The word *planned* is important, and these works describe short-term treatment that is intended to accomplish a set of therapeutic objectives within a sharply limited time frame. Planned short-term therapy should be distinguished from what might be called unplanned short-term therapy—that is, services that are brief because the client unilaterally terminates treatment.

RATIONALE FOR PLANNED SHORT-TERM THERAPY

Advocacy for planned short-term therapy flies in the face of a deeply ingrained mental health professional value system (Aldrich, 1968; Ursano & Dressler, 1977). In that value system, brief treatment is thought of as super-ficial, longer is equated with better, and the most influential and prestigious practitioners tend to be those who undertake intensive long-term therapy with a very few clients. Social workers expressed some early interest in planned short-term therapy but adopted the Freudian long-term model as they sought a rationale for their own professionalization (H. J. Parad & L. G. Parad, 1968; L. G. Parad & H. J. Parad, 1968). L. G. Parad (1971) has provided a compelling history of this value system and has shown that its origin can be seen early in the 20th century. Parad concludes her historical overview by noting that "while demands for service and other exigencies made it clear that the over-whelming majority of cases were short-term, the long-term intensive case has persisted as a therapeutic desideratum" (p. 129).

The reemergence of interest in planned short-term therapy has come about as a consequence of three factors—issues of efficiency and economy, changing concepts and theories of psychotherapy, and an accumulation of evidence that planned short-term therapy is *at least* as effective as long-term treatment. We will examine some of these evaluation studies at the end of this chapter.

Efficiency and economy

The efficiency and economy rationale for planned short-term therapy is stressed most notably by persons in the public sector. With the limitations in both financial and staff resources, a community mental health center, they argue, must derive the greatest possible effect from each one of the scarce therapeutic hours available to the public. Treatment will then be more feasible for larger numbers of clients (Avnet, 1965b). This conclusion is particularly cogent given the equivocal evidence of the effectiveness of long-term therapy (see, for example, Smith & Glass, 1977). Frances and Clarkin (1981) have, in fact, proposed the study of those clients for whom no treatment may be the prescription of choice. Hoffman and Remmel (1975) suggest that hourly fee assessments can be increased when the agency begins to assume that all applicants are potential short-term clients, since the total cost to the client for the episode of care can be reduced. These authors report a doubling of fee income over a three-year period in their family service agency after that assumption was adopted.

With the increasing demand for service, a planned short-term therapy orientation could result in the virtual elimination of waiting lists—a source of chronic tension for staff, clients, and for those people who hesitate to seek treatment because of their awareness of the existence of a waiting list. Finally, for many clients, whether because of economic or ideological considerations, planned short-term therapy is the only real alternative to no treatment at all (Avnet, 1965a, p. 22).

More recently, the private sector has also become interested in planned short-term therapy, but for a different set of reasons. First, serious consideration is being given to the reduction of third-party insurance reimbursement for outpatient psychotherapy as a consequence of the soaring cost of medical care. Second, new organizational forms of health care are being developed at a rapid rate. These models, such as health maintenance organizations or employee assistance programs, also offer the promise of reducing the cost of medical care. Central to these models is the provision of comprehensive health services to a family at a fixed cost per year. That is, such an organization profits by providing the minimum necessary care consistent with good health care practice. Third, primary care physicians are increasingly aware of the fact that they provide about two-thirds of all mental health services in the United States (Regier, Goldberg, & Taube, 1978) and that those services tend to be short-term. Thus, the mental health professional is, in a real sense, in competition with the primary care physician.

Changing concepts in psychotherapy

Recent changes in psychotherapeutic theory pertinent to the growing interest in planned short-term therapy include (1) acceptance of limited therapeutic goals, (2) emphasis in ego psychology on the client's strengths as well as weaknesses, (3) impact of behavior modification techniques, (4) increasing centrality of crisis theory in service-delivery-system planning, and (5) greater attention to current precipitating circumstances in contrast to past predisposing circumstances. These changes have resulted in making treatment more promptly available (Rosenbaum & Beebe, 1975, pp. 299–300), in the realization that when therapeutic time is limited, both client and therapist work harder and resistance as well as negative transference phenomena decrease (Applebaum, 1975, pp. 427ff.), and in exploring the possibility that planned short-term therapy may in some circumstances be the treatment of choice, aside from being less expensive (Ewing, 1978, p. 19; Hoch, 1965, pp. 53–54; Sifneos, 1967, p. 1069; Wolberg, 1965a).

The treatment-of-choice argument comes, in part, from the growing real-ization that most treatment is short-term, whether planned to be or not (Hoff-man & Remmel, 1975, p. 259; Hoppe, 1977, p. 307; H. J. Parad & L. G. Parad, 1968, p. 346; L. G. Parad, 1971, pp. 126–129) and that there is some potential utility in making it advertently short-term. Hoffman and Remmel suggest that "long-term psychotherapy is indicated . . . only if the client both wants and needs it. Experience shows that the overwhelming majority of the clients do not want it" (1975, p. 267; see also Cummings, 1977a, 1977b).

Mann states eloquently what a number of writers have noted: "There comes a point in the treatment of patients, whether in psychoanalysis or in psychotherapy, where time is no longer on the therapist's side insofar as the possibility of helping the patient to make further changes is involved, and where time serves far more the search by the patient for infantile gratification" (1973, p. xi).

Length of therapy and client satisfaction

There is no question that mental health professionals tend to view early and unilateral termination by clients as a sign of therapeutic failure and client dissatisfaction. It may, therefore, be reassuring to know that empirical studies of client satisfaction and length of treatment consistently fail to support this view.

Occasional reports have appeared in the literature during the past 30 years revealing how many clients in mental health and family casework agencies have one- or two-session episodes of care. Professional attitudes toward these single-contact episodes can be quickly discerned when it is noted that such clients are virtually always referred to as *dropouts*.

One finding is that such episodes are unusually common in lower social classes. Lazare, Cohen, Jacobson, Williams, Mignone, and Zisook (1972), sum-marizing the research of the prior 15 years concerned with outpatient treat-ment among persons in the lower socioeconomic class, noted that these stud-ies report dropout rates of over 50% after the first interview (see also Fiester & Rudestam, 1975). Lazare and colleagues concluded that "patients seemed to want the therapists to give practical advice, medications, and warmth—expectations that clearly differed from those of the therapists" (p. 882).

Social workers, particularly those identified with family service agencies, have long been interested in short-contact cases defined as those having a maximum of one planned intake appointment but including all telephone calls and letters (Frings, 1951). In 1948 the Family Service Association of America, surveying 64 cooperating agencies, found that about one-third of cases were closed after one in-person interview (see Shyne, 1957). To learn more about short-term cases in a family agency, Kogan (1957a, 1957b, 1957c) examined the records of all new clients in the Division of Family Services of the New York Community Service Society for one month in 1953. Of the 250 new cases, 56% were closed after one interview. Most of those closings were planned—that is, agreed on in advance by client and therapist. But 30% were unplanned—the client failed to keep subsequent appointments. Kogan was able to interview, in person or by telephone, 80% of these single-session clients between three months and one year after the case was closed. He had similar success in contacting cases with planned and unplanned closings. In addition, he analyzed therapist evaluations prepared at the time of case closings. Kogan's results are illuminating. In the majority of cases, therapists attributed unplanned closings to client resistance or lack of interest. Follow-up interviews with the clients, however, revealed that reality-based factors prevented continuance, and improvements in the problem situations may have accounted for a substantial proportion of these unplanned closings.

About two-thirds of all clients felt they had been helped—both among clients with planned closings and among those with unplanned closings. In contrast, therapists considered that clients were, in general, helped, but that those with planned closings were helped significantly more than those with unplanned closings. Therapists consistently underestimated the help that clients with unplanned closings judged they had received, and they consistently overestimated how helpful they had been to clients with planned closings.

Silverman and Beech (1979) managed to contact 47 persons out of a pool of 184 clients of a community mental health center who, in the previous year, had been seen only once and who were neither terminated nor referred elsewhere; that is, these clients had unilaterally terminated their contact with the center. Of these 47 persons, 70% expressed satisfaction with the services they had received, 79% reported that the problems that had brought them to the mental health center were solved (although only half of them attributed those solutions to the center), and the majority indicated that their expectations had been met. Thus, in the words of the authors, "the notion that dropouts represent failure by the client or the intervention system is clearly untenable" (1979, p. 241).

Littlepage, Kosloski, Schnelle, McNees, and Gendrich (1976) assessed client satisfaction by contacting 130 former clients out of the 349 who had terminated contacts with a community mental health center during 1974. These clients had had from 1 to 24 treatment contacts with the center. General level of satisfaction was high and was unrelated to number of contacts. Clients whose treatment terminated after only limited contact evaluated their experiences just as highly as clients who had had extended contact. Clients who dropped out of therapy did not evaluate their experiences differently from clients who attended their final scheduled therapy session. These authors concluded that their findings "are not consistent with the implicit assumption that persons with limited contacts terminate therapy because of dissatisfaction with the services" and that one should not "automatically assume that early client terminations reflect treatment failures" (p. 167).

In a more complex investigation, Fiester and Rudestam (1975) studied two public-sector mental health programs and contrasted clients who unilaterally terminated after the first or second session with clients who remained for three or more sessions, regardless of final disposition. Demographic information (including age, sex, education, socioeconomic status, and history of prior psychiatric care) and an array of pretherapy expectations and posttherapy reactions were collected before and after the first session. In addition, some demographic and professional background information was collected from all therapists. Results of these analyses were not the same in the two settings, a finding the authors attributed to differences in therapist characteristics.

In the facility where the therapeutic staff was older, more experienced, more affluent, and psychodynamically oriented, the clients who dropped out early and unilaterally tended more often to be lower-class people who felt they had been attentive to the therapist, whom they found to be helpful and serious, but who found themselves angry during the interview without being able to talk about it. In this setting, clients who terminated early tended to be dissatisfied with the services they had received.

In the other setting, where the staff was younger, less experienced, less doctrinaire, and of lower social class, very few clients who terminated early were dissatisfied Rather, most reported benefiting from their brief therapy. Clients described themselves as serious, in need of answers to questions, and desirous of an opportunity to express their emotions and resolve their problems. Furthermore, they tended to see the therapist as providing just what they needed. In this setting, early termination was not usually equated with failure. Dropout rate was unusually high, however, for seriously disturbed clients assigned to lower-status therapists, such as students, paraprofessionals, and mental health technicians.

The authors suggested that higher dropout rates among lower-class clients may take place primarily in settings where strict psychodynamic therapy is the treatment of choice—that is, that differential dropout rate is more closely related to therapist characteristics than to client characteristics. In the non-doctrinaire setting, "quite possibly, dropping out represents a problem primarily from the (rejected) therapist's perspective. This perspective is probably a corollary of clinical lore that asserts a direct relationship between length of treatment and patient improvement" (1975, p. 534).

Hoppe (1977) conducted a study of 106 former rehabilitation center clients who had all had prior histories of psychiatric hospitalization. Of these clients, 64 had terminated their association with the rehabilitation center unilaterally, by failing to keep scheduled appointments. The remaining 42 terminated by mutual agreement with their therapists. During the 18 months following their termination, clients were interviewed monthly and asked a series of short questions to find out whether they were working, were involved in a social life, were living independently, were paying rent, and had been rehospitalized since the last interview.

There were numerous differences between the two groups early in the 18-month period, but by the end of the study all differences had disappeared.

Hoppe concluded that the study "seriously questions the efficacy of the concept of 'dropping out' as a termination classification, and indicates that agencies may well be doing themselves a serious disservice by attaching negative connotations to dropout rates" (p. 313).

APPROACHES TO PLANNED SHORT-TERM THERAPY

There is as much variation in both the theory and practice of planned short-term therapy as in that of long-term therapy. Burke, White, and Havens (1979) divide short-term therapies into those that are *interpretive*, stressing the role of insight; *existential*, stressing the salutary effects of a brief, empathic encounter with a therapist; and *corrective*, stressing therapist-induced behavioral change. Straker (1977), among others, distinguishes between ego-supportive and anxiety-provoking forms of brief therapy. Butcher and Koss (1978) divide brief therapies into those that are psychodynamically oriented, crisis-oriented, and behavioral.

Evaluation studies have not found that certain types of brief therapy are superior to others (see Smith & Glass, 1977). Wolberg has made this point:

> The fact that the various kinds of short-term psychotherapy in the hands of competent therapists bring about approximately the same proportion of cures persuades one that the techniques and stratagems that are employed are among the least important elements responsible for improvement. The proposition is inviting that therapeutic maneuvers merely act as a means through which the therapist encourages the emergence of positive and the resolution of negative healing elements. . . . we tend to overemphasize technical virtuosity while minimizing the vital healing processes that emerge in the course of the helping relationship as a human experience. In many cases, insight acts merely as a placebo [1968, p. 353].

Yet, just as with long-term psychotherapy, an enormous amount of intellectual energy has gone into developing specific approaches to short-term therapy. Even if one type of therapy is not consistently superior to another, it is useful to examine these various approaches for at least two reasons. First, a certain approach might prove superior for certain problems, or certain types of clients, or under certain circumstances. If so, referrals or assignments to clinicians could be made more rationally than is typical in a mental health agency. Second, exposure to different approaches to planned short-term therapy might enable an individual clinician to develop a broader array of skills and thus to be effective with more diverse clients or problems.

Bellak and Small's emergency and brief psychotherapy

From 1958 until 1964—that is, largely before the start of the community mental health center movement—Bellak and Small (1965, 1978) established and were associated with the Trouble Shooting Clinic, a service of the Psychiatric Department of the City Hospital at Elmhurst, Queens, New York, that served as a 24-hour emotional first-aid station. During its six-year life, this clinic offered "immediate, walk-in care of emotional problems of minor or major degree, from advice to the lovelorn to care of acute psychoses" (1965, p. 141). Its rationale was both therapeutic and preventive, in the sense that minor problems could be prevented from becoming more severe and that helping a client deal with a problem might make it easier for that client to deal with a future problem without professional assistance.

   Goals of therapy.   Bellak and Small have come out of a conservative psychoanalytic tradition and have tried to show in their writings how psychoanalytic theory and therapeutic concepts can be used in providing brief and emergency psychotherapy. Rather than developing a separate theory, they argue that properly understood psychodynamic formulations can be successfully applied in brief psychotherapy. The term *brief* is to be understood as meaning between one and five or six therapy sessions of customary duration.

   Bellak and Small say that "the goal of brief psychotherapy is limited to the removal of or amelioration of specific symptoms: it does not attempt the reconstitution of personality except that any dynamic intervention may secondarily and, to a certain extent, autonomously lead to some restructuration" (1965, p. 9). Brief psychotherapy seeks to help a client continue to function, so that nature can continue its work of healing, and also, where indicated, to increase the client's self-supporting ability so that more extensive psychotherapy can be undertaken. Bellak and Small, while acknowledging that relatively brief psychotherapy may be sufficient to help some clients continue growing on their own, see it as capable of decreasing the sense of personal difficulty and increasing strength and adequacy of functioning so that improved earning power and improved motivation can lead the way to more substantial treatment. Where circumstances permit more prolonged treatment, Bellak and Small see few instances in which brief therapy would be preferable.

   Therapeutic techniques.   Bellak and Small's most important contributions to the practice of brief therapy are technical rather than theoretical. They see the steps in brief therapy as (1) identifying the presenting problem, (2) taking a detailed history, (3) establishing an understanding of the relation between that history and the presenting problem, (4) selecting and applying appropriate interventions, (5) working through the problem from differing perspectives, and (6) termination. They believe that this process can take place most successfully when the therapist is seen in a positive light as likable, reliable, understanding, accepting, hopeful, benign, interested, and helpful.

   Understanding the history and the details of the presenting problem is basic to developing formulations and intervention plans, and Bellak and Small allocate virtually all of the first interview to that task. They conceive of the history as comprising two parts—first, the history of the chief complaint and the life setting within which it arose and, second, a comprehensive developmental history of the client. If the history is skillfully obtained, it should be possible to understand the onset of the present problem in dynamic terms—that is, in relation to developmental and cultural events. The process of establishing cause-and-effect hypotheses is, for Bellak and Small, clearly within the psychoanalytic theoretical tradition and "requires every bit of intellectual and emotional equipment the psychotherapist can muster. . . . No unconscious process, no defensive reaction, no primitive quality in the human being can be alien to him" (1965, p. 49).

Bellak and Small describe the various intervention possibilities open to the therapist undertaking brief therapy. The central intervention is the imparting of insight through judicious interpretations. Other interventions, often just as important as the increase of understanding, include increasing self-esteem, providing the opportunity for catharsis (discharge of built-up emotions and tensions), helping clients suppress and restrain drives that are destructive to adjustment, assisting clients to distinguish between fantasy and reality, helping them become more sensitive to warning signals that originate both inside and outside them, providing clients with increased intellectual appreciation and understanding of salient issues they are facing, and providing reassurance and support.

The goal of brief psychotherapy is to strengthen the likelihood that more mature behavior will take place and that older, neurotic modes of adjustment will be extinguished. In brief therapy there is little time for the application of therapeutic gains in the therapeutic setting, but the client can continue to learn by applying the lessons of psychotherapy in real life.

Bellak and Small's comments about termination illustrate their own uncertainties about the definite benefits of brief psychotherapy: "In brief psychotherapy, the patient must be left with a carefully cultivated positive transference and a clear understanding that he is welcome to return. The maintenance of the positive transference avoids a sense of rejection in the terminating process and permits the patient to retain the therapist as a benign, introjected figure" (1965, p. 73; 1978, p. 106). Bellak and Small stress that although the client should be urged to apply the lessons of the therapy, it should be made clear that the therapist is available for additional help. The client should feel free to contact the therapist before future problems get out of hand and can be urged to provide periodic follow-up reports by letter or telephone.

A special strength of Bellak and Small's volumes is the discussion of the role of brief psychotherapy in specific psychiatric syndromes and life situations—depression, panic, depersonalization, acute psychotic states, acting out, severe somatic conditions, sexual dysfunctions, problems of the elderly, and stressful life events. In each instance, a variety of brief case histories are presented to illustrate the general therapeutic guiding principles.

For example, in acting out (the translation of inner conflicts into socially unacceptable or self-destructive direct behavior rather than into internalized symptoms), Bellak and Small suggest the following array of useful therapeutic techniques: (1) direct prohibition of certain relationships or behavior, (2) removing the client from the setting that precipitates the undesirable behavior, (3) prudent interpretation of the meanings of the behavior, (4) attempts to make the behavior unacceptable to the client, (5) intellectual presentation and discussion of the meaning of that behavior in that client, (6) prediction of acting-out behavior through an understanding of the factors that cause it, as a way of preventing the behavior, (7) encouragement of delay in acting-out behavior when outright prohibition seems impossible, (8) strengthening that aspect of the client's personality that wishes to control the behavior, that feels the behavior is undesirable, (9) helping the client think of today's behavioral temptations in the light of the immediate but easily forgotten past, (10) use of drugs to reduce anxiety, (11) enlisting the help of others to inhibit harmful acting out, (12) providing constantly available support and reassurance, and (13) reducing the inhibitions that prevent the client from successfully engaging in socially desirable behavior.

Malan's intensive brief psychotherapy

Malan (1963, 1976) wanted to call his brief therapy "radical" but, warned away from that term by its unfortunate connotations in America (Malan works in Great Britain), has chosen the word *intensive* to describe the kind of brief psychotherapy undertaken by his group at the Tavistock Clinic in London and the Cassel Hospital in Richmond. Regardless of what it is called, Malan wants the reader to understand that in the kind of brief therapy he practices the aim is "really to *resolve* either the patient's central problem or at least an important aspect of his psychopathology" (1976, p. 248). Malan's studies of brief therapy have been based on clients generally seen for 10 to 40 sessions, somewhat longer than is usually meant by the term *brief*.

Client characteristics.   Because successful brief therapy depends in part on client characteristics, Malan and his group have gone to considerable lengths to specify the criteria for acceptance or rejection of applicants. First, a potential client with any of the following clinical characteristics is rejected (because these conditions are often severe and disabling): serious suicide attempts, drug addiction, "convinced" homosexuality, long-term hospitalization, more than one course of electroconvulsive therapy, chronic alcoholism, incapacitating chronic obsessional symptoms, incapacitating chronic phobic symptoms, and gross destructive or self-destructive acting out (1976, pp. 67–68).

Second, clients are rejected if it is judged that any of the following conditions is quite likely to occur in therapy: inability to make contact, necessity for prolonged work in order to generate motivation for treatment, necessity for prolonged work in order to penetrate rigid defenses, inevitable involvement in complex or deep-seated issues that there seems no hope of working through in a short time, severe dependence or other forms of unfavorable, intense transference, and intensification of depressive or psychotic disturbance. The first three of these predicted conditions would preclude starting effective therapeutic work within the time limits imposed by the nature of the therapy; the next two would result in an inability to terminate; and the last would result in a depressive or psychotic breakdown (1976, p. 69).

If a prospective brief-therapy candidate is not rejected on the above grounds, he or she is accepted if both therapist and client can find an acceptable focus for the work to be undertaken and if the client has the apparent motivation to face the stresses of psychotherapy. Specifically, the therapist should be able to identify "some circumscribed aspect of psychopathology, formulated in terms of a basic interpretation, which it seems feasible to . . . work through in a short time" (1976, p. 256). In addition, it should be clear that clients have the capacity to think of their problems in psychological terms and that they are in accord with the therapist's formulation of a problem focus. Using this complex set of criteria, Malan's group rejected about one-third of the cases they considered for inclusion in their most recent clinical study of brief therapy. The selection process usually involved more than one interview and sometimes diagnostic psychological testing. It was necessary to assess the applicant's psychodynamic history, to see whether a therapeutic focus could be found, to test out the applicant's ability to accept and use interpretations, and to judge the level of motivation.

Therapeutic techniques.   Malan's techniques derive quite directly from psychoanalytic principles. That is, the strategic aim of psychotherapy, in Malan's view, is to bring into consciousness the emotional conflicts the client is struggling with and to help the client experience and clarify them. Such conflicts are thought of as the result of the anxiety brought about by the unsuccessful or uneconomical use of defenses to ward off an unacceptable impulse or intolerable feeling. Usually it is necessary to clarify the conflict in that order; that is, understanding the anxiety brought about by the failure of a defense makes it possible to bring the hidden feeling or impulse into consciousness.

Conflicts may display themselves in three main settings: in relation to important figures from the more remote past (most often parental figures), in relation to relatively current situations and persons (job or marriage, for example), and in relation to the therapist in the clinical interview itself. It is important to clarify the nature of the client's conflicts in all three settings, but this is somewhat simpler than it sounds because very often the same patterns of anxiety, defense, and impulse occur in each setting.

From a tactical point of view, the therapist is constantly acting on the basis of a judgment of (1) which component(s) of the impulse/defense/anxiety triad to interpret, (2) in which of the three settings it would be most therapeutic to examine any component of the conflict triad, and (3) how the most useful linking interpretations between settings can be made.

It is the ability to formulate the patient's problem in terms of this kind that gives the therapist the opportunity to exert very considerable control over the course of therapy. . . . Provided the initial formulation is correct, a good patient will follow these moves actively; that is, having received a partial interpretation, he will go on to complete it; and having received one interpretation in the sequence, he will spontaneously lead the therapist toward the next. This is part of what is meant by the "therapeutic alliance." It is the combination of a simple initial formulation, a responsive and well-motivated patient, and a therapist who intuitively understands these principles, that results in focal therapy [1976, p. 262].[1]

Malan brings the reader back to the importance of the therapeutic plan and the correct selection of clients: "The best way of keeping interpretations focal is to select focal patients in the first place and then to formulate a correct therapeutic plan" (1976, p. 263).

Malan's brief psychotherapy differs from traditional long-term therapy in three important respects. First, it has a limited aim—specifically, to work through a particular conflict or set of conflicts partially and then see what results follow; second, the client understands from the beginning that the number of sessions is limited; and third, the technique is focal in a remarkably single-minded manner because of the agreed-on therapeutic plan that guides the therapy as a whole (1963, pp. 208–210).

Wolberg's short-term psychotherapy

Reminding the reader that Freud practiced short-term therapy, Wolberg (1965c) outlines its advantages and suggests that its virtues have not been fully appreciated. But, he argues, short-term therapy requires its own methodology and the development of its own theoretical concepts. It is not simply less of traditional long-term therapy. In approaching these tasks, Wolberg discusses the essential compromises in short-term therapy in therapeutic goals, techniques, attitudes, and selection of cases. He then presents an impressive rationale and set of principles for what he calls "a flexible system of short-term psychotherapy" (1965c, p. 142).

Therapeutic goals.   Wolberg believes that abbreviated therapeutic goals must be accepted in short-term therapy. He mentions specifically (1) symptom relief, (2) restoration of prior level of functioning, (3) some understanding in the client of the factors operative in producing the problem for which help was sought, (4) beginning recognition of character traits that prevent a more satisfying life adjustment, (5) increased awareness of the role of early childhood experiences in establishing these character traits, (6) recognition of some of the relations between character traits and the current conflict, and (7) identification of some workable steps toward remediation. Among techniques that have special salience in short-term therapy, Wolberg identifies the placebo influence—that is, the role of faith in the agency providing help; the thera-

---

[1]From *The Frontier of Brief Psychotherapy: An Example of the Convergence of Research and Clinical Practice,* by D. H. Malan. Copyright © 1976 by Plenum Publishing Corporation. This and all other quotations from the same source reprinted by permission.

peutic value of the relationship itself; the virtue of unburdening and emotional catharsis; the helpfulness of suggestion and teaching; and finally, the unpredictable spontaneous forces and changes that arise from time to time with or without psychotherapy.

Client characteristics.   Wolberg proposes that conditions that might best respond to short-term therapy are those in which the goal is rapid restoration of homeostasis in an acute neurotic disorder, resolution of an acute upset in a chronic personality disorder, or personality reconstruction in persons unsuited for or unable to pursue long-term therapy. By contrast, conditions best suited for long-term therapy are those in which extensive personality reconstruction is the prime objective, dependency is so entrenched that prolonged support is essential, there are persistent and uncontrollable acting-out tendencies, or there is constant and unrestrainable anxiety.

Therapeutic techniques.   The most important needed changes in therapeutic technique that are entirely under the therapist's control include a higher activity level; open expressions of interest, sympathy, and encouragement; willingness to try a variety of therapeutic strategies rather than insisting on a single therapeutic approach; and a need to overcome (where it exists) the therapist's "prejudice of depth"—that is, the belief that discussing the past is necessarily more therapeutic than discussing the present, that discussing material of which the client is unaware is necessarily more therapeutic than discussing experiences that are conscious, and that discussing attitudes toward the therapist is necessarily more therapeutic than discussing attitudes toward other important figures in the client's life.

The indebtedness of Wolberg's system of short-term therapy to psychoanalytic concepts of personality development and of remediation is always clear. Wolberg makes important use of such concepts as dream interpretation, transference, the psychodynamic hypothesis, and resistance. But Wolberg also makes use of concepts that arise from learning theory, environmental analysis, and interpersonal psychology and, in addition, proposes that attention be directed to the establishment of life values and a life philosophy. That is, Wolberg's approach is itself an illustration of the responsible eclecticism that he suggests is needed by everyone doing short-term therapy.

The initial step in Wolberg's approach to short-term therapy is the rapid establishment of a working relationship through sympathetic listening, communicating understanding and self-confidence, reassuring clients who seem without hope, and taking an active role in structuring the therapeutic situation. While establishing a relationship, Wolberg tries to develop a diagnostic and psychodynamic formulation. In this process he draws heavily on psychoanalytic theories of personality development and psychopathology. In doing so, Wolberg acknowledges the contribution of Karl Menninger, who wrote "The special merit of psychoanalysis is that from the painstaking long-continued treatment of some individuals so much has been learned that is helpful in the shorter treatment of other individuals" (1963, quoted in Wolberg, 1965c, pp. 152–153).[2]

At about the time that the formulation of the client's problem begins to seem useful, the therapist and client must identify a specific problem area on which to focus. Often the focus is on the precipitating stressful situation. Sometimes it is on the most distressing symptom or symptoms. Less often the focus is on characteristics of the client/therapist relationship. Therapeutic techniques of particular importance to Wolberg include those actions that help clarify and interpret the client's behavior.

In addition, Wolberg helps his clients learn how to increase their self-understanding. He has identified five particular strategies. First, he suggests to clients that they relate their outbursts of tension, anxiety, and symptom increase to provocative incidents in the environment and to insecurities within the self. Second, he urges clients to become sensitive to the nature of circumstances that boost or lower feelings about themselves. Third, he encourages them to observe the vicissitudes in their relationships with other people. Fourth, he believes they should become more expert in understanding their own dreams and daydreams. Finally, he believes clients can become sensitive to those occasions when they fail to put their insights into action.

Like other authors, Wolberg believes that annual follow-up interviews are important, either in person, by telephone, or by a letter from the client outlining feelings and progress. Plans for the follow-up procedure are generally made as part of the termination phase of the therapy.

The therapist as educator.   Wolberg also believes clients can profit from knowing a few general principles that can assist in increasing life satisfaction. While values can change slowly in the course of long-term therapy, in short-term therapy Wolberg believes that therapists may be able to "expedite matters by acting in an educational capacity, pointing out faulty values and indicating healthy ones that the patient may advantageously adopt" (1965c, p. 183). Among these life principles that can be shared, Wolberg mentions a dozen that seem particularly salient to him, summarized here as a series of aphorisms.

1. What's past is past. Stop worrying about what happened long ago!
2. Learn to recognize when you are tense or anxious and try to identify the sources of these feelings!
3. A certain amount of tension and anxiety is normal in life!
4. All people have to live with a certain amount of anger and hostile feelings, and should learn to tolerate those feelings!
5. Expect to be frustrated from time to time in life, and learn to accept those experiences!

[2]From "The Technic of Short-Term Psychotherapy," by L. R. Wolberg. In L. R. Wolberg (Ed.), *Short-Term Psychotherapy*. Copyright © 1965 by Grune & Stratton, Inc. This and all other quotations from the same source reprinted by permission.

6. If you find something in your environment that needs changing, get started correcting it!

7. Some life circumstances are irremediable. When something can't be changed, learn to live with it!

8. When you see that you are being self-destructive, figure out what you're doing. Remember, you have the power to change your behavior!

9. Keep the demands you make on yourself within realistic and reasonable limits!

10. People are different. Just because there are some things other people can do that you can't doesn't make you inferior!

11. Life is to be enjoyed. Get all the pleasure you can out of it!

12. Value the opportunities you have to build better relationships with people with whom you interact. Try to see the world through their eyes!

Wolberg summarizes the stages that seem to occur in the resolution of an emotional problem in the process of short-term therapy:

> 1. The patient becomes reassured that he is not hopeless and that there is nothing so drastically wrong with him to prevent a resolution of his suffering. . . . 2. He develops some understanding of reasons for his emotional break-down and he becomes aware of the fact that he has had problems within himself that have sensitized him to his current upset. . . . 3. On the basis of his understanding, he recognizes that there are things he can do about his current environmental situation, as well as about his attitudes toward people and toward himself. . . . 4. He accepts the fact that there are and probably always will be limitations in his environment and in himself which he may be unable to change. . . . 5. He fulfills himself as completely as possible in spite of handicaps in his environment and in himself, at the same time that he promotes himself to as great degrees of maturity and responsibility as are within his potential [1965c, pp. 192–193].

Phillips and Wiener's structured behavior change therapy

Phillips and Wiener's (1966) approach to short-term therapy proceeds from their basic premise that the goal of all therapists is to produce significant behavior change as efficiently as possible. With this emphasis on prompt behavior change, they assert:

> Long-term therapy is not, in fact, the most desirable, not even for those who can afford it or who prefer it. It is not a matter of efficiency alone that makes us favor short- over long-term therapy. Instead, our belief is that structured therapy (which tends to be short-term) is better than long-term, conventional therapy for this reason: structured therapy is *purposely* as short-term as possible. By "purposely," we mean *structured to solve specific problems*—regardless of whether they are chronic and serious or only mildly disabling [1966, p. 2].

To Phillips and Wiener short-term therapy can do more than be supportive, provide guidance or the opportunity to discharge pent-up emotions, or fulfill dependency needs. They believe short-term therapy can produce substantial and persistent behavior change, and they believe the help most people need to develop more satisfying lives may be far more modest than therapists have been led to believe. In contrast to psychodynamic or nondirective therapies that emphasize characteristics of the person in understanding and modifying behavior, Phillips and Wiener's approach emphasizes characteristics of the external world and of the responses the person makes to it.

From this emphasis, many consequences follow. First, since the focus of interest is on behavior change, there is relatively little concern with the origins of a person's difficulties—that is, with the original stimuli for the problem. Second, after the therapist and the client have agreed on the objectives of the therapy, clients are taught to develop new responses to troublesome situations by changing their behavior, their environment, or both. Third, other people may be involved in the therapeutic process whenever they might be able to function as change agents. Fourth, with the emphasis on behavior change procedures, there is less need for traditional verbal, insight-oriented practices. Fifth, any and all problem-solving procedures are encouraged. Sixth, rather than allowing undesired behavior to occur so that it can be studied and extinguished, it is prevented from occurring whenever possible. Seventh, the general therapeutic task is to find, institute, and reinforce new desired behavior to substitute for the problem behavior. Eighth, behavior change, like all learning, can be expected to take place step by step rather than by sudden bursts of insight. Ninth, corrective measures are forward-looking and specific. The therapist's technical skills come into play in the process of identifying and promoting newly sought behavior patterns, with the use of such procedures as desensitization, operant conditioning, and aversive stimulation. Finally, there is no need for a language that is not tied directly to behavior—that is, for such concepts as diagnosis, anxiety, complexes, or the unconscious.

Phillips and Wiener take the position that since it is behavior change that the client is seeking, not only is the most direct approach to that goal the most efficient, but it might very well also be the best. Their ideas and approaches would be less applicable when behavior change is not the primary goal or not even a goal at all. Some therapists would argue that the goal of psychotherapy is to increase self-understanding and that changes that a client might make as a consequence of that increased understanding are of only secondary importance. But to the extent that behavior change is one of the major goals of psychotherapy, Phillips and Wiener's work provides an impressive justification for therapists to become skilled in the techniques of behavior analysis and behavior modification.

Lewin's brief confrontive therapy

Lewin's (1970) brief psychotherapy represents the application of a somewhat unorthodox view of the psychoanalytic theory of psychopathology to the process of helping clients quickly understand themselves better. Because the theory and the therapeutic strategy are inseparable, a review of those aspects of the modified theory that appear most salient in understanding the therapeutic process is necessary.

Theoretical background. Lewin's therapeutic strategy deliberately concentrates on superego issues—that is, issues of guilt, shame, and conscience, or what has been called "psychic masochism" (Bergler, 1949). This emphasis is based on the importance to Lewin of the process of introjection, the "process of incorporation of another person, usually a parent, into the child's self, the assimilation of another's personality" (1970, p. 13). Lewin believes that this process begins within the first year of life and that it can continue throughout adulthood. A previous introject can be extruded and replaced, although with increasing age the process becomes more difficult.

Lewin makes clear that it is not yet understood how the process of introjection takes place.

> How it is that one child takes as part of himself a loving, tender, accepting mother, while another child incorporates a cold, disapproving, rejecting aspect of that same mother, a totally exasperated parent, remains a mystery. The choice of introject does not necessarily follow the real, objective attitude of that mother. Position in the family occasionally dictates the choice; if the role of good introjected mother–good child has already been filled by a sibling, the child might well become the bad introjected mother–bad child. Most often, the child introjects that view of his mother that he feels he deserves. If there are aspects of himself of which he feels deeply ashamed or guilty, he is more likely to introject a disapproving, punitive mother [1970, p. 14].[3]

The importance of the nature of the introject to psychological well-being cannot be overemphasized. A good introject sustains us by constantly replenishing our capacity to love, our self-esteem, and our optimism. It allows us to be alone without being lonely. The child without a good introject may be schizophrenic. For such a child, loneliness is terrifying, regardless of life circumstances. While children with good introjects are happy within the limits imposed by their life situations, the children with bad introjects are in constant psychic pain.

Depending on the nature of the introject, shame and guilt can play vastly differing roles in a person's psychological functioning. Lewin writes:

> For the child with a good introject, shame and guilt serve constructive purposes. Shame, by producing anxiety when the child has not measured up to his ego ideal, spurs him to useful action. Guilt, by producing anxiety when the child has hurt others, encourages him to do better by them in the future. . . . for the child with a bad introject, shame and guilt serve no constructive purposes and become instead weapons for self-punishment and torture. Shame nags him with the humiliation of his debasement from his ego ideal and guilt flogs him for his wrong-

[3]From *Brief Encounters: Brief Psychotherapy*, by K. K. Lewin. Copyright © 1970 by Warren H. Green, Inc. This and all other quotations from the same source reprinted by permission.

doing. Neither shame nor guilt improve his actions in the future; they merely convince him that he is hopelessly ineffectual and bad [1970, p. 20].

As the reader might expect, Lewin sees the main goal of therapy as countering the client's psychic masochism, the internalized guilt and shame—as exposing and replacing the client's bad introject and disabling sense of right and wrong. The therapist sides with the client's ego, as it were, against the common enemy—a punishing and vindictive conscience. In this process, the therapist is active, confrontive, and, if necessary, critical. "Confrontations in brief therapy must be made in such a way that the patient sees them as helpful though painful. The doctor should emerge as a strong figure of assistance who is not afraid of, or repelled by, those traits of the patient about which he comments. The therapist represents both ego and healthy conscience" (p. 37).

Therapeutic techniques.   Perhaps the unusual feature of Lewin's therapeutic technique is his handling of negative feelings a client might have about the therapist—that is, what is commonly called the *negative transference*. Lewin writes:

> This method of brief therapy depends precisely on the development of initial negative transference. After all, people get sick from unpleasant feelings—envy, jealousy, greed, and anger—and those will surface immediately, if given a chance. The exposure of the patient's negative feelings toward him enables the therapist to confront the patient with his masochistic response to anger. . . . Almost invariably, patients react to any confrontation with anger, evident to the therapist *only in the manner in which the patient defends against expressing it openly to the doctor.* This is the characteristic masochistic maneuver of turning anger inward upon the self. The patient may flush, fall silent, cry, fumble with fingers, clench his fist, or show suppressed rage in some other fashion. At that point, the therapist confronts the patient, not merely with his anger, but with the patient's reluctance to express the anger openly out of fear of antagonizing the therapist, the figure upon whom the patient depends for help in his illness. He is asked, if he has so much conflict about his expression of anger at his doctor, a relatively unimportant stranger in his life, how much worse are his conflicts about his family and loved ones? [pp. 35–36].

The purposes of Lewin's brief psychotherapy are to restore the clients' functioning, to help clients understand how their conflicts have led to their self-destructive actions, and to suggest other ways of handling their conflicts. Insofar as it is possible, the therapy seeks to replace clients' punitive introjects with less pathological ones. Temporarily, the therapist's model of an introject is offered as a substitute. Success of the therapy depends, in part, on the client's ability to accept the substitute. Lewin comments, in discussing the evaluation of his brief psychotherapy, that the results are good and are generally comparable with the results of long-term therapy.

Lewin's book is rich in powerful clinical illustrations that exemplify very dramatically how the conduct of the clinical interview follows from the theoretical formulations just described.

Sifneos's anxiety-provoking short-term psychotherapy

Sifneos (1972, 1979) distinguishes two general types of psychotherapy based on an assessment of the client's current anxiety level. There is, according to Sifneos, an optimal level of anxiety—if anxiety is too high, it should be reduced in the therapeutic setting; if it is too low, it should be increased. Thus, Sifneos distinguishes between what he calls anxiety-suppressing and anxiety-provoking therapeutic styles.

Theoretical background. Therapy that is anxiety-suppressive seeks to "decrease or eliminate anxiety by use of supportive therapeutic techniques, such as reassurance, environmental manipulation, hospitalization, or appropriate medication" (1972, p. 45). Therapy that is anxiety-provoking is designed to increase anxiety in order to accomplish its more dynamic goals of emotional reeducation and the enhancement of improved problem-solving skills.

Both forms of therapy may be of varying duration. Sifneos distinguishes among crisis support (anxiety-suppressive therapy generally lasting less than two months); brief anxiety-suppressive psychotherapy, lasting between two months and one year; and long-term anxiety-suppressive psychotherapy, which might even last indefinitely and might most commonly be used to help seriously disturbed clients. Parallel distinctions are made for anxiety-provoking therapy. Crisis intervention is conceived as anxiety-provoking therapy lasting less than two months; short-term anxiety-provoking therapy may last between two months and one year. Psychoanalysis, according to Sifneos, is "anxiety-provoking psychotherapy of long-term duration" (1972, p. 71).

Therapeutic techniques. The therapeutic concept that sets Sifneos apart from other brief psychotherapists is anxiety provocation. Sifneos describes the concept in the following way:

> Out of a variety of presenting complaints the patient is asked to assign top priority to the one emotional problem which he wants to overcome. The therapist, who acts as both evaluator and teacher, can obtain, by skillful interviewing and history-taking, enough information from the patient to enable him to set up a tentative psychodynamic hypothesis to help him arrive at a formulation of the emotional conflicts underlying the patient's difficulty. Throughout the treatment he concentrates his attention especially on those conflicts in an effort to help the patient learn a new way to solve his emotional problem. To achieve these ends the therapist, over a short period of time, must create a therapeutic atmosphere, establish an alliance with the patient, agree with him as to the definition of the problem to be solved, and utilize the patient's positive feelings for him as the main therapeutic tool. He must use anxiety-provoking questions in order to obtain the evidence he

needs to substantiate or to modify his formulation. . . . he must stimulate the patient to examine the areas of emotional difficulty which he tends to avoid in order to help him become aware of his feelings, experience the conflicts, and learn new ways of solving his problem [1972, pp. x–xi].

An example will illustrate anxiety-provoking psychotherapy. (Pt = patient, Th = therapist.) A 25-year-old social worker expressed concern because she claimed to have forgotten what the area of concentration for her therapy was going to be. She went on as follows:

Pt: I know that it may be significant, but the funny thing about it is that I cannot remember what we agreed to talk about last week.

Th: Why is it funny?

Pt: I meant it in the sense that it was peculiar.

Th: But you used the word "funny." What's so amusing in forgetting what we decided to focus on during your therapy?

Pt: Well, it must have something to do with wanting some guidance of sorts. If I don't remember, then you will help me.

Th: Yet, how can I help you when I don't know as yet why you have the problems that bring you to the clinic.

Pt: That's true.

Th: So, there is a part of you which nevertheless wants me to do something which you know only too well I cannot do. Now, assuming that I tried to tell you what to talk about, how would you feel about it?

Pt: I'd like it.

Th: Part of you would like it, but how would the other part feel? The part that knows that I cannot do it?

Pt: A little silly.

Th: Meaning . . . .

Pt: (hesitating) . . . That you are a little silly, doing something like that when you really don't know.

Th: Precisely! So, wouldn't it be funny then to see your therapist do something silly?

Pt: In a way, yes.

Th: So the word "funny" was used appropriately.

Pt: I suppose so.

Th: Now that we have clarified this point, let's return to your lapse of memory.

Pt: The funny thing is that I have just remembered what we have agreed to concentrate on during my treatment.

Th: There are a lot of funny things going on today! [1979, pp. 63–64]

In this example, the therapist's style is clear—a high level of activity, gentle yet unrelenting exploration, active confrontation, clarification, and interpretation. With regard to overall technique, Sifneos characterizes therapist activity as concentrating on areas of unresolved emotional conflicts by the use of anxiety-provoking questions while avoiding involvement with deep-seated character defects, such as excessive passivity, dependence, or narcissism.

Client characteristics. Anxiety-provoking short-term psychotherapy makes serious demands on the client as well as the therapist. Accordingly, there are fairly explicit criteria by which to identify suitable candidates. In addition to the ability to tolerate increased anxiety, Sifneos identifies the following selection criteria: the client (1) must be of above-average intelligence, (2) must have had at least one meaningful relationship with another person during his or her lifetime, (3) must be able to interact with the mental health professional by the appropriate expression of some emotion during the interview and by showing some degree of flexibility, (4) must be able to voice a specific chief complaint, and (5) must be motivated for change, not just symptom relief, and must be willing to work hard during psychotherapy (see also Sifneos, 1979, pp. 22–39).

Evaluating motivation for psychotherapy is difficult, but Sifneos proposes that the assessment be made using the evidence that the prospective client has the ability to recognize that the symptoms are psychological in origin, appears to be introspective and honest, seems willing to participate actively in the therapeutic situation, is actively curious and willing to understand the self, is willing to explore, experiment, and change, has realistic expectations regarding psychotherapeutic outcome, and is willing to make reasonable sacrifices in the service of psychotherapy.

The selection criteria for anxiety-suppressive short-term therapy are fewer and less demanding than for anxiety-provoking short-term therapy. Sifneos suggests that suitability for this more supportive therapy might be judged by (1) ability to maintain a job, (2) a strong appeal for help to overcome an emotional difficulty, (3) recognition that the symptoms are psychological in origin, and (4) willingness to cooperate with psychotherapy.

Mann's time-limited psychotherapy

The critical word in Mann's (1973) time-limited psychotherapy is *time*. It is time, with its many meanings, that is not sufficiently understood, and it is the complex feelings toward the passage of time that help make the therapeutic relationship one of difficulty for client and therapist alike. Mann's work is based on an insistence that time be faced squarely and that it be used in the service of psychotherapeutic gain.

   Disadvantages of long-term therapy.   With the duration of psychotherapy left open, Mann has found, a "well-intentioned sabotage" (1973, p. x)
often takes place in clinical settings that are trying to see more clients by
shortening the length of treatment. Long-term psychotherapy with insufficiently or inaccurately defined treatment goals, argues Mann, "leads to a steady
widening of and diffusion of content. This creates a growing sense of ambiguity in the mind of the therapist as to what he is about, and . . . it surely
increases the patient's dependence on the therapist. The result is that patient
and therapist come to need each other, so that bringing the case to a conclusion
seems impossible" (p. x). Furthermore, as already mentioned, Mann argues
that there comes a point in the treatment of patients when time is no longer
on the therapist's side.
   To counteract this nontherapeutic state of affairs, Mann has experimented
with a procedure that might allow helping larger numbers of clients. He has
established a short-term psychotherapy limited to exactly 12 treatment hours
with flexible distribution and duration of visits but with a fixed ending date
agreed to in advance by both therapist and client.

   Theoretical background.   Mann views attitudes toward time develop-
mentally. During childhood, time seems infinite—the future seems forever
beyond reach. In adolescence, the limits of time are discovered—decisions
have to be made, they cannot be put off. The older we get, the more real and
inexorable becomes the passage of time. The child lives in the special paradise
of timelessness. With maturity comes a growing realization of the limits of
time and of the ultimate separation of death that time brings. Mann argues
that there is a sense of childlike timelessness within the unconscious of all
human beings and that all short forms of psychotherapy revive these complex
feelings about time both in the therapist and in the client.
   Thus, there are a child time and an adult time, and time-limited psychotherapy addresses both. Mann writes: "The greater the ambiguity as to the
duration of treatment, the greater the influence of child time on unconscious
wishes and expectations. The greater the specificity of duration of treatment,
the more rapidly and appropriately is child time confronted with reality and
the work to be done" (p. 11).

   Therapeutic techniques.   At the initial session, the therapist tries to identify
the single most important unresolved issue being faced by the client and seeks
agreement from the client that that issue will be the focal point of the treatment. The issue chosen for investigation is viewed both in terms of its historical, or genetic, role and in terms of its current, or adaptive, role in the client's
personality. In selecting the focal issue to work on, Mann draws heavily on
psychoanalytic theory of personality and psychopathology. He believes that
the number of such central unresolved issues is small and comments at some
length on the four most important issues—independence versus dependence,
activity versus passivity, adequate self-esteem versus diminished or lost self-

esteem, and unresolved or delayed grief. He gives examples of such summary statements presented to clients for their consideration.

> I gather from all that you have told me that the greatest problem facing you at this time is your very deep disappointment with yourself to find yourself as you are at this time in your life [1973, p. 18].
>
> Your major difficulty is that you feel inadequate and chronically depressed as a result of your need to challenge and to pacify men who are important to you [p. 20].
>
> Because there have been a number of sudden and very painful events in your life, things always seem uncertain, and you are excessively nervous because you do not expect anything to go along well [p. 20].

Mann has found that the series of 12 treatment sessions often divides itself into roughly equal thirds. During the first three or four meetings, there is often rapid symptomatic improvement. Mann suggests that this phenomenon can be understood as "consisting mostly in a surge of unconscious magical expectations that long ago disappointments will now be undone and that all will be made forever well, as they should have been so long ago" (p. 33). During the middle phase of the therapy, the client's initial enthusiasm begins to wane. Symptoms may return, and pessimism about what will be achieved in treatment can be seen emerging. During the ending phase of the treatment, the client's reaction to termination becomes the focus of discussion, and it is now that the definitive work of resolution will take place. Separation from the therapist stands in direct symbolic relationship with all previous losses and separations, and resolution of this separation is the key to the therapeutic effect. Mann cautions that "it is absolutely incumbent upon the therapist to deal directly with the reaction to termination in all its painful aspects and affects if he expects to help the patient come to some vividly affective understanding of the now inappropriate nature of his early unconscious conflict" (p. 36).

Resolving previously unresolved losses is the critical goal in Mann's time-limited psychotherapy. That is, Mann views life as (in part; to be sure) a series of unresolved separations from persons, such as parents, toward whom feelings are complex and often contradictory. The four universal conflict situations identified earlier express ways that human beings experience loss. "It is as though each individual feels that he needed something more of the sustaining object when he was deprived of that object. If only he were able to go back in time to review negotiations with that object so that he could gain what he had not previously" (p. 27). Mann's time-limited psychotherapy is designed precisely to provide the opportunity to resolve those previous losses.

Farrelly and Brandsma's provocative therapy

Provocative therapy (Farrelly & Brandsma, 1974) is an aptly named form of relatively short-term therapy (average number of interviews is 20–25 with a range of 2–100) practiced by its originator, Frank Farrelly, since 1963. Farrelly, a psychiatric social worker, expresses his indebtedness to Carl Rogers, with whom he worked at Mendota State Hospital, Wisconsin, in the study of client-centered therapy with chronic schizophrenics, for helping him appreciate the importance of developing an empathic understanding of patients. But Farrelly moved past the role of client-centered therapist as he slowly discovered that "the more passive, receptive, traditional role of the therapist" (1974, p. 20) was not for him. Farrelly discovered that when he "threw therapy out the window" (p. 19) and began telling clients how he found himself reacting to them, they began to improve. That is, Farrelly had come to the conclusion that empathic understanding, warm caring, and genuine congruence were rarely enough and, even when effective as a therapeutic strategy, were far too slow. Furthermore, Farrelly found that this conclusion was as valid for private- as for public-sector clients and as appropriate for neurotics as for psychotics.

Origins of provocative therapy.   Farrelly found that another strategy worked well with his clients: he could help clients develop stronger egos if he sided with their punitive superegos.

> While in the 91st interview with the patient whom I'll call "Bill," I "stumbled" onto what felt like a crystalization of these previous experiences. Because I had not yet integrated my learning experiences and was a member of the project, I felt somewhat constrained to use a client centered approach with this patient. I had been essentially communicating three basic ideas to him 1) You are worthwhile and of value; 2) You can change; and 3) Your whole life can be different. He, in turn, had been persistently communicating back to me three complementary responses: 1) I am worthless; 2) I'm hopeless and can never change; and 3) My life will always be one long psychotic episode and hospitalization. It was becoming increasingly clear that empathic understanding, feedback, warm caring, and genuine congruence were simply not enough and were getting us nowhere. At this point I "gave up" and said to him, "Okay, I agree. You're hopeless. Now let's try *this* for 91 interviews. Let's try agreeing with you about yourself from here on out."
>
> Almost immediately (within a matter of seconds and minutes, not weeks and months), he began to protest that he was not *that* bad, nor *that* hopeless. Easily observable and measurable characteristics of his in-therapy behavior started changing. For example, his rate of speech markedly increased, his voice quality changed from a dull, slow motion, soporific monotone to a more normal tone of voice with inflections and easily noticeable affect. He became less over-controlled and showed humor, embarrassment, irritation, and far more spontaneity [1974, p. 26].

Assumptions, hypotheses, and goals.   In examining provocative therapy retrospectively, Farrelly and Brandsma have been able to identify ten assumptions that govern their behavior as therapists. In summary form, these assumptions are as follows:

1. People change and grow in response to challenge.
2. Clients can change if they choose to do so.

3. Clients have far more potential for achieving adaptive, productive, and socialized modes of living than they or most clinicians assume.
4. The psychological fragility of clients is vastly overrated both by themselves and by others.
5. Clients' maladaptive, unproductive, antisocial attitudes and behaviors can be drastically altered, however severe or chronic.
6. Adult or current experiences are at least as significant as childhood or previous experiences, if not more so, in shaping client values, attitudes, and behaviors.
7. The client's behavior with the therapist is a relatively accurate reflection of his or her habitual patterns of social and interpersonal relationships.
8. People make sense; the human animal is exquisitely logical and understandable.
9. The more important messages between people are nonverbal.
10. The expression of therapeutic hate and joyful sadism toward clients can markedly benefit them.[4]

Two central hypotheses govern the behavior of a therapist practicing provocative therapy. First, *"if provoked by the therapist (humorously, perceptively, and within the client's own internal frame of reference), the client will tend to move in the opposite direction from the therapist's definition of the client as a person"* (p. 52). Second, *"if urged provocatively (humorously and perceptively) by the therapist to continue his self-defeating, deviant behaviors, the client will tend to engage in self- and other-enhancing behaviors which more closely approximate the societal norm"* (p. 52).

The goals of provocative therapy are to help clients (1) affirm their self-worth, (2) be appropriately assertive, (3) defend themselves realistically, (4) respond to reality adaptively, and (5) communicate their own feelings in personal relationships freely and authentically.

Therapeutic techniques.   For the provocative therapist to achieve these goals, Farrelly and Brandsma believe in using virtually any tactic—"obvious lying, denial, rationalization, invention (e.g., of 'instant research'), crying and zany thinking" (p. 57). Farrelly and Brandsma write: "Figuratively therapists are often bound by Marquis of Queensbury type roles while patients use the psychological equivalent of knee to the groin and thumb in the eye. The outcome of such a contest is not often in doubt—to the ultimate detriment of the patient" (p. 57). Here is an example of provocative therapy in action:

Pt.   (Loudly and furiously): Goddamn you! If you don't stop talking in that snotty, sarcastic way of yours, I'm going to quit therapy and not pay your bill!

---

[4]From *Provocative Therapy*, by F. Farrelly and J. Brandsma. Copyright © 1974 by Meta Publications. This and all other quotations from the same source are reprinted by permission.

Th.   (With an alarmed, anxious, pleading expression): Please, *don't*! I need
          the money! (Slumps dejectedly in chair, holding forehead in hand, in a
          depressed, choked tone of voice.) Oh well, I'll just have to tell June and
          the kids no Christmas again *this* year.

Pt.   (A kaleidoscope of emotions crossing his face: anger, laughter, suddenly
          placating): O.K., O.K., damn you, I know I need you more than you need
          me, but damn it, Frank, won't you please just . . . [1974, p. 69].

The therapist plays devil's advocate; sides with the negative half of the
client's ambivalent conflicts; urges the client to continue deviant and pathological behavior (for plausible reasons); verbalizes the client's worst self-doubts,
thoughts, and fears; absurdly and ludicrously encourages the client's symptoms; and lampoons, ridicules, and burlesques the client's attitudes, always
trying to provoke the client to give at least equal time to the positive, joyful,
and growth-producing experiences in life. This orientation is reminiscent of
Watzlawick's assertion that "jokes have a disrespectful ability to make light of
seemingly monolithic world orders and world images. This may help to explain
why it is that people who suffer from emotional problems are half over them
once they manage to laugh at their predicament" (1978, pp. 55–56).

The therapeutic process.   Clients typically pass through four stages in
provocative therapy. First, "the client is precipitously provoked into a series
of experiences that tend to leave him astonished, incredulous, uncertain and
even at times outraged. He experiences a marked clash of expectational systems; his expectations of the therapist's role are not only disconfirmed but are
almost reversed" (Farrelly & Brandsma, 1974, pp. 131–132). Second, "the client
typically decreases his protestations regarding the therapist's behaviors, begins
to recognize that he and not the therapist must change, and starts reorganizing
his expectational system toward the therapist. . . . There may emerge the
feeble beginnings of the five types of desired behaviors that constitute the
goals of provocative therapy. And finally this stage is characterized by a marked
diminishing if not total extinction of psychotic defenses if these were initially
present" (p. 135).

In the third stage, there is considerable clarification and movement. "The
hallmark of this stage is the client's congruent and increasingly firm protestations that the therapist's definition of him is a skewed, inaccurate one based
on a distorted reading of inadequate samplings" (p. 137). The fourth stage is
one of consolidation and integration. "The client is now protesting significantly less if at all about the therapist's definition of him as a person. If he
does protest, he does it impatiently or humorously and is increasingly confident in his present self's adaptive and coping capacities" (p. 137).

Farrelly and Brandsma's techniques tend to force their clients to prove
how healthy they are, if only to prove how wrong their therapist is. It is clear
that the provocations in this therapy are accompanied by a strong underlying

sense of good will and that the strategy of helping clients get well by pointing out, tongue in cheek, how wonderful it is to be sick can be effective if undertaken judiciously.

Erickson's brief strategic therapy

Milton Erickson, trained in psychology and psychiatry, was active in the field of psychotherapy primarily in the practice of clinical hypnosis. In addition, however, he developed a unique and original style of brief psychotherapy based largely on concepts derived from his understanding of hypnosis. Jay Haley has presented Erickson's work and underlying theories in a volume (Haley, 1973) that is, in the main, a casebook. Cases are described within the framework of family therapy, a field in which Haley is expert. The book, read and approved by Erickson, is based on a 15-year collaboration, and details come from many hours of recorded conversations between Haley and Erickson. It is perhaps unnecessary to add that Haley is a great admirer of Erickson. He has tried Erickson's methods with success and believes many psychotherapists can adapt these methods to their own styles.

Erickson has left an extraordinary intellectual and clinical legacy. In 1966, Haley, along with a number of colleagues, established the Brief Therapy Center at the Mental Research Institute in Palo Alto, California. Erickson's ideas spread through Haley to Watzlawick and his associates (Haley, 1963; Watzlawick, 1978; Watzlawick, Weakland, & Fisch, 1974) and to Rabkin (1977), among others.

Haley has used the word *strategic* to describe Erickson's therapeutic style. Haley writes:

> Therapy can be called strategic if the clinician initiates what happens during therapy and designs a particular approach for each problem. . . . in strategic therapy the initiative is largely taken by the therapist. He must identify solvable problems, set goals, design interventions to achieve those goals, examine the responses he receives to correct his approach, and ultimately examine the outcome of his therapy to see if it has been effective. . . . Strategic therapy is not a particular approach or theory but a name for those types of therapy where the therapist takes responsibility for directly influencing people [1973, p. 17].[5]

Strategic therapy is thus directive and active in character—a logical extension of hypnotherapy, in which the therapist generally initiates all that is to happen. But Erickson thinks of hypnosis far more broadly than a procedure whereby a person is "put to sleep" and given suggestions. For Erickson, *hypnosis* refers to a type of communication between people, a process between people. Hypnosis shares goals and procedures with other forms of therapy and, in particular, includes two types of directives. First, clients are asked to do something they can voluntarily do—for example, sit or lie down, look at a

---

[5]From *Uncommon Therapy: The Psychiatric Techniques of Milton H. Erickson, M.D.*, by J. Haley. Copyright © 1973 by W. W. Norton & Co., Inc. This and all other quotations from the same source are reprinted by permission.

certain spot, concentrate on a certain image or idea. Second, clients are asked to behave in ways that are not under their voluntary control—for example, feel better, free-associate, see something that isn't there, turn off a physiological process. Like all forms of therapy, hypnosis is based on a voluntary relationship, yet one tinged with hesitancy and resistance. Thus, hypnotists, just like other therapists, must deal with resistance, must motivate clients to cooperate, and must use a certain amount of persuasion.

Many of Erickson's specific techniques are unusual, and Haley has singled out several of them for special comment. Erickson is often able to deal with resistance by labeling it as cooperation—that is, by working with rather than against it. If a couple fight continually in spite of good advice to the contrary, he is likely to direct them to have a fight, but he will specify the place or the time, thus causing a change in their behavior. Erickson will often direct a client to engage in one of a large class of behaviors, knowing that the specific suggestion will not be readily accepted. The client will choose to engage in another behavior, but still in the desired class. For example, Erickson may want clients to exercise and will instruct them to engage in a particular exercise that they do not find acceptable. As a consequence, clients will choose another, more congenial exercise for themselves. Erickson will sometimes encourage a client to relapse, when the client has been improving "too rapidly." He might say, for example, "I want you to go back and feel as badly as you did when you first came in with the problem, because I want you to see if there is anything from that time that you wish to recover and salvage" (Haley, 1973, p. 31). Such instructions almost always prevent a relapse. Erickson will often encourage a response by inhibiting it—for example, encouraging a silent family member to speak by interrupting him for a period of time whenever he looks as if he is about to say something. Erickson frequently communicates in metaphor and by analogy. Haley writes:

> If Erickson is dealing with a married couple who have a conflict over sexual relations and would rather not discuss it directly, he will approach the problem metaphorically. He will choose some aspect of their lives that is analogous to sexual relations and change that as a way of changing the sexual behavior. He might, for example, talk to them about having dinner together and draw them out on their preferences. He will discuss with them how the wife likes appetizers before dinner, while the husband prefers to dive right into the meat and potatoes. Or the wife might prefer a quiet and leisurely dinner, while the husband, who is quick and direct, just wants the meal over with. If the couple begin to connect what they are saying with sexual relations, Erickson will "drift rapidly" away to other topics, and then he will return to the analogy. He might end such a conversation with a directive that the couple arrange a pleasant dinner on a particular evening that is satisfactory to both of them. When successful, this approach shifts the couple from a more pleasant dinner to more pleasant sexual relations without their being aware that he has deliberately set this goal.

Erickson's willingness to accept working within metaphors applies not only to verbal interchange but even to persons who live a metaphoric life. Such a style of life is typical of schizophrenics, and Erickson assumes that with a schizophrenic the important message is the metaphor. For example, when Erickson was on the staff of Worcester State Hospital, there was a young patient who called himself Jesus. He paraded about as the Messiah, wore a sheet draped around him, and attempted to impose Christianity on people. Erickson approached him on the hospital grounds and said, "I understand you have had experience as a carpenter?" The patient could only reply that he had. Erickson involved the young man in a special project of building a bookcase and shifted him to productive labor [1973, pp. 27–28].

Rabkin (1977) has applied the phrase *reverse psychology* to Erickson's therapeutic techniques. More recently, Watzlawick, impressed with both the recent research and theory regarding the two-brain theory (our left brains being concerned with speech, writing, counting, and reasoning; our right brains being concerned with concepts, totalities, configurations, abstractions, and emotions), has written about Erickson's therapeutic techniques as "blocking the left hemisphere" (see Watzlawick, 1978, pp. 91–126).

The most radical aspect of Erickson's approach is his apparent complete uninterest in helping a client discover the causes of the problem.

> His style of therapy is not based upon insight into unconscious processes, it does not involve helping people understand their interpersonal difficulties, he makes no transference interpretations, he does not explore a person's motivations, nor does he simply recondition. His theory of change is more complex; it seems to be based upon the interpersonal impact of the therapist outside the patient's awareness, it includes providing directives that cause changes of behavior, and it emphasizes communicating in metaphor [Haley, 1973, p. 39].

Watzlawick, Weakland, and Fisch write: "Everyday, not just clinical, experience shows not only that there can be change without insight, but that very few behavioral or social changes are accompanied, let alone preceded, by insight into the vicissitudes of their genesis" (1974, p. 86).

Focused single-session therapy

Focused single-session therapy (Bloom, 1981a) examines the concept of planned short-term therapy by deliberately creating and evaluating the limiting case—an encounter designed to provide a significant therapeutic impact in a single interview. Whether intentionally or not, a large proportion of therapeutic encounters consist of but a single interview. Focused single-session therapy intentionally attempts to complete a meaningful unit of psychotherapy in one interview.

Single-session encounters are remarkably common. Not only is their frequency underestimated, but more important, their therapeutic impact appears to be underestimated as well. Such encounters appear to have positive consequences whether their main objective is therapy or evaluation, and as Rubin and Mitchell (1976) report, interviews whose primary purpose is research may have profound clinical impact on subjects as well. To the extent that the deliberate use of single therapeutic interviews can be appropriately implemented, we may be able to increase our ability to help an entire community of clients without requiring a parallel increase in personnel or funds.

Most of my experience in focused single-session therapy has taken place in our local community mental health center, where, for a couple of months at a time, I spend one-half day per week seeing clients who are referred to me. There have been two series of such clients. The most important difference between the two series was the length of the sessions. In the first series, sessions were one hour long; in the second, I decided to make up to two hours available for each interview. This change was inaugurated because in the first series I had often been unable to limit the intervention to one session. In fact, on the average, I saw each client in the first series for two separate interviews. In the second series, all cases were satisfactorily concluded in a single session that lasted up to two hours.

After introducing myself, getting the client's permission to tape-record the interview, and explaining my volunteer status at the mental health center, the contractual agreement I made with each client was that I was assuming that a single appointment would be sufficient. If, at the end of the interview, we both felt another appointment was necessary, we would schedule it for the following week. If not, I would give the client my card and invite him or her to call me if there was a need to get in touch with me for any reason—with a problem or a progress report, for example. Finally, I said that if the client did not contact me in a couple of months, I would call to see how he or she was getting along. I have called every one of the clients I saw, in this very primitive type of evaluation, and have heard the following report: nearly all are doing well; nearly all found the intervention helpful; and with two exceptions, they have not sought additional professional help.

I believe that any reasonably skilled therapist would get the same results. I also believe that we all sell or give our time, our most precious resource, far too easily and that we can all accomplish far more in brief therapy than we realize, if we are deliberate and plan well.

Here are a dozen technical principles of focused single-session therapy that seem valid to me. All of them are presented very tentatively. All are subject to revision, and I am sure many will be extensively modified as I gain additional experience.

1. *Identify a focal problem.* It is my hope in every focused single-session therapy to listen hard enough and explore skillfully enough to be able to identify a piece of psychological reality that is pertinent to the client's presenting problem, below the client's initial level of usable awareness, and yet acceptable to the client in the form of an interpretation or observation. In doing so, I am careful not to focus too early or foreclose too quickly. The success of the session seems to depend on my ability to identify and focus on one salient and relevant issue.

Identifying a focal problem is considerably easier if one has a workable theory of personality and psychopathology that can serve as a template through which the process of active listening can take place. Any theoretical perspective would be satisfactory. My own training is psychodynamic, and so the theories and concepts I bring into the therapeutic encounter derive from that perspective. Marmor (1968, p. 5) has described that perspective very succinctly in a statement that summarizes for him the essence of the psychodynamic approach—

> the recognition that human behavior is motivated; that the nature of this motivation is often largely concealed from awareness; that our personalities are shaped not only by our biological potentials, but also by experiential vicissitudes; that functional disturbances in human cognition, affect, and behavior are the result of contradictory and conflictual inputs or feedbacks; and that early developmental experiences are of particular significance in shaping subsequent perceptions and reactions in adolescence and adulthood.

2. *Do not underestimate clients' strengths.* I think of the therapy session as having the potential for breaking through an impasse in the client's psychological life, so that the client can resume the normal process of growth and development. I count on clients' abilities to work on an identified issue on their own, particularly if I can be helpful in identifying what that issue might be. I count on clients' ego strengths and on their abilities to mobilize those strengths.

3. *Be prudently active.* Most people who write about planned short-term therapy seem to agree that it requires of the therapist a higher level of activity than long-term therapy typically does. I have found it useful to be more active than I have been accustomed to being, but active in specific ways. I ask questions rather than make statements. I try not to make speeches or to lecture. I do virtually no self-disclosure. I avoid asking questions that have yes or no answers. When necessary, I give information, but in the context of the client's presenting problem, and I keep it simple. I use the client's language, making sure first that I understand what is meant by the key words and phrases he or she uses.

4. *Explore, then present interpretations tentatively.* In my interpretations, I try to do all the necessary exploration first and then tentatively present an idea in such a way that it is persuasive yet may be disagreed with without jeopardizing my potential effectiveness. I say "Do you think it is possible that . . ." or "Have you ever wondered why . . ." or "I wonder whether . . ." Knowing when and how to label or confront or interpret is partly a matter of experience, partly a matter of style. Reading the previous reviews of various approaches to planned short-term therapy should convince you that there is a very broad range of therapeutic strategies and styles.

5. *Encourage the expression of affect.* I encourage and explicitly recognize the expression of affect and use it as a way of pointing to important life events

or figures: "It's okay to cry" or "That really upsets you, doesn't it?" Similarly, when it seems timely, I point out incongruities in affect: "You're laughing, but there doesn't seem to be anything to laugh about." In my experience with focused single-session therapy, I have found no more effective technique than explicit and accurate recognition of the feelings the client is carrying around.

6. *Use the interview to start a problem-solving process.* I try to identify important life figures in relation to unresolved issues and start or encourage a process of getting some of that unfinished business taken care of. "Have you ever told your mother that when you were a little girl, you used to be so frightened of her?" "Have you ever talked with your sister about that?" "Do you think your father could shed some light on why you used to do that?" "Does your mother know how upset you are about her divorce?" This effort gives the single session some increased longevity by attempting to internalize a process that can continue for a period of time.

7. *Keep track of the interview.* There is a tempo, a pacing, to a two-hour interview. It is enough time so I do not feel rushed; yet, I have to stay aware of the passing time and keep planning how to use it. Sometimes I make a few notes to myself, jotting down topics I want to make sure I talk about. More often, I don't need to keep notes, but either way, it is important to estimate how much time will be needed to discuss a particular topic and to make sure there is a reasonably good match between the needed and the available time.

There is also the issue of the phases through which the interview passes. I can identify the introductory material, the middle development of important themes, the planning period, and the gradual closing of the interview. I tend to judge how much or how little anxiety clients bring with them to the interview and how much seems to be generated by the interview. I act accordingly, now exploring in a way I know will raise anxiety, now modulating the anxiety, now introducing humor, now being very serious—all in an effort to keep anxiety at its optimal level: enough to assure progress but not so much as to be disabling.

8. *Do not be overambitious.* I try not to do too much. If I can find just one issue, just one idea, that is useful to the client, the intervention can be successful. My experience, from listening to both my own and others' interviews, is that it is very hard for clients to make real use of more than two or three ideas in a single interview. As a consequence, the choice of which ideas to elaborate on when exploring an issue is very important. In addition, it is important to keep the ideas simple. My personal rule of thumb is that if I cannot express a fundamental issue of concern to the client in ten words or fewer, I do not understand the issue.

9. *Keep factual questions to a minimum.* I avoid collecting demographic information or doing a traditional mental-status examination. It is my experience that the answers will nearly always be forthcoming without my having to ask the questions. I rarely ask age or number of siblings or information about parents or children. Such questions can be intrusive, and the most

important information will emerge in the normal course of the interview. Sometimes it is useful to ask for identifying information as a way of reducing a momentarily excessive level of anxiety, but except for this occasion, the quest for demographic information about the client and significant people in the client's life seems a poor use of time.

10. *Do not be overly concerned about the precipitating event.* Focused single-session therapy is not crisis intervention, and so I feel no necessity to identify a crisis or event that precipitated a client's coming to the mental health center. Many clients seem not to know exactly why they came in. So I simply begin an interview by asking "What can I do to be helpful?" The client has come in because something is wrong for which help is needed, not because he or she has a regular appointment at that time every week. Since the client has inaugurated the therapeutic encounter, the therapist has every right to expect the client to get to work, to describe the problem, and to begin moving toward its resolution. No interview has more leverage in this regard than the first interview, and that leverage is further enhanced by the fact that both client and therapist know it is likely to be the only interview.

11. *Avoid detours.* I have had to learn to avoid attractive detours and to remain single-minded about what I am trying to accomplish. There are numerous occasions in every intervention when I find myself wishing I could explore some little phrase for just a few minutes, but such diversions have nearly always turned out to be errors. Initially, of course, I have no idea where I am heading, and so I keep all my options open. I try to narrow the domain of inquiry in proportion to what I am learning about the client, and I do not single out a particular issue or conflict to concentrate on until I have every reason to believe it is an appropriate target for investigation and clarification. Not only is there no time to explore side issues, but such exploration detracts from the effectiveness of the therapy.

12. *Do not overestimate a client's self-awareness.* Finally, I am continuing to learn not to overestimate how much clients know about themselves. Clients may be totally oblivious of something about themselves that seems perfectly obvious to me and probably to everyone who knows them. I have had clients scream at me that they are not angry and tearfully tell me they are not sad. Although clients are, in one sense, expert on what is going on inside them, they are very often unable to label, acknowledge, or effectively use that knowledge. Increasing a client's useful self-awareness, even in only one critical area, can have an important impact on the adequacy of his or her functioning. In working toward that objective, an accurate appraisal of what clients do and do not know about themselves is critically important.

Brief contact therapy

Short-term therapy can be brief not only in having few sessions but also in that each contact may be considerably shorter than is ordinarily thought of as desirable. Koegler (1966) argues for the use of brief contact therapy in outpatient treatment settings. By *brief contact therapy* Koegler means a series of short talks with an authority figure, perhaps accompanied by medication. In brief contact therapy the interview is never longer than half an hour and frequently shorter. Koegler considers the greatest benefit of an interview to occur during the first 15–30 minutes.

In proposing brief contact therapy, Koegler notes that

> psychiatry is the only medical specialty in which the patient sees the doctor for a fixed period of time, regardless of the patient's needs. The patient is stretched or shortened to fit the psychiatrist's procrustean time-couch. Psychiatric patients arrive and leave at fixed times; and a psychiatrist whose patients are permitted to overstay their allotted time is thought to have "guilt about money" by his colleagues. Patients soon become accustomed to the system, too, and woe be it to the therapist who stops the session two minutes short [1966, pp. 141–142].

Koegler cites several advantages of the move toward the shorter therapy session. Greater numbers of clients could be accommodated. Psychiatric service would be made more economical and, therefore, more accessible. In addition, Koegler feels that briefer interviews would be more appropriate for clients who have low verbal ability or who are psychotic or prepsychotic.

In brief contact therapy, the therapist tries to aid clients to arrive at a solution of their emotional difficulties and to achieve some relief of their emotional pain, within the framework of the therapist's training and orientation. The therapist adjusts the emphasis of the therapeutic contacts to the client's cultural background and needs. The therapist's basic orientation and personality characteristics are no different than in regular therapy, although the emphasis is more likely to be on the here and now.

Castelnuovo-Tedesco (1967, 1970) has experimented with a maximum of ten 20-minute interviews, particularly in the context of training primary care physicians who must learn how to incorporate a psychotherapeutic orientation into their relatively busy medical practices. Mandell (1961) has suggested a 15-minute hour.

Dreiblatt and Weatherley (1965) conducted two studies to examine the effect of even briefer contacts with hospitalized psychiatric patients. In their first study, a group of 44 new patients in a Veterans Administration hospital was divided into three subgroups after an initial evaluation of self-esteem and anxiety level. There were no significant differences among the three groups on initial test scores. During the two-week program, one group received regular ward care; the second group, six 5–10-minute contacts in addition to normal ward care; the third, twelve 5–10-minute contacts in addition to normal ward care. Contacts were made at various times of day and were quite informal. They usually began with an open-ended question and were carried out in a friendly, chatty manner.

Self-esteem and anxiety measures were repeated at the end of the program. Not only did the two brief contact groups show a significant increase in self-esteem, but they both had significantly shorter periods of hospitalization than the control group. In addition, the group receiving twelve brief contacts showed a significant reduction in anxiety.

In a second study, these authors organized the brief contacts so that they were provided by four different staff members. In addition, they varied the nature of the brief contact by arranging for one experimental group to talk about their symptoms, a second group to talk about social matters unrelated to symptomatology, and a third group to be contacted to help with a contrived ward task. All experimental groups received six contacts per week. Again, there was a normal-ward-routine control group. In total, 74 new patients were involved in the second study.

The general usefulness of the brief contacts was confirmed. Among the brief contacts, those patients who discussed issues unrelated to their symptoms seemed to gain most, and those who were contacted to help with a ward task gained least. The authors concluded that "brief contact therapy can have a markedly beneficial effect upon hospitalized psychiatric patients. . . . The beneficial effects of brief contacts are best understood as a product of an implicit message which they convey to the patient. The message is an ego-enhancing, supportive one; it tells the patient that he is accepted as a person" (1965, p. 518).

EVALUATION OF PLANNED SHORT-TERM THERAPY

There is a substantial literature examining the clinical effectiveness of planned short-term therapy. Some of this literature is nonquantitative or based on very small samples (for example, Gottschalk, Mayerson, & Gottlieb, 1967; Kaffman, 1963; Lewin, 1970, pp. 245–261; H. J. Parad & L. G. Parad, 1968; L. G. Parad & H. J. Parad, 1968; Sifneos, 1972, pp. 124–143; Strupp, 1980a, 1980b, 1980c, 1980d). In addition, a literature on short-term marital, family, and group therapy is emerging (for example, Aiello, 1979; Budman, Bennett, & Wisneski, 1980, 1981; Budman & Clifford, 1979; Budman, Demby, & Randall, 1980; Daley & Koppenaal, 1981; Donner & Gamson, 1968; Holloway, 1979; Lewin, 1970, pp. 164–197; Rabkin, 1977, pp. 181–207; Sabin, 1981; Sadock, Newman, & Normand, 1968; Schwartz, 1975; Small, 1979, pp. 140–147, 157–165; Sundel & Lawrence, 1977; Wolf, 1965).

An impressive number of evaluation studies of planned short-term therapy are based on fairly large samples and were designed to contrast short-term and time-unlimited outpatient and inpatient care by randomly assigning clients to short-term or time-unlimited care and then following them for some period after completion of the therapy in order to assess outcome. In addition, a sufficient number of evaluation studies have been reported so that reviews of these studies have already appeared (Butcher & Koss, 1978; Malan, 1963, pp. 15–36; Meltzoff & Kornreich, 1970; Phillips & Wiener, 1966, pp. 27–58;

Small, 1979, pp. 324–345). This section will examine some of these studies in detail (see also Keilson, Dworkin, & Gelso, 1979; Sloane, Staples, Cristol, Yorkton, & Whipple, 1975).

Outpatient studies

In one of the earliest systematic evaluations of short-term therapy, Phillips and Johnston (1954) contrasted 16 cases in a child guidance clinic who were assigned to short-term therapy (ten interviews or fewer) with 44 cases assigned to conventional therapy. Outcome was judged from written case records, consultation with therapists, and one-year follow-up interviews with mothers. A significantly greater proportion of the cases assigned to short-term therapy were judged to have improved. Furthermore, even though judgment bias was "more apt to be against short-term treatment because of its newness and its challenge to old assumptions" (p. 272), in 12 of the 44 conventionally treated cases, outcome was judged to be a failure, while in all of the 16 short-term cases, the treatment was thought to have been at least partly successful.

From 1959 to 1962, Group Health Insurance, Inc., a fee-for-service physicians' insurance plan in New York and New Jersey, conducted a study of the feasibility of offering short-term psychiatric treatment to a sample of 76,000 of its members. During the study, 1115 adults and children received benefits consisting of up to 15 individual therapeutic interviews with one of 1200 participating psychiatrists. At the time of discharge, 76% of these clients were judged by their therapists to be improved or recovered. Two and one-half years later, a follow-up survey revealed that 81% of the patients reported substantial recovery or improvement (Avnet, 1965a, 1965b). Interestingly, although patients' ratings tended to be unrelated to length of treatment, psychiatrists were uncertain or pessimistic regarding about half the clients who had been seen for fewer than six interviews and far more optimistic about clients seen longer.

In 1963, Malan reported his first clinical outcome study. He contrasted the conservative view of planned short-term therapy outcome—"Results are essentially palliative and consist of 'symptom removal' only. Deeper changes should not be attempted, and can be brought about only by long-term methods"—with the radical view of planned short-term therapy—"There is no essential difference between the therapeutic results of brief and long-term methods. Quite far-reaching changes are often possible" (1963, p. 16; see also Shoulberg, 1976). Malan concluded that "the result of this study was unequivocal support for every aspect of the radical view of brief psychotherapy" (1976, p. 20).

In 1976, Malan reported on a replication of his study. With regard to the results of that replication, he noted:

> The previous finding is conclusively confirmed that with carefully selected patients the radical rather than the conservative view is correct . . . that is, that relatively disturbed patients can be helped toward permanent major changes. . . . The con-

servative view of brief psychotherapy—according to which only patients with the most mild and recent illnesses can be helped, the technique should be superficial and should not involve transference interpretations, and the results are only palliative—has been disproved, and should disappear from the literature, together with the view that the *only* patients suitable for brief psychotherapy are those in crisis [1976, pp. 54–55].

Muench (1965) contrasted outcome results in three groups of college students seen in a college counseling center (35 students per group). At the initial interview, students were assigned to either time-limited therapy of 8–19 sessions with a prearranged termination date or to time-unlimited therapy. This latter group was subdivided at the time of termination into a short-term group (fewer than 8 sessions) and a long-term group (20 or more sessions).

Subjects were seen by one of 12 experienced psychotherapists who "attempted to develop a close interpersonal relationship with their clients tending toward greater self-understanding and self-acceptance" (p. 295). Each therapist saw clients in each of the three groups. The Rotter Sentence Completion Test and the Maslow Security-Insecurity Inventory were administered before and after therapy. The three groups had no significant initial differences in test scores. Both the short-term-therapy and the time-limited-therapy groups improved significantly from pre- to posttest. No improvement was found in the long-term-therapy group. No significant intertherapist differences in success rate were found. Muench concluded that "psychotherapy, limited to certain designated time periods appears to be economic, not only in terms of total staff time, but also in terms of client progress in therapy" (1965, p. 298).

Another study, with similar findings, was reported by Reid and Shyne (1969). An experimental group of 60 intact families was seen in planned short-term treatment (a maximum of eight interviews within a period of three months) at the Community Service Society of New York. A comparison group of 60 families was seen in treatment that continued for up to 18 months. While 64% of the open-ended cases showed improvement, 84% of the planned short-term cases did. Furthermore, the gains in the short-term group were as long-lasting as those made by the continued-treatment families.

Rosenthal and Levine (1970, 1971) compared the outcomes of time-limited and time-unlimited psychotherapy with children. They randomly assigned 66 children to either brief therapy (a maximum of eight contact hours within a maximum of ten weeks) or long-term therapy (time and contact hours unlimited). A variety of therapists, with several therapeutic orientations and from several mental health professions, treated children under both time-limited and time-unlimited conditions. Evaluations of outcome were made three months, six months, and one year after treatment had begun. In addition to clinical evaluations, judgments of improvement were obtained from parents and teachers. In the long-term-therapy group, 79% showed marked improvement at the end of one year, during which time the average length of therapy had been about 40 weeks. In the brief-therapy group, 76% showed marked improvement at the end of one year, during which time the average length of therapy had been only 8 weeks. There are difficulties in a study of this kind in knowing what the phrase *marked improvement* means and whether the judges of the outcome of short-term therapy used the phrase in the same way as the judges of the outcome of long-term therapy. Still, the similarity of the figures is remarkable; no difference in therapeutic effect was found, even though one group received five times as much therapist time as the other.

Sucato (1978) contrasted the problem-solving process in 14 clients assigned to planned short-term service (PSTS) and 14 clients assigned to continued service (CS), all of whom were receiving casework services for family-related problems. The short-term service was limited to eight interviews within a maximum of 3 months. Continued service permitted an unlimited number of interviews over a maximum of 18 months.

On the basis of a careful analysis of three selected tape-recorded interviews from the beginning, middle, and closing phases of the therapy, Sucato concluded that

> with the absence of a structured time limit, CS is less likely to encourage control behavior or active attempts at problem solution in the first three months of service and is more likely to repeat orientation than to progress to a control phase. Conversely, PSTS's structured time limit and focus encourage the steady decline of orientation after phase I in order to make way for an increase in evaluative behavior in phase II, which decreases after midpoint along with orientation, to make way for the increase of control behavior in the last month of short-term service [1978, pp. 257–258].

Sucato further concluded that problem solving occurs more readily in short-term therapy than in long-term therapy and that therapists can be sensitized so that they can facilitate problem-solving activities when working with clients.

There is also a literature on the effectiveness of single outpatient therapeutic interviews. A small number of successful single-session-therapy case histories (sometimes including verbatim transcripts of portions of the interview) have appeared in the literature. In chronological order, these case histories include Freud in the 1890s (Breuer & Freud, 1895/1957, pp. 125–134), Tannenbaum (1919), Groddeck in 1927 (Groddeck, 1951, pp. 90–95), Reider (1955, pp. 116–118), Kaffman (1963, pp. 223–225), Rosenbaum (1964, p. 511), Gillman (1965, pp. 603–604), Seagull (1966), Lewin (1970, pp. 88–93), Scrignar (1979), Sifneos (1979, pp. 70–73), and Bloom (1981a). These case histories are invariably presented as a way of illustrating how clients occasionally make significant changes in their lives as a consequence of a single therapeutic intervention.

These case histories do not, of course, substitute for more objectively conducted empirical research studies. A few such studies have been reported, however, and they uniformly support the conclusion that a single interview can have significant therapeutic impact.

Getz, Fujita, and Allen (1975) sought evaluations of a single interview with a paraprofessional during a crisis from a sample of 104 persons who had made one-time use of a night crisis-intervention service connected with a community-hospital emergency room. Clients were contacted 6 to 12 months after their interview at the crisis program. (This sample comprised only 39% of persons who were eligible to be included in the study. The remaining 61% could not be located, for one reason or another.) The clients generally felt that the crisis-intervention service had been very helpful, exceeded in helpfulness only by the support provided by significant others in their lives. Degree of helpfulness was clearly related to the presenting problem; clients whose complaint was depression or anxiety found crisis counselors twice as helpful as clients whose problems involved drug abuse or psychosis. The authors concluded that "timely intervention in crisis situations may have long-lasting effects on particular kinds of problems" (p. 143). They also reported no difference in client assessment between counselors who were well-trained graduate students and those who were community volunteers, and suggested that planners of similar programs need not feel hampered if they lack a pool of well-trained "professional" volunteers.

Malan, Heath, Bacal, and Balfour (1975) conducted two- through eight-year follow-up studies of 45 adult neurotic clients who were seen for one consultation but had never had psychotherapy. Before the follow-up interview, none had been interviewed by a psychiatrist more than twice in their lives. These authors found that one-quarter of the patients had improved symptomatically, and another quarter had also improved dynamically, a type of improvement the authors call "genuine." From their careful clinical assessments, the authors concluded that "these single diagnostic interviews had some powerful therapeutic effects" (p. 122). Three of these clients had, in fact, written to their interviewing psychiatrist, saying they felt better as a consequence of acquiring insight into their difficulties. These findings forced the authors to realize that they "had not been studying spontaneous remission at all, but one-session psychotherapy" (p. 122).

Edwards, Orford, Egert, Guthrie, Hawker, Hensman, Mitcheson, Oppenheimer, and Taylor (1977) randomly assigned 100 male married alcoholics to two treatment groups in London after an initial three-hour physical, psychological, psychiatric, and social-work assessment of the couple. Males were between ages 25 and 60 and free of severe physical disease, psychosis, or gross brain damage. In the treatment group, both husband and wife were offered an initial counseling session, followed by medical, psychiatric, and social-work services; in addition, the husband was introduced to Alcoholics Anonymous, and inpatient services were made available as needed. The treatment period lasted one year. In the advice group, the entire intervention consisted of the initial counseling session, in which both husband and wife participated.

Progress was assessed monthly throughout the one-year period by brief interviews that social workers conducted with the wives. All the patients were seen by a psychiatrist at the one-year anniversary of the intake assessment. As might be expected, there were dramatic differences in the amount of help obtained from all sources, both within and outside the project. Edwards et al. (1977) wrote that "although some advice-group patients sought help from other sources, and some treatment-group patients engaged in only a rather minimal degree of contact with the Clinic, the over-all between-group differences remained at a level which can leave no doubt that two very different types of therapeutic engagements are being compared" (p. 1012).

The findings can be briefly summarized. The authors could find no substantial differences between the two groups at the time of the one-year follow-up in terms of amount of alcohol intake, subjective ratings of the drinking problem, social adjustment, or other difficulties. Significant improvement was shown by 39% of the advice group as against 26% of the treatment group.

Most interesting were the patients' views on what had been most helpful to them during the year. In both groups, the three factors most commonly judged responsible for improvement were unrelated to the treatment program: first, changes in external reality (for example, work conditions, work settings, or housing); second, the single-session intake interview; and third, changes in self-appraisal or mood. The authors indicated there was no persuasive evidence that the latter intrapsychic changes were related to the therapeutic program.

Perhaps the most provocative findings reported in the literature are those linking a single therapeutic interview with dramatic subsequent reductions in the use of medical care. There is already a substantial body of literature showing that brief therapy can have this effect (for example, Goldberg, Krantz, & Locke, 1970; Jameson, Shuman, & Young, 1978; Jones & Vischi, 1979; Mumford, Schlesinger, & Glass, 1982; Rosen & Wiens, 1979), but to demonstrate it following a single interview is startling indeed.

Cummings and Follette (Cummings, 1977a, 1977b; Cummings & Follette, 1968; Follette & Cummings, 1967) undertook a series of studies to investigate the role of psychotherapy in reducing medical care utilization in a prepaid-health-plan setting. In such settings, they found, clients could easily somatize emotional problems and thus overutilize medical facilities. They estimated that "60% or more of the physicians visits are made by patients who demonstrate an emotional, rather than an organic, etiology for their physical symptoms" (Cummings, 1977a, p. 711).

Among the groups they studied was a sample of 80 emotionally distressed patients who were assigned to receive a single psychotherapeutic interview. They found, totally unexpectedly, that one interview, with no repeat psychological visits, reduced medical utilization by 60% over the next five years as a consequence of resolving the emotional distress that was being reflected in physical symptoms.

Two other studies provide additional, equally startling findings. Goldberg and colleagues (1970) studied the effects of short-term outpatient therapy on utilization of medical services. Their sample consisted of 256 persons enrolled in the Group Health Association prepaid medical program in Washington, D.C., who had been referred and found eligible for and in need of outpatient psychiatric care. In the year following referral, this group showed an average reduction of 31% in physician visits and 30% in laboratory and X-ray visits from the previous year. But this reduction was independent of whether those referred for care had actually received it. In fact, the reduction in physician visits was 23% among those who had had ten or more sessions of psychotherapy and 30% among those who had had between one and nine sessions, but 39% among those who had had no psychotherapy at all.

Rosen and Wiens (1979) examined the same issue at the University of Oregon Health Sciences Center. Four groups of patients were compared: (1) those who received medical services but were not referred for psychological services, (2) those who were referred for psychological services but never kept their scheduled appointments, (3) those who were referred for psychological services but received only an evaluation, and (4) those who were referred and who received both an evaluation and subsequent brief psychotherapy. Groups 1 and 2—that is, those who received no psychological services—showed no subsequent reduction in the utilization of medical care, including number of outpatient visits, emergency-room visits, days of hospitalization, diagnostic procedures, and pharmaceutical prescriptions. Groups 3 and 4, those receiving only an evaluation or an evaluation and brief psychotherapy (averaging seven interviews), showed significant reduction in the utilization of medical care, but the group receiving only the evaluation showed the most consistent reduction in, among other things, medical outpatient visits, pharmaceutical prescriptions, emergency-room visits, and diagnostic services.

The one fact that links the findings of all these studies is that a single contact, virtually regardless of its purpose, appears to have salutary consequences. That is, it appears to make no demonstrable difference whether the contact is designed to be primarily evaluative or therapeutic.

In summary, planned short-term outpatient therapy appears to be at least as effective as traditional long-term therapy. Butcher and Koss (1978) concluded their review of the effectiveness of brief therapy by noting that "comparative studies of brief and unlimited therapies show essentially no differences in results. Consequently, brief therapy results in a great saving of clinical time and can reach more people in need of treatment" (p. 758). There seems hardly any question that planned short-term therapy has been shown to be sufficiently effective to justify actively continuing to experiment with its use. L. G. Parad, speaking from the point of view of the field of social welfare, has provided a summary statement that is equally pertinent for psychology or psychiatry:

> For a variety of interlocking reasons—manpower shortages, demands for massive community mental health services, dissatisfaction with waiting lists, studies in goal-limited therapy, research on coping behavior and crisis phenomena—we are

now witnessing a dramatic resurgence of interest in short-term approaches. Ours claims to be a pragmatic profession. If the level of outcome effectiveness evidenced in the recent studies is further substantiated in future large-scale experimental research, it would be logical to infer that short-term treatment should be the basic therapeutic approach for all but a relatively small selected group of applicants for family agency and child guidance services [1971, p. 145].

Inpatient studies

Psychiatric hospitalization was once routinely thought of as requiring years, if not a lifetime. But length of hospitalization for psychiatric disorders has been steadily decreasing over the past quarter-century. In Maryland, for example, between 1948 and 1968 the proportion of admissions into state mental hospitals who were discharged within a month rose from 7.8% to 41.0%, and the proportion discharged within six months rose from 14.6% to 69.4% (Gorwitz, 1969). United States figures for 1971 indicate that nearly 40% of inpatients admitted into public mental hospitals were discharged within one month (Meyer & Taube, 1973). In 1975, median length of hospitalization of psychiatric patients who were discharged was 8.1 days for public general hospitals and 13.6 days for nonpublic general hospitals (Faden & Taube, 1977).

In short-stay general hospitals (those in which average length of hospitalization for all patients does not exceed 30 days), patients with diagnosed mental disorders have, since 1974 at least, an average length of hospitalization of about 11 days—a figure that is remarkably similar to the figure for patients without mental disorders (Graves & Lovato, 1981). Thus, a very substantial number of psychiatric patients are hospitalized for brief periods, in part because of the special benefits discussed in Chapter 1 (Changes in Institutional Psychiatric Care) that are thought to result from such hospitalizations (Gruenberg, 1974; Mendel, 1967).

Caffey, Galbrecht, and Klett (1971) contrasted three inpatient programs in 14 Veterans Administration hospitals to which 201 schizophrenic men were randomly assigned: (1) standard hospital care, (2) standard hospital care followed by a one-year outpatient aftercare program, and (3) an accelerated 21-day hospital program followed by one year of outpatient aftercare. Even though the standard-care groups were hospitalized three times as long as the accelerated-care group, there were remarkably few differences among the groups during the one-year follow-up period. All three groups improved during hospitalization. Patients in the longer-hospitalization groups were less symptomatic at discharge than patients in the short-hospitalization group, but these differences were no longer in evidence either 6 or 12 months after discharge. Rehospitalization rates did not differ significantly among the three groups during the year following discharge, nor did the level and nature of community adjustment.

Glick, Hargreaves, and Goldfield (1974) compared outcomes for two groups of schizophrenics hospitalized at the Langley Porter Neuropsychiatric Institute in San Francisco. The 141 patients were randomly assigned to one of two treatment conditions: short-term (21–28-day) treatment oriented around crisis resolution and symptom relief and long-term (90–120-day) treatment that emphasized psychotherapy and major rehabilitative measures. Level of functioning was repeatedly assessed through interviews and a variety of scales completed by patients, relatives, and hospital staff members. Assessments focused on global outcome, course of posthospital treatment, reduction of symptoms, family functioning, use of leisure time, and work functioning.

At the preliminary one-year follow-up evaluation, based on about half of the sample, the long-term patients appeared to be functioning better, although they had had significantly more outpatient psychotherapy and more antipsychotic medication following discharge than the short-term group.

In a second evaluation (Glick, Hargreaves, Raskin, & Kutner, 1975), detailed information on the inpatient phase of treatment was examined for the total group. Short-term patients generally were found to have improved more quickly, but long-term patients functioned more adequately at the time of discharge.

Two years after the study began, Hargreaves, Glick, Drues, Shaustack, and Feigenbaum (1977) found that differences between short-term and long-term patients were no longer significant, although there was consistent evidence that long-term hospitalization was particularly effective for patients with good prehospital functioning but not for patients with poor prehospital functioning. Long-term patients were continuing to receive more antipsychotic medication, regardless of prehospital level of functioning, but were no longer receiving more outpatient psychotherapy than short-term patients.

These researchers undertook this evaluation in part in order to examine the hypothesis that long-term hospitalization may be harmful. Although their long-term group was hospitalized a maximum of only four months, they concluded that "long-term subjects do not function worse in the community than do the short-term subjects" (Hargreaves et al., 1977, p. 310). Since the objection to long-term hospitalization tends to be raised regarding hospitalizations of years rather than months, examination of the potential negative consequences of long-term hospitalization will undoubtedly have to be continued. More important for our purposes is the fact that long-term clients, according to these studies, do not function any better in the community than short-term clients.

Herz, Endicott, and Spitzer (1975, 1976; Endicott, Herz, & Gibbon, 1978) compared three treatment approaches to which a total of 175 newly admitted inpatients were randomly assigned: (1) brief hospitalization (often less than one week, and averaging 11 days) followed by transitional day care as needed ($N = 61$), (2) brief hospitalization followed by outpatient care as needed ($N = 51$), and (3) standard hospitalization (averaging 60 days) with discharge to outpatient care at the therapist's discretion ($N = 63$). The patients all had families who were willing to care for them after hospitalization.

The three groups were initially comparable on all measures of past and present psychopathology, role functioning, family burden, and most demo-graphic characteristics. Patients and their families were evaluated at 3 weeks and at 3, 6, 12, 18, and 24 months after admission.

All three groups of patients improved on almost all measures of adjust-ment, and they showed no significant differences in amount of improvement at any of the observation points of the study or in readmission rates. Briefly hospitalized patients were able to resume their vocational roles sooner and were less of a financial burden to their families. The authors found "few dif-ferences in psychopathology, role functioning, or effects on the family between groups. When differences did occur, they tended to favor the brief groups" (1978, p. 708).

Over the two-year period, the standard group had a significantly greater average number of inpatient days than either of the brief groups, even when day care was included in the brief/day-care group. From the beginning, brief-hospitalization patients consistently received less antipsychotic or other med-ication (reducing both direct cost and negative drug-related side effects). Costs to the family (for example, percentage of eligible patients not working at the six-month evaluation) and to the community (for example, percentage of fam-ilies on welfare at the two-year evaluation) were both substantially greater for the standard-hospitalization group.

Swartzburg and Schwartz (1976) contrasted therapeutic outcome over a four-year period on a brief-treatment (three to five days) inpatient unit with experiences during the fifth year, when the unit was moved, converted to a more traditional long-term locked ward, and staffed by personnel who were unfamiliar with the concepts that had led to the initial development of the brief-treatment unit. Nearly 1900 patients were admitted to these programs during the five-year period.

Demographic characteristics of the patients did not change with the change in treatment approach, nor did distribution by diagnosis. The brief-treatment inpatient program was just as successful as the more traditional program in getting patients out of the hospital and keeping them out.

In a series of studies, a group at the Hillside Medical Center in New York (Mattes, Rosen, & Klein, 1977; Mattes, Rosen, Klein, & Millan, 1977; Rosen, Katzoff, Carrillo, & Klein, 1976) contrasted short-term hospitalization (less than 90 days) with unlimited-stay hospitalization (averaging 179 days) by ran-domly assigning 173 patients to these two conditions and following them for a three- to four-year period. Treatment while in the hospital was essentially the same for the two groups, except that the short-term patients more com-monly had group therapy.

At discharge, short-term patients were significantly more improved in both cognitive and affective symptoms. At the three- to four-year follow-up, the two groups were doing equally well, although long-term patients had been rehospitalized significantly more often than short-term patients during the follow-up period. The authors concluded that long-term hospitalization "should be avoided whenever possible since, compared with shorter hospitalization, it does not lead to greater benefit in any of the evaluated areas of adjustment and, in fact, with some patients it appears to predispose to more and longer rehospitalization" (Mattes, Rosen, & Klein, 1977, p. 387).

In summary, short-term hospitalization appears to be as effective as long-term hospitalization. Riessman, Rabkin, and Struening (1977), reviewing a similar group of studies that had contrasted brief and standard psychiatric hospitalizations, concluded that the evidence

> provides support for the . . . hypothesis that the effects of brief hospitalization are essentially equivalent to those of standard hospitalization. . . . These investigations cumulatively indicate that groups of patients hospitalized for an average of 3 to 60 days do not significantly differ from those with longer average hospitalizations with respect to symptoms, social functioning, global adjustment, or the risk of rehospitalization either at discharge or within the next 2 years. These findings appear to be consistent across diagnostic groups and across hospitals characterized by marked differences in treatment philosophy, patient-staff ratio, and other factors [pp. 8–9].

CONCLUSIONS AND OVERVIEW

In the beginning of this chapter, reference was made to the limited effectiveness of traditional psychotherapy. In their review of nearly 400 controlled evaluations of counseling and psychotherapy, Smith and Glass concluded that after treatment "the typical therapy client is better off than 75% of untreated individuals" (1977, p. 752). To turn this statement around, after treatment the typical therapy client is worse off than 25% of untreated individuals. That is, one out of every four untreated individuals would be worse off if treated.

Although psychotherapy is probably better than no psychotherapy, its lack of more firmly established effectiveness should give practitioners and educators pause. The evaluation research literature strongly suggests that far too much time is devoted to preparing students for a form of treatment that has such equivocal effectiveness and far too little to the search for more effective treatments. Planned short-term therapy seems a likely candidate for a more effective as well as more efficient treatment.

In addition, the studies of planned short-term therapy reviewed here have profound social-policy and economic implications. These findings argue for a substantial modification of the reimbursement policies by third-party insurers for much psychotherapy. For example, the entire cost of psychotherapy (up to some dollar maximum, to be sure) could be reimbursed for the first two or three interviews, with perhaps 50% of the cost reimbursed for the next two or three. The burden of proof for requesting reimbursement beyond this normal maximum could rest with the psychotherapist and a peer-review procedure.

Many mental health practitioners seem to subscribe to two beliefs that are virtually unknown in the rest of the healing arts: first, it will take a long time to get better; and, second, once you are better, you probably will never need to come back. Most human service providers hold an alternative point of view, one that seems more persuasive in the context of planned short-term therapy: first, let us try to help you as quickly as possible; and, second, something might very well go wrong in the future, in which case come back and we will try to help you once again.

With this latter orientation, commitment to the client can be seen from a very different point of view from that typically considered by the mental health professions. Rabkin (1977) described the short-term therapy orientation to that commitment very well:

> Under the best of conditions, relationships with professionals other than psycho-therapists are not regarded as terminating at all. They are seen as intermittent. For example, the accountant, lawyer, family doctor, or barber may have permanent relationships with clients and perhaps their families, although the actual face-to-face contacts occur only for specific tasks or problems. Particularly in relationships of confidence, as in the case of the accountant and the physician, the tie may last a lifetime [p. 211].

Planned short-term therapy can be an effective and responsible form of psychotherapy if we remember that the relationship between client and therapist or between client and agency can be lifelong but intermittent.

CHAPTER

3

Crisis
Intervention

The concept of the personal crisis, long utilized by novelists and playwrights, has during the past 30 years increasingly attracted the attention of mental health professionals. A crisis is provoked "when a person faces an obstacle to important life goals that is, for a time, insurmountable through the utilization of customary methods of problem-solving. A period of disorganization ensues, a period of upset, during which many different abortive attempts at solution are made. Eventually, some kind of adaptation is achieved, which may or may not be in the best interests of that person and his fellows" (Caplan, 1961a, p. 18).

The management of personal crises has become of great interest to community mental health workers—first, because all of us undergo crises at various times in our lives, and how these crises are resolved often has implications for our emotional well-being. Second, it is the basic premise of crisis-intervention theory that mental health services provided during a period of crisis have the potential to be far more efficient than services provided at any other time. It is thought that during a crisis—a relatively short period lasting perhaps six to eight weeks—a person is unusually receptive to clinical intervention. This belief has been instrumental in increasing the emphasis of community mental health programs on prompt, brief clinical contact, often in emergency situations, as opposed to long-term psychotherapy that the client may have to wait for. If brief contact during crises is at least as effective as longer therapy after a time on a waiting list, developing a crisis-intervention strategy will enable mental health centers to reach greater numbers of clients with greater impact and greater speed and will thus increase productivity without increasing costs (Bloom, 1969).

A third reason for the growing interest in crisis intervention has to do with prevention. Initial adverse reactions to crises are rarely true psychiatric disorders, but if such reactions persist, they may become disabling. Hence, effective crisis-intervention services may reduce the incidence of psychiatric disability. A crisis presents an opportunity for growth as well as an opportunity for regression. Successful resolution of a traumatic crisis may make a person stronger and healthier, better able to deal with future crises should they develop, and more resistant to the negative effects of future crises. By this line of reasoning, psychological well-being may be little more than the consequence of a history of successful crisis resolutions. That is, mental health may, at any particular moment, be fully defined as the summation of crisis resolutions thus far in the person's life—a kind of batting average based on the success of crisis resolutions to date.

This chapter describes the concept of crisis and the origins of crisis-intervention programs. Then the body of ideas collectively known as crisis theory is presented. Three special types of crisis-intervention programs are examined—programs that call on the police to intervene in family conflicts, programs that provide services at times of mass population phenomena that could become crises, and programs that provide crisis-intervention services over the telephone. Finally, efforts to evaluate the effectiveness of crisis-intervention programs are summarized and analyzed.

TRAUMAS AND STRENS

Often, what at first seems a traumatic crisis later becomes viewed as a blessing in disguise. In fact, the word *stren* was coined by Hollister (1967) to designate those experiences in an individual's life that build strength into his or her personality. Finkel (1975) asked college students to describe in detail episodes in their lives that constituted either traumas or strens. Two-thirds of the 40 undergraduates reported episodes that were initially viewed as traumas but subsequently viewed as strens. About one-third of the traumatic events were in this category. Finkel concluded that

> the initial . . . interpretation of the event was replaced by a new evaluation and interpretation. The event and oneself now seem different. This process can be differentiated from intellectualization, rationalization, denial, or reaction formation, where part of the painful reality is denied or selectively distorted. The new view of self after the conversion process is not devoid of flaws and weaknesses; to the contrary, mistakes, hurts, insecurities, dependency, and fear are painfully acknowledged. What does emerge are attributes (e.g., the discovered ability to cope, adapt, learn, grow, and become self-reliant and independent) which produce a greater sense of strength, depth, maturity, sensitivity, honesty, and self-confidence [1975, p. 176].

Finkel suggests that the conversion process is primarily cognitive—that one appraisal of the event is replaced by another that is broader and more optimistic than the first—and that most of these reappraisals occur two weeks to four months after the original traumatic event.

In a replication of Finkel's work, Beaver, Buck, and McWilliams (1979) repeated his methodology with a sample of 68 students at another university. In addition to determining whether the same general results would be obtained in another setting, these authors attempted to expand the construct validity of the concept of trauma-stren conversion by identifying personality and cognitive-process characteristics that might differentiate converters from nonconverters.

At least as many students in this sample reported trauma-stren conversions as in Finkel's study, and the distribution of reports of occurrences of traumas, strens, and conversions was the same. No significant relations were found between the proportion of significant life experiences that were categorized as conversions from traumas to strens and any of the personality or cognitive measures used in the study. Beaver and colleagues noted that their sample contained so few nonconverters that statistical tests of the differences between converters and nonconverters were somewhat suspect. In addition, they believed the concept of trauma-stren conversion is probably somewhat oversimplified. For example, it is important to distinguish between a true conversion involving reevaluation of an event's importance and an event that had both traumatic and strenful elements at the same time. Nevertheless, the existence of the trauma-stren conversion phenomenon seems established.

ORIGIN OF CRISIS THEORY

Virtually all reviews of the field of crisis intervention (see, for example, Bolman & Bolian, 1979; Butcher & Maudal, 1976) date the beginning of interest in the field to a paper by Erich Lindemann (1944) that has been one of the most influential papers in the history of community mental health. Lindemann, then affiliated with the Department of Psychiatry at Harvard Medical School and with the Massachusetts General Hospital, was active in providing psychiatric help to families of victims of an extraordinary disaster. On the evening of November 28, 1942, a fire swept through a large, crowded nightclub in Boston—the Cocoanut Grove—and 493 people perished. In this kind of emergency situation, only the briefest kind of psychotherapy was possible; yet, Dr. Lindemann was able to help the survivors and at the same time study the process of acute grief and conceptualize how his efforts were or were not helpful to people in the management of their grief. His paper is a model of superb clinical reporting and analysis.

First, he described the remarkably uniform reactions to grief, which included sensations of bodily distress occurring in waves lasting from 20 minutes to an hour, feelings of tightness in the throat, choking, and shortness of breath, a need for deep sighing, an empty feeling in the abdomen, lack of muscular power, and intense subjective distress that was described as tension or psychological pain. Lindemann noted that the survivor soon learned that these waves of discomfort were precipitated by a variety of events, such as mentioning the deceased, visiting with relatives, or receiving expressions of sympathy and that survivors tended to avoid these stimulating events at any cost. Survivors also had a slight sense of unreality, a feeling of increased emotional distance from other people, and an intense preoccupation with the image of the deceased. Another strong preoccupation was with feelings of guilt. The survivors accused themselves of negligence, of failure to do right by the victim. There was a loss of warmth in relationships with other people; the survivors experienced feelings of hostility and anger that surprised and disturbed them. Survivors were restless and unable to sit still, and they seemed compelled to talk; yet, they seemed unable to initiate and maintain organized patterns of activity. They lacked zest, and activities that were formerly performed almost automatically now seemed to require enormous effort. The loss of the loved one led to a strong dependency on anyone who would stimulate the survivor to initiate any activity.

Next, Lindemann described the course of events that normally followed the initial grief reactions. These events led ultimately to a psychological separation from the deceased, a readjustment to a world in which the deceased was no longer present, and the formation of new relationships. He found that the major obstacle to successful resolution of the crisis was an unwillingness to express the intense emotional distress connected with the experience. Lindemann found that if he could facilitate the expression of grief, there would follow a rapid relief of tension and a constructive development of plans for the future. To achieve this goal required an average of eight to ten interviews over four to six weeks. Morbid grief reactions, in contrast, included postponement of grief reaction and such distorted reactions as overactivity without a sense of loss, development of symptoms previously displayed by the deceased, development of psychosomatic disorders, conspicuous alterations in relationships with friends and relatives, extreme hostility toward specific persons, including the physician, and an agitated depression, with tension, insomnia, feelings of worthlessness, self-accusation, and suicidal impulses.

Lindemann also developed some ideas about how a mental health professional could assist in the management of grief: by helping people express their grief; by attending to underreactions as well as overreactions; by helping the survivor find new patterns of rewarding interaction, review his or her relationship with the deceased, and verbalize feelings of guilt; and by prescribing appropriate medication. All these actions went far beyond the more traditional responses practiced since time immemorial—comforting the survivor, invoking divine will, and offering the promise of a later reunion with the deceased. Most societies are organized so that certain roles legitimately include crisis-intervention activities. In Western countries, the roles of the police, physicians, and the clergy include such activities, and mental health professionals have made some efforts to train these persons to intervene more comfortably and more effectively in the variety of crises that they see in the course of their normal role performance.

Most of the fundamentals of crisis theory were articulated in this single, brief paper, and Lindemann's attention then turned to extending the implications of his analysis into the development of community-based, prevention-oriented mental health programs, such as the Human Relations Service of Wellesley, Massachusetts, which he later headed. He felt that unsuccessful crisis resolution could precipitate significant psychiatric problems and that all mental health practitioners, as well as members of the clergy and workers in social welfare agencies, could assist in crisis resolution by offering psychological first aid following any crisis. Among the crises identified and investigated since this first study are premature birth of a child (Kaplan & Mason, 1960), kindergarten entry (Klein & Ross, 1958), relocation from slum housing (Fried & Lindemann, 1961), psychiatric hospitalization of parents (Irvine, 1964), unwed motherhood (Bernstein, 1960), suicide of a friend or family member (Farberow & Shneidman, 1961), retirement (Bell, 1975), and widowhood (Silverman, MacKenzie, Pettipas, & Wilson, 1975).

In a test of crisis-theory predictions concerning retirement, Bell (1975) interviewed 114 men just before retirement and again some months later, by which time they had been retired an average of about six months. On the basis of his analysis of crisis theory, Bell hypothesized that retirement would cause the men to report a decrease in life satisfaction. This hypothesis was confirmed. A related hypothesis was that there would be a significant disruption in interactions with kin, in involvement with voluntary organizations such as church or civic clubs, and in interaction with close friends and neighbors. This prediction was not confirmed. Next, Bell suggested that where such interactions did show disruption, there would be a decreased sense of satisfaction with life. This prediction was also not confirmed. Two final predictions were disconfirmed—first, that life satisfaction following retirement would decrease most in those persons who had a strong preretirement commitment to the work role and, second, that those same retirees would have a strong desire to return to the work role after retirement.

Thus, the general assertion that a crisis (in this case, retirement) can result in decreased life satisfaction was found to be true, but predictions regarding the specific bases for that reduced sense of life satisfaction were not supported. The author did suggest that a third series of interviews, some time later, might have yielded confirmation of some of these predictions. Most important to glean from this study, however, is the realization that crisis-producing events affect people differently and that a greater understanding of the effects of such events may require individual case studies and individualized predictions.

DISTINCTIONS BETWEEN CRISIS INTERVENTION AND PLANNED SHORT-TERM THERAPY

Although crisis intervention can be viewed as a type of planned short-term treatment (Ewing, 1978), planned short-term treatment can be undertaken independently of whether a crisis appears to be present (Malan, 1976, pp. 11–16). Moreover, whereas a principal goal of crisis intervention is to restore the precrisis level of functioning, planned short-term therapy aims at the more ambitious goal of increasing the level of psychological functioning and adjustment beyond that earlier level (Marmor, 1979; Straker, 1977). Stuart and Mackey (1977) propose a useful distinction among three somewhat overlapping terms in the context of the general formulation "*Reaction* is a function of *Stress* plus *Person*." They suggest that in emergency treatment the focus is on the reaction; in crisis intervention the focus is on the stress; and in short-term treatment the focus is on the person.

Castelnuovo-Tedesco (1970) distinguishes between crisis intervention and brief psychotherapy on the basis of etiological concepts, reserving the term *brief psychotherapy* for efforts to deal with internal conflict and the term *crisis intervention* for efforts to deal with external stress.

Marmor (1979) distinguishes among emergency care (see also Gerson & Bassuk, 1980), crisis intervention, and short-term dynamic psychotherapy, which seem to him to represent three points on a single continuum:

> Emergency care is concerned with the provision of immediate relief or help to a person who has decompensated in the face of internal or external stress and is coping poorly. The goal of crisis intervention is to reduce or remove the stress situation and/or help the patient deal with it more effectively. In short-term dynamic psychotherapy we are dealing with individuals in conflict, not necessarily in crisis, although a crisis situation may be involved. The goal in short-term dynamic psychotherapy is primarily on modifying the patient's coping abilities and only secondarily on relieving stress [p. 154].

Stuart and Mackey (1977) identify the same three points on the continuum of therapeutic intervention:

> An emergency for a patient is a subjective state in which he feels he cannot deal with the situation without immediate help. . . . While an emergency is experienced by the patient as an inability to cope, a crisis is the time of great change or impending change, requiring unfamiliar responses. In a crisis, great stress is placed on an individual or a family system that previously functioned in a certain way. There is a demand for reaction as changes force the system to make some kind of adjustment. Often there appears to be no satisfactory response available, and ineffectual or regressive behavior becomes apparent. . . . In crisis intervention the central element is the stress, while in short-term therapy the focus is primarily on the person. . . . The goal of short-term psychotherapy is not merely alleviation of symptoms, but also examination of patterns of behavior [pp. 528–529].

Crisis intervention and planned short-term therapy have certain attributes in common as well. Ewing (1978) has identified some of these similarities. While acknowledging that crisis-intervention techniques can be used for other purposes, such as suicide prevention, and that short-term therapy need not take place only during crises, Ewing observes that "by far the most popular use of crisis intervention is as a form of psychotherapy" (p. 5). Paraphrasing an earlier definition of psychotherapy (Meltzoff & Kornreich, 1970), Ewing defines crisis intervention as "the informed and planful application of techniques derived from the established principles of crisis theory, by persons qualified through training and experience to understand these principles, with the intention of assisting individuals or families to modify personal characteristics such as feelings, attitudes, and behaviors that are judged to be maladaptive or maladjustive" (pp. 6–7).[1]

Ewing believes that crisis intervention is a form of short-term psychotherapy, and his definition makes that point very clearly. One need only take the additional step of suggesting that a crisis is present whenever anyone requests mental health services (as Schwartz, 1971, and Wolkon, 1972, have done) to forge the final link between the two important concepts of short-term psychotherapy and crisis intervention. Ewing notes that Caplan (1964) stresses that a crisis is not in itself a pathological state but rather a "struggle for adjustment and adaptation in the face of problems that are for a time insoluble" (1978, p. 14). In particular, Ewing's ideas about psychotherapy during times of crisis derive from the belief that at those times people are more interested in being helped and more responsive to such help than at times of more stable functioning. Furthermore, Ewing believes that successful outcomes of crises result mainly from actions by the subject and interventions by others at the time of crisis rather than such antecedent factors as prior experience, personality characteristics, or even the nature of the problem.

CRISIS THEORY

Types of crises and types of crisis-intervention programs

Crises have traditionally been divided into two major types, and the classification of crisis-intervention programs is related to this typology. First, there is a category of crises typically called *accidental, situational,* or *unanticipated* (see Parad, 1965, pp. 73–74; Schwartz, 1971). Examples are death of a family member, illness, accident, surgery, loss or change of jobs, and marital disruption. These crises are all characterized by periods of acute disorganization of behavior or affect precipitated by a stressful and somewhat unpredictable life experience. The second type of crisis, called *maturational, developmental,* or *normative,* is characterized by periods of acute disorganization of behavior or affect, precipitated by a transition from one developmental phase to another (Datan & Ginsberg, 1975). Examples are entering kindergarten, high school, or college, becoming engaged, marrying, becoming a parent, and retiring. These crises are all predictable and thus lend themselves to the development of comprehensive intervention services (see also Baldwin, 1979).

Datan and Ginsberg (1975) classify normative crises into three types—crises in individual development, such as role transitions during adolescence

[1]From *Crisis Intervention as Psychotherapy,* by C. P. Ewing. Copyright © 1978 by Oxford University Press. Reprinted by permission.

or at retirement, or death; crises in the family life cycle, such as marriage or parenthood; and crises in the social system, such as those involving the work role or aging as a societal issue. Interventions often focus on the development of increased competency to deal with the transition in question. Thus, discussion of interventions for normative crises is often synonymous with discussion of social competency and social-skills building, covered in Chapter 7. This chapter will concentrate on crisis intervention in unanticipated or emergency situations.

The most important consequences of identifying types of crises are the implications for how and where crisis-intervention programs should be organized, staffed, and housed. A community interested in developing services to meet the needs of persons undergoing situational crises will have to determine where and how often these crises occur and what needs are predominant in the victims. Even more fundamental is the challenging task of identifying the types of phenomena that constitute potential crises—a task few communities undertake. Contrasting the frequency with which potentially critical events take place with the frequency with which intervention services are provided might yield some clues to the magnitude of unmet needs. If you were interested in developing crisis-intervention services for persons who had lost or were about to lose a family member through death, you might well station yourself near the admitting office of the local general hospital, keep in close contact with morticians, or read the obituaries. If you wished to develop crisis-intervention services for persons undergoing marital disruption, you would need to keep up on divorce decrees or work closely with attorneys, the clergy, or other groups of persons who might know of individuals currently undergoing that kind of stress. To develop supportive services for persons who have lost their jobs, a facility might work in close collaboration with both public and private employment services or with employers contemplating layoffs.

Locating people undergoing developmental crises is somewhat easier. Eighth- or ninth-grade students constitute the population about to make the transition to high school. High school seniors include many of the persons planning to enter college. To find women who are about to face the so-called empty-nest syndrome, one has only to identify those high school seniors who are the youngest children in their families. Mothers of these seniors constitute the population at risk. Working with heads of large companies, one could meet persons within six months or a year of retirement and develop special programs for them.

The course of emotional crises

Caplan (1964) has identified four phases that are characteristic of crises. First, the situation calls forth habitual problem-solving responses. Then, failure to resolve the problem results in a rise in tension and a feeling of upset and ineffectuality. Next, the person tries emergency and novel methods of problem resolution. Finally, if these methods have failed, distortion of reality, resignation, or unmanageable tension may result, with subsequent disorgan ization of personality.

Taplin (1971) has reviewed the literature on psychological crises and has identified the major assertions commonly made about them. First, life is a succession of crisis events, or stresses, that occur in the normal maturational/ developmental, social-learning process. Second, crises have a definite course in time, causing different amounts of personal disruption or strain at different points in their evolution. Third, crises are more accessible to intervention at their peak. Fourth, they may be resolved in adaptive or maladaptive ways. Fifth, a history of successful crisis resolutions increases the probability of successful crisis resolutions in the future. Sixth, assistance in crisis does not have to come from specially trained professionals. Seventh, aspects of the current situation play an important part in sustaining a crisis, and changing the situation the person currently faces can significantly affect the course of a crisis. Eighth, the onset of a crisis usually involves an identifiable precipitating event, generally a situational or interpersonal one.

Baldwin (1979) has identified ten corollaries of crisis theory that are help-ful in understanding emotional crises. There is some overlap between these corollaries and Taplin's list of assertions about crises just reviewed. First, "Because each individual's tolerance for stress is idiosyncratic and finite, emotional crises have no per se relationship to psychopathology and occur even among the well-adjusted."[2] Second, "Emotional crises are self-limiting events in which crisis resolution, either adaptive or maladaptive, takes place within an average of four to six weeks." Third, "During a crisis state, psychological defenses are weakened or absent and the individual has cognitive and/or affective aware-ness of material previously well-defended and less accessible." Fourth, "Dur-ing a crisis state, the individual has enhanced capacity for both cognitive and affective learning because of the vulnerability of this state and the motivation produced by emotional disequilibrium." Fifth, "Adaptive crisis resolution is frequently a vehicle for resolving underlying conflicts that have in part deter-mined the emotional crisis and/or that interfere with the crisis resolution process." Sixth, "A small external influence during a crisis state can produce dispropor-tionate change in a short period of time when compared to therapeutic change that occurs during non-crisis states." Seventh, "The resolution of an emotional crisis is not necessarily determined by previous experience or character struc-ture, but rather is shaped by current and perhaps unique socio-psychological influences operating in the present." Eighth, "Inherent in every emotional crisis is an actual or anticipated loss to the individual that must be reconciled as part of the crisis resolution process." Ninth, "Every emotional crisis is an interpersonal event involving at least one significant other person who is

[2]From "Crisis Intervention: An Overview of Theory and Practice," by B. A. Baldwin. In *The Counseling Psychologist*, 8(2), 43–52. Copyright 1979. Reprinted by permission.

represented in the crisis situation directly, indirectly, or symbolically." Tenth, "Effective crisis resolution prevents future crises of a similar nature by removing vulnerabilities from the past and by increasing the individual's repertoire of available coping skills that can be used in such situations" (Baldwin, 1979, pp. 45–47; see also Aguilera & Messick, 1974; Darbonne, 1967; Halpern, 1973; Lukton, 1974; Parad, 1971; Viney, 1976).

Given these assertions, it is easy to see why the long waiting list, detailed diagnostic study, case conference, and assignment to a therapist for long-term, once-weekly psychotherapy have given way in many community mental health centers to encouraging people to seek help immediately when they find themselves in a critical period in their lives and to offering prompt and brief clinical assessment and intervention.

There is a question of how much clinical expertise is required for successful crisis intervention. According to Taplin (1971, p. 5), "The humanity of significant others may be both sufficient and necessary for assistance in crisis." Bellak and Small, in contrast, assert that "brief and emergency psychotherapy is . . . properly a specialty for the experienced practitioner, and one that requires full use of his capacities" (1965, p. 6).

Crisis duration.   Because crises are presumed to be relatively brief, it is especially important to locate persons in crisis so that needed services can be delivered expeditiously. In one of the few published studies examining crisis duration, Lewis, Gottesman, and Gutstein (1979) administered a group of psychological tests to 35 patients undergoing surgery for a suspected malignancy, and to a comparison group of 35 patients undergoing surgery for less serious illnesses, on five occasions starting the night before surgery.

These authors developed a composite summary statement of crisis theory: "An unexpected event causes severe psychological discomfort that cannot be resolved by ordinary coping strategies. New methods of coping are attempted, and if these also fail, the result is anxiety, depression, helplessness, and a loss of self-esteem. After 8 weeks or less, the psychological aspects of the crisis are resolved, either adaptively or maladaptively, although the precipitating event may still be present" (1979, p. 128).

The authors found that the cancer group was significantly more anxious and depressed than the comparison group, and for a longer time, and that the cancer group had significantly lower scores on a measure of internal locus of control (that is, the extent to which people feel in control of their fate). The repeated testings suggested that the crisis state lasted longer than the 6–8 weeks postulated by crisis theory but that it was shorter than 7 months (the time of the last testing). At that time, the cancer group reported less anxiety, less depression, and less of a sense of crisis.

General crisis-intervention techniques.   A number of literature reviews suggest crisis-intervention axioms and techniques that anyone undertaking such interventions should keep in mind (see, for example, Baldwin, 1979;

Caplan & Grunebaum, 1967). First, it is suggested that the best way to utilize professional time and effort is to schedule frequent contacts with the client during the brief period of the crisis rather than weekly interviews over an extended period. Second, crisis intervention should support the integrity of the family and prevent its fragmentation, so as to preserve its capacity to assist the family member in crisis. Third, undue dependence on the mental health professional should be prevented. The professional can control this by providing active interventive help during the crisis and by dealing with current realities rather than with historical antecedents of the problem. Fourth, the effort should be to facilitate the client's mastery of the problem by giving information and hope, which will assist the client in confronting and dealing with the crisis. Fifth, outside supports should be sought and provided wherever possible. And, sixth, the goal of crisis intervention should be to help the client deal affirmatively with the current situation, regardless of his or her prior history of success or failure in crisis resolution, rather than to achieve a personality reorganization.

Ewing (1978) postulates six essential and overlapping stages in the process of crisis intervention as psychotherapy: (1) problem delineation, (2) evaluation, (3) contracting, (4) intervening, (5) termination, and (6) follow-up. The goal of problem delineation is to "define a fairly specific problem area toward which the intervention may be directed" (p. 95). To achieve this objective, the therapist has to develop a trusting relationship with the client, a process usually referred to as developing *rapport*. Clients often have multiple difficulties and may be only dimly aware of some of them. Accordingly, the therapist may need to review the major dimensions of the client's life history and identify any recent life changes or stresses. Most crisis therapists agree, suggests Ewing, that "without a clearly defined problem-focus, effective crisis intervention cannot proceed" (p. 95).

The stage of evaluation (during initial contact between client and therapist) should involve an assessment of the client and of the current life situation. Ewing suggests that the evaluation should include the basic demographic facts (age, family and marital status, residence, education, occupation, and so on); previous and current psychotherapeutic history and involvement; accessibility to intervention; psychological functioning (appearance, behavior, speech characteristics, thought and perception, appropriateness and nature of mood and emotionality); motivation; and a general description of precrisis adjustment.

The process of contracting with the client should include specification of the problem focus, time limits for the intervention, whether other persons should be involved in the psychotherapeutic process, and the individual responsibilities of the client and therapist. Intervention also develops during the client-therapist initial contact, but becomes dominant after completion of the first three stages. Ewing identifies nine tactics: (1) listening and encouraging verbalization, (2) identifying and using the support of friends and family, (3) using other institutional and agency supports and services, (4) advocacy on the client's behalf, (5) sensitive yet pointed confrontation, (6) providing factual information, (7) exploring alternative coping mechanisms, (8) judicious advice and suggestion, and (9) assigning carefully selected homework tasks.

Since the initial contracting already includes the issue of length of treatment, the process of termination actually starts when the treatment starts. Even though treatment is very short, termination can be difficult. Some clients insist on continuing beyond the agreed-on completion date. Others signal their difficulties by terminating prematurely and without notification. As Ewing suggests, "The termination of any meaningful relationship may be expected to evoke strong sentiments" (1978, p. 115).

Finally, Ewing suggests that some type of follow-up to determine the client's condition and progress, even if only by telephone, is a necessary component of short-term treatment. It can take place a month or two after termination and can serve important evaluative, educational, and clinical functions.

Ewing's views are unusually important because they underline a special point rarely stressed enough. All mental health programs and professionals, public or private, provide a certain amount of crisis intervention. Yet it is not uncommon for mental health professionals to believe, sometimes implicitly, that psychotherapy can begin only after the crisis is over. Ewing urges the practitioner to look to crisis intervention itself as a golden opportunity to do significant short-term psychotherapy.

> Certainly there are CMHC's [community mental health centers] utilizing crisis intervention as psychotherapy. The bulk of CMHC immediate services, however, are oriented toward emergency evaluation or triage rather than crisis intervention. These services, though sometimes advertised as crisis intervention, often amount only to brief evaluation followed by discharge or referral to traditional services such as hospitalization or outpatient evaluation/treatment. Thus, they serve as a means for *screening* rather than actually *treating* clients. As Beigel and Levinson (1972) observe, this screening and referral function is in itself an important and often essential aspect of CMHC emergency services. But, as they also note, if CMHC emergency personnel are trained in and encouraged to use crisis intervention, "then the definitive care for many patients can be handled within the emergency service, and referral is not needed." In the long run, much of the future of crisis intervention as psychotherapy may rest upon the extent to which CMHC administrators and clinicians accept this suggestion and utilize crisis intervention as a primary treatment modality [1978, pp. 86–87].

The last few years have seen a number of other presentations of the techniques of crisis intervention. Morrice (1976) has described the therapeutic techniques used in a variety of crisis-intervention programs in Great Britain, Golan (1978) has described social-work approaches to crisis situations, and Puryear (1979) has prepared a practical guide to crisis intervention.

In addition, several scholarly articles have described specific settings in which crisis-intervention services have been provided. Among these are the work of Kinney, Madsen, Fleming, and Haapala (1977) on helping families in crisis; Jaffe, Thompson, and Paquin's (1978) report on how mental health personnel work closely with the police to respond to family crises; Silverman's (1978) description of a crisis-intervention service for the mates and families of rape victims; and Fraser and Froelich's (1979) description of the crisis worker in the court system.

FAMILY CRISIS INTERVENTION BY POLICE OFFICERS

Among the most innovative approaches to crisis intervention have been the programs training police officers in family crisis intervention. These programs were initially developed by Bard and his colleagues in New York City (Bard, 1970; Bard & Berkowitz, 1967, 1969). Bard, who was himself a policeman before becoming a mental health professional, and Berkowitz noted that "police officers in today's society are realistically involved in many interpersonal service functions for which traditional police training leaves them unprepared" (1969, p. 209) and that, in particular, "while troubled middle- and upper-class families may invoke the help of lawyers, clergymen, and marriage counselors of the various behavioral disciplines, lower-class families tend to call only on the police at times of crisis. Half of the calls for assistance to an urban police department may involve family crises or other complaints of a personal or interpersonal nature" (1967, p. 315).

Bard and Berkowitz noted that perhaps 90% of a police officer's duties are unrelated to crime control or law enforcement, that homicides and serious assaults are far more likely to occur within a family than between strangers, and that officers responding to family disturbances are often injured or killed. Driscoll, Meyer, and Schanie (1973) suggest that because most nuclear families are geographically isolated, when a family "has exhausted its internal resources and methods for handling conflict, its members often have no place to turn but to public arbitration. . . . the mental health system in most communities is not responsive to this type of problem, it is seldom available 'round-the-clock on short notice, and many family conflicts involve violence. All this sets the problem squarely on the shoulders of the police" (p. 63).[3]

Bard and his colleagues were instrumental in calling to the attention of the general public the fact that the police are, if one can judge by how they spend their time, first and foremost front-line human service workers and that they receive very little training or reward for this work. With this in mind, these psychologists sought to develop and evaluate a training program to assist the police in serving this human service function with the highest possible level of skill. Bard and Berkowitz concentrated their efforts on training the police for their role in family crisis intervention.

[3]From "Training Police in Family Crisis Intervention," by J. M. Driscoll, R. G. Meyer, and C. F. Schanie, *Journal of Applied Behavioral Science*, 1973, 9, 62–82. This and all other quotations from this source are reprinted by special permission of the N.T.L. Institute of Applied Behavioral Science.

Their project took place in an Upper West Side Manhattan precinct, primarily residential in character, that houses about 85,000 lower-class and lower-middle-class residents, mostly Black and Puerto Rican. Bard and Berkowitz, working with graduate students in the Psychology Department of the City College of the City University of New York, selected 18 volunteers out of a total of 220 police officers in the precinct, enough to make it possible for two men to be on duty 24 hours a day, 365 days a year. The men had all had at least three years of patrol experience, were interested in higher education and professional advancement, and showed aptitude and motivation for the project goals. All 18 men were trained together in a one-month, 160-hour (full-time) training program. Then, for two years, they served, one pair to a shift, in a radio patrol car reserved for family crisis work. During this two-year period, the 18 men received both individual and group consultation. During the first 20 months after the training phase, the Family Crisis Intervention Unit (FCIU) intervened in more than 1400 domestic disturbances in more than 900 families.

A neighboring police precinct with a somewhat similar population composition was selected to serve as a comparison setting. It was hypothesized that the experimental precinct would show decreases in the number of family-disturbance complaints and recurring complaints by the same families; in homicides and assaults, particularly among family members; and in injuries sustained by the police.

In their preliminary presentation of the project findings, Bard and Berkowitz (1969) noted that the FCIU was having a positive effect on community attitudes toward the police, that no complaints had been made against members of the FCIU for improper performance of duty, that the men had performed with distinction and high morale, that the training they had received had enhanced their skills as policemen, and that not a single injury had been sustained by a member of the FCIU in handling a family disturbance.

When the final project results were announced (Bard, 1970), it became clear that not all the project objectives had been achieved. There was no decrease, in the experimental precinct, in the number of family-disturbance complaints, recurring complaints by the same families, or homicides. But there was a decrease in the number of assaults within families, and the record of no injuries to trained officers was maintained. In contrast, two members of the regular police force had sustained injuries in family disputes, as had one officer in the control precinct.

Driscoll and his colleagues argued that the design of the Bard study prevented a direct and unconfounded evaluation and that "while the reduction of crime incidence is obviously a worthy goal, the problems inherent in the use of crime statistics as indices of success of a police training project invite near-certain failure. Two major problems . . . seem to have been differential reporting and the operation of variables extraneous to the project that may have been much more powerful than the effects of the project itself" (1973, pp. 66–67). Driscoll and his colleagues suggested that, as an alternative evaluation strategy, data be collected at a point much closer to the crisis-intervention setting. They hypothesized that if citizens in experimental and control precincts were asked their reactions to police officers who had intervened, citizens in the experimental precinct would report higher levels of rapport between themselves and the officers, greater involvement on the part of the officers, more satisfaction with and regard for the police, and greater acceptance of the police. Furthermore, trained officers could be expected to report increased understanding of the problems with which they were dealing, increased acceptance by citizens, greater receptivity of citizens to their suggestions, a decrease in the necessity for force, an increase in their effectiveness, and a generally positive reaction to the new techniques and to the training program.

These researchers administered a training program in Louisville, Kentucky, patterned after the Bard program, and then placed six two-man crisis teams in the field for a six-month period. During this time, radio dispatchers assigned domestic-trouble calls to these trained intervention teams whenever possible but, when not possible, to untrained teams. During the six months more than 400 domestic-trouble calls were answered, 31% of them by trained officers.

Data collected from clients and from officers support the proposition that trained police officers function more adequately than untrained officers. Driscoll and colleagues conclude that "there appears to be reasonable assurance that the Bard model of crisis intervention training, with some adaptation, can produce more satisfactory and effective family crisis interventions by police officers" (1973, p. 81).

Training of police officers in crisis intervention and conflict management has become an increasingly accepted part of their preparation throughout the United States, and efforts to evaluate the effects of this training on attitudes and performance are continuing (see Mulvey & Reppucci, 1981, for example). In addition, the literature on family violence is growing very rapidly (see, for example, the annotated bibliography on violence in the home published by the U.S. Department of Health, Education and Welfare, 1974).

CRISIS INTERVENTION AND MASS POPULATION PHENOMENA

In recent years, the concepts of crisis theory and crisis intervention have been applied to mental health care in times of natural disaster or in settings involving large numbers of people. There is a long-standing interest in describing natural disasters and in documenting behavior during mass crises (see Moore, 1964, for example), but the concept of developing intervention services to deal with the crisis on a planned, mass basis is relatively new.

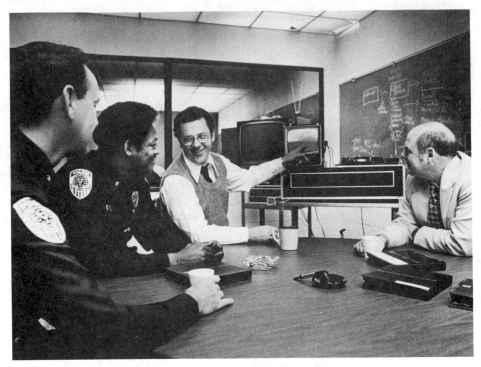

As part of their training in crisis intervention, these police officers discuss with James Driscoll a videotaped simulated family crisis. *(Photo courtesy of Carl Maupin, University of Louisville Public Information Office.)*

Crises during mass events

Reports of crisis-intervention programs' experiences during events involving large numbers of persons have a reassuring similarity. For example, Lowy, Wintrob, and Dhindsa (1969) have described their experiences with psychiatric emergencies during Expo '67 in Montreal. Millions of visitors attended Expo '67, and many were exposed to undue stress and fatigue associated with crowding on highways as well as at the fair, long lines for many services, problems in securing lodging, and the irritations of travel. Lowy and his colleagues anticipated the attendance of a certain number of drifters, thrill seekers, eccentrics, and criminals at the fair and sought to determine the incidence and severity of psychiatric disorders. To accomplish this, they examined the records of one of the four general medical clinics located on the grounds of Expo '67. Physicians and nurses at these clinics managed a wide range of disorders and referred to the hospital only those patients who could not be satisfactorily treated at the clinic.

Of the approximately 10,000 patients who came to this particular clinic during the six months the fair was open, 256 could be reliably diagnosed as having psychiatric problems. Most were under age 35, female, and Canadian, and nearly 80% had symptoms that could be classified as neurotic or psycho-somatic. Only 10 of the 256 cases appeared to be psychotic, and only 38 were referred to the hospital emergency room. The authors noted that "although preparations were made to manage large numbers of psychiatric casualties, these failed to materialize" (p. 969). Furthermore, their findings in Montreal were consistent with the experiences of medical authorities at both the Brussels World's Fair of 1958 and the New York Fair of 1964–65.

Carpenter, Tamarkin, and Raskin (1971) describe their experiences in pro-viding emergency psychiatric services during the march on Washington of November 13–15, 1969, in which an estimated 400,000–500,000 persons par-ticipated. The authors anticipated that ordinary hospital emergency facilities would be strained by this enormous and sudden population increase and that the problem would be even more complex because the new population would be unfamiliar with the location of existing medical facilities and suspicious of conventional services. Finally, it was anticipated that there would be an espe-cially high incidence of drug-related problems. Accordingly, a medical/psy-chiatric facility was established in a church basement a mile from the dem-onstration area. In addition, there were many medical/psychiatric volunteers, both at this facility and at several first-aid stations established along the march route.

In total, 30 patients were evaluated during the three days of the clinic's operation. Half appeared not to have drug-related problems. A survey of all greater-metropolitan-Washington emergency rooms and psychiatric inpatient facilities turned up 5 additional patients. These authors came to the same general conclusion as the group in Montreal—psychiatric problems were far less frequent and severe than expected. The authors noted that

> it was commonly expected that the great influx of young people over a three-day period would result in large-scale drug abuse, with considerable social tension and personal distress. Reports circulated in medical circles that government offi-cials had undertaken contingency planning for mass drug casualties. A stark contrast exists between this expectation and what occurred. . . . It is surprising, then, that in spite of adverse conditions such as crowded and insufficient housing, unpleasantly cold and wet weather, extensive travel, and lack of sleep, there were so few psychiatric emergencies [pp. 1331–1332].

Kahn (1980) described the anticipatory efforts of the Lake Placid Olympic Organizing Committee (LPOOC) to deal with crises that might befall athletes or visitors to the 1980 Winter Olympics. The LPOOC had established a Stress Center at the local American Legion post.

> The center was supposed to alleviate the general public's woes and also, the LPOOC announced, to counsel athletes "in handling the trauma of defeat and coping with the exhilaration of victory." But when I dropped by there, reportori-ally, a couple of days before the closing ceremony, I was told that not a solitary

athlete had yet materialized. . . . Indeed, the center had greeted only eight or ten visitors a day, and the only one it had had to soothe was a drunken spectator who, between snorts, had been overheard muttering threats of suicide [p. 67].

A very different type of group phenomenon was reported by Sank (1979), who described how the mental health staff of the George Washington University Health Plan dealt with the aftermath of the 39-hour takeover of 154 hostages by the Hanafi Muslim sect in three Washington, D.C., locations on March 9–11, 1977. The staff of the health plan was particularly involved in this takeover because many persons held captive were members of this health maintenance organization.

The treatment format was short-term, crisis-oriented, broad-spectrum group behavior therapy. Treatment began within a week after the hostages' release and was available to all hostages regardless of insurance coverage. About half the hostages were seen in treatment. Sank reported that "the victims gained a sense of comfort from the assurance that they were being followed professionally from the outset" and that "there was the pleasant surprise that this Health Plan was seeking them out, regardless of their insurance affiliation" (1979, p. 337). The treatment program, which appeared to be remarkably effective, had several distinctive features:

> First, a strategy of primary prevention was employed. Initially, only a few of the hostage victims experienced any unpleasant effects from the ordeal, except for exhaustion. The Practice felt confident, however (and their prediction was borne out), that there would be an emotional fallout from the experience. They set about employing a treatment program focused on minimizing the effects of the trauma. They attempted to teach coping and support skills to the victims to assist themselves, their colleagues, and their families. The Practice instituted a community-based approach to treatment. They acted on the belief that the most powerful tool available to them was the natural support system provided by past and future associations at the work place. Consistent with this belief in mutual support, they set about fostering it through group treatment, work-site-based treatment, and the retention of an already existent supportive atmosphere. They reinforced openness, the solicitation of caring, and an eager positive response to these requests [p. 337].

Perez (1982) has described and analyzed the organizational, social, and clinical issues that had to be dealt with in providing mental health services to the Cuban immigrants who arrived in Florida during the 1980 sealift. In particular, Perez described the work of the hastily formed interdisciplinary team who attempted to meet the needs of several hundred minors who found themselves placed among several thousand adults in one of the refugee centers. Perez concluded:

> Ultimately, like most therapeutic interventions, the provision of ventilation, catharsis, and an honest, concerned and open relationship proved to be critical. A need was observed for a setting in which experiences and feelings could be freely and openly explored. Many minors shared feelings of abandonment by families or

guilt at having left a loved one behind. Most experienced considerable ambivalence over their decision to leave Cuba and come to the U.S. However, the discussion of feelings among the population of minors had previously not been acceptable. The simple provision of an open setting in which these feelings could be discussed proved quite helpful to many [p. 43].

The 1971 Los Angeles earthquake

Let's now examine the experiences of mental health professionals who have mobilized their resources to deal with natural disasters. On February 9, 1971, an earthquake hit the Los Angeles area and was unusually severe and damaging in the San Fernando Valley. Blaufarb and Levine (1972) have described the crisis-intervention techniques they used to help families deal with this traumatic event. The director of clinical services at the San Fernando Valley Child Guidance Clinic made a radio broadcast offering services of the clinic to frightened parents and children. Telephone contact was made available, and the clinic staff readied itself to provide group crisis-intervention services.

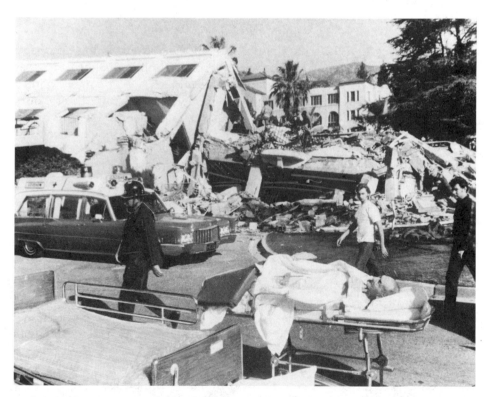

This Veterans Administration hospital collapsed during the earthquake that shook the Los Angeles area in 1971. The patient you see was evacuated, but many others died. (Photo courtesy of Wide World Photos, Inc.)

Some 800 parents took advantage of the offer and phoned, most needing only reassurance that they were reacting appropriately. Nearly 300 families participated in group crisis-intervention services during the next five weeks, about 85% of the families attending only one session. In reviewing these clinic contacts, Blaufarb and Levine noted that the most common problems reported in children were fear of going to sleep in their own rooms, inability to sleep through the night, a wish to sleep with their parents, fear of remaining alone in one part of the house even though the mother was in another part of the house, and fear of leaving the mother in order to play with other children. These problems all indicated severe separation anxiety and "represented the children's attempts to maintain contact with parents who provide safety and security" (p. 18).

The clinic staff tried to reduce the anxiety level of both parents and children and to provide an opportunity for the sharing of experiences among earthquake victims. Although there were no resources to undertake a formal evaluation of the crisis services, Blaufarb and Levine feel that "crisis intervention is an effective technique for alleviating the negative effects of psychological trauma on those persons who have experienced a natural disaster" (p. 19).

The 1972 Buffalo Creek disaster

On February 26, 1972, a dam constructed by the Buffalo Mining Company in West Virginia gave way, unleashing more than a million gallons of water and mud into Buffalo Creek Valley. The water's impact lasted no more than 15 minutes at any one point in the 18-mile-long valley, and within three hours the water and mud had washed into the Guyandotte River at the foot of the valley. Yet everything in the path of the flow was destroyed; 125 persons were killed and 4000 left homeless. A group of 65 social scientists and mental health professionals, mainly from the University of Cincinnati, were retained by the attorneys for 625 persons who brought legal action against the conglomerate owning the mining operation, and in 1974 the plaintiffs agreed to a settlement of $13.5 million, of which more than $6 million was for "psychic impairment"—a term devised to describe the social, vocational, and personal disability from psychological causes arising from the disaster and its aftermath (Erikson, 1976a, 1976b; Lifton, 1976; Lifton & Olson, 1976; Newman, 1976; Stern, 1976a, 1976b; Titchener & Kapp, 1976; Titchener, Kapp, & Winget, 1976).

A team of raters assessed the degree of psychic impairment of the 625 plaintiffs and concluded that 2% had no impairment, over 20% had minimal impairment, over 70% had moderate to severe impairment, and 1% were considered totally disabled. Thus, these judges found that negative psychological consequences were nearly universal and that they were often persistent, still affecting many survivors two years after the disaster. Even taking into account that these mental health professionals were part of an adversary system and that their findings might therefore be somewhat suspect, it seems clear that this disaster had very serious consequences for the survivors.

The scientists associated with this project described these consequences, tried to explain why they had come about, and proposed what seemed to them to be potentially effective interventions. Titchener and his colleagues (1976) found that the consequences of the disaster could be grouped into, first, the acute effects of the disaster's impact, second, symptoms that persisted months and even years later, and, third, pervasive character, attitude, and life-style changes (see also Rangell, 1976).

Among the acute effects, they noted memory disturbances, insomnia, nightmares, irritability, and occasional panic. The more persistent, chronic symptoms included continuing anxiety, phobias, depression, increased smoking and drinking, and loss of interest and enjoyment in sexual relationships, socializing, and sports activities such as hunting and fishing. Finally, character changes included diminished trust in others and lower valuation of self, a sense of guilt and shame about surviving, unresolved grief not only over the loss of family and friends but also over the loss of a way of life, and a pervasive sense of hopelessness and meaninglessness. This complex constellation of transitory and persistent symptoms has been called the *survivor syndrome*.

Lifton (1976) asserted that the effects of the disaster had been so extensive that no one exposed to it had escaped them. He divided the survivor syndrome into five elements: (1) virtually indelible memories and images of death and

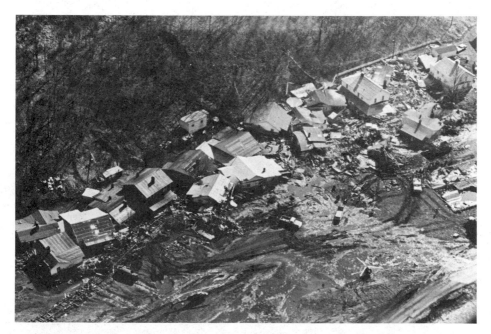

This photo, taken in the Buffalo Creek Valley after the February 1972 flood, suggests the extent of the upheaval in the lives of the survivors. *(Photo courtesy of Wide World Photos, Inc.)*

anxiety about death and disaster, (2) guilt over having lived while others died, (3) a numbing or diminishing of feelings—apathy, withdrawal, depression, and general constriction in living, (4) impaired human relationships, often involving a simultaneous need for and suspicion of close contact with others, and (5) a need to find some acceptable formulation of one's own disaster experience.

Turning now to the reasons that this particular disaster had such profound consequences, Lifton (1976) suggested its suddenness, lack of warning, and terrifying quality, the recognition that this disaster was caused by people (people for whom the residents of Buffalo Creek had little esteem), the continuing economic dependence of the survivors on the people responsible for the disaster, the geographic isolation of the community, with the resulting strong attachments to home, family, and friends and weak attachments to support systems outside the community, and, finally, the completeness of the destruction of the community, with all the consequences that entailed in terms of difficulties in providing adequate help.

These social scientists proposed some suggestions for effective interventions. The survivors required extensive help in rebuilding their psychological as well as physical community, and they needed to do it on the basis of their own ideas. Medical and psychological services were required, again planned in collaboration with the survivors. The survivors needed to be given support in and recognition for the difficult tasks they faced. They needed to be helped to find meaning in the experience, in part by being provided opportunities to share their experiences and resulting wisdom with others not directly involved in the experience. And the survivors needed some explicit education about what could be expected as normal reactions to the disaster.

The 1972 Pennsylvania hurricane and flood

On June 23, 1972, Hurricane Agnes brought heavy rains into eastern and central Pennsylvania, causing the greatest amount of property damage of any natural disaster in American history. The Susquehanna River, whose normal flood height is 22 feet, crested at 40.6 feet, broke through dikes, and overflowed banks for several hundred miles. Although only seven lives were lost during the flooding, property damage exceeded $1 billion, more than 100,000 people were directly affected by the flood, and between 20,000 and 30,000 lost their homes. In the city of Wilkes-Barre, population 35,000, only three businesses remained open. Families and community services were severely disrupted. At one point, more than 20,000 persons were declared missing. Once the physical dangers had passed, attention turned to the psychological dangers. Richard (1974) prepared a preliminary report of the massive effort to provide crisis-intervention services to a very large population. He wrote:

> For these flood victims the disruption of family patterns, lack of familiarity with the new physical environment, loss of familiar neighbors, the corner grocery store, the neighborhood school and church precipitated severe disequilibrium and

concomitant emotional and behavioral reactions for most families. . . . Other major areas of concern included the anticipated need for extended crowded living conditions in motels or mobile homes; lack of personal finances to remodel or buy a permanent dwelling; disruption of normal community care-giving service patterns; and the acute "sense of loss" of past traditions, customs, habits, interpersonal contacts and personal property [pp. 211–212].

Soon after the initial flood-recovery operations were underway, representatives from a variety of Pennsylvania agencies met with the National Institute of Mental Health and developed four one-year contracts, representing a total expenditure of approximately $1 million, to train outreach workers, implement two crisis-intervention projects, and perform an evaluation of the projects. The overall project was begun on August 10, 1972, only seven weeks after the flood. Its goals were to "provide preventive, interventive and restorative human services to flood victims through the use of trained indigenous paraprofessionals working in the community and neighborhoods" (Richard, 1974, p. 213).

During the first eight months of the project, local staff members were trained and nearly 1500 cases were opened, a third of these during the first five weeks. Problems encountered by these flood victims were varied, with emotional difficulties, the most common problem, making up 19% of the total. The outreach project continued until April 1975 in order to meet area residents'

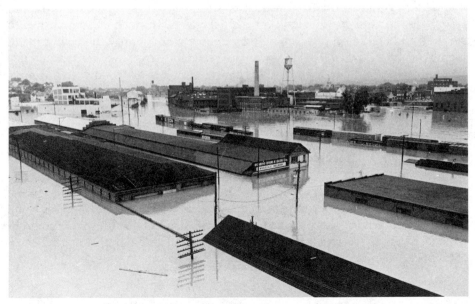

This photograph, taken in June 1972, shows the extent of the flooding that accompanied Hurricane Agnes. *(Photo courtesy of the U.S. Department of Housing and Urban Development.)*

needs. During its latter phases, this 32-month-long project developed linkages with the local community mental health center, as an increasing proportion of presenting problems were emotional. Outreach counselors recorded over 25,000 individual client contacts.

Heffron (1977) has provided a retrospective assessment of these crisis-intervention services. His comments are particularly valuable because they take into account the experiences gained in a number of other disasters as well.

> For over two decades the disaster-related literature has proposed that there are a number of relatively specific, time-limited periods of disaster, each with concomitant individual emotional reactions. The Agnes experience, in general, supports this belief. Individual victims did exhibit identifiable psychological responses which tended to characterize certain phases of the disaster and the recovery process. Furthermore, according to other reports, these reactions appear to be relatively consistent from disaster to disaster. . . . The available evidence leaves little doubt that disasters trigger emotional crises in the victims [pp. 107–108].

Heffron provides a number of general recommendations to decrease the impact of a disaster and to facilitate the adjustment process. First, disaster intervention programs should adopt a preventive approach to working with victims, helping them focus on their problems and resolve whatever issues seem to be most pressing. Second, crisis workers should provide an opportunity for disaster victims to ventilate their own feelings, since so many of them feel overwhelmed and unable to deal realistically with the situation. Third, community stereotypes related to the concepts of mental health and mental illness may influence the success of a disaster intervention program. In general, victims do not look on themselves as in need of mental health services and will reject offers of help by people who identify themselves with mental health agencies. Fourth, to be most effective, crisis workers should use an aggressive outreach approach, bringing services to the disaster victims rather than waiting for them to seek help. Finally, Heffron suggests that crisis workers involved directly in disaster intervention programs should be sensitive not only to the emotional needs and reactions of the victims but also to the potential stresses on the helpers.

The number of people who were spared emotional disorders because of the active intervention by the outreach staff will never be known. The evaluators of the project concluded, however, that there was little question that it was important and that it performed useful and needed services for flood victims. Furthermore, the project helped focus national attention on the problems faced by disaster victims (see also Newman, Chapman, Deegan, & Wescott, 1979; Ollendick & Hoffmann, 1982).

The 1974 Indiana tornadoes

Mental health crisis-intervention services were provided for the victims of the tornadoes of April 3, 1974, in the resort community of Monticello, Indiana. In contrast to what happened in Pennsylvania, Zarle, Hartsough, and Ottinger (1974) found it difficult to secure resources quickly to mount a crisis-intervention program, and nearly four months elapsed between the time negotiations began for financial support and the time state and federal agencies responded. As the Pennsylvania planners had done, this group chose to train indigenous community volunteers to provide the bulk of the crisis-intervention services. This report, like the report by Richard (1974), described the program for training the local residents who would be providing the direct services. In addition, Zarle and his associates (1974) described the phases in the development and implementation of the mental health crisis-intervention project: (1) identifying the need for a mental health response, (2) establishing contact with local agencies in the disaster area, (3) obtaining sanction from local agencies to form an umbrella of sponsoring community groups to look for funds and to develop an intervention program, (4) identifying personnel resources inside and outside the disaster area, (5) identifying and soliciting necessary financial and physical resources, (6) developing a training program for paraprofessional disaster-recovery workers, (7) implementing the training program, and (8) implementing the project and planning for follow-up and for identification of long-term community needs (see Zarle et al., pp. 313–315).

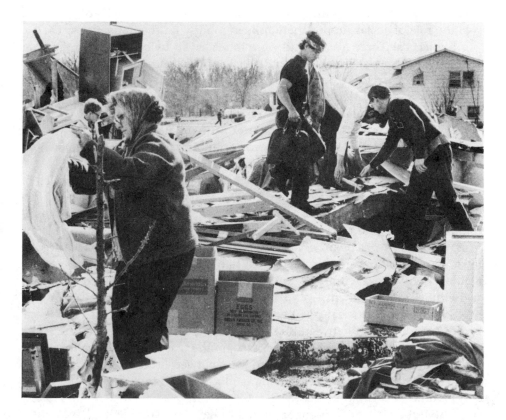

Residents pick through the remains of their homes to find belongings after the onslaught of the 1974 Indiana tornadoes. *(Courtesy of Wide World Photos.)*

The 1979 Three Mile Island accident

The Three Mile Island nuclear reactor accident occurred in early 1979, and controversy still rages regarding its ultimate negative effects on nearby residents. In addition to the psychological effects of the accident itself, there may very well have been adverse effects due to the fact that 60% of the population in the area was evacuated for some period of time after the accident before being allowed to return to their homes. The National Institute of Mental Health funded an investigation of changes in the mental health of three groups thought to be at unusual risk—mothers of preschool children living within 10 miles of the reactor, mental health agency clients living within the same radius, and workers at the nuclear power plant.

Bromet, Parkinson, Schulberg, Dunn, and Gondek (1982) had no pre-accident data on nearby residents or workers. They chose instead to examine samples of mothers, mental health agency clients, and nuclear plant employees, and to contrast these groups with similarly selected samples of persons living near a comparison site featuring a nuclear reactor that had not suffered any accident. The investigators were interested in three issues: (1) What were the consequences of prolonged stress? (2) What changes in mental health resulted from the additional stress of the anniversary of the accident? (3) What was the role of social support networks in modifying the impact of stress?

Subjects at Three Mile Island were interviewed twice—8–9 months after the accident, and again three months later on the first anniversary of the accident. Comparison group subjects were also interviewed twice with equivalent time intervals. During the initial interview, demographic information about the sample was collected as well as information about social support, current symptomatology, current job stress, and mental health during the past year. Similar information was gathered at the time of the second interview, and in addition a measure of life-time mental health was obtained.

Important differences were found to exist between the two samples of mothers with preschool children. Mothers at Three Mile Island were functioning under more stress and reported significantly more psychiatric symptoms during the year after the accident than comparison group mothers, particularly in measures of anxiety and depression. Those mothers who were the most symptomatic were those who had had psychiatric histories prior to the accident, who lived within five miles of the reactor, and who were pregnant at the time of the accident.

In the case of nuclear plant employees, only small differences in mental health were detected between those working at Three Mile Island and those in the comparison area nuclear plant. Also, in the case of mental health agency clients, few differences were found to exist between those clients who lived near Three Mile Island and the comparison group (Bromet, Parkinson, Schulberg, Dunn, and Gondek, 1982).

Thus, the nuclear accident appeared to have measurable negative consequonces on the mental health of mothers as long as one year after the accident, although the role played by the existence of prior psychiatric disability was not insignificant. In the case of nuclear plant employees and mental health system clients, on the other hand, no significant negative consequences were found, indicating that, for them at least, no measurable 'anniversary' effect was to be found.

The 1981 Kansas City hotel disaster

In the case of the Kansas City hotel disaster, Gist and Stolz (1982) have described the response of the mental health community following the sudden collapse in July 1981 of two aerial walkways that spanned the lobby of the Hyatt Regency Hotel, resulting in the deaths of 113 persons and injuries to more than 200 others. Because nearly all of the killed or injured were local

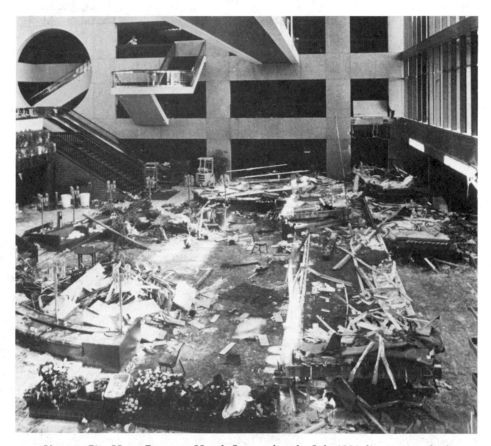

Kansas City Hyatt Regency Hotel. Scene after the July 1981 disaster in which 113 people were killed when the second and fourth floor catwalks collapsed onto the dance floor. (*Courtesy of Wide World Photos.*)

residents, the impact of the crisis extended to the entire community. It was estimated that, counting rescue workers and family and friends of those killed and injured, more than 5,000 persons were at risk of developing negative reactions to that crisis.

In this instance it was difficult to develop a prompt and effective professional response. The seven community mental health centers that served Kansas City had no coordinated crisis response plan, and there were no guidelines to help the mental health centers. A community-wide response was developed, however, within 72 hours of the tragedy by a collaborative effort of the community mental health centers, the local mental health association, the Red Cross, and the local regional office of the federal Department of Health and Human Services. That response included three components—the creation of support groups at each of the mental health centers, the development of a training program for mental health professionals and for ordinary citizens who would be a major source of support in the community, and a mental health information and education campaign that was distributed by the mass media.

It was estimated that more than 10% of the at-risk population contacted a community mental health center for assistance. But later requests for direct clinical services for delayed adverse reactions were far fewer than would have been anticipated on the basis of the existing literature. Thus, Gist and Stolz believe that longer-term negative consequences of this tragedy were diminished by "the efforts of the Kansas City mental health community and media to provide coordinated, aggressive prevention programming immediately after the disaster" (1982, p. 1139).

In a recent review of studies of mental health needs in time of disaster, Zusman (1976) outlined the difficulties in conducting definitive epidemiologic research in this area. This research should be able to show whether more people are disabled after the disaster than would be expected in the same population had there been no disaster. Furthermore, the research should be able to indicate what proportion of the exposed group is affected and how these people differ from the unaffected people.

There are severe difficulties in obtaining these basic data. First, there are rarely any predisaster baseline data, and so there is no basis for comparison with postdisaster experience. Second, the population is typically so disrupted during and after a disaster that adequate follow-up studies are almost impossible, with the result that it is not possible to determine who is affected and who is unaffected by the disaster. Finally, human service systems are usually so busy after a disaster that their policies regarding whom they will treat, and how, must change. Accordingly, when a researcher finds an increase in the number of treated cases after a disaster, it is impossible to know whether this represents a true change in the rate of illness or whether the change is due to changing admission policies in the agencies in question.

We have already seen that certain settings have been found to produce far fewer casualties than expected. Zusman (1976) reported that most incidence measures of mental disorders rose during the period immediately after Hurricane Agnes. But comparable figures collected after Hurricane Carla, which inundated southeastern Texas in 1961, showed a substantial decrease (see Moore, 1964, pp. 134–137). Indeed, one of the most intriguing questions yet to be answered unequivocally is whether disaster produces an increase in psychopathology—that is, whether a natural disaster constitutes a crisis. Penick, Powell, and Sieck (1976) found that three-fourths of the 26 victims interviewed five months after a 1973 tornado retrospectively reported increased psychological discomfort, including anxiety and nervousness. Their findings are tentative and are based on a very small sample (only 26 persons who had incurred substantial personal property damage, although they report that, in the town of Joplin, Missouri, where the tornado struck, approximately 24,000 persons out of a total of 40,000 suffered some kind of property damage). These results, however, are similar to those reported in the Buffalo Creek disaster. Quarantelli (1957) and Dynes and Quarantelli (1968), in contrast, found, in surveying disaster reports, that most people do not panic in the face of disaster, that people in disaster areas frequently go out of their way to help total strangers, that survivors show considerable initiative and rarely rely on public assistance, that there is relatively little looting, and that antisocial behavior and major crimes often decrease. In another study, Greenley, Gillespie, and Lindenthal (1975) found a significant *reduction* in psychological distress in residents of an area after a race riot.

As this brief review suggests, there may be appropriate roles for mental health professionals and paraprofessionals in crisis-intervention activities during and after natural disasters, but it is not yet clear what these roles are. In a recent review of crisis and disaster research from the sociological perspective, Quarantelli and Dynes (1977) concluded that there is almost no likelihood of mental illness in the wake of the typical major disaster. However, truly massive catastrophes, such as the Buffalo Creek disaster, may be exceptions to this general conclusion. The federal government is supportive of crisis-intervention efforts, not only ideologically but financially as well, and has published a field manual for human service workers in major disasters (U.S. Department of Health, Education and Welfare, 1978a), a description of crisis-intervention programs for disaster victims in small communities (U.S. Department of Health, Education and Welfare, 1979a), a description of emergency mental health problems following aircraft accidents (U.S. Department of Health and Human Services, 1981a), and a manual for child health workers in major disasters (U.S. Department of Health and Human Services, 1981b). There are a multitude of unanswered questions, of course, but the next several years should witness the development of a nationally available training capacity along with a set of evaluated technical procedures for providing crisis services in times of disaster.

TELEPHONE CRISIS SERVICES

One innovative crisis-intervention program in the United States is the telephone-based service, often called the *hotline*. Such services, often staffed by paraprofessional workers, typically operate at times when traditional helping services are not readily available, often functioning 24 hours a day, seven days a week. Some telephone crisis services are organized to meet the needs of a special population, such as suicidal persons (McGee, 1974) or widows (Abrahams, 1972), but many try to provide advice, information, and referral for anyone who calls with a problem (see Bleach & Claiborn, 1974).

Telephone crisis-intervention services have a substantial history. Sixty years before the beginning of the modern telephone crisis-intervention movement

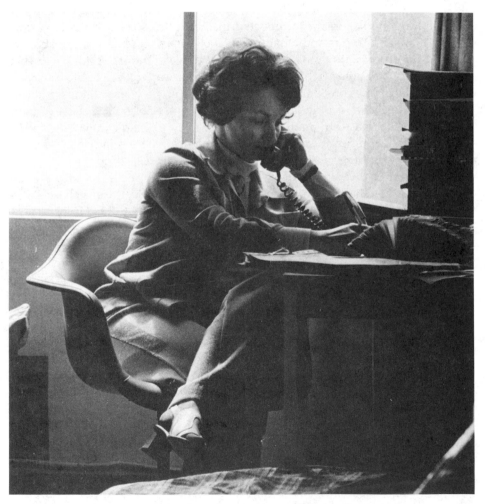

A suicide-prevention-center counselor at work. *(Photo by Gaylord Hill.)*

in the United States (at the Los Angeles Suicide Prevention Center), the National Save-A-Life League had established a 24-hour telephone answering service for suicidal people in New York City (McGee, 1974).

McCord and Packwood (1973) have surveyed community crisis centers, which they define as community service organizations whose primary function is telephone counseling or listening. In their survey, 253 centers met this definition. Most were very new, having been established since 1966. Most were open on a 24-hour basis, and the average center received over 100 calls each day. Their survey provides useful information on staff selection, training, and supervision, financing, and costs. A useful review of legal and procedural aspects of telephone emergency services has been prepared by Brockopp and Oughterson (1972).

The staff of the Los Angeles Suicide Prevention Center has developed a comprehensive training program for preparing staff to respond to crisis telephone calls. This group pioneered the technology of telephone crisis management, developed a procedure for rapidly assessing the degree of seriousness, or *lethality,* of the suicide threat, and showed that a telephone crisis service was feasible. The publications of this group should be carefully examined (see McGee, 1974, especially pp. 295–300).

The following excerpt from an actual call received by the Los Angeles Suicide Prevention Center illustrates the intensity of feeling in a suicidal person calling for help and how a skillful staff member can deal with such a call. Identifying information has been omitted. This excerpt represents about half of the entire conversation, which lasted about an hour. The location of omitted material is indicated by three asterisks.

Caller: Hello. Can you offer anything to someone on skid row or should he just die?

SPC: How old are you?

Caller: Twenty-seven.

SPC: All right. I'm the director of the Suicide Prevention Center here. Can you tell me what the nature of the problem is?

Caller: Well, I'm twenty-seven years old, in good health; I was, up until three years ago, a television studio engineer. For the past few years, I've gone through a wife, about eight jobs. Let's see; New York, Detroit, Chicago, Los Angeles, and a couple of small cities. I've reached a point where I just don't see—well, to use a medical term, the prognosis is negative. There is nothing left. My family is finished; everything.

SPC: A young man usually takes alcohol to go down that fast. Is that what's been with you?

Caller: Alcohol, women, gambling; you name it, I've had it. I've tried alcoholism, I've tried religion, I've tried the works. I've tried missions; they don't work. I've tried AA; it doesn't work. You tell me. If you can think of one good sane reason—

SPC: Have you tried psychiatry?

Caller: Well, let's face it. I—a man who is just about barely able to make his own living, it's rather difficult to go to a psychiatrist, unless you go to a—well, I spent a couple of weeks in Bellevue, and it didn't impress me very much. That was for drinking and a number of other—

SPC: Suicide attempts?

Caller: No.

SPC: No. Have you ever done anything to yourself? Self-destructive action?

Caller: Well, once when I had a fight with my wife, but it wasn't a suicide attempt. It was just a—I don't know what the heck it was.

SPC: What did you do?

Caller: I went across my wrist with a rather sharp knife, but devil, I should have known where my own radial artery was; I'm well educated. But that was quite a few years ago.

SPC: You probably were ambivalent about the thing; still in relationship with your wife and all. Do you have any children?

Caller: One, but this was, as I say, a few years ago and—

SPC: Where is that child now?

Caller: In New York; Albany, New York. We're divorced. This thing is finished. It's been finished for three years, it's dead.

SPC: I see. Well, how long have you been here in L.A.

Caller: Oh, about three weeks now. I've been getting by on different kinds of labor. It isn't the question of—well, I'm not exactly in an enviable position financially, but any able-bodied man is certainly not going to go without a place to sleep or a meal or anything like that in any major city. That's not the reason. The reason is when I see in front of me quite a few more years of the same life I've had, that doesn't look very good.

SPC: Wasn't any of this fun? Weren't there any kicks in all this gambling, women, and all that?

Caller: There were kicks, but ninety-nine percent of the time I was struggling for existence, living in sleazy hotels, hung over doing work that—well, I'm not proud; I can't say the work was beneath me, but doing work far beneath my talents, so far beneath what I should be doing; living like a dog. I'm living like a dog right now.

SPC: You need some help; I can see that. How did you get in touch with us or hear about us?

Caller: Well, I—again, I have heard about that there are in cities things— social agencies of this type. I just looked it up in the telephone directory.

SPC: I see.

Caller: But, mainly, I don't think that there is anything wrong with me mentally. Maybe I'm crazy, but I don't go around doing anything insane. I haven't been arrested in the past three years for anything. But, as I say, a man who has—I was once a television studio engineer in New York. I'm in perfect health, twenty-seven years old, and I'm living the life of a—well, I know winos on skid row that are probably happier than I am right now. I don't see any other choice, and if you can tell me one possible other choice, well, I'll be happy to hear it. Nobody likes to end his own life, but if I am faced, and I think any intelligent person, as it appears to me right now—I'm faced with many, many more years of the same stuff and I'm sick of it. And even the kicks I've had, or—the spunk has gone out of them. I can't even go on drinking anymore.

*   *   *

SPC: You just get yourself so far and then you'd probably quit and get back into a mess again.

Caller: Right. In other words, if someone were to hand me a hundred-dollar bill right now, I don't know what the devil I'd do with it, but whatever it is, it would probably be further harm to me.

SPC: Drink it, and things like that.

Caller: On the other hand, if someone were to say, well, we have a job for you . . . here's a good job and we'll take care of you until you make payday, . . . I'd probably last about six or seven weeks on it. It's happened before. Maybe, at the very outside, two or three months, and then whammo.

SPC: Now, what sort of injuring method do you have in mind? What would you do to yourself?

Caller: Probably the quickest and most painful way. There's plenty of tall buildings and I'm a fairly good swimmer. I guess I'd have my choice between the two.

SPC: I see.

Caller: Just swim out as far as I can swim, or climb to a high place and go off. I'm in no way afraid of heights. I've climbed antenna towers when I worked for the broadcasting industry. I don't know. Maybe I'd chicken out, but I don't think so, because I can't see any further hope.

SPC: Right now you're in town here, and there is nobody that knows you and nobody cares. Is that the situation?

Caller: I haven't got one person in the city of Los Angeles and in the United States of America and in the entire world that I think gives one good damn whether I live or die except from a professional standpoint. You might say, well, that that's the reason I haven't given you my last name or exact location, as I dare say the police would be interested in stopping me; that's their job.

SPC: That's true.

Caller: That's what I mean. You might be interested in preventing my demise, but again, that's your job. What I'm trying to find out is, is there one good reason why I shouldn't.

SPC: Well, the good reason—the only one good reason is that possibility that you have got a mental illness of a sort, or a severe neurosis rising out of your confused and unstable background, and that you could lick it and stabilize yourself, and get some more pleasure out of life and some self-respect, is the only thing.

Caller: But how do you lick something like that?

*   *   *

Caller: And, also I feel that psychotherapy—then maybe I'm wrong, it's suggestion more than anything else and I'm just not that suggestible.

SPC: Well, . . . I wouldn't say that. Therapy has been—actually, it's geared to the capacity and the need of the person who is having the therapy; for many types of people, therapy is the chance to clear their mind and a chance to get some distance from their own problem and to analyze it with an attitude free of some of the complications that you have. You do have quite a bit of guilt and quite a bit of self-criticism, and I imagine that does complicate trying to analyze your problem. An indefinable thing should be more clearly definable.

Caller: I've tried to apply all the intelligence that I have to finding out just exactly what was wrong with me and correcting it. I've had every chance in the world. I've had every break in the world, and here I am in Los Angeles flat on my tail. In other words, oh, I still am well dressed. I manage to get a few days' work in, but for all practical purposes, broke and without anyplace to go, and faced with a choice of going back to skid row or taking my own life, and I think—if you had this choice, what would you do?

SPC: Well, there seems to be more to it than that. I'd say there is a lot more to your life than just those two choices. As long as you assume that you are stuck in your pattern, then I suppose those are the only two choices you have, but to me, viewing it as an outsider, I think it's just ridiculous that a guy should be stuck in his pattern. I've seen so many people blast themselves loose from their pattern so many times that it is a matter of understanding your pattern and getting some distance from your anxiety, so that you can see where you put the proper effort to change it; change the pattern.

Caller: But how? I seem to—

SPC: Well, I should say something like this. I don't—here, we get four, five, six calls a day from people like yourself; all sorts of people in trouble. In your case, you're the kind of a situation here which—with enormous resources. We really run into people who are at the end of their rope; older people, sick people, unhealthy people. What you are is a healthy neurotic, just like all the rest of us; only your pattern is one that society doesn't reward at all, and so your self-destructive pattern—some people with a neurosis, like maybe your twin brother, overwork and they get ulcers later in life, but they have money. I'd say that you need psychotherapy, psychiatric therapy, outpatient therapy for your neurosis, and I'd suggest you come on in and talk with me to start it out.

Caller: Well, how does a skid row bum get psychotherapy?

SPC: Let's discuss that.[4]

The important features to note in this conversation are the obvious anguish of the caller, the suicide prevention center staff member's interest in helping the caller, the skillful exploration of the caller's problem, the staff member's ability to empathize with the caller's distress, the staff member's directness and honesty regarding his task and that of the police, the staff member's effort to assess lethality, and the staff member's successful effort to convert the caller's sense of hopelessness and despair into one of some hope—successful partly because he worked with the caller to develop a concrete plan of action.

Since most callers to telephone hotline services are anonymous, evaluating the appropriateness and effectiveness of the advice, information, and referrals provided by staff is not easy. In recent years, however, an interesting strategy for evaluating such efforts has developed—namely, the use of simulated clients, whose calls are tape-recorded and analyzed. Such calls are generally made with the knowledge and consent of the staff of crisis centers, but staff members have no way of knowing whether a particular call is genuine or simulated. Since experimental calls constitute but a tiny proportion of all calls, staff members have no choice but to treat all calls as genuine.

Apsler and Hodas (1975) had two callers, a male and a female, telephone a 24-hour hotline in Boston that normally receives more than 275 calls a day, to ask about getting help for a dental problem. Although such a request lacks the drama of a suicidal person's cry for help, it is typical in its call for information and referral. The caller described himself or herself as a 23-year-old resident of a Boston suburb, employed in Boston, without much money, who needed dental care. The researchers knew beforehand that 21 local sources of dental services were available to hotline counselors and 5 of those sources were specifically appropriate for the presented problem. The callers kept track

[4]Reproduced by special permission of the Los Angeles Suicide Prevention Center.

of whether the questions that were asked were of the type that could lead to a correct referral, whether a full and appropriate referral was made, and the degree to which the staff member who answered the phone was helpful and polite.

A total of 21 calls were made, one on each of the 21 shifts during a one-week period. A total of 13 calls received one or more correct referrals; 12 calls received one or more incorrect referrals. Only 9 calls received one or more correct referrals *and* no incorrect referrals. The report of this evaluation study includes, in addition, information about counselor effectiveness and manner as well as a discussion of ethical considerations in research of this kind.

In a more complex study, Bleach and Claiborn (1974) arranged for 96 simulated crisis calls to four Washington, D.C., hotlines serving high-school- and college-age populations. The callers, six female undergraduates, asked for help with four problems—pregnancy, loneliness, parent difficulties, and drug-related conflicts. Each caller, after an initial period of training, called each hotline with each problem only once. Calls were rated on three scales that measured amount of information given, two scales that measured style in which information was given, and single scales measuring empathy, warmth, and genuineness of the telephone counselor. All counselors knew of the study in advance and had agreed to participate. At the end of the study, results were shared with the four hotline staff members.

The authors found that the scales measuring empathy, warmth, and genuineness, one of the amount-of-information scales (accuracy of information), and one of the style-of-information-giving scales (quality of alternatives given) were very highly correlated, so that these five scales actually formed one dimension. Counselor-style scales tended to differ across hotlines but not across problems. Information-scale scores tended to differ across problems. It was possible to identify the most satisfactory hotline by this procedure and to identify the particular ways in which hotlines could provide more effective services for each of the problems presented.

These two studies illustrate how researchers can evaluate telephone crisis services without invading the caller's privacy or destroying the credibility of the service. Both studies suggest that if data collection and feedback are handled sensitively, staff can be expected to welcome such evaluations.

King (1977) sought information from 66 college students who had made use of the telephone counseling program on their campus in an Alabama university. These students formed about 2% of the student population. Almost none of the students in this sample indicated that they were in any kind of psychotherapeutic relationship. The vast majority of students reported that the telephone counseling had been helpful—for females more so than males. Female callers who spoke with male counselors expressed the greatest satisfaction with the experience. Counselors were generally characterized as intelligent, warm, understanding, honest, effective, active, caring, professional, close, and helpful. In the context of the generally good reports users made of this service, it is instructive to note that this almost totally volunteer service received about 4000 calls a year and had a total annual budget of $4000.

Rosenbaum and Calhoun (1977) have reviewed the use of telephone hotlines as part of a crisis-intervention service. They estimate that, as of 1977, over 600 such services were in existence in the United States, serving more than 10 million people a year. Most hotlines operate 24 hours a day, seven days a week; most are staffed, at least in part, by both professionals and nonprofessionals who work without pay; most accept calls from anyone with any need; and most offer advice, information, and referral services. Rosenbaum and Calhoun conclude their review by noting:

> Intuitively, the concept of the hotline is a good one. It provides a relatively economical method of dispensing helping services to greater portions of the community than could be reached by conventional services. It utilizes a large, potentially invaluable source of manpower, the volunteer nonprofessionals, enabling a minimum number of professionals, serving in administrative and consulting capacities, to serve a maximum number of people. The hotline makes help, information, advice, comfort, and counseling available around the clock, most importantly when most agencies are normally closed. It is a free service regardless of the caller's socioeconomic status, yet it is without the welfare or charity stigma. It offers anonymity and freedom from both legal and bureaucratic "red tape" which makes it invaluable in areas such as drugs, sex, birth control, abortion counseling, suicides, and many adolescent problems. The hotline transcends geographical barriers where seconds can make a life or death difference and offers an acceptable form of help to many persons who would not ordinarily come into a helping agency. The hotline appears so valuable that, in the absence of any hard evidence to the contrary, most people are content to assume that it offers an effective service. It is in this atmosphere that hotlines have become what is perhaps the fastest growing helping service in the country [p. 337].[5]

The authors believe that the hotline has potential not only as an effective therapeutic strategy but also for primary prevention. They believe that "research is needed to determine which variables are therapeutically effective and how the hotline service can be improved" (p. 338).

TRAINING OF CRISIS COUNSELORS

A number of efforts to train mental health workers in crisis-intervention helping skills have been reported (Carkhuff, 1973; Goldstein, 1973; Ivey, 1971). Most of these studies show that the training results in significant increases in effectiveness. Well-developed helping skills are important in effective telephone counseling services, and use of these skills extends to more traditional psychotherapeutic settings as well.

---

[5]From "The Use of the Telephone Hotline in Crisis Intervention: A Review," by C. P. Rosenbaum and J. F. Calhoun. In *Journal of Community Psychology*, 1977, 5, 325–339. Reprinted by permission.

Perhaps the most fully developed of these training programs has been the work of Danish and Hauer (1973a, 1973b). Danish, D'Augelli, and Brock (1976) have identified eight types of verbal responses that helpers typically use—content reflections, affect reflections, closed (yes or no) questions, open-ended questions, direct efforts to change attitudes and behavior, presentation of alternatives, expressions of self-involvement, and self-disclosure. Of these types of statements, Danish and Hauer believe that effective helping skills involve more content and affect reflection, more use of open-ended questions, fewer closed questions, and less effort to influence or advise.

Danish, D'Augelli, and Brock developed a 25-hour, ten-session training program organized around (1) understanding one's own helping needs, (2) using effective verbal and nonverbal behavior, (3) using self-involving behavior, (4) understanding the communication of others, and (5) establishing effective helping relationships. In their first study, they provided training to a sample of 126 trainees, mainly undergraduates. They were able to show that (1) types of verbalizations by trainees could be reliably judged and coded, (2) amount of content and affective reflection could be increased significantly, and (3) use of closed questions as well as efforts to influence and advise could be decreased significantly. In spite of their efforts, they were unable to produce a significant increase in the use of open-ended questions.

In a later study, D'Augelli and Levy (1978) contrasted trainees whose helping skills were evaluated not only before and after their training program but also two months later with a group of volunteers who had received no helping-skills training and who conducted one interview. Initial helping-skills scores did not differ materially between the trained and untrained groups. Most of the skills learned during the training sessions were maintained, though not at the same level as immediately after the training program had been completed. Use of open-ended questions again showed no increase as of the time of program completion but had increased substantially by the follow-up study two months later.

Ehrlich, D'Augelli, and Danish (1979) examined the relative effectiveness of six counselor verbal responses. Ninety female undergraduates volunteered to play the role of a client in a simulated helping interaction. An advanced undergraduate female student acted as the counselor in the simulation. Six scripts were prepared that contained 30 counselor/client exchanges. The scripts differed only in terms of the counselor verbal responses. Each script included only one type of verbal response—content reflection, affect reflection, closed questions, open-ended questions, efforts to influence, or provision of alternative modes of behavior or thought.

Twenty of the client statements were prepared in advance. For the other ten, the student playing the role of client could say anything she wanted to. Thus, "client" and "counselor" each read her own script in which all the counselor's statements and all but ten of the client's were prepared in advance. To avoid nonverbal cues, a screen separated the two participants.

The role-played interview lasted 10–15 minutes. Clients then completed a questionnaire that assessed their perceptions of the counselor's expertness, attractiveness, and trustworthiness. In addition, judges scored the ten free responses that each client made in terms of response length, proportion of words used that denoted affect, use of self-referent pronouns, and time orientation. It was hypothesized that the more successful the exchanges between client and counselor, the longer would be the free responses, the greater would be the proportion of words denoting affect, the greater would be the use of self-referent pronouns, and the more the client would talk in the here and now.

In general, reflections of affect were most effective in yielding desirable client behavior and were also given the highest ratings by clients. Reflections of affect were especially effective in encouraging clients to discuss feelings. Thus, training programs that advocate the extensive use of continuing responses, particularly the reflection of affect and of open-ended questions, appear to be correct.

D'Augelli, Handis, Brumbaugh, Illig, Searer, Turner, and D'Augelli (1978) contrasted the verbal helping behavior of experienced and novice telephone counselors using the Danish, D'Augelli, and Brock helping-skills verbal-responses category system. There were very few differences between the two groups of counselors in their verbal helping behaviors when dealing with telephone calls. Perhaps the most impressive finding was the high positive correlation between the number of counselor reflective comments (either content or affect) and how long the clients spoke.

In a related study, O'Donnell and George (1977) contrasted four groups of telephone counselors on the basis of ratings on empathy, concreteness and specificity, genuineness, confrontation of discrepancies, ability to link problem statements with the nature of the client/counselor interaction, use of problem-solving strategies, and use of community resources. The ratings were made by judges who worked from tape recordings of phone calls by 40 simulated clients, each of whom made one call to the telephone counseling service. Forty counselors were studied—community mental health center professional staff members, experienced volunteers, inexperienced but trained volunteers, and a control group of ten college students who had expressed no interest in volunteering for the telephone counseling service.

The control group scored significantly lower than all other groups on total effectiveness, significantly lower than the mental health professionals on concreteness, and significantly lower than the mental health professionals and experienced volunteers on use of community resources. The control group scored lower, but not significantly so, than all other groups on empathy and genuineness. But perhaps most interesting was the finding that no significant differences were found among mental health professionals, experienced volunteers, and trained but inexperienced volunteers. Thus, some combination of training plus motivation to be of help to others appears to be associated with overall helping effectiveness. The authors concluded that "carefully selected and trained volunteers can function as effectively as professional staff in providing supportive and emergency telephone services for distressed callers and community mental health center clients" (pp. 10–11).

The training program for counselors in the Telephone Counseling and Referral Service (TCRS), a campus-community crisis-intervention program in Tallahassee, Florida, emphasizes identification of the problem or problems, recognition and exploration of feelings, survey of past coping attempts, and exploration of alternatives. Thus, its objectives are very similar to those developed by Danish and Hauer. The TCRS training program requires eight hours per week for ten weeks. Kalafat, Boroto, and France (1979) contrasted telephone helping behavior among three groups—untrained volunteers, newly trained volunteers, and veteran, trained telephone counselors who had been working in the TCRS for at least six months. These researchers also used simulated telephone calls made by trained experimental callers, but in this case the counselors knew that some calls during a specific time period would be simulations, though not which ones. Kalafat and colleagues found significantly higher technical functioning by the veterans, lower functioning by the newly trained volunteers, and still lower functioning by the untrained volunteers. In addition, they found that more experienced counselors were judged as significantly more empathic (see also DeVol, 1976; Doyle, Foreman, & Wales, 1977; Engs & Kirk, 1974; Getz et al., 1975).

GENERAL ASSESSMENT OF CRISIS-INTERVENTION PROGRAMS

To test the efficacy of intervention at times of crisis, one must identify a sample of people in crisis. One may contrast outcome in a subgroup exposed to intervention procedures with outcome in a subgroup not exposed to such procedures. Outcome in both subgroups may be compared with that in a noncrisis group. But whether or not a noncrisis group is used, the identification of the group in crisis should be sufficiently unambiguous so that it is the *intervention* that is clearly the subject of study. Failure of intervention procedures should not be attributable to misdiagnosis of the crisis state. This diagnostic problem exists, in part, because, as Auerbach and Kilmann have indicated, "as construct, *crisis* has no established core of meaning or formal theoretical base" (1977, p. 1189).

In an effort to develop an increased understanding of the definitional aspects of the crisis concept, I prepared a series of 14 brief vignettes, each describing a single stressful event in the life of a central character (Bloom, 1963). Eight experts in the field of crisis theory, all members of the staff of the Community Mental Health Program at the Harvard School of Public Health, were asked whether each event constituted a crisis for the central character and, if so, why. The vignettes were constructed so that five separate dimensions were varied, more or less independently of one another: presence or absence of a known precipitating event, sudden or gradual onset of symptoms, internal tension recognized or unrecognized by the central character, visible or nonvisible behavioral disorganization, and rapid or slow conflict resolution. The judges were asked to check "yes," "no," or "don't know" in response to the question whether the event constituted a crisis. The following are examples of the stories used.

Story B

Mr. Jones slammed on the brakes but not in time to avoid hitting the boy who had dashed out in the street in front of his car. Before he could even open the door of the car, he felt nauseated and very frightened. He managed, almost blindly, to reach the front of the car but found himself unable to do anything to assist the moaning teen-ager who was badly cut and bleeding. When help arrived, Mr. Jones was in a dazed condition, unable to talk coherently about the accident but aware that he was tremendously disturbed. Fortunately, the boy's injuries seemed much more severe than they actually were, and he recovered with no permanent injuries. Although Mr. Jones was found not to be legally responsible for the accident—and the boy whom he hit fully admitted that it was not Mr. Jones' fault—it was months before Mr. Jones was able to talk about the accident and drive his car comfortably.

Story M

Mr. Jones' peculiar behavior had begun very gradually. At first he seemed to become forgetful, then simply "off on another planet" most of the time. When Mrs. Jones would try to call it to his attention, she found him completely unaware of his actions. Then one day he just disappeared. There was simply no trace of him for nearly a week, when he was found by a United States Customs officer returning to New York on a flight from Europe. He was arguing with the officer about paying duty on a guitar he had bought in Spain, and he had attracted quite a crowd. He was very belligerent and the officer, suspecting he was not well, called the police—who in turn called an ambulance. In the ambulance Mr. Jones suddenly seemed to realize who and where he was and, after satisfying the medical authorities that he was well, was released. He was home again the next day, virtually back to normal.

Story N

The day after Mrs. Jones was killed in a plane accident, Mr. Jones reported for work on time just as he had done more or less regularly for the past several years. The office staff were rather surprised to see him, particularly since Mrs. Jones' death had been so tragic—and they had been so much in love. The staff remarked to each other how well he was reacting to the tragedy and how no one could ever have guessed that so terrible a thing had happened so recently. Mr. Jones' boss was particularly understanding and tried to induce him to take time off, but Mr. Jones seemed willing to work and was as friendly and relaxed as ever. Weeks later

Mr. Jones remarked that his wife's death had been a blow to him, but life had to go on. He said that he had never felt any serious discomfort or any real difficulty in carrying on his normal activities.[6]

The task was clearly a complex one for the judges. For only 5 of the 14 stories were the crisis judgments unanimous. For the remaining 9 stories, "yes" percentages ranged from 20 to 86. In 4 of the stories, the "yes" percentages were between 40 and 63. "Don't know" percentages ranged from 0 to 50. In only 5 stories were there no "don't know" judgments.

Of the five manipulated variables, presence or absence of a precipitating event was significantly related to the judgment of crisis: a crisis was judged to have occurred significantly more often when a precipitating event was known than when it was unknown. A second dimension, speed of resolution, was also significantly (but less significantly) related to the crisis judgment. Resolutions that required between one and two months were more often judged to be the consequence of a crisis than were resolutions that required less than a week.

One story—Story N—was composed in such a way that a known precipitating event was not followed by symptoms (either internal or external) of any kind. Six of the eight judges made a judgment about the presence or absence of a crisis in this event, and all six judged that a crisis had occurred.

These results would seem to indicate that, in practice, a crisis is defined primarily in terms of a precipitating event and secondarily in terms of a slow resolution. Known precipitating events are generally judged to lead to crisis if there is no reaction *or* if there is a reaction of any kind and resolution requires a month or more. The judges' comments suggest that mental health professionals view situations in which the resolution is rapid as illustrations of appropriate responses to reality situations. Reactions of any kind that appear when there is no known precipitating event are likely to be considered psychiatric disorders rather than crises.

The single variable affecting the crisis judgment most strongly appeared to be the existence of a precipitating event. On this basis, one could simply define the crisis state as what follows certain specified events. This is an appealing but oversimplified operational solution to the task of definition; these judges did not seem to be acting on the belief that crises inevitably follow certain events. If one does not define crisis solely by the occurrence of some event in a person's life, then one must be able to distinguish between those people for whom the event results in a crisis state and those people for whom it does not. The present findings suggest that this kind of discrimination may not now be possible. Until further refinement of the crisis concept is undertaken, assessing the effectiveness of intervention efforts will be difficult.

Polak, Egan, Vandenbergh, and Williams (1975) mounted a crisis-intervention program for surviving family members that went into effect immediately after a relatively sudden death. Families who had recently and suddenly lost a member were randomly assigned to a treated group ($N = 39$) or to an untreated control group ($N = 66$). Another control group—56 families in which no deaths had occurred during the previous two years—was also studied. The three groups were matched for age, socioeconomic status, education, and residential location. Outcome measures, administered 6 and 18 months after the death, were self-report questionnaires and psychiatric evaluations.

The first report of this study presents an analysis of information collected at the 6-month follow-up. The results indicate, first, that family members in both bereaved groups showed poorer functioning in several areas than the nonbereaved. Specifically, bereaved persons showed significantly more pathological emotional expression and depression and significantly greater problems in family, intrapersonal, interpersonal, and social functioning. Second, the crisis-intervention program did not improve coping behavior or lower the incidence of medical or psychiatric illness or of disturbed social functioning in bereaved families.

In a later follow-up of the participants in their study, Williams and Polak (1979) reported that their earlier conclusions were unchanged—their preventive intervention service had little or no impact. These authors concluded:

> . . . A short-term crisis service that involved person-centered cathartic approaches and was offered by mental health professionals had little or no impact upon post adjustment of family survivors. In fact, inspection of the multiple correlation analyses suggests that the short-term crisis service may have delayed or actually interfered with the more traditional time-honored bereavement process practiced in the United States. There is evidence to suggest that the application of crisis techniques is effective in the treatment of major mental illnesses, particularly when the person and family either seek help or are pressured to seek help. . . . The current results, however, suggest that such techniques are less applicable to the treatment of normal persons or families who do not actively seek help and who are experiencing a normal life crisis [p. 44].[7]

Regarding ways of improving the effectiveness of crisis-intervention services that seek to be of assistance in times of grief, the authors suggest:

> The data clearly indicate that sudden death does have a major impact upon family survivors and close bereaved relatives. The first phase of this impact is manifested by an increased risk of ill health . . . coping behavior problems . . . and social-personal functioning difficulties. . . . This first phase lasts about 1 year and gradually gives way to the second phase of the impact, characterized by a concentration

---

[7]From "Follow-up Research in Primary Prevention: A Model of Adjustment in Acute Grief," by W. V. Williams and P. R. Polak. In *Journal of Clinical Psychology*, 1979, 35, 35–45. This and all other quotations from the same source are reprinted by permission.

on more pragmatic problems centered around finances and quality of life assets.
. . . It appears that any intervention service, in order to be effective, would have
to take into account the interactive nature of environmental stresses and family/
individual determinants. In this respect, prevention may be achieved more effectively by focusing upon basic education of the public of facts that involve major
life crises and loss and the utilization of natural care givers. The professional then
becomes a consultant and educator rather than intruder [pp. 43–44].

Unfortunately, two major design errors make it difficult to interpret these
results. First, the bereaved and nonbereaved groups differed dramatically in
social and personal adjustment prior to the project, the nonbereaved families
having significantly better adjustment. Second, the treated and untreated
bereaved groups differed significantly initially, with far more deaths by suicide
and a far higher degree of suddenness of death characterizing the treated
group. That is, the procedure for assigning bereaved families to a treated or
untreated group failed to be random, and the nonbereaved families did not
constitute an adequate comparison group on a number of critical dimensions.
The authors did compensate, in part, for these initial differences by perform-
ing a variety of special statistical analyses, but such statistical procedures are
far less satisfactory than more successful initial matching of experimental,
control, and comparison populations.

In another effort to evaluate the effectiveness of a crisis-intervention program, Gottschalk, Fox, and Bates (1973) contrasted two groups of 34 persons,
all of whom came voluntarily to a crisis-intervention clinic in Orange County,
California. The 68 persons were assigned randomly either to a group receiving
immediate intervention therapy or to a group being put on a waiting list. All
subjects were interviewed and assessed at the time of their petition for help,
and all but 7 of them were interviewed again six weeks later. Of the measures,
the most important in measuring program effectiveness were a measure of
psychiatric morbidity, measures of ego strength and weakness, an index of
social alienation and personal disorganization, and a measure of optimism
and positive outlook. Subjects assigned to the immediate-treatment group
received brief crisis psychotherapy within one hour of the initial evaluation
and subsequently received from one to six treatment sessions with a mental
health professional. In addition, medications were prescribed for those patients
who needed them.

At the six-week follow-up interviews, it was found that some patients
assigned to the treatment group had not appeared for treatment ($N = 7$) and
that some patients assigned to the waiting list had obtained treatment elsewhere ($N = 12$). In addition, 5 waiting-list patients and 2 treatment-group
patients could not be located and were lost to the study. The critical analysis
contrasted the 24 patients who had actually not received treatment, regardless
of their initial group assignment, with the 37 patients who actually received
treatment, again without regard to their original group assignment. No significant differences were found.

The most consistent and significant correlate of posttreatment psychiatric morbidity, in both groups, was the pretreatment psychiatric morbidity score ($r = + .58$ in the treatment group and $+ .46$ in the waiting-list group). Patients in the treatment group showed improvement but no more than those who remained on the waiting list. However, the switching from waiting-list to treatment group after original random assignment was of such a nature that those patients who ended up in the treatment group had higher initial levels of psychiatric morbidity than those who ended up in a no-treatment situation. It is thus possible that, by this process of self-selection, patients in more need of treatment managed to obtain it, while those in less need, and possibly with the better chance of improvement without treatment, chose not to obtain it. The authors suggest, as other possibilities, that the initial assessment interview, conducted by a researcher who did not assume the role of a therapist, may have been as effective as specific crisis-intervention therapy and that crises may resolve themselves within six weeks regardless of whether anything is done to facilitate the process.

Finally, the authors indicate that two areas of investigation were not explored in their study—first, the degree of comfort and ease of crisis resolution with and without crisis-intervention services and, second, the extent to which crisis-intervention services result in improved coping mechanisms in later life crises. With regard to this latter point, the authors state: "We know of no controlled studies that have sought to demonstrate decisively that this important goal of crisis therapy has ever been attained; but we believe, on the basis of impressionistic longitudinal clinical observations, that experienced psychotherapists are capable of achieving such goals" (p. 1111).

The fact that the Polak and Gottschalk studies failed to verify one of the most influential theories of community mental health—namely, that brief intervention at the time of crisis may be more helpful than longer treatment after the crisis has passed—should illustrate the fact that it may be at least as difficult, if not more difficult, to evaluate crisis-intervention programs as to evaluate psychotherapy (see, for example, Bergin & Garfield, 1971, and Strupp, 1973). In addition to all the problems that make evaluating the outcome of psychotherapy so complex, another difficulty exists when evaluating crisis-intervention services—namely, the necessity of defining a crisis. Polak, in his research, defined a crisis in terms of a particular precipitating event; every family in which there was a sudden death was defined as being in crisis. Gottschalk and his colleagues allowed patients to define themselves as being in crisis, regardless of the nature (or absence) of a known precipitating event.

Caplan (1962) has suggested that people in crisis are unusually open to help and that "from a preventive psychiatric point of view, this is a matter of supreme importance; because by deploying helping services to deal with individuals in crisis, a small amount of effort leads to a maximum amount of lasting response" (p. 82). Whatever else may be required to test this provocative hypothesis, relevant life events must be unambiguously definable as either crises or noncrises. The success of studies of attempts to intervene and influence the outcome of such life experiences will depend partly on the adequacy of this fundamental definition.

In reexamining the Polak and Gottschalk crisis-intervention evaluation studies, it is possible to pose a series of questions that can give some direction to further research efforts. First, what evidence is there that a sudden death constitutes a stressor for the surviving family members? The answer to this question, one might argue, is self-evident; just ask anyone who has lived through such an experience. But the question, in order to yield a useful answer, needs to be couched in more specific terms. What are the demonstrated consequences of sudden death for the survivors? One research study pertinent to this question is MacMahon and Pugh's (1965), examining suicide rates in the widowed. Suicides were unusually frequent during the first year of widowhood. Thus, these researchers demonstrated that death is a stressor for surviving family members by showing an unexpected incidence of a certain behavior in a certain family member during a particular time period. If sudden death is to be viewed as a stressful life event, then the negative effects on survivors must be well documented by numerous such studies focusing on particular populations, behaviors, or time periods. Even more important, however, is the fact that these specific documented negative consequences may well suggest specific rather than general strategies of crisis intervention and specific data that should be collected in order to assess the value of a crisis-intervention program.

Second, Gottschalk and his colleagues suggest that effective crisis intervention can take place in a very broad array of settings. Since biblical times, every organized religious group has had its own method of crisis intervention following a death in a family. Friends gather and provide a substantial amount of comfort and support. All this suggests that in Polak's control group there surely was a significant amount of crisis intervention being provided. Perhaps Polak and his colleagues failed to show a positive outcome in their experimental crisis-intervention service because their service did not constitute a significant increment over and above the traditional powerful familial and religious interventions that were taking place in the control group. This line of reasoning suggests that crisis-intervention services might best be introduced in settings where there are no services traditionally provided in the culture or where people at risk are frequently not reached by these traditional services.

Third, Polak's study suggests the possibility that families in which there is poor personal and social adjustment may be unusually vulnerable to crises. This unusual vulnerability may help explain why Polak was unable to match bereaved and nonbereaved families on prior personal adjustment, while they were able to match them for age, socioeconomic status, and so on. If family or personal characteristics are associated not only with the outcome of crisis-intervention services but with whether crises occur to begin with, the issues involved in evaluating crisis-intervention services are complex indeed.

Fourth, the Gottschalk study makes a strong case for the argument that people in need of help somehow manage to obtain it, although sometimes in unconventional ways. Furthermore, their study suggests that the best predictor of psychiatric morbidity after crisis intervention is psychiatric morbidity before crisis intervention and that, whether or not subjects participate in a crisis-intervention program, those persons with the greatest amount of initial symptomatology have the highest level of symptomatology at some later time. Applying these findings to the Polak study suggests that those persons in the crisis-intervention group who did not feel the need for the special services available to them simply did not take advantage of those services and that those bereaved families in the control group who needed supportive services generally managed to obtain them. As a consequence, then, the outcomes in the two groups would not be expected to differ. Evaluating this hypothesis would require a larger data base in order to be able to analyze the relationship between outcome and utilization of crisis-intervention services, holding constant the initial level of disability.

Fifth, it is possible that crisis-intervention-service outcomes might need to be evaluated uniquely for each program participant and that crisis-intervention services might need to be developed uniquely on the basis of a diagnostic assessment of each case. It might be overly simplistic to propose that all the subjects in an intervention program will exhibit their improvement in a similar way. Crisis-intervention programs might need to specify the particular set of goals they are trying to achieve for each subject and then evaluate the outcome in terms of that unique set of objectives.

Finally, there is one important difference between the Gottschalk and Polak subject populations. The patients in the Gottschalk study defined themselves as in need of psychiatric care. In contrast, Polak's subjects had no such self-definition. Crisis theory and crisis management call for deliberate intervention at times of stress, of course, whether or not the consequences of that stress are seen as psychiatric in character. But evaluation of crisis-intervention programs will probably need to keep this dimension in mind, since the nature of services to be provided and goals to be achieved will likely be a function of whether or not the stress is seen as having psychiatric components and consequences.

More recent evaluations of crisis-intervention programs appear to have yielded far more positive findings. Donovan, Bennett, and McElroy (1979) evaluated the effectiveness of a short-term crisis group that met twice a week for four weeks. They noted that

> the crisis group candidate is someone who has experienced the acute onset of significant symptoms—i.e., sleeplessness, inability to work—in connection with a definable precipitating event or stress. This patient is not psychotic, homicidal, or suicidal, and he is willing to attend 8 semiweekly sessions over a 4-week period. . . . The group focuses on the present, especially the problem that provoked the individual's crisis reaction. There is only secondary emphasis on the group process.

The therapists are active and directive; the overall group tone is warm, supportive, and task-oriented. There is little reliance on medication [p. 906].[8]

Effectiveness was assessed by contrasting scores on scales measuring anxiety, depression, and ego strength that were obtained initially, just after the end of treatment, and one year later. A total of 86 persons attended four or more sessions of the crisis group, and 43 of these completed the one-year follow-up questionnaire. Losses of subjects were attributed mainly to clients' moving out of the community.

During the treatment period, scores on the anxiety and depression scales were significantly reduced and scores on the ego-strength scale increased significantly. As much improvement took place between the end of treatment and the follow-up as during the treatment period itself.

Noting that "the crisis group appears surprisingly effective despite its brevity" (p. 909), the authors proposed the following explanation:

> The cohesiveness of the group culture and the knowledge that others are in similar difficulties and want to help seem the key to the treatment. It is important here to recall how insignificant the patients felt the therapists to be as change agents in comparison to fellow patients. Interested and involved group members seem to replace the lost or disappointing person who often has abandoned the patient and precipitated the crisis. The presence of people who are terminating therapy, having solved many of their problems, and who can realistically advise and encourage newer patients is no doubt important. They socialize new patients into the group culture. The timeliness and intensity of the intervention, which comes at the height of the crisis when the feelings are strongest and which occurs twice weekly for 1½ hours per session, probably are also important [p. 909].

Gordon (1978; Gordon & Kilpatrick, 1977) studied the effectiveness of a two-hour group counseling session for men who accompanied women undergoing legal abortions. Twenty-three men were randomly selected to participate in these sessions, in groups of three to seven persons, and a control group of 23 men in the same circumstances who were not invited to such a crisis-intervention service was also studied.

Data for the crisis-group participants were collected before and after the group experience; data for the control group were collected when its members arrived at the abortion clinic and again two hours later. On both occasions, measures of state anxiety (transitory anxiety that tends to vary from day to day) were obtained as well as a set of items measuring attitudes toward abortion and its perceived safety.

The authors found that state anxiety decreased significantly among men in the crisis-intervention group. In addition, these men rated the abortion and

---

[8]From "The Crisis Group—An Outcome Study," by J. M. Donovan, M. J. Bennett, and C. M. McElroy. In *The American Journal of Psychiatry*, Vol. 136, pp. 906 and 909, 1979. Copyright, 1979, the American Psychiatric Association. This and all other quotations from the same source are reprinted by permission.

its safety more positively after the group meeting than before, whereas ratings by the untreated control subjects were more negative at the second testing than at the first.

Gordon concluded that the intervention had been effective in helping the men. "The effectiveness of such a short counseling session may be accounted for, at least in part, by an individual's increased susceptibility to psychological help during a period of crisis. . . . The group crisis-counseling approach based on crisis intervention theory of community mental health appears to be an effective means of helping a formerly psychologically neglected population" (pp. 245–246).

Three studies have recently shown that outreach services provided at times of psychiatric crises can significantly reduce the use of hospitalization as a principal treatment modality. Spaulding, Edwards, and Fichman (1976) found that, in some diagnostic groups, hospitalizations of less than 48 hours were an effective alternative to traditional long-term hospitalization for enlisted male naval personnel undergoing acute psychiatric crises. They measured treatment success by assessing occupational effectiveness for a two-year period following the crisis intervention. These authors concluded:

> The short-term hospitalization effectively screens individuals that do not require a long-term psychiatric hospitalization. Further, it allows those in crisis a period of time to reestablish their values and coping mechanisms. The results clearly indicate that short-term hospitalization can return more men to serve effectively in their assignment than long-term treatment. . . . For personality disorders, brief hospitalization places less emphasis on illness as a technique for avoiding stress. The adjustment reactions of either adolescence or adult life can benefit by brief intervention focusing on regrouping, reality structuring, and compassionate care and concern [p. 460].

Sundel, Rhodes, and Ferguson (1978) described the establishment of a 20-bed crisis-intervention unit that provided, along with referral to community mental health centers or other community agencies, alternatives to admission to state-hospital wards. Length of hospitalization on the crisis-intervention unit did not exceed one week.

In studying the problems of patients admitted during a one-month period, Sundel and colleagues found among many of them "serious stress as a result of situational factors associated with unemployment, lack of formal education, low income, and detachment from their families and a lack of social support systems. Such problems of living can more appropriately be handled by other human service agencies. These findings indicated the need for systematic efforts to involve the staff of those agencies in the assessment, referral, and disposition of individuals seeking services" (p. 570).

Long-term hospitalization was avoided for more than 40% of patients referred for admission, in some cases by using the short-term crisis-intervention unit followed by referral to community agencies. In about two-thirds of these patients referred for admission, referral to community agencies was sufficient, that is, the crisis intervention unit was not needed at all.

Delaney, Seidman, and Willis (1978) were able to show that an active outreach crisis-intervention program could reduce hospital admissions dramatically. Two-person teams visited with persons judged to be in need of mental treatment as soon as petitions for hospitalization were filed. Whenever possible, prospective patients were seen in their own homes along with members of their families.

First, these mental health personnel determined whether the crisis was one in which a mental health agency could be helpful. If another agency or program was thought to be more suitable, referral was made. If it was determined that mental health services were needed, they were arranged, with a preference for local, outpatient, brief, and voluntary settings rather than distant, inpatient, long-term, and involuntary settings.

The authors summarized the principles governing their actions by noting that "our active crisis intervention efforts concentrated on keeping inappropriate referrals out of the mental health system, assisting those individuals in obtaining the appropriate and needed material and psychological resources, and aiding those judged in need of mental health treatment to obtain beneficial services in line with the principles of the community mental health movement (e.g., local, brief, outpatient)" (p. 40).

The authors contrasted admission rates into the state mental hospital from their catchment area with rates from a geographically and demographically similar area without equivalent crisis-intervention services, over a four-year period starting two years before the services began. They were able to show a dramatic decrease in admission rates from their area coincident with the start of their program. The authors concluded that their program "was successful in reducing the number of state hospital admissions diagnosed as mentally ill" (p. 42).

In another examination of crisis intervention, Bunn and Clarke (1979) contrasted level of anxiety before and after brief counseling for relatives who arrived in a hospital emergency admitting ward with a seriously ill or injured patient. They also compared those findings with similar measures obtained from a noncounseled group. During the counseling session, averaging 20 minutes, the therapist tried to be supportive and empathic and encouraged the relatives to express their feelings and concerns about the crisis. Despite the brevity of this crisis-intervention effort, significant decreases in anxiety were found in the experimental group, contrasted with the group receiving no counseling. The authors concluded that "at the time of admission, relatives of patients do exhibit very high levels of anxiety and that crisis intervention in a hospital emergency admitting ward can reduce these very high levels of diffuse and generalized anxiety. . . . Further studies might profitably examine the long term course of anxiety for both kinds of clients—the patients and the relatives who accompany the patient to the hospital" (p. 194).

CONCLUSIONS AND OVERVIEW

The enormous appeal of crisis-intervention theory lies in the hope that, by following its principles, the limited number of community mental health center staff members can increase their impact on the community quite dramatically. There seems little question that a very small number of interviews, skillfully conducted during a time of crisis, can have profound and long-lasting effects. Crisis-intervention techniques are fairly well developed. The basic theoretical and conceptual foundations for crisis intervention are in place, and a number of publications oriented toward training crisis counselors have appeared. Extraordinary innovativeness has repeatedly been shown in the application of these concepts to nontraditional settings. There is a clear professional commitment to the recruitment and training of crisis counselors, as well as to undertaking responsible evaluations of the effectiveness of crisis intervention.

Auerbach and Kilmann (1977) have critically analyzed many crisis-intervention outcome research studies. Too few studies of crisis-intervention programs conducted in psychiatric settings include suitable control groups or appropriate follow-up evaluative procedures. However, "the biggest obstacle to drawing meaningful conclusions from research in this area is the failure . . . of researchers to specify operationally, in terms of process variables, what is taking place when crisis intervention techniques are being applied. Future studies should systematically vary selected treatment factors and control others, and assess the interactive effects of treatment with client variables on outcome measures that logically extend from the goals of therapy" (p. 1203).

Several studies have examined the effectiveness of crisis intervention as a function of (1) immediacy of intervention and (2) the client's adaptability. Greer (1979) found some evidence that intervention immediacy is influential— especially when immediacy is defined not in terms of time between crisis and the start of intervention but rather in terms of characteristics of the client, such as anxiety or other symptomatology. Similarly, there is some evidence that characteristics of the client before the crisis are among the best prognosticators of crisis outcome. Most of these client characteristics are measures of prior psychiatric history, such as prior psychiatric hospitalization or suicidal behavior. In general, Greer found that past responses to stress are an influential determinant of outcome.

Outcome has also been examined as a function of characteristics of the therapeutic encounter, particularly the extent to which emotional support is provided and the extent to which an active problem-solving orientation is maintained. Studies that tended to confirm the effectiveness of these therapeutic techniques were those that focused on therapeutic process rather than on self-reported descriptions of therapeutic technique by counselors.

Greer notes that "the most prominent implication of the extant research is that we are still, by and large, unaware of the general and specific conditions which are predictive of favorable crisis outcome" (1979, p. 64). He makes the following observations about the research literature: First, there is some evidence that certain therapeutic techniques that have value in standard psychotherapy have similar value in crisis therapy. Second, there is some evidence of improvement during crisis therapy, but not much evidence for the superiority of therapy that is characterized specifically by its timeliness, supportiveness, or directiveness. Third, research needs to be undertaken examining the role of socioeconomic factors, the family, and individual cognitive and developmental factors in crisis-therapy outcome. Fourth, research studies will be improved to the extent that there is clearer agreement about criteria of success. Fifth, educational procedures might be just as effective as therapeutic procedures and may have an additional advantage of being able to influence client expectancies and thus crisis outcome.

Greer concludes his review by noting that the

> treatment of persons in crisis furnishes a unique research opportunity. . . . it usually involves highly focused activity on the part of both therapist and client in a brief span of time with diminished significance on extra-therapeutic variables. . . . crisis resolution truly provides a succinct period in which to investigate some basic units of individual change. It is conceivable that some of these basic elements are part and parcel of the same framework that determines personal growth and change in general. In this time of community mental health reassessment, the light that this can, in turn, shed on implications for preventative efforts would be welcomed [p. 67].

Two developments seem possible in the near future. First, the result of the crisis-intervention orientation can be to view each individual therapeutic session as a self-contained unit, in which the counselor deliberately identifies a piece of therapeutic work that needs to be done and is pertinent to the crisis and then proceeds to do it. At the end of the interview, the client can be invited to return whenever necessary, but there is no provision for regular appointments. It seems clear from the reviews in this as well as the preceding chapters that this orientation may well be suitable for a substantial proportion of the clients in a community mental health center, though certainly not for all. A related task for the future is to develop training programs to improve clinical skills in providing effective crisis-intervention services not only promptly but also briefly.

A second, perhaps more complex task will be to learn how to make outreach crisis-intervention services more effective. More research is necessary to identify high-risk groups who can be helped and to develop effective services. It is not simply a matter of trying to be helpful—that effort is laudable but not enough. Yet, optimism about the ultimate effectiveness of crisis-intervention services seems warranted, particularly when they are seen as part of an effort to build a greater sense of competence and mastery in all members of the community.

CHAPTER

4

Mental Health
Consultation

$\mathbf{M}$ental health consultation is the major
form of *indirect service* associated with the community mental health movement. Consultation is an indirect service in that the mental health consultant
does not ordinarily work directly with a client. Rather, the consultant interacts
with a *consultee* or group of consultees (such as teachers, the clergy, or public
health nurses) who themselves provide services directly to clients.

The term *consultation* has long been used in medical practice to mean the
employment of an outside medical expert to assist in formulating a diagnosis
and treatment plan for a particular patient (see Meyers, 1981). In the mental
health field, the term has taken on a somewhat different and restricted meaning. Mental health consultation has been defined as "a process of interaction
between two professional persons—the consultant, who is a specialist, and
the consultee, who invokes the consultant's help in regard to a current work
problem with which he is having some difficulty and which he has decided
is within the other's area of specialized competence" (Caplan, 1970, p. 19).
The "current work problem" may be the consultee's difficulty handling a particular client or group of clients or the development of a program for serving
all clients with a certain problem.

A more recent definition by MacLennan, Quinn, and Schroeder (cited in
Mannino, MacLennan, & Shore, 1975) is somewhat different: "Mental health
consultation is the provision of technical assistance by an expert to individual
and agency caregivers related to the mental health dimension of their work.
Such assistance is directed to specific work-related problems, is advisory in
nature, and the consultant has no direct responsibility for its acceptance and
implementation" (pp. 4–5). This definition emphasizes the technical nature
of the assistance provided by the consultant and seems to deemphasize the

sense of professional equality between consultant and consultee suggested by Caplan's definition.

It is important to distinguish consultation from other mental health activities with which it is sometimes confused and with which it has some overlapping characteristics. Consultation can be distinguished from *supervision* on the grounds that (1) the consultant may not be of the same professional specialty as the consultee, (2) the consultant has no administrative responsibility for the work of the consultee, (3) consultation may be irregular in character rather than continuous, and (4) the consultant is not in a position of power with respect to the consultee. Consultation can be distinguished from *education* on the basis of (1) the relative freedom of the consultee to accept or reject the consultant's ideas, (2) the lack of a planned curriculum, and (3) the absence of any evaluation or assessment of the consultee's progress by the consultant. Consultation also needs to be differentiated from *psychotherapy*. In psychotherapy, there is a clear contractual relationship between an individual designated as a patient and another individual designated as a therapist. In this relationship, the patient acknowledges the existence of personal problems and allows the invasion of his or her privacy in order to resolve these problems. No such contractual relationship exists between consultant and consultee. The goal of consultation is improved work performance rather than improved personal adjustment. The consultant and consultee are in a peer relationship, and each expects his or her privacy to be honored. Consultation should, finally, be distinguished from *collaboration*. Consultation carries no implication that the consultant will participate with the consultee in the implementation of any plans. The task of the consultant is to assist the consultee in meeting his or her work responsibilities more effectively (see Bindman, 1959, and Mannino et al., 1975, pp. 8–9).

The primary goal of the consultant is to have a positive but indirect effect on a client population by improving the work skills of the consultee who works directly with that population. The rationale for mental health consultation is the belief that mental health personnel cannot hope to interact directly and meaningfully with all the people who need help and that one solution to this problem is to identify agencies that work directly with segments of the population and to try to assist these agencies in providing more effective services (see Bloom, 1969).

MacLennan, Quinn, and Schroeder (cited in Mannino et al., 1975) suggest that consultation activities might have any of the following objectives: referral or management of an individual, family, or group; management of the consultee's feelings about a client; assistance with administrative and staff organization and relationships; assessment of the nature and etiology of mental health problems and the need for new or modified programs; advice on the planning, development, and evaluation of research, training, or service programs; and transmission of knowledge and skills in treatment, training, research, administration, evaluation, and preparation of written and audiovisual materials.

In their introduction to a monograph on consultation research, Mannino and Shore said consultation "is a major, if not the major, technique and focus of community psychology, community psychiatry, and community mental health" (1971, p. 1). These authors believe consultation is important because (1) it allows large segments of the population to be reached by relatively few people, (2) it provides a means for teaching mental health principles to other community service professionals, (3) it can develop, in various kinds of community agencies and programs, an awareness of mental health problems and the resources necessary to deal with them, (4) it may be one solution to the problem of shortages of skilled mental health workers, and (5) it can build and maintain the competence of human service providers who are too far from the mental health arena to be aware of new knowledge.

BASIC MENTAL HEALTH CONSULTATION CONCEPTS

Types of mental health consultation

Although the field of consultation is not nearly so well articulated as the field of psychotherapy, several conceptualizations of it have been developed. The seminal taxonomy of types of consultation was developed by Caplan (1963), who divides consultation into four varieties. The first he calls *client-centered case consultation*. Its primary goal is to help the consultee deal with the presented case. To achieve this goal, the consultant uses his or her specialized skills and knowledge to help the consultee assess the client's problem and to recommend how best to deal with the problem. The second variety of consultation Caplan terms *consultee-centered case consultation*. In this type, the consultant identifies the consultee's difficulties in handling the case and remedies these difficulties, whether they stem from insufficient skill, knowledge, self-confidence, or objectivity. This type of consultation offers the promise of increased consultee effectiveness in a wide variety of professional encounters in the future. In the third variety of consultation, *program-centered administrative consultation*, the consultant's primary goal is to suggest some actions the consultee might take in order to develop, expand, or modify a clinical or agency program. Here the consultant draws not only on general mental health skills but also on his or her understanding of the functioning of social systems and of the principles of mental health program administration. Finally, in *consultee-centered administrative consultation*, the consultant identifies difficulties within the consultee that limit his or her effectiveness in instituting program change.

Each of these types of consultation involves a different level of intervention and has an identifiable target (the client, the consultee, the delivery system) and an identifiable goal (behavior change in the client, enhanced performance in the consultee, or change in the delivery system). Nagler and Cook (1973) suggest that the decision about what level to intervene at as a consultant is, in part, based on ideological grounds related to how one thinks about and analyzes social problems. They say that a consultation service could be organized to be clinical and case-oriented; consultees would be taught to focus on individual maladjustment and remediation. Alternatively, a consultation service could be system-oriented and could focus on identifying problems that could be solved by changing agency policies or environmental conditions. In a related paper, Perlmutter and Silverman (1973) point out the conflict between those who view consultation as treatment and those who view it as prevention. They suggest that two very different ideologies and sets of skills are involved in these two types of consultation.

Applying these concepts to the analysis of a school consultation program, Nagler and Cook (1973) found that there was a heavy emphasis on case consultation (75% of all contacts), in which school personnel were assisted in coping with students who were judged to have problems. Accordingly, no significant institutional or systemwide changes could be anticipated. In the absence of a consultation service designed to help school personnel achieve social change in their work system by reducing institutional inadequacies, the authors argue, the rate of psychological casualties in the school system will not significantly decrease, even with the benefit of the mental health consultation program. They urge that more attention be paid to the ideological positions that underlie consultation programs in general and that decisions about the targets and goals of a consultation program not be left entirely in the hands of persons who have a stake in maintaining the existing agency program and philosophy.

Signell and Scott (1971) describe a model of consultation that is more interactional than the earlier case- and consultee-centered models. These authors suggest that mental health consultants have gradually involved themselves with a broader array of caregivers and have become increasingly concerned with primary prevention and with families, large reference groups, and the social environment—in other words, with systems as well as with individuals. In contrast to the earlier view of the mental health consultant as somewhat detached, more current theory sees the consultant as an active change agent— a source of hope by personal example and an active participant in interactions with consultees and their clients.

In an overview of consultation models, Dworkin and Dworkin(1975) identify four specific models (one of which is consultee-centered case consultation) and distinguish among them along the dimensions of (1) the implied or explicit definition of consultation, (2) the self-perception of the consultant, (3) the target population, (4) the motivation of the client system, (5) the mode of entry of the consultant into the system, (6) the goal of consultation, (7) the role of the consultant in problem diagnosis, (8) the techniques used by the consultant, (9) when and how the consultation relationship is terminated, and (10) how the consultation process is to be evaluated.

In addition to the consultee-centered model, Dworkin and Dworkin identify (1) the group process model, in which consultation is viewed from a humanistic, interpersonal framework wherein the consultant facilitates the client system's motivation and ability to identify, analyze, and solve its problems, (2) the social action model, in which the consultant uses his or her "understanding of political power distributions and organizational skills to identify, recruit, and train indigenous leaders who can, in turn, help their constituency of 'oppressed' people to obtain a power base in an identified social system" (p. 153), and (3) the ecological model, in which the consultant "develops intervention strategies for an ecosystem"—for example, a school system including the administrators and elected school board.

Consultants operating under these models use different techniques:

> The consultee-centered consultant helps the consultee, where appropriate, by (1) pointing out, through example, parable, anecdote, or metaphor, how the consultee's lack of professional objectivity is contributing to the problem; (2) giving the consultee missing data; (3) helping the consultee develop and improve skills; and (4) providing ego support. The group process consultant utilizes a variety of group techniques . . . including (1) sensitivity training groups, (2) reflection, (3) authentic feedback, [and] (4) role playing. . . . The techniques of social action consultants involve (1) identifying and recruiting indigenous leadership, (2) surfacing and exaggerating system crises, (3) organizing the constituency, and (4) developing and implementing appropriate strategies and tactics for transferring power to the constituency. Ecological consultants utilize theory, research, and naturalistic observation to generate data for planning and recommending interventions. Because of the variety of individual and environmental needs which exist in an ecosystem, the consultant recommends multileveled interventions, anticipating potential side-effects, and assessing the impact of implemented programs [p. 155].[1]

Woody (1975) differentiates between process consultation, in which the "consultant tries to understand the consultee's phenomenological world" and behavioral consultation, in which "behaviors are observed and the observational data are analyzed to establish the reinforcement contingencies" (p. 278). The process consultant tries to help the consultee clarify his or her own thinking and determine his or her own goals by means of a nondirective relationship. In contrast, the behavioral consultant recommends techniques to modify the behavior of the target person, gives expert advice, and accepts a directive and supervisory role. Woody examined the distinction between process and behavioral consultation by contrasting replies to a questionnaire about response style administered to consultants, by comparing success in maintaining effective consultation relationships, and by examining the techniques for producing

---

[1]From "A Conceptual Overview of Selected Consultation Models," by A. L. Dworkin and E. P. Dworkin, *American Journal of Community Psychology*, 1975, 3, 151–159. Reprinted by permission of Plenum Publishing Corporation.

change taught in training programs specializing in one or the other form of consultation. The analysis supported the hypothesis that there are two distinct consultation models. Regarding response styles, for example, behavioral consultants were significantly more directive and enforcing and significantly less clarifying, probing, and reflective than process consultants.

Cooper and Hodges (1983) have identified three basic models of mental health consultation—educational, individual process, and systems process. In the educational model, the consultant conceptualizes the consultee's difficulty as due mainly to lack of skill or knowledge. Intervention is oriented toward imparting information or helping with skill building through behavioral modeling (see, for example, Keller, 1981; Kuehnel & Kuehnel, 1983). In the individual process model, the consultant conceptualizes the difficulty as due to the consultee's attitudes, motivations, intrapsychic conflicts, or personal style. Intervention focuses on eliminating defensive processes or facilitating personal growth (see, for example, Heller & Monahan, 1983). In the systems model, the consultee's difficulty is seen as due to characteristics of the organization or community to which both the client and the consultee belong. Intervention focuses on modifying channels of communication, distribution of power, support, and influence (see, for example, Schmuck, 1983).

One area of mental health consultation that is particularly common is *organizational consultation*. Although most organizations receiving consultation are private agencies or businesses, a growing amount of consultation is being provided to public or nonprofit human service delivery organizations as well. Goodstein (1978) proposes that all forms of consultation can be conceived along three axes—the intervention techniques being used, the focal issues that justify the consultation, and the desirable unit of change, whether the individual, the group, the organization, or the larger social system. Focal issues include four major types—power and authority issues, morale and cohesion issues, norms and standards of behavior, and establishment of goals or objectives.

Goodstein identifies five strategies that are probably the only techniques that have been developed for intervening in the affairs of others regardless of the target of the intervention or the nature of the problem for which intervention is being sought. These intervention strategies are *acceptant* (expressions of support, empathy, positive regard), *catalytic* (efforts to increase the rate at which information is acquired and processed), *confrontational* (attempts to identify inappropriate, invalid, or unjustified assumptions governing the consultee's performance), *prescriptive* (giving directions and advice), and *educational* (providing theories or principles by which the consultee can deal with the current as well as future problems).

Goodstein says that the acceptant strategy can aid the client through "sympathetic listening, empathic understanding, and the clear communication of positive regard for the client who is experiencing psychological discomfort"

(1978, p. 32).[2] Catalytic interventions are aimed at "helping clients gain a better understanding of the situations in which they find themselves by gaining additional information or by verifying existing data" (p. 33). In catalytic consultation the consultant collects data about the client and feeds the data back to the client. "The data can be collected somewhat less formally through interviews and direct observation or more formally through the administration of formal questionnaires and survey instruments. This latter kind of survey feedback is perhaps the most widely practiced kind of organizational consultation currently being conducted" (p. 33).

In confrontational interventions, "the consultant hopes to unravel the underlying values by which the client has been operating and, when appropriate, help the client face the unreality of these values. The client, as most of us, has been previously unable to see that some of his or her deeply held values are inappropriate because of rationalization, denial, justification, projection, and all the other defense mechanisms we use to maintain our self-esteem" (1978, pp. 34–35). A prescriptive intervention for an individual might involve "a behavioral change plan for making a supervisor more accessible to his or her subordinates, a training [regimen] to increase a parent's effectiveness, a behavior [regimen] to promote dieting, and so on" (p. 36). For a group, the prescription might be "moving a juvenile gang out of the street into the community center or teaching a family how to budget its financial resources. Arbitration, particularly compulsory arbitration, is a prescriptive solution to intergroup conflict" (p. 36). Finally, an educational intervention implies that the knowledge base of the consultant is shared with those who need it, in order to free them to use the consultant's knowledge without requiring his or her direct help.

Within this context, Goodstein has examined ways of understanding organizations, as well as issues related to entry into the organizational system (see also Pipes, 1981), organizational problem diagnosis, and consultative interventions.

Individual and group consultation

The concept of group consultation implies more or less regular meetings of one consultant with a group of consultees. Just as an interest in group psychotherapy appeared shortly after the emergence of the field of individual psychotherapy, so has an interest in group consultation emerged. And just as group psychotherapy is viewed as having two virtues—its economy and its special effectiveness with interpersonal problems—so too is group consultation seen as having virtues different from those of individual consultation.

---

[2]From Goodstein, *Consulting with Human Service Systems,* © 1978. Addison-Wesley, Reading, Mass. pp: 32, 33, 34, 35, 36. Reprinted with permission.

In an early report of a group consultation program, Altrocchi, Spielberger, and Eisdorfer (1965) described their case-seminar approach. In the case-seminar method, a consultee is asked to present to the group a problem case for which he or she had responsibility. The consultee is encouraged to select a case of general interest to the group. The case presentation is supplemented by some firsthand exposure of the consultant to the consultee/client relationship—either observation of it or an interview of the client about it. This firsthand contact gives the consultant additional information for case discussion and assists the consultant in helping the consultee prepare the case presentation for the group. In these case seminars, the authors have noted, the first meetings of a newly formed group often involve a testing-out phase in which bizarre or "impossible" cases or cases involving members of minority or profoundly disadvantaged groups are presented. They also note that early presenters tend to be the least defensive and most competent members of the consultee group and that consultee groups differ with respect to initial cohesiveness, resistance to discussing their professional work, and how rapidly they proceed from the introductory stage of group building to the more productive and creative stage of group problem solving.

According to Altrocchi and his colleagues, the group consultant must function simultaneously as teacher, group leader, clinician, and facilitator of communication among community agencies; it is obvious that these authors see effective group consultation as a demanding task.

Tobiessen and Shai (1971) contrasted the reactions of consultees who had met individually with a mental health consultant and consultees who had met in a group with a mental health consultant. They administered a follow-up questionnaire to elementary school teachers who had been consultees in eight elementary schools that had been divided into two groups; in four schools weekly individual consultation was offered, and in four schools weekly group consultation was offered. The eight schools were in four school districts. Each district contained an individual-consultation and a group-consultation school, and the two schools were similar in size and nature of student population. Furthermore, the same consultant provided the individual and the group consultation in each school district. The consultation appears to have been of a case-oriented variety, and the programs were in existence for an entire school year.

With regard to reported improvement of the problem children discussed during the consultation sessions, there was no difference attributable to type of consultation. Almost half the children were reported to show some improvement, and half were said to show no improvement. No comparable information was presented on the rate of improvement of problem children in the absence of consultation. Regarding teachers' reports of the usefulness of consultation, again no differences appeared that could be attributed to the type of consultation. The most frequent response was that the consultation was moderately useful, and more teachers reported that the consultation was very useful than reported that it was not useful at all. One specific objective of the consultation program was to provide teachers with general information about normal and abnormal child development. The group-consultation approach was significantly more successful in achieving this objective than the individual-consultation approach and was significantly more successful in generating discussion and exchange of ideas among teachers in the school— another specific objective. In general, those teachers who had had more contact with consultants, whether in group or individual sessions, reported higher general usefulness of the consultation. Group consultation thus seems to be a more effective and efficient use of consultants' time than individual consultation.

Theme interference and theme-interference reduction

Perhaps the most innovative concept that has been developed to assist the mental health consultant is theme-interference reduction (Caplan, 1970; Hirschowitz, 1973). Caplan defines *theme interference* as "a symbolic inhibition of free perception and communication between consultee and client and a concomitant disorder of objectivity" (1964, p. 223)—in other words, a lack of objectivity in the consultee because of his or her own characteristics. Theme interference may be accompanied by some degree of emotional upset, ranging from relatively mild tension to a marked crisis response. "The consultee usually ascribes his discomfort to his difficulties with the client, onto whose case he displaces feelings of anxiety, hostility, shame, and depression, which can be seen by the consultant to be partly or even primarily originating in his personal life or in his involvement with the social-system problems of his institution" (Caplan, 1964, p. 223). Such theme interferences obviously reduce the consultee's effectiveness in working with clients, and the technique of theme-interference reduction used by the mental health consultant is designed to modify the line of reasoning the consultee is following as well as the consultee's feelings, both of which serve to maintain the theme interference.

The history of the concept of theme-interference reduction is extremely interesting. The concept was developed relatively late in Caplan's work and replaced an earlier consultation technique, called *unlinking*. Caplan viewed the consultee as a person vulnerable to just as wide a variety of reality distortions and anxieties as anyone else and just as prone to carry over some of those irrational distortions into the work setting. An elementary school teacher, for example, deeply troubled by self-doubts because of uncertainty about his or her own intellectual abilities, might be unusually prone to see intellectual retardation in pupils and then to give up trying to teach them, in the belief that such children are constitutionally unable to learn. There are two distinguishable aspects to this state of affairs. First, the consultee believes a particular student to have limited intellectual ability—a belief that may or may not be valid. Second, the consultee believes it is hopeless to try to teach children

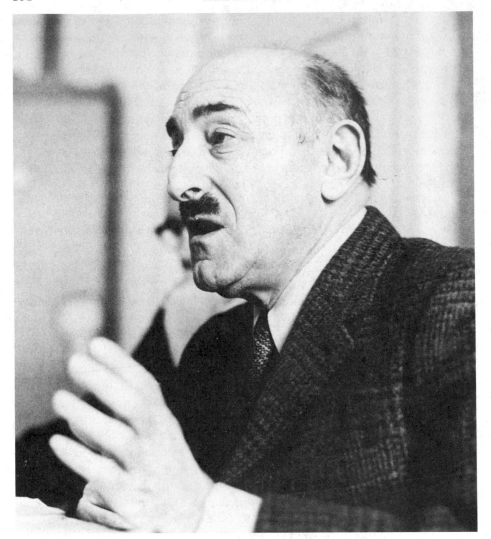

Gerald Caplan, originator of some of the most influential concepts in the field of community mental health. *(Photo by Brian Dowley.)*

of limited intellectual ability, because they cannot learn—a belief that also may or may not be valid.

Caplan's initial proposal for how a mental health consultant might deal with this general kind of problem, which he believed was very common, was to influence the consultee to change his or her perceptions of the client—a process he termed *unlinking*. Notice that even if this process works, the second belief—that mentally retarded persons cannot learn—is untouched. Accordingly, as Caplan found, even if this consultation strategy worked, it would be only a matter of time before the teacher would find another pupil to be of limited intellectual ability. Thus, the technique of unlinking was abandoned as being a major consultation error, even though the consultee often gained some temporary relief and the client in question was often helped.

Caplan then turned to the second aspect of the consultee's belief system. Accepting the premise that the client may be mentally retarded, the consultant tries to deal with the consultee's belief that such persons cannot profit from an education. It is this belief that is referred to as the theme interference. When the consultant persuades the consultee to reexamine the evidence on which this belief is based and to consider other possible outcomes, given that mental retardation exists, he or she is engaging in theme-interference reduction. Such a technique can change the consultee's attitude about pupils with intellectual limitations and thus change how the consultee deals with an entire category of pupils.

Consultation and systems theory

The interest in mental health consultation has brought with it an interest in systems theory. Since all consultees and clients are embedded in multiple and overlapping social organizations, efforts to change their behavior or attitudes must take into account this larger system network in order to be effective. In a broader sense, it is generally believed that the roots of most mental disorders reside "not just within the individual but also in disturbances within this dynamic network of interacting systems" (Marmor, 1975). The fundamental premise of systems theory is absolute interdependence—that is, that components of every system influence and are influenced by one another in complex and often surprising ways. The British poet Francis Thompson, in the poem "The Mistress of Vision," described this interdependence when he wrote "Thou canst not stir a flower without troubling of a star." Recognition of this interdependence is important in those engaged in psychotherapy; in those engaged in consultation, it is critical.

In its most general sense, a *system* is "a set of interacting units with relationships among them" (J. G. Miller, 1971, p. 281; see also Hall & Fagan, 1956). The field referred to as *general systems theory* deals with the common properties of systems across all levels—from single cells to total societies. The systems within which people function are *open* systems, characterized by boundaries that are permeable and that allow energy, material, and information to enter and leave and living things to grow, learn, and reproduce. A system is more or less stable in structure and has a history and a set of functions, some of which are reversible (such as an illness that can be successfully treated) and some of which are irreversible (such as birth or death). Since stress within any part of a system can have effects throughout the system, it follows that reducing stress at some point in a social system can have positive consequences for the mental health of a great many individuals within the system. W. B. Miller (1973) has alerted consultants to the fact that their consultees are embedded in systems that may include subsystems and that may themselves be nested within larger systems. Each of these systems is made up of component elements, or units, which are in dynamic interaction, and is surrounded by boundaries that separate it functionally from other systems. Systems may be concrete and real—for example, a person or a family—or may be abstract—for example, the id/ego/superego system of psychoanalytic theory. Systems may develop and change over time and may be described in terms of their state at some particular moment. They may also be described in terms of their disposition, or potential to function in certain ways under certain circumstances. Many systems, and most living systems, tend to resist change and to set up forces to oppose or resist the threat of change. The term *stress* is used to describe the threatened changes, and the term *strain* is used to describe the system's resistant forces.

As an example of how systems theory can be applied, W. B. Miller considers psychiatric consultation in a general-hospital setting. A common question in this setting is whether a patient's symptoms are of organic or psychological origin. Faced with this question, the consultant to the hospital staff must first understand the patient in the context of interdependent psychological and physiological systems. Second, the consultant must understand such dyadic (two-member) systems as patient/doctor and patient/nurse and such triadic (three-member) systems as doctor/nurse/patient. Third, the consultant must develop an appreciation of suprasystems, such as the hospital and the family, in which the patient is embedded. Thus, the consultant's task is multidimensional; the consultant must be aware of and able to evaluate the position of the patient in the various systems in order to decide which systems are most important to the patient at any given moment.

CONSULTATION SERVICES IN
COMMUNITY MENTAL HEALTH CENTERS

An indication of the time devoted to consultation services can be obtained from a survey of federally funded community mental health centers conducted by the National Institute of Mental Health (see Bass, 1974). A questionnaire was distributed to the 325 funded comprehensive community mental health centers operating in 1973. One section of the inventory requested information on consultation and education activities during February 1973. More than three-quarters of the mental health centers completed this section.

Analysis of the responses showed that an average of 5.5% of total staff time was devoted to consultation and education activities, as compared with, for example, 32.2% devoted to inpatient care, 20.6% to outpatient care, 13.7% to partial hospitalization, and 4.8% to emergency services. Comparing these results with the results of a similar survey undertaken a year earlier revealed a decrease in the proportion of time devoted to consultation and education. One reason is that these activities do not ordinarily generate revenues from those persons or agencies who make use of them in proportion to the time devoted and therefore tend to be cut back. Only 0.3% of total mental health center revenue was obtained from consultation services. Some variability was found among mental health centers in time invested in consultation. Half of the responding centers reported between 2.6 and 8.4% of staff time devoted to consultation, and 90% reported between 0.9 and 18.9%.

Case consultation took up 47% of the total consultation effort, program consultation 31%, and staff development or continuing education the remaining 22%. Over one-third of the total amount of consultation was provided to schools (see Conoley, 1981), 10% to welfare agencies and to alcohol- and drug-abuse prevention agencies combined, and about 9% each to law enforcement personnel, medical facilities, and other health facilities. Not only are schools the most common consultees, they are also the largest source of revenue for mental health centers from consultation. The one-third of the total consultation time devoted to schools yields about two-thirds of all revenues obtained from consultation services.

Although the preceding survey found some small regional differences within the United States in the proportion of staff time devoted to consultation, it found no major differences as a function of the rural/urban dimension or as a function of the affluence of the catchment area. Perlmutter (1979) has described the consultation and education activities in rural mental health centers in the East Central United States. In contrasting 13 rural mental health centers with 30 nonrural centers in the same geographic area, Perlmutter found fewer well-organized consultation programs in the rural areas and generally poorer leadership.

Consultation programs in rural community mental health centers were often in precarious condition. Mental health centers were thought of as serving the severely psychiatrically impaired; much stigma was attached to mental illness; many important members of the community were uninformed on mental health issues; and many staff members had an exceedingly traditional orientation to mental health services, sometimes even preferring inpatient to outpatient care when a choice could be made. Rural mental health centers appeared to be dominated by the medical model, with virtually exclusive interest in the provision of therapeutic services. Many centers lacked support from their parent organization or governing board. Finally, there seemed to be a chronic sense of distrust between rural mental health centers and county government. Under these circumstances, consultation programs were not faring well at all.

According to Perlmutter, breaking out of this state of affairs will require educating the local community as well as the professionals in the community

about the benefits of mental health consultation programs, carefully nourish-
ing support wherever it can be found, educating members of policy-making
boards of directors of mental health centers, working particularly actively with
the medical community, and reducing rancorous conflict wherever possible.

AN EXAMPLE OF MENTAL HEALTH CONSULTATION

In one of the earliest publications describing and giving examples of mental health consultation, Kazanjian, Stein, and Weinberg (1962, pp. 10–11) provide a very useful excerpt from a session between a mental health consultant
and a speech-therapist consultee, along with illustrations of the thought
processes of the consultant. This exchange provides an excellent example of
the mental health consultant in action in consultee-centered case consultation.
Few published verbatim accounts of the consultation process exist. The general
absence of detailed case material highlights the fact that problems exist in the
training of mental health consultants.

Consultee-1.   *A youngster I have seen for more than a year in speech therapy has
made very little progress, and I don't know what to do about her.*

Consultant-1.   *Can you tell me something about the child?*
Hypothesis. Consultee sounds discouraged. What is her conflict about?
What are her expectations? *Reasoning.* Further information needed to test
consultant's initial hypothesis of discouragement. *Note.* It is obtained
indirectly by asking about the client.

Consultee-2.   *She is a 10-year-old youngster who was barely able to pronounce a
one-syllable word when she first came to me. One of the clinics in the city
recommended her for speech therapy. They evidently felt that she could profit from
speech work. The clinic is still seeing her in psychotherapy, and plans to continue.
They said she wasn't retarded, but in over a year I haven't been able to get her
beyond words of more than two syllables. I hate to give up, but I don't feel I can
work with her any longer. What do you think I ought to do?*

Consultant-2.   *She sounds discouraging.*
Hypothesis. Child disturbed, speech difficulty severe, probably related to
emotional problems—how? Conflict coming into clearer focus—consultee has desire to give up—but she also needs to hang on—why? She
seems to question the clinic's statement about retardation. *Reasoning.*
Consultant empathizes with the feeling that he assumes the client elicits
in the consultee. Also the consultant attempts to validate his original
hypothesis, that is, that consultee felt discouraged. *Note.* Validation of
the hypothesis is done by talking about the client. If the consultee feels
"understood," it will permit her to elaborate further on her conflict. Consultant deliberately avoids suggesting what the consultee ought to do.
Suggestions are made, but it is too early in the session to make one. If

the "core anxiety" is to be understood, consultant needs to play for time. Further, frequent suggestions by the consultant tend to promote undesirable dependency.

Consultee-3. *Believe me, she is, but at times she tries so hard I just don't have the heart to give her up. Yet I wonder, am I doing her an injustice?*

Consultant-3. *What did the clinic say about her?*
Hypothesis. Hypothesis of discouragement is reinforced. Dynamic material emerges that seems to be related to consultee's identification with the client. This suggests possible reason for consultee's opposing needs, that is, to hang on to or to give up with the client. *Reasoning.* Seeking further diagnostic information; that is, did the clinic give additional data? If so, what is the consultee's perception of the clinic's expectations of her?

Consultee-4. *They said there was no organic reason why she can't talk normally. The clinic thinks she is autistic. Is speech characteristically slow for this kind of child?*

Consultant-4. *Yes, sometimes it takes many years before one sees any appreciable change in a child who has been diagnosed as having such a disorder.*
Hypothesis. None. *Reasoning.* Since the child was diagnosed as autistic, consultee's discouragement is based on reality. Consultant imparts factual information consistent with clinical knowledge, which can reduce irrational self-expectations, super-ego demands, and so forth. Further, the consultant makes appropriate use of his clinical experience to establish his role as an expert in the area of mental health.

Consultee-5. *Well, you know, there are some days that are just wasted; I just don't get through to her. That's when I feel like giving up.*

Consultant-5. *That's understandable. Other speech people with whom I have worked have told me how helpless, and at times angry, they feel when they are working very hard to help someone who isn't responding; let alone appreciate what is being done.*
Hypothesis. As a result of the positive consultation relationship that has been established, the consultee has been helped to express her feelings with much less defensiveness. *Reasoning.* Accepting and discussing specific feelings such children have caused in others is helpful in reducing anxiety in the consultee; that is, others with similar experiences have felt as she does. *Note.* That a comparison is made which is designed to be supportive, but is about what others have felt, rather than a statement directed toward the consultee's expressed feelings.

Consultee-6. *That is exactly the way I feel. There are some days I want to send her home.*

Consultant-6. *Can you do that?*
Hypothesis. "Core anxiety" revealed. Consultee's feelings are out in the open, but she appears uncertain about her proposed action. Dynamically,

one suspects she wants the consultant to assume responsibility for her contemplated action. *Reasoning.* Consultant deliberately avoids deciding for consultee or taking on the role of her administrator. Further, a question of this order helps the consultant learn about the amount of autonomy the consultee is permitted within her particular institution.

Consultee-7.   *Yes. Do you suppose that would be okay?*

Consultant-7.   *I don't know why not.*
   Hypothesis. This question is interpreted to mean, will the consultee's action be harmful to her client; also, can she dare permit herself relief from her super-ego demands. *Reasoning.* Here consultant takes a stand based on available clinical information about the consultee and client. Primary purpose is to relieve consultee of super-ego demands and possibly irrational guilt. Implicitly, the consultant's attitude during this entire session and explicitly the above statement he made to the consultee reinforces the consultee's belief that she is not inadequate if she takes action based on an awareness of her own limitations for frustration. Experience has taught us that when the "core anxiety" is reduced, consultee's ego is free to approach even the most difficult problem again, but more rationally. *Note.* Decision to continue with this child still remains with the consultee.

Consultee-8.   *Tell me, do you think my continuing with her will have an ill effect on her?*

Consultant-8.   *In what way?*
   Hypothesis. The shift in the kind of question asked and its content meaning ("Can my work with this child hurt her?") resulted in part from the consultee's recognizing that the consultant had accepted the very difficult problem with which she was confronted, and had conveyed the feeling that he understood its concomitant frustration. This transition in the content of the consultee's question also suggests that she is now toying with the notion of continuing her work with the child. The statement may also contain an element of guilt. *Reasoning.* Explores hypothesis of guilt.

Consultee-9.   *Well, you know, maybe I was expecting too much of her. At times, I have really had to put on the pressure, but of course, I have never worked with a child before who has had such a severe speech problem.*

Consultant-9.   *It sounds as if you have already done quite well with her. If you plan on continuing with her you can expect slow progress.*
   Hypothesis. Consultee probably expects too much of herself. Information is sketchy, but perhaps guilt is related to her "pressuring" child. *Reasoning.* Supportive statement. Restatement of clinical reality.

Consultee-10.   *Do you think I should?*

Consultant-10.   *That's really for you to decide. But as her emotional problems improve, your work with her should prove more helpful and effective.*

Hypothesis. The recurrent request for an external decision. *Reasoning.* Separating out again who is responsible for what order of decision. It also implies confidence in her to make her own decisions. At the same time, the consultant imparts clinically valid information that will help the consultee to decide [pp. 10–11].[3]

This vignette illustrates a number of principles that Kazanjian and his colleagues have found useful in their consultation practice (1962, pp. 5–7). First, consultation is an indirect service; primary contact is with the consultee rather than with the client. Second, the consultant should try to make general questions specific (examples: Consultant-1; Consultant-8). Third, it is appropriate to talk about a consultee's feelings or motivation but not about the consultee's personality dynamics or conflict (examples: Consultant-2; Consultant-5). Fourth, the consultant should permit the consultee to solve his or her own problem (example: Consultant-6). Fifth, the consultant can make use of his or her own feelings to bring into focus the feelings the client might engender in the consultee (example: Consultant-5). Sixth, the consultant should try to identify the emotional core of the consultee's problem (example: Consultee-6; Consultant-6). Seventh, the decision for consultee change should rest with the consultee (example: Consultee-10; Consultant-10). Eighth, when the consultant comes from a higher-status profession than the consultee, the consultant should avoid downgrading the profession of the consultee or putting the consultee on the defensive regarding his or her professional identity. Ninth, the consultant is not responsible for the consultee's professional adequacy. Tenth, the consultant should work in the here and now and avoid attempting to help the consultee understand the present in the light of the perhaps unconscious past. And, finally, the consultant should facilitate constructive communication between consultee and client.

This excerpt from a consultation session should serve to illustrate the skills and sensitivities needed by a mental health consultant. In many ways the practice of mental health consultation is more complex and demanding than the practice of psychotherapy; it seeks to have an impact indirectly, through intermediaries, rather than directly with a client population. Accordingly, one might expect that the training needed to become a skilled mental health consultant is far more arduous than that needed to become a skilled psychotherapist. For reasons that are not altogether clear, however, such training does not seem to be offered. Most persons functioning as mental health consultants have little or no special training and receive little or no ongoing supervision in their work as consultants.

---

[3]From *An Introduction to Mental Health Consultation,* by V. Kazanjian, S. Stein, and W. L. Weinberg. Public Health Monograph No. 69. Washington, D.C.: U.S. Government Printing Office, 1962.

EXAMPLES OF CONSULTATION PROGRAMS

Adler (1972, 1977) has provided a very useful description of a five-year history of the provision of mental health consultation services in a community mental health center. Adler views the mental health system as a set of four concentric circles. The innermost is the personal network, which includes the individual's family, friends, and neighbors. The next is the caretaker network, which includes such community institutions and professionals as public schools, work settings, health service delivery systems, and the clergy. The next is the professional mental health network—that is, formally designated mental health institutions and professionals. Finally, the outermost circle is the out-of-community network, including prisons and state mental hospitals. This view of the community's human services network is similar to that developed by Bower (1972).

Within this formulation, Adler says that the original community mental health center concept emphasized eliminating the outermost, out-of-community network and strengthening the mental health professional network. Only mental health consultation, as originally conceived, seemed to be directed at the caretaker network, in its efforts to increase the capacity of community caretakers to prevent, recognize, and manage problems in the settings where those problems actually occur.

After five years of program development and implementation in the field of mental health consultation, Adler reported that in the efforts of the mental health center to provide indirect services to caretaker agencies, stresses developed within the center with those components involved in providing direct services to clients. These stresses were resolved, in part, by the development of a direct-service program by the mental health consultation staff that focused on prevention. Such services included identifying and helping children who were not thriving in school, developing school-sponsored discussion groups with high-risk adolescents, and direct services to members of the community with mental health problems who came to the attention of the police. In addition, the consultation and education staff began providing skill-building services directly to the community, such as a tutoring and therapeutic play program for young underachievers from a disadvantaged community, developmental stimulation programs for infants and toddlers, and educational programs for parents of preschoolers. Many of these programs were begun under the sponsorship of the community mental health center but later became autonomous and independently supported.

Adler found that the original conceptualization of two kinds of services in community mental health centers—direct and indirect—was inadequate; there was, in reality, a continuum of services. This realization was crucial to the development of their consultation programs. In Adler's words:

> Dichotomies may be adequate to conceptualize the activities of psychiatrically oriented centers where only narrowly conceived treatment concerns are addressed,

and they may still serve in centers where work with community structures of the Caretaker Network occurs isolated from clinical issues. However, once into the interface area, traditional distinctions between "direct" and "indirect" service, between treatment and prevention, between consultation and service no longer hold. They not only cannot be separated, they often cannot be distinguished [1977, p. 123].

Pyle (1977) has described the development of consultative services to public school facilities in the community served by his mental health center. The consultation program was teacher-centered and was conceived of as a reciprocal relationship between peers who shared in the process of system diagnosis. The consultant served mainly as a facilitator and negotiator. Pyle wrote: "The consultant has a role in teaching diagnostic and problem-solving skills, but it is generally counterproductive for a consultant to attempt to solve the problem by him/herself" (p. 193).

Pyle has identified five principles that seem important in the successful development of a consultation program in the schools. First, the consultant should make it clear that difficulties in coping with the complex human inter-actions in the classroom are common and normal. Second, most teachers want to improve their classroom environment but need help in identifying what to improve and how to improve it. Third, the classroom teacher is an expert in understanding the emotional climate of the school, and the consultant draws on that understanding in learning about the relevant interpersonal networks outside the classrooms. Fourth, teachers must learn to understand the class-room environment, share in the diagnosis of classroom problems, and be actively involved in any ongoing change program. Finally, the consultant must be skilled in establishing productive interpersonal relationships, since credi-bility will be strengthened as the consultant becomes better known to the consultee.

Cherniss (1977) has provided an unusually interesting case history of an unsuccessful effort by a community mental health center to establish a school consultation program. The proposed program was discussed within the men-tal health center. About six months later, letters of invitation were sent to teachers, but it took so long to obtain an adequate response level that by the time it was possible to schedule meetings with interested teachers, the poten-tial consultation staff was no longer able to participate. At this point the project was abandoned.

Diagnosing the difficulties in getting this consultation program off the ground, Cherniss suggested, first, that there were problems in the staff mem-bers' approach to the schools: they had failed to involve the teachers, their target population, in their planning; they were unwise in characterizing the program as mental health consultation, since that could be thought of as an offer to provide mental health services for the teachers; and they seriously underestimated the time that would be required to inaugurate the program. In addition, Cherniss identified some difficulties within the mental health center itself. Its decentralized nature made it easy to start programs but difficult to sustain them, since very little active institutional support was available. Preventive services had far lower urgency in the thinking of the center's administrative staff than direct clinical services. Finally, Cherniss, who was planning the consultation program, was only part-time at the center and thus had little organizational status or authority.

From this experience as well as from experiences that have emerged elsewhere in the development of new consultation programs, Cherniss derived the following generalizations, among others: (1) recipients of proposed services must be involved in their early planning, (2) programmatic innovations can thrive only in settings where special mechanisms are developed to sustain them, and (3) creators of innovative programs will be successful to the extent that those persons are central to the functioning of the agency. On the basis of these experiences, Cherniss has concluded that systems-oriented, preventive programs, such as the one he tried to start, would do better if they were based not in a community mental health center but in an autonomous institution whose mission would be preventive rather than therapeutic.

Baizerman and Hall (1977) believe it would be useful to view mental health consultation as a political process; that is, establishing a consultation program is a bargaining process in which "expertise, organizational position, and personal and organizational reputation are the currency of the bargaining between consultant and consultee; and in which each actor attempts to maximize his currency at a minimum cost" (p. 143). From this point of view it may be easier to understand the experiences Cherniss reports. Baizerman and Hall write, for example, "The consultant is 'of' his agency, and hence may feel, may act, and may be seen by others (for example, the consultee) as a member of an agency. Herein lies the source of the notion in our definition that organizational position and organizational reputation are some of the units of currency in consultation" (p. 144). Cherniss's part-time status in his community mental health center may have resulted in his having a poor organizational reputation and thus poor bargaining power in the process of establishing the school consultation program. Similarly, teachers and the school system may have felt that they had too little to gain in terms of expertise to enter into a relationship that would be costly to them, if only in time and energy.

Kaseman and Anderson (1977) have described the development and first-year history of a consultation program for the local clergy. This program appears to have been quite successful, and it is therefore important to note that the program was established at the request of the clergy, who were interested in learning about family therapy and who were concerned about their own local clergy organization, which did not seem to be thriving. There were 23 full-time members of the clergy in the community, and 60–70% of them were actively involved in the consultation and educational program.

Following the expression of interest in such a consultation program, a task force was created that included representative members of the clergy and of the community mental health center staff. As a consequence of its meetings, a brief questionnaire was distributed to all clergy members in the community to identify their needs. The most commonly mentioned problems they found themselves confronting in the community were child-rearing questions, divorce, and alcoholism. They also expressed interest in how to be more helpful in working with families with an impending or recent death, an adolescent runaway, or need for a referral to other community resources. In addition, the local clergy association was seen as weak and ineffective. On the basis of this analysis, the task force established four goals: (1) to develop a more effective local clergy association, (2) to develop the pastoral counseling skills of the local clergy, (3) to develop community-based groups through the local clergy that could provide social support for people in need in the community, and (4) to develop a coordinated counseling program for the clergy to use with parishioners and other community residents.

Mental health center staff provided consultation on ways of strengthening the clergy association, provided six two-hour seminars on clergy roles and on pastoral counseling, helped develop social support groups for socially isolated middle-aged persons in the community and for persons with prior psychiatric histories, and worked toward development of a collaborative counseling program.

One year later, the clergy association seemed to be functioning well. Pastoral counseling skills were improving, social support groups were thriving, and clergy members were effective in starting new groups as needed. Work was still progressing on the coordinated counseling program. At the same time, the community mental health center felt it had gained much in the process of working with the clergy. Kaseman and Anderson summarized their experiences by noting that the program, "which has involved a minimum time commitment on the part of the agency task force, has been viewed as having positive results by the clergy, the community, and the agency. In addition to its stated goals, the program has also been influential in improving clergy-agency relationships, in creating a better understanding of respective roles, and in effecting a more collaborative understanding of community mental health" (1977, p. 91).

ASSESSMENT OF CONSULTATION PROGRAMS

There is a compelling quality to the concept of consultation as an indirect service. To the extent that consultation is effective, it can be a powerful strategy for extending mental health services by working through caretaking agencies. But, to be proved effective, consultation has to be evaluated in terms of its effect on the client population. It may not be sufficient to document merely that consultees find the consultation experience helpful or stimulating or enlightening without demonstrating a subsequent effect on clients.

It would seem, then, that an effective consultant needs to have both substantial competence in the areas of concern to the consultee and certain general personality traits. These traits should include the capacity to be permissive and accepting, the ability to share ideas constructively, the ability to relate effectively to other people, personal warmth, and an awareness of the subtleties of interpersonal relationships. No research has yet been reported in which the effectiveness of consultation has been related to these two sets of attributes. It would seem only logical, however, that an effective consultant/consultee relationship would demand both of them. Personal sensitivity would allow the consultant to help the consultee develop increasing access to his or her own feelings. Subject-matter skills would allow development of alternative ways of viewing the problem.

Resistance to consultation

Establishing mental health consultation programs often requires overcoming agency or institutional resistance. Berlin (1979) has identified four major types of resistance—inertia, active opposition, planned ineptitude, and feared loss of power. Inertia appears to be made up of "anxiety about any change which is felt by many members and its potential threats to particular entrenched positions. Change also imperils old methods of dealing with common problems. The threat of new learning often results in verbal acquiescence to suggestions for change but no real action to promote change" (p. 120).

Regarding active opposition as a type of resistance, Berlin writes: "Forces for change can be regarded as foreign bodies that are surrounded by a variety of entangling regulations and hierarchical layers, each of which needs to examine and approve any change and thus encapsulate these forces. The delays and the vagueness about where the plan stands in an organization tend to wear people out and make any organizational change too difficult to effect" (pp. 120–121).

As for resistance by ineptitude, Berlin notes that an administrator can agree to some form of change but can place the responsibility of implementing the change in the hands of totally inept subordinates and others who are committed to the status quo. Finally, Berlin suggests that certain administrators can deliberately mobilize parts of the organization to oppose a change when they themselves cannot acknowledge that they are in opposition to it.

If mental health consultants are to be effective in instituting organizational change, then they must, according to Berlin, have a thorough knowledge of the institution they seek to modify, have close working relationships with staff members throughout the organization, have an analytic approach to understanding the obstacles to change, understand the organization's typical ways of dealing with crisis, and establish effective alliances in the community and in the organization as well as effective bridges between the community and the organization.

Cautions about consultation

Gottlieb (1974) has expressed concern that although mental health consultation has been thought of as an important strategy for primary prevention in the community, it may in fact work at cross-purposes with primary prevention. Gottlieb suggests, first, that mental health consultation may defeat the purposes of primary prevention because it may focus the consultee on issues of assessment and treatment of clients, thus generating cases for treatment rather than increasing the consultee's tolerance of social deviance. Second, as Berlin (1979) has noted, mental health consultation may need to function within an organization that is refractory to change. That is, whereas individual consultees may be interested in changes in their ways of functioning, the task of the mental health consultant may be defined as helping the staff work better within the constraints imposed by the organization and the system of agencies of which the organization is a part. Gottlieb says that "the preventive potential of mental health consultation is limited when the organization itself is not defined as the consultee's client" (1974, p. 5).

Third, Gottlieb asserts that much mental health consultation is provided on the assumption that community caretakers are not functioning effectively as health-enhancing resources. In fact, argues Gottlieb, "such an assumption not only ignores the research which points to the high utilization and efficacy of these persons prior to their involvement with mental health professionals, but it also disregards the possibility that such involvement may weaken or destroy the natural, informal mode of helping which they have been practicing" (1974, p. 5). Gottlieb believes that naturally occurring support systems and deliberately created self-help groups and voluntary associations have a very strong preventive potential and that the mental health consultant may inadvertently weaken or destroy these natural help-giving community processes.

Consultation outcome studies

To assist community mental health centers in evaluating their consultation programs, Mannino and MacLennan (1978) reviewed how consultation services were monitored and evaluated in nearly 80 settings. They found that information being collected could be grouped into three categories: (1) information on the community being served, such as assessment of needs, survey of available resources, or characteristics of the population, (2) characteristics of the consultation program, such as target groups, frequency of contacts, financing, program descriptions, progress reports, or use of staff, and (3) outcome data, such as measures of consultee satisfaction, subjective judgments by consultants, or goal-attainment measures.

It is virtually impossible to develop an effective consultation program without knowing a good deal about the community being served. Mannino and MacLennan concluded that "often the only way to begin is by asking the professionals questions about the nature of the community they work in. Generally this must be done by asking very concrete questions about different aspects of the community, e.g., what are the schools like? How many are there? Where are they located? What kinds of people live in the community? Where do they work? How many and what kinds of churches are in the community, and so forth" (1978, p. 9).[4]

Monitoring consultation programs requires a systematic approach to program description. Mannino and MacLennan said that "such information is useful for planning purposes, modifying programs, designing training programs, and determining qualifications of staff. It can also help to determine whether or not the program is reaching those target groups or areas most in need of help. In addition, the information can be useful in relation to program review in order to determine whether the program is accomplishing what it set out to do" (pp. 22–23).

Finally, the effectiveness of consultation programs must be evaluated. Mannino and MacLennan suggested that

> approaches vary in technical sophistication, evaluative levels, and inherent problems related to reliability, validity, and the isolation of cause and effect relationships. . . . If incorporated into a permanent system of recordkeeping and monitoring, they can provide useful information about the extent to which program objectives are met. When viewed as part of the larger information process, they allow one to look at relationships between population characteristics and needs, program structure and processes, and program effect. This kind of information is needed by program managers and administrators to guide them in planning and managing consultation and education services in an intelligent and systematic manner [pp. 32–33].

In a study of factors influencing the outcome of consultation, Robbins, Spencer, and Frank (1970) undertook a pilot study with a sample of 143 persons from local health departments and voluntary agencies throughout the United States who had applied for grants under the United States Public Health Service Community Health and Facilities Act. These authors sought to determine whether there was a significant relationship between success in obtaining grant support and the use of consultation during the process of preparing the grant proposal. They found that there was a significant but moderate relationship. The authors next studied 35 consultations in California in detail, using questionnaires prior to consultation sessions, observation and tape recordings of the consultation sessions, questionnaires afterward, and a follow-up interview with each consultee two or three weeks later. Using a variety of measures of outcome, including consultee satisfaction and evaluation of the follow-up interviews, the authors were able to show that outcomes were better (1) the more prepared the consultant was, (2) the more interested the consultant was

---

[4]From *Monitoring and Evaluating Mental Health Consultation and Education Services*, by F. V. Mannino and B. W. MacLennan. DHEW Publication No. (ADM) 77–550. Washington, D.C.: U.S. Government Printing Office, 1978.

in the project, (3) the more supportive the consultant was, (4) the more familiar the consultees were with the consultants prior to the consultation, and (5) the higher the agreement among the participants on the purposes of the consultation. One of the most provocative aspects of the findings was that consultee satisfaction was related almost exclusively to variables that had little to do with consultant competence. Rather, the consultant qualities of interest, support, and familiarity were the ones that yielded consultee satisfaction. Signell and Scott (1971) suggest the same conclusion when they state "It is consistent with emerging consultation philosophy that content itself is less important than process" (p. 298). Clearly needed at this point are studies to determine whether personal attributes of the consultant allow the consultation to be effective even if the consultant has little or no competence in the substantive area of consultation.

Levine and Brocking (1974) assessed the effectiveness of nine novice graduate-student consultants by collecting ratings from 81 consultees who were undergraduate nursing students assigned to work in public health nursing offices. Consultees felt that the most valuable aspect of the consultation was the opportunity it provided to discuss their feelings about their cases. The consultants reported that they became much more aware of the impact on the family of illness, aging, and death of a family member and the importance of the consultee nurses' provision of emotional support to families coping with these problems.

Given the complexities of the consultation process and the often overly general statements of consultation program objectives, it should not be surprising that few well-controlled studies evaluating either consultee or client outcomes have been reported. But the studies that have been done warrant careful analysis. MacLennan, Montgomery, and Stern (1970), in providing an overview of the task of evaluating consultation services, write:

> All indirect services, such as consultation and training, affect both their immediate recipients and those the recipients serve. Consultation has impact at four main levels: directly in the consultee system; directly on the individual consultee; indirectly on the quality of mental health delivery to alleviate mental health problems in the client population; and indirectly on the individual client. Overall program evaluation should be concerned with all these levels, although at any one time, evaluation may concentrate on any of these aspects [p. 34].

In introducing a chapter on evaluation of consultation programs, Caplan (1970) writes:

> I have emphasized the necessity to evaluate the goal achievement of consultation, in order that the consultant might become aware of the differential effectiveness of various techniques that he uses in particular situations, so that he may improve his skills and learn to operate in a more consistently helpful manner. There are two aspects to such an evaluation. First, the consultant must record . . . an account of the consultation predicament and of how he appraised and dealt with it. . . .

Secondly, the consultant must develop some method by which he can assess whether and to what extent his particular technical response to the consultee's behavior achieved the desired result in improving the consultee's job performance and accomplishment. . . . Fundamentally, the goal of consultation is that the mental health of a client or a client population will be improved as a direct result of improved behavior of a consultee or group of consultees produced by the intervention of the consultant. Ideally, the technique used by the consultant should be specified and related to a change in the mental health of the clients that would not otherwise have occurred. The latter implies using some form of control group design—for example, a matched group of clients being dealt with by a matched group of consultees who do not receive the type of consultation being evaluated. Assuming the study group shows demonstrable, and if possible measurable, changes in mental health not shown by the control group, these changes should be ascribable to the altered operations of the consultees, which should in turn be of a nature that they can be linked with the intervention of the consultant. This implies demonstrating a chain of interlocking factors—that is, consultant intervention, change in consultee perceptions and attitudes, change in consultee-client behavior, resulting in change in client behavior and performance [pp. 294–295].[5]

The painstaking efforts of Caplan and his colleagues to evaluate their own theme-interference-reduction consultation illustrate the difficulties inherent in such evaluations. Their consultation program was organized in the 12 health centers of a city health department, and the consultees were the public health nurses who covered the city out of these district health centers (see Caplan, 1970, pp. 301–329). Over the three-year period of the study, 112 nurses were employed in the centers, of whom 86 made use of the consultation service. Consultation was on an intermittent basis; usually, a nurse saw a consultant for two or three successive visits and then not again for several weeks or months. A total of 331 clusters of such consultation visits, each called a consultation unit, were identified. Thus, each participating nurse averaged slightly less than four consultation units—a total of nearly six sessions.

The first question was whether it was possible to make reliable judgments about the presence or absence of the technique of theme-interference reduction from the detailed notes prepared by consultants after each consultation. The procedure appears to have been to select one consultation unit for each nurse and to ask two judges to rate that unit according to whether theme-interference reduction had taken place. Several pairs of judges were used, and in general it appears as if the judges agreed in about 75% of the cases. Since one would expect 50% agreement by chance, it seems clear that the concept of theme-interference reduction has some validity but that methods for identifying the concept operationally need considerable improvement. After this study, judges worked together to reconcile their differences and arrived at an

---

[5]From *The Theory and Practice of Mental Health Consultation*, by Gerald Caplan, © 1970 by Basic Books, Inc., Publishers, New York. Reprinted by permission.

agreement about each consultation unit, including those units not examined in the reliability study. Of the 331 consultation units, theme-interference reduction was judged to have taken place in 143 instances. In 57 of these 143 cases, the two judges' independent assessments were identical, and in 86 consensus was arrived at after the judges discussed their differences. These figures lend even greater urgency to the need to develop more reliable indicators of theme-interference-reduction consultation.

In addition to indicating the presence or absence of this particular type of consultation, judges made other assertions about the consultation—for example, whether its character was primarily educational or supportive and reassuring. These other judgments were made with even less consistency; judges disagreed more often than chance would dictate. Accordingly, most of the final determinations of characteristics of consultation units other than theme-interference reduction were made by consensus.

It must be understood that consultee nurses were not randomly assigned to a type of consultation. The type of consultation they received was determined by each consultant in an unsystematic way. Thus, in evaluating these data, it must be kept in mind that whether theme-interference-reduction consultation took place might be closely associated with a variety of characteristics of the consultee nurses, such as, obviously, the presence of theme interference or, less obviously, competence or mental health.

The first of the series of studies that Caplan reports shows that judged objectivity increased significantly more often in consultees who had received theme-interference reduction than in those who received other types of consultation. Caplan continues the analysis of the objectivity study to show that the nurses who scored lowest on objectivity at the start of the consultation unit were the ones most likely to receive theme-interference-reduction consultation. It is possible that consultation of any kind is unusually effective in situations in which consultees have initially low objectivity and thus that the finding linking theme-interference-reduction consultation with increased objectivity is spurious. What is required is a study in which consultees of varying initial levels of objectivity are systematically assigned to various types of mental health consultation.

In another study, Caplan and his colleagues presented a fictitious case history for interpretation both at the start and at the end of the data-collection period to the 86 participating consultees and to 71 nurses who did not ask for consultation or who worked in a neighboring community in which there were no mental health consultation programs. The groups were in no sense matched and differed quite dramatically in age, education, and length of service. Again the dependent variable was objectivity, and in this study the results were clearly negative—that is, those nurses who had had theme-interference-reduction consultation did not improve any more than did the control nurses. Regardless of group, those nurses with lowest initial levels of objectivity improved most. Part of the difficulty in interpreting this finding results from the fact that the measure of objectivity used in this project has a very low ceiling; the higher the initial score, the less the opportunity for improvement.

The description of this research is a model of self-critical reporting. The evaluation task is obviously formidable, and Caplan and his colleagues are quite cognizant of the preliminary nature of their findings. As they acknowledge, their research fails to demonstrate more than that a first step in the amelioration of defective attitudes of consultees toward their clients may have been taken. They were not able to study changes in consultee/client interactions or consequent improvements in client mental health (see Caplan, 1970, pp. 324–325), and they are not optimistic that such studies can be successfully undertaken.

In another early effort to evaluate a consultation program, Schiff and Kellam and their associates (Schiff & Kellam, 1967; Kellam & Schiff, 1967; Kellam, Branch, Agrawal, & Ensminger, 1975; Kellam, Branch, Agrawal, & Grabill, 1972; Schiff, 1972) developed a consultation service in a Black subcommunity of Chicago. The consultees were teachers and administrators in elementary schools and parents of the clients, and the clients were first-grade students. Twelve public and parochial elementary schools in the community were grouped into six matched pairs; one member of each pair served as a control, the other as the experimental school. The consultation program included weekly meetings between consultation program staff and members of the school hierarchy, including all first-grade teachers, classroom meetings between first-grade teachers and children, and meetings of the parents of all the first-grade children. The first-grade population was selected as the target because the community felt that young children were its first priority, because first-grade children were the youngest group that could be reached in totality, because the transition from family to school is a critical adaptational task, because the first-grade population was available for longitudinal study, and because the effects of working with this group had the potential for spreading throughout the institution. A final reason for working with this group in this community was that, in the judgment of teachers, nearly 70% of the children were mildly, moderately, or severely maladapting.

The experiment was begun in the fall of 1964 and involved about 1000 children in the intervention program and another 1000 in the control schools each year. Rather than collecting longitudinal data, the authors periodically collected from teachers adaptation ratings of first-grade children only.

> The results of the brief intervention program during the school year 1964–65, showed an increase in maladaptation by June of 1965 in the intervention schools, as compared to control schools, as indicated by end-of-year ratings. . . . Ratings made in the fall of 1965 on the *new, untreated 2,000 first graders* showed that a similar difference still existed between the intervention schools and the control schools. . . . The difference between the levels of adaptation in the control and intervention schools was also seen in the early ratings made on the *new, untreated 1966 first graders*. Our conclusion, therefore, is that the first measured impact of

the intervention program was a change in the standards of the teachers in the intervention schools in the direction of greater expectations [Kellam & Schiff, 1967, pp. 85–86].

The authors reported that the end-of-year ratings for the school year 1965–66 showed a significant shift toward greater adaptation in the intervention schools, while the control schools moved toward greater maladaptation.

The data presented by these authors show adaptation levels of first-graders at the start of three consecutive school years in both the control and the intervention-program schools. In the intervention-program schools, initial adaptation levels, which were very similar to those in control schools the first year, fell the second year and rose the third, ending at approximately the same level as they started. Since the data came from three separate groups of students, it is not possible to determine whether the fall in adaptation level was due to the rising expectations of teachers or to a real fall in adaptation level of the second group of children compared with the first group. It appears that adaptation level rose and then fell in the control schools and fell and then rose in the intervention schools, but it is not clear from the authors' report whether final adaptation levels differed significantly from initial levels.

The authors also describe a technique for assessing psychiatric symptoms that is entirely separate from the assessment of adaptation level and provide data suggesting that there is reasonably good agreement between these two measures. The highest agreement in ratings was between the psychiatric measure of clinical status and teachers' ratings of social contact—that is, of shyness, friendliness, aloofness, and so on. Psychiatric ratings were not significantly associated with teachers' ratings of authority acceptance, cognitive achievement, or ability to concentrate.

Another study evaluating the effects of consultation on clients of consultees as well as on consultees themselves was reported by Bolman, Halleck, Rice, and Ryan (1969). At the University of Wisconsin, biweekly small-group consultation was provided to about 25 upper-division students who served as student advisers in a residence hall housing about 1100 freshman and sophomore men and women. The control group consisted of the students in another residence hall, housing about 800 similar students. The authors found that in the experimental residence hall there was a significant increase in grade-point averages from the first to the second semester. The virtue of the control-group design can be seen in the fact that the same increase was noted in the residence hall where no consultation was provided. In the absence of a control group, it would have been tempting to account for the increased grade-point averages on the basis of the consultation being provided to residence-hall advisers. As it is, more likely explanations are dropping out by students who did poorly during the first semester and such factors as increased motivation, improved study habits, and increased comfort and familiarity with the university.

In addition to studying academic attainment, the authors examined the frequency of contacts students made with a variety of university agencies.

Again, no difference was found between the students in the experimental and the control residence halls. The authors believe that one of the reasons for the lack of significant positive consequences of their consultation program was that "the group meetings had served to bring into the open a latent conflict between dormitory housefellows and administrative personnel," which served to "neutralize any positive gains in knowledge or sensitivity by the housefellows, in that the application of such gains required administrative measures which were impaired by the lack of common goals" (Bolman et al., 1969, p. 513). As this study seems to document, the process of consultation within a complex agency system is far from simple and can have negative as well as positive reverberations throughout the system.

In an exploratory study of attitudinal changes in a group of 20 police-officer consultees and 14 doctoral-student and psychiatric-resident consultants, Zacker, Rutter, and Bard (1971) administered a series of adjective checklists and other scales before the first of the 14 weekly consultations and again near the end of the consultation period. Police officers experienced no significant changes in their attitudes. In contrast, consultants saw police as less aggressive by the end of the consultation period, although high in authoritarianism throughout the period. By the end of the consultation period, police officers were seen in a more favorable light and the police system in a less favorable one by the consultants. Changes in police-officer functioning during interpersonal conflicts were not measured. Perhaps the most informative aspect of this study was the fact that the consultees affected the attitudes of consultants, not vice versa. This finding underlines the interactive quality of the consultant/consultee relationship.

Ulmer and Kupferman (1970) evaluated the outcome of psychiatric consultation provided by one part-time, fee-for-service consultant to a private, vocationally oriented casework agency in Los Angeles during a ten-year period. Moed and Muhich refer to such a consultant, unattached to the agency being provided the consultation, as "disembodied" (1972, pp. 236–237). The consultation was predominantly client-centered. The consultant attempted to make specific recommendations for changes in the consultee's actions that might be helpful to the client. Evaluation data came from reports by consultees. There was no evidence that a consultee became more skillful in recognizing or treating emotional disorder as a consequence of the consultation, that consultation was helpful in assisting clients to get jobs, or that the professional development of consultees was markedly enhanced. In general, this consultation effort appears to have had little value.

In another study, Marchant (1972) administered counseling to a group of fourth- and fifth-grade students, case consultation to the teachers of another group, a combination of counseling and consultation to a third group, and neither counseling nor teacher consultation to a fourth (control) group. Four groups of 10 to 12 students each were selected on the basis of teachers' reports of behavior problems. During the five-week treatment period, each counselor or consultant visited each school twice weekly. At the end of the five weeks, each teacher again completed the report form used at the start of the study to identify problem behavior. Marchant found that, among all students combined (including those in the control group), there was a significant gain in adjustment scores from pretest to posttest; the gain was least in the control group. Furthermore, when the three experimental groups were contrasted, there were no differences among them in effectiveness. Thus, consultation was significantly better than no intervention, but so were counseling and a combination of counseling and consultation. Marchant concluded that "the techniques used in this study have been shown to have relatively immediate, short-term impact. . . . It might be helpful to note that teachers of children in the counseling only group expressed dissatisfaction at not being more involved in the counseling process. In that the counselor should provide services to children and teachers, a counseling and consultation method for working in the elementary school seems preferable" (p. 7).

In a review of empirical studies assessing the effects of consultation, Mannino and Shore (1975) conclude that "the evidence appears to indicate that consultation as a technique of intervention does have a positive effect" (p. 17).[6] These authors reviewed a large body of literature. Of the total of 35 studies they examined, nearly 70% demonstrated positive change of some kind. According to Mannino and Shore,

> There is much to suggest that progress is being made in the evaluation of consultation . . . although such progress has been slow. However, minor gains are preferable to major fallacies. We see a need for more studies in depth that could attempt to delineate process variables and relate these to outcome variables. Also, we continue to see the need for multivariate studies to study different levels of change in relationship to other factors, such as how the consultees' views and expectations of consultation affect outcome, or how experienced consultants and inexperienced consultants have different effects. In the final analysis, the more we can delimit the population studied, specify the activities performed, and use multilevel outcome variables, the more meaningful, and therefore more valuable, should be the results [pp. 17–19].

It is worth examining these 35 studies in slightly greater detail. First, of the 35 studies, 22 dealt with mental health, psychological, or psychiatric consultation. The others were less pertinent to the evaluation of mental health consultation. Of the 22 studies, 8 were unpublished. Of the 9 studies reported since 1971, 6 were unpublished. Thus, the more recent studies tended to be unpublished and, at the same time, as Mannino and Shore suggest, of better quality. For example, of the 14 published studies, only half used any type of control or comparison group, while all the unpublished studies used control

---

[6]From "The Effects of Consultation: A Review of Empirical Studies," by F. V. Mannino and M. F. Shore, *American Journal of Community Psychology,* 1975, 3, 1–21. This and all other quotations from this source are reprinted by permission of Plenum Publishing Corporation.

or comparison groups. In the published studies, 78% of the tested consultation effects were positive; in the unpublished studies, 56% were. Thus, there is some suggestion that the more recent, and better-controlled, studies yield poorer results. At the same time, it is always difficult to evaluate unpublished studies. Many are doctoral dissertations and have yet to pass the tests of methodological and substantive scrutiny imposed by journal reviewers.

Mannino (1981) has recently updated his overview of evaluation studies in the field of mental health consultation. As for the studies that seek to legitimize mental health consultation as a valid method of community mental health practice—that is, studies that seek to add to our knowledge base or to validate mental health consultation methods—Mannino believes that there has been a dramatic increase both in number and in quality during the past several years. The increase in quality is found in the more common use of control or comparison groups, in the development of several dependent measures of outcome, and in the careful description of the consultation method being evaluated.

Among studies that examined impact on consultees, about 60% found the consultation resulted in significant positive change. Among studies that examined the indirect impact of consultation on clients, nearly 40% showed significant positive change. Mannino concluded that "there are a number of studies of a variety of consultation approaches which have demonstrated some degree of effectiveness. It is only through continuing to accumulate evidence of this kind that we can establish a base of data attesting to the validity of consultation as a method of practice" (p. 150). Mannino's general views about the usefulness of mental health consultation can be seen in the conclusions from his review of recent evaluative research:

> Mental health consultation continues to be one of the most useful approaches to community mental health practice. Its relevance covers each of the levels of public health prevention, i.e., primary, secondary, and tertiary, and extends even further to the promotion of mentally healthy environments and communities. At times, even secondary and tertiary consultation activities include latent primary preventive and promotional effects. It is such factors as these that contribute to the potential worth of mental health consultation. To be sure, they also contribute to the exceedingly complex research problems which make it so difficult to document its validity as a practice method. Yet, if we are to advance the field, it is crucial that such efforts continue [1981, pp. 153–154].[7]

CONCLUSIONS AND OVERVIEW

The usefulness of consultation as a community mental health technique is being increasingly supported. Consultation has enormous appeal among mental health professionals, and substantial time is currently allocated to this

---

[7]From "Empirical Perspectives in Mental Health Consultation," by F. V. Mannino. In *Journal of Prevention*, 1981, *1*, 147–155. Copyright 1981 by Human Sciences Press. Reprinted by permission.

activity by mental health professionals working in community mental health centers. The field of mental health consultation is conceptually rich. In addition to the writings of Gerald Caplan, dealing with both conceptual and practical issues in mental health consultation, reports of group consultation have been presented by Altrocchi and his colleagues (1965) and by Spielberger (1967), and important overviews of the field have been published by Kazanjian, Stein, and Weinberg (1962), Cohen (1966), Altrocchi (1972), Grady, Gibson, and Trickett (1981), and, most recently, Cooper and Hodges (1983).

The problems inherent in documenting the positive effects of mental health consultation on clients are great; if it is difficult to demonstrate unequivocally the effectiveness of psychotherapy, how much more difficult it must be to demonstrate the effectiveness of an approach that asks a mental health consultant to assist an intervening person in providing more effective help to another set of persons. Yet, the potential of mental health consultation remains high. Some forms of client-centered consultation appear to be effective. Program-centered administrative consultation is often successful (Goodstein, 1978; Libo & Griffith, 1966; Scheidlinger, Struening, & Rabkin, 1970), and consultation is increasingly being viewed as a two-way interaction in which consultants also learn about the consultees and their clients. As Signell and Scott suggest, "Consulting in the interaction model means being changed by the consultees and clients whom one seeks to change" (1971, p. 298).

One must not dismiss a consultation program that has a measurable positive impact only on consultees. Such programs may very well increase job satisfaction and improve morale, increase productivity, and decrease turnover in a consultee group, and these goals may be quite legitimate in their own right. Thus, evaluation of consultation services depends, as do evaluations of any other community mental health service, on an explicit statement of program objectives. If the ultimate purpose of the consultation is to increase the well-being of the clientele of a consultee or group of consultees, then the evaluative effort has to examine client status. If, however, the purpose of the consultation is to effect change in consultees, evaluation can concern itself exclusively with measures of consultee characteristics relevant to program objectives.

These comments about consultation program objectives are important in the context of evaluation because much of the evaluation literature concerns itself with the changes in consultees. Yet consultation was originally envisioned as a major technique for preventing client mental health problems. Yolles (1969), when he was head of the National Institute of Mental Health, described the process whereby mental health consultation was included as an tial program component of a community mental health center.

As the months of planning went by, it became increasingly apparent that no mental health program could meet the needs of the people unless it began to prevent mental illness and improve the mental health of populations as well as of individual people. But even with increased support to finance training of core mental health professionals, communities could not develop such preventive services. What was needed then surely was for other helping professionals in the schools, the courts, the churches, and the social and welfare agencies to secure mental health consultation and education in adapting what they considered to be their own primary functions to the mental health needs of those residents of a community who came first to them for help. It was with this realization that consultation and education services were included as essential under eligibility regulations of the Mental Health Centers Act. *For the first time, provision of preventive services became mandatory in a publicly supported mental health program* [p. 14].[8]

The implications of this statement seem clear. Mental health consultation was seen primarily as a strategy for preventing mental disorders. Thus, in the early days of the community mental health movement, the terms *consultation* and *prevention* became virtually synonymous. Not only are these terms not synonyms, but, to the contrary, consultation and prevention are quite independent of each other. That is, mental health consultation may have as *one* of its objectives the prevention of psychological disorders through development of a consultative relationship with teachers or the clergy. But mental health consultation has a number of other objectives—providing case-management assistance to human service providers who are dealing with clients who are already psychologically disabled or providing assistance to organizations to help them function more effectively or efficiently. Neither of these two objectives has any significant relation to prevention. Similarly, although mental health consultation may be *one* of the techniques used in achieving prevention-oriented program objectives, a number of other techniques (see Chapter 5) totally unrelated to consultation may also be appropriate for achieving goals of prevention.

It is crucial to keep the distinction between mental health consultation and prevention firmly in mind: mental health consultation is a *process;* prevention is an *objective* or *goal.* As to its merit, although evidence of the indirect effects of mental health consultation on clients is slowly accumulating, it would probably be accurate to conclude that at present its effectiveness with consultees is more firmly established.

[8]From "Past, Present and 1980: Trend Projections," by S. F. Yolles. In L. Bellak and H. H. Barten (Eds.), *Progress in Community Mental Health* (Vol. 1). Copyright 1969 by Grune & Stratton, Inc. This and all other quotations from this source are reprinted by permission.

3

Prevention of Mental Disorders

The three chapters in this section deal with concepts and activities central to the prevention of mental disorders. Chapter 5 introduces the most important basic concepts that need to be understood for a useful grasp of prevention as a set of values and techniques, and examines the new field of risk-factor research. Chapter 6 deals with stressful-life-event theory and reviews the literature linking such events to both physical and emotional disorders. The chapter also illustrates the usefulness of stressful-life-event theory for the design and implementation of preventive intervention programs. Chapter 7 presents an overview of the field of mental health education, a major approach to prevention, and demonstrates its utility by providing a number of examples of educational programs in action.

CHAPTER

5

Basic Concepts in Prevention

Until very recently, it was generally believed that at any given moment 10% of the population was at least partly disabled by an emotional or psychiatric disorder. Indeed, the phrase "one out of ten" has long been the rallying cry of citizen advocates for expanded services for the mentally ill. Yet, tragically, in spite of the continually increasing capacity of the American mental health service delivery system to provide care, it is now estimated that 15% of the American population suffer from some form of emotional disorder and that, of these 32 million persons, nearly 7 million receive no care of any kind (Regier, Goldberg, & Taube, 1978).

It is an important public health axiom that most illnesses are controlled by prevention rather than by treatment. In the United States, at least, there seems to be no alternative other than to conclude that emotional disorders will not be controlled until more resources are put into programs that prevent such disorders before they start.

Interest in the prevention of emotional disorders is growing rapidly, and Albee (1980) has suggested that this growth has many of the characteristics of a revolution, one that will challenge both the authority of the mental health establishment and the current disproportionately large allocation of mental health resources to treatment for persons who are already emotionally disordered.

Although the rationale for expanded preventive programs seems unobjectionable, the issues that are raised as one discusses prevention can quickly become very complex and often controversial. It is important to clarify these issues because this complexity results partly from inadequate understanding of some basic concepts in the field of prevention (Caplan, 1961b, 1964; DeWild, 1981).

President Kennedy's interest, cited earlier, in the prevention of mental disorders can be seen as part of a long tradition in thinking about psycho-pathology. In 1922 Adolf Meyer wrote: "Communities have to learn what they produce in the way of mental problems and waste of human opportunities, and with such knowledge they will rise from mere charity and mere mending, or hasty propaganda, to well-balanced early care, prevention and general gain of health" (cited in Brand, 1968, pp. 22–23). In 1931, Harry Stack Sullivan wrote: "Either you believe that mental disorders are acts of God, predestined, inexorably fixed, arising from a constitutional or some other irremediable sub-stratum, the victims of which are to be helped through an innocuous life to a more or less euthanastic [sic] exit . . . *or* you believe that mental disorder is largely preventable and somewhat remediable by control of psychosociological factors" (cited in Brand, 1968, p. 28).

Interest in prevention as an alternative to treatment has, of course, a far longer history. In the 12th century, the Spanish philosopher Maimonides described the eight degrees of charity.

> The *first* and lowest degree is to give, but with reluctance or regret. This is the gift of the hand but not of the heart. The *second* is to give cheerfully but not proportionately to the distress of the sufferer. The *third* is to give cheerfully and proportionately, but not until solicited. The *fourth* is to give cheerfully, propor-tionately, and even unsolicited, but to put it in the poor man's hand, thereby exciting in him the painful emotion of shame. The *fifth* is to give charity in such a way that the distressed may receive the bounty, and know their benefactor. The *sixth*, which rises still higher, is to know the objects of our bounty but remain unknown to them. The *seventh* is still more meritorious, namely, to bestow charity in such a way that the benefactor may not know the relieved persons, nor they the names of their benefactors. The *eighth* and the most meritorious of all, is to anticipate charity by preventing poverty; namely, to assist the reduced fellow man, either by considerable gift, or a sum of money, or by teaching him a trade, or by putting man in the way of business, so that he may earn an honest livelihood, and not be forced to the dreadful alternative of holding out his hand for charity [cited in Cohen, 1927].

Interest in prevention of emotional disorders may currently be increasing as part of the trend toward giving more attention to prevention in general. Interest in preventing infectious and nutritional diseases has always been high, and it seems to be growing. The 1979 report of the Surgeon General of the United States Public Health Service on health promotion and disease preven-tion (U.S. Department of Health, Education and Welfare, 1979b) noted that death rates from tuberculosis, diphtheria, poliomyelitis, infant mortality, and heart disease, among other causes, have all fallen in recent years, while life expectancy has increased by 2.7 years in the past decade. Although these gains are due, in part, to improvements in sanitation, housing, nutrition, and immunization, more recent gains are due to measures people have taken to help themselves—changes in life-styles resulting from a growing awareness of the impact of certain habits on health. The report notes that Americans are deeply interested in improving their health and that the increasing attention being paid to exercise, nutrition, environmental health, and occupational safety all testify to this increasing interest in health promotion and disease prevention. The report concludes that "with the growing understanding of causes and risk factors for chronic diseases, the 1980s present new opportunities for major gains. Prevention is an idea whose time has come. We have the scientific knowledge to begin to formulate recommendations for improved health. And, although the degenerative diseases differ from their infectious disease predecessors in having more—and more complex—causes, it is now clear that many are preventable" (1979b, p. 7).

In the first volume of the *Annual Review of Public Health* (Breslow, Fielding, & Lave, 1980), the editors noted in their preface that after some years during which a preventive strategy was not thought possible against such major causes of mortality as cardiovascular disease and cancer, prevention has once again become an important aspect of public health thinking. This change is due to several factors. First, our knowledge base has increased significantly, particularly regarding such disorders as lung cancer and other lung diseases, dental caries, and cardiovascular disease. Second, much of that knowledge base has been successfully applied so that mortality and morbidity rates have been reduced—for example, the death rate from lung cancer among British physicians after they began to quit smoking, the morbidity from dental caries after the introduction of fluorides into public water supplies, and the earlier and better management of high blood pressure as a way of reducing the disability and death rate from that disorder. A third factor has been the increasing public awareness of controllable hazards to health. For example, even though some people still smoke cigarettes, by 1975 nearly nine out of ten persons believed that smoking endangers health. Furthermore, a very large number of smokers had tried to quit, and many had succeeded.

HISTORICAL CONTEXT OF DISEASE PREVENTION

A review of medical history shows that preventive activities have been significantly more successful than treatment services in reducing the prevalence of most diseases. This is true for both the infectious and the nutritional diseases and, one hopes, will be found true for the vast number of chronic conditions, among which can be counted the mental disorders. Long before the acceptance of germ theory, in the 18th and early 19th centuries, European and American sanitarians and humanitarians had singled out odors and odor-producing accumulations of filth as the causes of all disease and proposed a massive clean-up campaign and sewage-disposal system as a disease preventive. The emphasis on cleanliness and on the eradication of *miasmas*, or noxious odors, had enormous consequences. By 1800, maternal mortality had dropped to one-seventh of its 1750 level; typhoid fever, yellow fever, tuberculosis, typhus, cholera, and infant mortality all were sharply reduced, without the benefit of germ theory. It is not generally known that Florence Nightingale started the nursing profession during the Crimean War (1853–1856) as a protest against germ theory. She wrote:

> I was brought up . . . to believe that small-pox, for instance, was a thing of which there was once a first specimen in the world, which went on propagating itself, in a perpetual chain of descent. . . . Since then I have seen with my own eyes and smelt with my nose small-pox growing up in first specimens either in close rooms or in overcrowded wards where it could not by any possibility have been "caught" but must have begun. Nay, more, I have seen diseases begin, grow up, and pass into one another. I have seen, for instance, with a little overcrowding continued fever grow up; and with a little more, typhoid fever; and with a little more, typhus, and all in the same ward or hut [pp. 14–15].[1]

Miasma theory held that soil polluted with waste products of any kind gave off a "miasma" into the air, which caused many major infectious diseases of the day. According to this theory, which dated from the writings of Hippocrates, these "poisonous substances" rose up from the earth and were spread through the winds. People living near swamps, and thus particularly vulnerable to marsh gases, were thought to develop fever from these gases—a fever that came to be known as *malaria* (bad air).

The miasmatist believed the way to prevent disease was to modify the environment—to remove the sources of the miasma. The early miasmatists declared war on all refuse quite indiscriminately. Accumulated manure was considered just as dangerous as a cesspool that was contaminating a supply of drinking water. The public health movement had its beginnings with these early environmental and sanitary engineers, who sought to prevent disease by removing and preventing the accumulation of filth.

It must be remembered that sanitary conditions were unbelievably bad in the mid-19th century, particularly in those urban areas to which large numbers of immigrants were attracted in order to work in factories that were being established with the start of the industrial revolution. Rosen (1958) described these crowded urban areas in England from the point of view of a public health historian.

> The infrequency of sewage and garbage removal, as well as the neglected state of the courts and alleys around which the houses were built, gave rise to the practice of using them as places of deposit for all the residents of a given court. As a result, there was scarcely a court that was not occupied by a communal cesspool or dunghill. Houses in the poorer districts had no water closets, and many had no

---

[1] From *Florence Nightingale and the Doctors*, by Z. Cope. Copyright © 1958 by J. B. Lippincott Company. Reprinted by permission.

privies. These conditions were not restricted to the homes of the working classes, but they were worst there. In "Little Ireland" in Manchester, there were two privies to 250 people. Nearby Ashton had one district with only two privies for 50 families, and such instances could easily be repeated for other communities. Instead of water closets or privies, there was a "necessary," a kind of tub that had to be emptied every morning. Even with this facility, the situation was grim. In one Manchester district the needs of some 7000 people were supplied by 33 "necessaries," that is, supplied after a fashion. Since there was in most cases no access to the back yard except through the house, all the dirt and filth had to be carried through rooms, passageways, doorways, and over pavements, which were defiled as a result. This cloacal inferno was even intensified by the rapid migration during the 1840's of thousands of starving Irish who streamed through the port of Liverpool to huddle in the cellars and hovels of factory towns and cities like Birmingham, Bristol, Leeds, Manchester, and others.

The overcrowding in these dwellings can be imagined. Manchester had 1500 cellars where three persons, 738 where four, and 281 where five slept in one bed. In Bristol there were 2800 families, of whom 46 percent had one room each. Liverpool had 40,000 people who lived in cellars and 60,000 in close courts as described. These figures must be seen against the background information that out of a population of 223,054 in the 1841 census, 160,000 belonged to the working classes. In short, more than 70 per cent were workers and more than 60 per cent of these lived in crowded, dirty, insanitary conditions [pp. 205–206].[2]

The odors that emanated from these quarters must have been unbearable, and miasma theory undoubtedly made very good sense to those members of the community who became interested in sanitary reform. Dubos (1959) described the events that were taking place in the 1850s.

To a group of public-minded citizens guided by the physician Southwood Smith and the engineer Edwin Chadwick, it appeared that, since disease always accompanied want, dirt, and pollution, health could be restored only by bringing back to the multitudes pure air, pure water, pure food, and pleasant surroundings. This simple concept was synthesized in the movement "The Health of Towns Association," the prototype of the present-day voluntary health associations throughout the world. Its aim was to "substitute health for disease, cleanliness for filth, order for disorder, . . . prevention for palliation, . . . enlightened self-interest for ignorant selfishness, and bring home to the poorest, . . . in purity and abundance, the simple blessings which ignorance and negligence have long combined to spoil—*Air, Water, Light!*" [pp. 124–125].

Although miasma theory has given way to the germ theory of disease and to the doctrine of contagion, its effectiveness should not be minimized. Shryock (1949), contrasting the effectiveness of the miasmatists in disease prevention with the effectiveness of doctors in disease treatment, noted that

[2]From *A History of Public Health,* by G. Rosen. Copyright 1958 by MD Publications, Inc. Reprinted by permission.

the conviction that the quickest way to improve the health of the poor was through sanitation received statistical verification during the 1850's when various British towns showed marked mortality declines following the establishment of sanitary controls. . . . At the same time that sanitation promised so much, direct medical care of the poor seemed to promise little. . . . It is no wonder that lay reformers . . . had more confidence in what mathematics could do for the poor than they had in medicine [p. 41].

As we will see, one of the concepts currently used by mental health professionals seems analogous to the pre-germ-theory view of disease—namely, that disorders are caused by noxious elements in the environment (stresses) and that much emotional disorder can be eliminated by removing the stresses or increasing the population's resistance to them.

SOME USEFUL PUBLIC HEALTH CONCEPTS

In viewing the development of any disease, it has been found useful to consider three components that in combination have been shown to explain the disease process. First, one needs to understand relevant characteristics of the vulnerable individual, or *host*—his or her general health, past history, genetic makeup, vitality or robustness, level of fatigue, and so on. Second, one needs to identify the relevant characteristics of the *environment*—its physically or psychologically stressful aspects. Finally, one needs to identify an *agent*—that modality or sequence of events by which stressful aspects of the environment become internalized so as to result in some identifiable disease or disorder. For example, in studying malaria, scientists have been able to determine that there is differential vulnerability to this disease process, that the agent is a specific type of mosquito, and that this particular mosquito breeds in certain swampy areas in the tropical and subtropical regions of the world. Malaria or any disease can be prevented, at least theoretically, by significant modification of the potential patient, the agent, or the environment. Thus, efforts to eradicate malaria should be successful if they involve increasing people's resistance to the disease, rendering the mosquito sterile or eliminating mosquito breeding grounds. In fact, this last method has been and is being successfully used.

Using the same conceptual framework, one can look at factors that produce automobile accidents. Driving when tired, driving when drunk, and driving too fast are all characteristics or behaviors of the driver that have been shown to increase the risk of automobile accidents significantly. The automobile itself, as the agent, has been identified in a variety of studies as responsible for many accidents, and characteristics of the road surface or weather or light have been shown to be environmental factors associated with automobile accidents. Efforts to reduce the incidence of automobile accidents have been aimed at all three types of factors.

Basic definitions

In the control of any disorder—emotional or physical—two types of interventions exist. The first type seeks to reduce the number of persons suffering from the disorder—that is, to reduce the *prevalence* of the disorder. The second type seeks to reduce the severity or discomfort or disability associated with the disorder. Programs designed to reduce severity, discomfort, or disability are formally known as *tertiary prevention* but are better known as *rehabilitation*. With lifelong disorders, rehabilitation programs generally have little effect on prevalence. Indeed, a well-run rehabilitation program may actually increase the prevalence of these disorders by increasing life expectancy. Unfortunately, given our current knowledge, many emotional disorders appear to be lifelong or nearly lifelong and thus cannot be significantly reduced in prevalence through rehabilitation programs.

Because the prevalence of any disorder is a function of its duration and the rate at which new cases are produced, two approaches to reducing the prevalence of a disorder are commonly used. The first seeks to reduce prevalence by reducing the duration of the disorder, usually through the development of some form of early casefinding combined with the prompt application of effective treatment. This approach is formally called *secondary prevention*. Secondary prevention efforts are preventive only in that systematic early casefinding brings with it the possibility of reducing the duration of the disorder.

Should a technique for the early identification of some disorder be applied without the concomitant development of more effective treatment procedures, a paradoxical increase in prevalence of that disorder would occur. Gruenberg has commented that "without an effective treatment, early diagnosis only provides more work for clinicians without changing the prevalence of the disorder" (1980, p. 1323). For example, the duration and prevalence of diabetes have increased because of improved techniques for early detection. A similar increase has occurred for Down's syndrome as a consequence of the development of antibiotics, which have significantly reduced the death rate from secondary causes among persons with that syndrome (Gruenberg, 1977).

The alternative approach to prevalence reduction is to reduce the rate at which new cases of a disorder develop. This approach seeks to reduce prevalence by reducing *incidence* and is formally designated as *primary prevention*. This is the concept that most closely matches the lay use of the term *prevention*. Effective primary prevention programs actually prevent disorders from occurring or reduce the likelihood that a disorder will occur in a particular population (Adam, 1981; Perlmutter, Vayda, & Woodburn, 1976).

The concept of primary prevention requires that the intervention take place in a population free of the disorder. It might be appropriate to consider the development of a primary prevention program for schizophrenia aimed at a sample of neurotics, but as long as it is thought that acute and chronic schizophrenia are part of a single continuum, it would be incorrect to suggest that effective treatment services provided for acute schizophrenics constitute a primary prevention program for chronic schizophrenia. Such programs, though critically important, are in fact secondary prevention; that is, they seek to reduce the duration of a disorder already present. However, physical rehabilitation and consciousness-raising programs for postmastectomy patients can quite legitimately be considered primary prevention for emotional disorders (Goldston, 1977).

Disease prevention and health promotion

Some disorders can be prevented by highly specific procedures—procedures that do not appear to be effective in preventing anything other than that specified disease. Malaria can be prevented by destroying the breeding grounds of a particular type of mosquito. There is no evidence that any other disease is thereby prevented. Drinking fluoridated water dramatically reduces the incidence of dental caries. No other disorder is reduced by fluoridated water. Although the mechanisms that give rise to a specific disease or disorder may not be completely understood, many diseases can be prevented by the application of such procedures, and as will be seen, this disease-specific prevention strategy has been very effectively used for several psychiatric disorders.

The disease-prevention paradigm that has governed research and intervention programs during the past two centuries can be outlined as follows:

1. Identify a disease of sufficient importance to justify the development of a preventive intervention program. Develop reliable methods for its diagnosis so that people can be divided with confidence into groups according to whether they do or do not have the disease.
2. By a series of epidemiological and laboratory studies, identify the most likely theories of the path of development of that disease.
3. Mount and evaluate an experimental preventive intervention program based on the results of those research studies.

This, in somewhat oversimplified form, is the paradigm we assume whenever we think about the prevention of a specific disorder. The paradigm has been remarkably effective for a broad array of communicable diseases—smallpox, typhus, cholera, typhoid fever, plague, malaria, diphtheria, tuberculosis, tetanus, and more recently, sexually transmitted diseases, rubella, and polio—and an equally impressive list of what are now known to be nutritional diseases: scurvy, beriberi, pellagra, rickets, kwashiorkor, endemic goiter, and dental caries.

All these diseases have one attribute in common. For each, there is an identified necessary, though not always sufficient, biological precondition for its appearance—lack of thiamine or niacin, protein deficiency, invasion of a particular bacillus, lack of fluoride, and so on. Because of this necessary precondition, we can talk about the "cause" of a particular disease. In keeping

with this tradition, active research has been underway for some time to identify the biological bases of specific psychiatric disorders.

In contrast, a variety of nonspecific practices, such as providing crisis-
intervention services or social support during times of stress, may have a
positive effect on health in general and may, in fact, prevent a variety of forms
of disordered behavior. Those practices that have a generally salutary but
unspecifiable effect on health are called *health promotion* (McPheeters, 1976).
Eisenberg defines *health promotion* as those activities that "contribute to resistance to disease, even when the disease agents are not known or beyond
control" (1981, p. 5).

One of the most influential documents dealing with ways of improving
the general level of health in a population was prepared by the Canadian
Minister of National Health and Welfare (Lalonde, 1974). It dealt with both
disease prevention and health promotion strategies. In this report, Lalonde
introduced the concept of the *health field* and its four components: human
biology, environment, life-style, and health care organization.

Human biology refers to aspects of health that are developed within the
human body and are related to the organic nature of the individual, including
genetic makeup. *Environment* refers to those matters outside the body over
which the individual has little if any control and which can affect health.
Included in this category would be food and water purity, air pollution, safe
disposal of sewage, noise control, and road and vehicular safety.

Life-style refers to decisions people make about their own behavior, over
which they have considerable control, that can affect their health—for example, overeating, smoking, abuse of alcohol and other drugs, insufficient exercise, or careless driving. Finally, *health care organization* refers to the quality,
quantity, and distribution of health-related services in any community.

Using the health-field concept, one can examine morbidity or mortality
rates to determine to what extent these rates could be reduced. For example,
it has been estimated that 75% of traffic deaths can be accounted for by pathological life-styles, 20% by the environment, and 5% by defects in the health
care organization. Similarly, it has been estimated that self-destructive life-
styles account for about half of all deaths that occur before age 70 and that
20% of these premature deaths can be attributed to just two life-style habits—
cigarette smoking and excessive use of alcohol.

Since the publication of this Canadian report, there has been a growing
interest in examining life-styles and their role in illness and in premature
death. As part of this interest in health promotion, mental health professionals
are beginning to examine various aspects of life-styles to ascertain their role
in predisposing people to emotional disorders or in precipitating such disorders in vulnerable populations. The explicit objective in this examination is to
develop programmatic strategies for preventing emotional disorders before
they start.

Types of prevention programs

Catalano and Dooley (1980) have proposed dividing primary prevention programs into those that are proactive (having the goal of avoiding the risk factor altogether) and reactive (having the goal of preparing people to react effectively to unavoidable risk factors). Thus, proactive strategies seek to prevent specific stressors, while reactive strategies attempt to enhance coping strategies in dealing with stressors once they have occurred. A proactive strategy, for example, might be to try to reduce the number of divorces by programs for improving marital happiness. A reactive strategy would be to help people adapt more successfully to divorce so that it would not be such a shattering experience. It is Catalano and Dooley's view that far more can be done proactively to prevent mental disorders than is generally believed.

One can select the recipients of preventively oriented programs in several ways. One approach has been to aim preventive programs at the *total population* in a defined geographic area. Programs of water purification and sewage disposal are communitywide in their impact. Mental health education efforts using the mass media are aimed at the total community. A second method is what might be called the *milestone* approach. A preventive service is provided to the members of a community when they reach a particular, predefined point in their life histories—sometimes a point thought to constitute a turning point— or when they undergo some particular stressful life event. For example, in the mental health field, the transition from being a preschooler to starting school has been viewed as such a turning point. Accordingly, a major intervention program at the Woodlawn Mental Health Center in Chicago (Kellam et al., 1975) involved all first-grade children in the area this center serves. Anticipatory guidance techniques, consultation, and crisis intervention can all be used in milestone programs.

A third approach has been to identify groups of persons at *high risk* of developing the behaviors that the program is designed to prevent. Because industrial health studies have shown the harmful respiratory effects of engaging in certain forms of mining or the dangers to the eye involved in using a grindstone, preventive measures such as wearing face masks or goggles are usually required. Similarly, crisis-intervention services could be instituted for all preschool or school-age children facing such hazards as the death of a parent or a sibling. Consultation could be provided to attorneys of persons petitioning for a divorce, on the basis of evidence linking marital disruption with subsequent psychiatric disability. Anticipatory guidance services could be made available to workers getting ready to retire or to homemakers whose youngest child is within a few months of graduating from high school and leaving home. Identification of such turning points can proceed by informal observation or from the analysis of changing role-performance requirements in the developing person. Identification of high-risk groups most usually proceeds, however, from epidemiological investigations that seek to discover the personality characteristics significantly associated with the development of certain psychiatric disorders.

Bolman and Westman (1967) identify three major categories of preventive services: *person-centered, family-centered,* and *society-centered* programs. Among person-centered programs, because Bolman and Westman are particularly interested in the mental health of children, they concentrate on identifying programs for reducing the incidence of casualty before or soon after birth, programs for children with special defects (for example, the mentally retarded and blind), programs oriented toward the child/parent relationship, programs oriented toward hazardous events in childhood, and programs oriented toward the child in school. With regard to family-centered programs, Bolman and Westman illustrate programs oriented toward intact families, culturally deprived families, families in crisis, and families undergoing disorganization. As community-centered or society-centered programs, the authors mention mental health planning projects, community development and community organization activities, education, and social action. Although Bolman and Westman help identify new directions in preventive intervention, it is useful to remind ourselves that we do not now systematically provide those preventive services that have demonstrated effectiveness, such as well-baby clinics, nutritional services, or genetic counseling.

In a related paper, Bolman (1967) outlines an array of preventive psychiatric programs that might be offered for children. His outline includes 15 program types, ranging from identifying and treating maternal disease before birth of the child, to preventing or minimizing the damaging consequences of such childhood crises as hospitalization or loss of a parent, to the provision of adequate facilities for recreation, group experiences, and so on for schoolchildren. If one were to add to this array those programs that seek to reduce stress in adults who have recently experienced a stressful event, such as a natural disaster, combat, divorce, or retirement, the list of preventive programs would be very close to complete. Other reviews of preventive intervention programs can be found in Roberts (1968), Bower (1969), and Flanagan (1971).

MacMahon, Pugh, and Hutchison (1961), in discussing the evaluation of community mental health programs, distinguish between the evaluation of accomplishment—testing the hypothesis that "a certain practice, if successfully carried out within specified limits, has a measurable beneficial outcome in the group on whom it is practiced" (p. 964), and the evaluation of technique—finding out whether "a supposedly therapeutic or preventive practice is in fact being carried out" (p. 964). This distinction is important because it forms a very useful basis for classifying preventive intervention services. One category includes those programs whose effectiveness has not yet been documented. In this case, the fundamental question is whether the program works— that is, achieves its objectives. The other category includes those programs whose effectiveness has already been established. In this case, one wants to determine whether all people who could benefit from the program are in fact receiving it.

In viewing these preventive strategies, it is useful to keep in mind that, like water purification or swamp spraying, a program emphasizing community change can significantly influence the entire population. Person-oriented programs are somewhat more limited in their breadth of influence, although, like smallpox vaccination, they may be enormously effective. When one takes a broad ecological view of mental disorders and their prevention, it is easy to become a generalist and to agree with Rogers's argument that "general preventive measures directed at the determination and control of the underlying patterns of environmental relationships will prove more efficient and effective in the long run than so-called specific measures" (1962, pp. 759–760). Sanford makes the same point:

> Where our concern is with people who are not yet disordered we dispense with the assumption of various diseases each with its specific causes which can be discovered and removed, and . . . accept fully the organismic view of the person. . . . If we do this last, it will become clear that any planned action affecting a person's welfare must take into account his complexity and potentialities for further development, and that the goal of full development should take precedence over goals of preventing particular forms of disorder [1972, p. 462].

PREVENTABLE PSYCHIATRIC DISORDERS

There is by now a well-established knowledge base regarding the role of specific intervention in preventing specific psychiatric disorders. The American Public Health Association (1962) has identified six categories of mental disorders that are preventable, in part because they are all disorders of known etiology. Although these disorders do not form a large proportion of all mental disorders, nearly all result in chronic brain syndromes, many are lifelong in their effects, and they represent an enormous cost to society as well as to the victims and their families (Gruenberg, 1980; Kornberg & Caplan, 1980).

Diseases caused by poisoning

The first group of preventable disorders is those caused by poisoning. These disorders are typically subdivided into acute poisoning, the result of intentional or accidental ingestion of drugs, inhalants, or solvents; and chronic poisoning, caused by prolonged exposure to industrial toxins or prolonged use of medications or addicting drugs. Over 250,000 chemicals and drugs can be poisonous, including, for example, acetone, arsenic, barbiturates, carbon monoxide, cyanides, DDT, kerosene, morphine, and turpentine. Poisonings account for about 3000 deaths every year and another 3000 survivors who are left with chronic brain syndromes. Prevention requires changes in the environment, in life-styles, and in the health care system—specifically, more prudent prescribing, dispensing, and storage of drugs, more careful control over drug prescriptions and their renewal, reduced exposure to industrial poisons, better safety standards in industrial and agricultural settings, better labeling of industrial and household products, and prompt and accurate diagnosis and medical treatment. Health education can play an important role in achieving these objectives, as can changes in laws and regulations and the development of a network of readily accessible poison-control centers.

Diseases caused by infections

The second category of preventable disorders is those resulting from infectious agents that can invade the central nervous system and leave permanent brain damage. Infections during the fetal period, such as those caused by rubella, syphilis, and toxoplasmosis, can produce severe mental retardation, epilepsy, perceptual and cognitive defects, and difficulty in impulse control. Rubella can be prevented by administering gamma globulin to women who have not previously had the disease. Successful treatment of syphilis in the mother prevents the development of fetal syphilis. Prompt treatment of toxoplasmosis can prevent the transmission of the disease during pregnancy.

Infectious diseases during childhood, such as pertussis, influenza, measles, meningitis, mumps, and tuberculosis, can also produce permanent brain damage that can lead to defects in sensory, motor, and intellectual development. Many of these infectious processes can be prevented by immunizations; yet, substantial proportions of young children are not completely immunized against these diseases (Eisenberg, 1981, pp. 9–10).

Genetic diseases

Some preventable disorders are brought about by a genetic process. Among these conditions are Tay-Sachs disease, phenylketonuria, galactosemia, tuberous sclerosis, and Huntington's chorea. The severe mental retardation produced by phenylketonuria and galactosemia can be prevented by special diets. For most genetic disorders, carriers can be identified or risks estimated on the basis of family studies, and genetic counseling can help reduce the number of vulnerable children.

Nutritional diseases

Other preventable mental disorders are produced by nutritional deficiencies, including beriberi, Wernicke's encephalopathy, kwashiorkor, pellagra, and anoxemia. These prolonged nutritional deficiencies during childhood appear to have a general impact on mental development and increase the risk of mental retardation, epilepsy, and a variety of perceptual and cognitive disorders. In addition, there is considerable evidence that general nutritional deficiencies increase vulnerability to infections. Dietary supplementation combined with nutritional education can prevent many of these disorders.

Diseases caused by injuries and systemic disorders

The fifth category of preventable mental disorders is those caused by injuries to the central nervous system, including falls, gunshot wounds, and vehicular accidents. The incidence of such injuries can be dramatically reduced by making the sources, such as guns, less readily available, by encouraging the use of protective equipment, such as motorcycle helmets and seat belts, and by improving the safety of motor vehicles and roads. Finally, there are a number of preventable or treatable general systemic disorders that can produce chronic brain syndromes, such as erythroblastosis fetalis, hyperthyroidism, cretinism, intracranial masses, toxemia of pregnancy, and prematurity.

The case of motorcycle helmet use laws

Current studies of the effectiveness of motorcycle helmets in reducing both injury and mortality rates are unusually interesting because the laws governing their use are in a very fluid state. A very large proportion of the survivors of motorcycle accidents have what are called *organic mental disorders* in which structural damage to the brain with permanent residual impairment in the form of dementia (loss of intellectual abilities) or delirium (clouded consciousness) has occurred. In addition, these studies are worth examining because they illustrate the controversy that is often generated in the discussion of prevention when health-related values appear to be in conflict with economic considerations and values related to personal liberty.

More than 4000 persons were killed and 350,000 injured in motorcycle accidents in 1977, representing a rate seven times that in automobile accidents. Head injuries are the major cause of such deaths and are far less frequent among persons wearing protective helmets than among those not wearing them. As a consequence of earlier findings like these, when federal funds became available in 1967 for state highway safety programs, states were required to enact motorcycle helmet use laws in order to qualify for those funds. By 1975 virtually all states had enacted laws requiring motorcycle riders to wear helmets, and studies of the effectiveness of these laws showed that both mortality rate and degree of severity of nonfatal injuries subsequently decreased. Fatalities fell by about 30% (Watson, Zador, & Wilks, 1980). That is, there was an annual reduction of more than 1000 in motorcycle fatalities and of many times that number in nonfatal injuries.

In 1976 the U.S. Congress removed the financial penalty for noncompliance with the helmet-law provisions, influenced in part by the lobbying of organizations such as the American Motorcyclist Association that are opposed to this requirement. Between 1976 and 1978, 26 states repealed their motorcycle helmet use laws. Studies in those states showed substantial increases in motorcycle fatalities and injuries following the repeal of these laws. In 1979 nearly 5000 motorcyclists died in crashes (Watson, Zador, & Wilks, 1981).

Watson and colleagues (1980) found a 38% increase in motorcycle fatalities in those states in which helmet laws had been repealed when contrasted with geographically and demographically similar states in which the laws had not been repealed. Of the 26 states where the helmet law was repealed, fatality rates increased in all but three. Noting that the mortality rate was twice as high among unhelmeted as among helmeted riders, Watson and colleagues concluded that "the repeals of motorcycle helmet laws have been one of the most tragic decisions made recently in the USA from the standpoint of public health" (1980, p. 583). In a related study, Muller (1980) ascertained that more than $60 million could be saved annually if all motorcyclists were to wear helmets. In spite of these studies, current efforts to reenact motorcycle helmet use laws at the state level are generally unsuccessful.

Current status of disease prevention in psychopathology

At least two forms of psychiatric disorders have been virtually eliminated in the past 50 years. In both cases, the disorder was the consequence of a physical disease process, and elimination of the disease resulted in elimination of the psychiatric disorder. The first is a disorder called *psychosis with pellagra.* Pellagra is a disease caused primarily by a deficiency of niacin in the diet, and with the increase in proper attention to dietary intake, the associated psychoticlike symptoms have virtually disappeared. The second is *general paresis,* an organic psychosis secondary to the syphilitic infection. With the successful ability to prevent and treat primary syphilis came a reduction in the incidence of this psychiatric disorder. In the 1920s, 8–10% of patients admitted to state mental hospitals were suffering from general paresis. Now these older patients are dying, and almost no patients with this diagnosis are being admitted. This reduction is a direct consequence of the decrease in the incidence of syphilis and of earlier and better treatment of the disease when it is diagnosed (Kolb, 1968b, pp. 231–242).

Preventable conditions that are not being completely prevented include fetal rubella, Down's syndrome, phenylketonuria, Huntington's chorea, and a variety of organic brain syndromes due to poisons, industrial and environmental contamination, and improper use of medication and other drugs.

With respect to diseases we now know how to prevent, additional investigations are required only when it appears that effective procedures are not being applied. That is, for example, when we do not know why, in view of the clear effectiveness of seat belts in reducing automobile accident injuries, drivers and passengers persist in failing to wear them, or why a substantial proportion of people are not immunized against diseases such as measles that can sometimes have profoundly harmful effects on central-nervous-system functioning.

The knowledge base pertinent to the primary prevention of psychiatric disorders is being expanded by the field of risk-factor research. Such research has not yet made sufficient progress so that the list of preventable emotional disorders can be expanded beyond what has already been presented. It is to risk-factor research, however, that attention is being directed in the hope that additional emotional disorders will soon become preventable. A recent report dealing with the current status of risk-factor research (Regier & Allen, 1981) includes reviews by Garmezy (1981) on children at risk for schizophrenia, by Kety and Kinney (1981) on adult schizophrenia, by Hirschfeld and Cross (1981) on depression, by Prange and Loosen (1981) on affective disorders, by Marks (1981) on anxiety, and by Martin and Guze (1981) on personality disorders.

Regarding children at risk for schizophrenia, a number of potential risk factors have been identified, although far more research on each factor will be necessary for sufficient certainty about its causal role. The risk factors that are now suspected include birth complications, postpartum psychiatric disturbance in the mother, adoption and foster placement, and certain aspects of attentional dysfunction, particularly the ability to sustain attention under conditions of distraction.

There is evidence of substantial genetic risk for adult schizophrenia. In addition, it has been suggested, though not yet established, that obstetrical complications such as prolonged labor, season of birth, prenatal maternal stress, infectious processes, and dietary factors may also increase the risk of schizophrenia.

Risk factors for depression appear to be psychosocial rather than biological, and suspected factors include such variables as sex, age, social class, and marital status. That is, depression is more common among older people, females, the poor, and people with disrupted marriages. In addition, depression appears to be associated with frequent stressful life events and with a weakness in the extent of personal resources.

For personality disorders, the evidence suggests some hereditary predisposition. In addition, the possible role of psychosocial factors is under study by a number of investigators.

In addition to these summary reports, two recent summaries have appeared regarding possibilities for prevention of childhood psychopathology. The two conclusions differ remarkably. Schwartz and Johnson (1981) have concluded that

> the primary prevention of childhood psychopathology remains a largely unfulfilled hope. Nonspecific educational programs for children and for their parents, while seemingly worthwhile, have not been related to the prevention of any form of childhood psychopathology. Schizophrenia and the other psychoses of childhood are not well enough understood to be prevented, although the various high-risk research programs hold some hope for the future. Delinquency, a costly and important social problem, has been the focus of a great deal of effort that has led to little noticeable change in its incidence. It would seem that high-risk studies may be of use in clarifying some of the potentially modifiable causes of delinquency as well [p. 384].

Erickson's (1982) summary statement provides a very different conclusion. She writes: "The possibility of preventing a substantial percentage of behavior and developmental problem cases has become increasingly feasible.

Identification of etiological factors, genetic counseling, prenatal diagnosis, and early postnatal physical and behavioral assessment all contribute toward a reduction in the number of cases or the severity of children's behavior disorders, or both" (p. 310).

These two summary statements differ in part because they focus on different aspects of the task of primary prevention. The latter statement deals much more with those aspects of childhood psychopathology that appear to be preventable.

RATE CALCULATIONS IN EPIDEMIOLOGY

Incidence, prevalence, and duration

As has been indicated, the three principal measures of interest to epidemiologists are incidence, prevalence, and duration. These measures not only are of importance in their own right but are used in the assessment of risk factors. Calculation of incidence rates is particularly difficult for psychological disorders because it is extremely difficult to determine when such disorders begin. Accordingly, to provide an initial illustration of how such rates are calculated, data on leukemia will be examined.

Tables 5–1 and 5–2 show the calculation of measures of incidence, prevalence, and duration. These tables provide information on acute and chronic leukemia for the five-year period 1948–1952 in the white population of Brooklyn, New York. In 1950 that population was 2,525,000. Keep in mind that these statistics were collected before the development and widespread use of antileukemic drugs. Five-year survival rates are now 40% for chronic leukemia, 15% for acute leukemia in adults, and 55% for acute leukemia in children ("Cancer: A Progress Report," 1981).

Table 5–1 shows there were 7 patients alive on January 1, 1948, who had previously been diagnosed as having acute leukemia. During the next five years, 410 new cases were found. Of this total of 417 cases, 395 patients died during the study period and 15 were lost track of, leaving 7 still alive at the end of the period. With regard to chronic leukemia, 129 patients were alive on January 1, 1948, who had been diagnosed previously, and 366 new cases were diagnosed during the next five years. Of this total of 495 cases, 384 patients died and 30 were lost track of during the study period. At the end of the study period, 81 were still alive.

The *prevalence* of acute leukemia on January 1, 1948, was 7 cases. The rate is thus 7 cases per 2,525,000 total population, or 2.77 cases per million. Selection of the size of the standard population (in this case, 1 million) is arbitrary; the rate of 2.77 per million is the same as .227 per hundred thousand or .00277 per thousand. Similarly, the prevalence of chronic leukemia on January 1, 1948, was 129 cases per 2,525,000, or 51.09 cases per million. These figures, in addition to similarly calculated prevalence rates for 1950 and 1952, are shown in Table 5–2.

TABLE 5–1.   Acute and chronic leukemia in the white population of Brooklyn, New York, 1948–1952.

	Acute leukemia						Chronic leukemia					
Year	Alive at beginning of year	New cases	Total	Deaths	Lost trace of	Alive at end of year	Alive at beginning of year	New cases	Total	Deaths	Lost trace of	Alive at end of year
1948	7	69	76	54	7	15	129	79	208	50	8	150
1949	15	91	106	86	3	17	150	83	233	71	5	157
1950	17	83	100	73	3	24	157	90	247	90	6	151
1951	24	99	123	101	1	21	151	61	212	84	7	121
1952	21	68	89	81	1	7	121	53	174	89	4	81
Total	84	410	494	395	15	84	708	366	1074	384	30	660

Adapted from *Epidemiologic Methods*, by B. MacMahon, T. F. Pugh, and J. Ipsen, copyright 1960 by Little, Brown and Co., and from *Epidemiology: Principles and Methods*, by B. MacMahon and T. F. Pugh, copyright 1970 by Little, Brown and Co. Reprinted by permission.

TABLE 5-2. Prevalence, incidence, and duration of acute and chronic leukemia, derived from Table 5-1

Measure	Type of leukemia	
	Acute	Chronic
Prevalence, 1948 (per million)	2.77	51.09
Prevalence, 1950 (per million)	6.73	62.18
Prevalence, 1952 (per million)	8.32	47.92
Incidence, 1948 (per million)	27.33	31.29
Incidence, 1950 (per million)	32.87	35.64
Incidence, 1952 (per million)	26.93	20.99
Average prevalence, 1948–1952 (per million)	6.65	56.08
Average incidence, 1948–1952 (per million)	32.48	28.99
Average duration, 1948–1952 (in years)	0.21	1.93
Average duration, 1948–1952 (in months)	2.46	23.21

Annual *incidence* rates are calculated in the same manner. The number of new cases diagnosed during the year is converted into a rate per standard population unit. During 1948, for example, 69 new cases of acute leukemia were identified, or 27.33 cases per million. During 1948, 79 new cases of chronic leukemia were diagnosed, or 31.29 cases per million. These and other incidence rates are shown in Table 5–2.

Because the incidence and prevalence rates tend to show substantial annual variation, it is useful to calculate average rates. From Table 5–1 it can be determined that the average number of acute leukemia patients alive at the start of each year was 16.8—that is, 84 divided by 5. Thus, the average prevalence was 16.8 cases per 2,525,000, or 6.65 cases per million. Similarly, the average number of persons diagnosed each year as having acute leukemia was 82—that is, 410 divided by 5. On this basis, one can calculate that the average incidence was 82 cases per year per 2,525,000 population, or 32.48 cases per million. Similarly, the average prevalence of chronic leukemia can be calculated at 56.08 cases per million, and the average incidence can be calculated at 28.99 cases per million per year.

Finally, one can calculate the average *duration* of the two conditions by using the formula $P = I \times D$. For acute leukemia, substituting 6.65 for P and 32.48 for I yields a value for D of .20 years, or 2.4 months. For chronic leukemia, using the same procedure, one can calculate that the average duration was 1.93 years, or 23.2 months. Obviously, one could calculate duration directly by following all known cases until their termination. This direct method yields more accurate results, but it is also far more time-consuming and therefore more costly, and except under special circumstances it will not yield results dramatically different from those obtained with this simple equation. Among

these patients, for example, special follow-up studies revealed that the actual
average duration of acute leukemia was 2.4 months and of chronic leukemia
20 months.

Similar calculations for stays in state and county mental hospitals are
shown in Table 5–3. These calculations yield important information about
hospital use but should not be thought of as indicating actual incidence, prevalence, or duration of mental disorders. Unduplicated hospital admissions
during a given year (called *additions*) can be thought of as analogous to incidence. Total number of inpatients in residence at the end of a given year can
be thought of as analogous to prevalence. Average duration of hospitalization
has been calculated using the same formula as was just used in estimating the
duration of acute and chronic leukemia.

As seen in Table 5–3, incidence was fairly stable over the period 1971–
1977, while prevalence steadily decreased. Accordingly, it should not be surprising to learn that average duration of hospitalization decreased from 7.8 to
4.6 months during this seven-year period. It should be remembered that the
use of the equation to calculate duration is valid only to the extent that one is
dealing with a stable situation. In dealing with mental hospital statistics, the
situation is not stable: prevalence is significantly decreasing each year. The
extent of this instability can be seen in the fact that average length of hospitalization for patients admitted into state and county mental hospitals in 1975
was less than 1 month (see Rosenstein & Milazzo-Sayre, 1981).

Admission rates can also be calculated for various demographic subgroups.
The results of such calculations are shown in Table 5–4 for sex and age and
in Table 5–5 for marital status and sex (see Rosenstein & Milazzo-Sayre, 1981,
for additional details). In these calculations, the numerator is the actual number of patients admitted during 1975, and the denominator is an estimate of
the total population in that same demographic category—that is, the number
of people in the demographic category at risk of being admitted into psychiatric facilities.

TABLE 5–3. **Incidence, prevalence, and calculated duration data for state
and county mental hospitals, 1971–1977**

	1971	1973	1975	1977
Additions (incidence)	474,923	422,530	433,529	414,507
Inpatients at end of year (prevalence)	308,983	248,518	191,395	159,405
Average duration (in months)	7.81	7.06	5.30	4.61

From *Provisional Patient Movement and Selective Administrative Data, State and County
Mental Hospitals, by State: United States, 1977,* by M. J. Witkin. Statistical Note No. 156.
Washington, D.C.: U.S. Government Printing Office, 1981.

TABLE 5–4. Admission rates per 100,000 population[a] to selected mental health facilities[b] by sex and age, United States, 1975

Age	Total, both sexes	Male	Female	Ratio male-to-female rate
Under 18	988.6	1169.0	801.2	1.5
18–24	2298.7	2432.9	2172.9	1.1
25–44	2726.8	2589.5	2855.9	0.9
45–64	1597.1	1748.4	1458.7	1.2
65+	785.4	793.5	779.8	1.0
Total, all ages	1690.5	1767.8	1618.3	1.1

[a]Population estimates used as denominators for rate computations are from *Current Population Reports*, Bureau of the Census, Series P-25, No. 614.
[b]Includes the inpatient psychiatric services of state and county mental hospitals, private mental hospitals, VA neuropsychiatric hospitals, VA general hospitals with separate psychiatric units, and nonfederal general hospitals with separate psychiatric units; the outpatient psychiatric services of free-standing clinics plus those affiliated with other mental health facilities; and federally funded CMHCs.

Figures such as those in Tables 5–4 and 5–5 can provide very useful information about groups in the population that appear to be especially vulnerable for admission into mental health facilities. For example, Table 5–4 makes it clear that young adults are far more likely to be admitted into mental health facilities than people in any other age group and that males under age 18 are substantially more vulnerable than females under 18. Table 5–5 reveals the excess risk of admission for separated and divorced persons, regardless of sex.

Measures of risk

Epidemiologists are interested in such questions as who becomes ill, why, and what can be done to reduce the risk of illness. One of the goals of the field of epidemiology is to find a modifiable risk factor—that is, a risk factor that can be manipulated through social or individual action so as to lower the incidence of a disease, a disorder, a disability, or death (Gruenberg, 1981).

Two measures of risk can be identified. The first, *attributable risk*, is the rate of a disease or disorder in a population of exposed persons that can be attributed to the exposure—that is, the rate among exposed persons from which is subtracted the rate among unexposed persons. Table 5–6 shows the risk of lung cancer associated with cigarette smoking. The death rate from lung cancer is 2.27 per 1000 among heavy smokers and 0.07 per 1000 among nonsmokers. Thus, the attributable death rate is 2.20 per 1000 (MacMahon & Pugh, 1970, p. 233). In other words, of all deaths from lung cancer among heavy smokers, 2.20 out of 2.27 (or 97%) can be attributed to smoking.

Using such risk calculations, one can calculate what the reduction in death rate would be among the exposed population if the exposure were terminated. For example, the risk of death from lung cancer among all smokers (not just

TABLE 5–5. Admission rates per 100,000 population to public or private psychiatric hospitals by marital status and sex, United States, 1969–1975

Year	Type of hospital	Sex	Marital status				
			Never married	Married	Separated/divorced	Widowed	Total
1969	public	M	757.6	169.8	2012.6	1046.9	310.2
		F	398.8	119.4	712.3	359.7	195.4
1970	public	M	438.8	132.6	2975.9/2167.6	629.6	331.3
		F	242.1	124.8	1065.5/758.6	249.2	212.2
1970–1971	private	M	927.4	271.8	1904.9	416.1	422.5
		F	524.6	300.8	907.6	543.1	357.7
1975	public	M	501.1	122.1	1712.4	355.6	318.5
		F	216.8	81.7	595.1	152.6	159.7

From "Marital Disruption as a Stressor: A Review and Analysis," by B. L. Bloom, S. J. Asher, and S. W. White. In *Psychological Bulletin,* 1978, *85,* 867–894. Copyright 1978 by the American Psychological Association. Reprinted by permission.

TABLE 5-6. Relative and attributable risks of death from selected causes associated with heavy cigarette smoking by British male physicians, 1951-1961

Cause of death	Death rate[a] among nonsmokers	Death rate[a] among heavy smokers[b]	Relative risk	Attributable death rate[a]
Lung cancer	0.07	2.27	32.4	2.20
Other cancers	1.91	2.59	1.4	0.68
Chronic bronchitis	0.05	1.06	21.2	1.01
Cardiovascular disease	7.32	9.93	1.4	2.61
All causes	12.06	19.67	1.6	7.61

[a]Annual death rates per 1000.
[b]Heavy smokers are defined as smokers of 25 or more cigarettes per day.
From Doll and Hill, in *British Medical Journal*, 1:1399-1410, 1460-1467, 1964. Reprinted by permission.

heavy smokers) is 0.65 per 1000. Since the death rate among nonsmokers is 0.07 per 1000, the attributable death rate from lung cancer among all smokers is 0.65 minus 0.07, or 0.58. Therefore, one can conclude that the death rate from lung cancer would be reduced by 89% (0.58 divided by 0.65) among all smokers were they not to smoke. If one knew what proportion of a particular population smoked, one could then predict the total number of lives that would be saved in that population from lung cancer if there were no smoking.

The second type of risk that is frequently of interest is called *relative risk*. Relative risk is the ratio of the rate of some disease among an exposed population to that among an unexposed population—that is, the rate among the exposed population divided by the rate among the unexposed population. Drawing once again on the data on cigarette smoking and lung cancer, it can be calculated that the risk of death from lung cancer is 32 times as high among heavy smokers as among nonsmokers (2.27 divided by 0.07).

If one is interested in preventing a particular disease or disorder, the measure of relative risk will give more valid information on which a preventive intervention program could be mounted. The measure of attributable risk, however, gives a good indication of what the impact of a successful preventive intervention program might be on mortality in the population being studied.

EPIDEMIOLOGY AND THE IDENTIFICATION OF HIGH-RISK GROUPS

Epidemiology is the study of the distribution and determinants of disease prevalence. In studying the distribution of a disease or a disorder, we are involved in the field of *descriptive epidemiology*. In studying its determinants, we are interpreting its distribution in order to identify possible causal factors.

When data that allow evaluation of these possible causal factors are collected, one can speak of the field of *analytic epidemiology*. When such analyses lend themselves to trial programs designed to study the power of our causal explanations, we have entered the field of *experimental epidemiology*. Thus, descriptive epidemiology shades into demography and human ecology. Analytic epidemiology is related to applied (field-study) research, and experimental epidemiology is sometimes indistinguishable from program evaluation.

From the time of Hippocrates through the era of the European sanitarians, into the modern era of germ theory and nutritional theory, the epidemiologist has noted that diseases have not been randomly distributed over time, places, and persons and has sought to identify causal factors by analyzing these differences in distribution. One after another, the great infectious and nutritional diseases have succumbed to the clinical and environmental research of the epidemiologist, bacteriologist, and nutritionist, until today it can be asserted that techniques are available for the prevention of virtually every major infectious and nutritional disease.

The challenge in the field of the infectious and nutritional diseases at present is in the fact that, in spite of our understanding of the microbiology and physiology of these disorders, they continue to be *endemic* (always present to a greater or lesser extent in a particular area) or *epidemic* throughout most of the world. The contribution of the epidemiologist has already been made. The fate of these diseases now rests in the hands of the social scientist. The causal connection between iodine deficiency and exophthalmic goiter, for example, is crystal clear, yet, in many places in southeast Asia, goiter, with its resultant sapping of productivity, intellect, and life expectancy, remains endemic, and its eradication is struggled against by its very victims because of the belief that, without a large goiter, a Burmese or Laotian or Cambodian woman may not be considered a desirable marriage prospect. Beriberi—a nutritional disease endemic in the Philippines—can be prevented simply by ceasing to remove the hulls and outer layers of rice before eating. Yet an extraordinarily resistant strain of folklore has arisen around this yellowish outer layer that makes this simple preventive measure literally unpalatable. As we just saw, the role of cigarette smoking in the etiology of lung cancer is extraordinarily powerful; about 90% of the deaths attributed to lung cancer could be prevented by stopping cigarette smoking. Yet it is clear that this solution, though simple, is not easy.

The great unfinished work of epidemiologists is in the chronic diseases, including coronary artery disease, cancer, and the mental disorders. Although mental disorders are rarely fatal, as a group they are responsible for more long-lasting misery than any other pathological health condition. It is the search for causes of these conditions that now largely occupies the epidemiologist.

Until quite recently, people who studied the factors associated with mental disorders tended to concentrate their efforts on what are termed *predisposing* factors, such as parent loss or other specific traumas in childhood. But the long time intervals between such events and their presumed consequences have made it virtually impossible to identify any such factors with certainty.

The past decade or two has witnessed a shift in emphasis away from considerations of predisposing factors in mental illness toward a concern with *precipitating* and *perpetuating* factors. This shift has set the tone for much that is innovative in the community mental health movement. The literature on precipitating proximal factors in the occurrence of mental disorders was reviewed by Reid (1961) and, more recently, by B. S. Dohrenwend and B. P. Dohrenwend (1974).

Little is known about the process by which events in the environment lead to mental disorders, but evidence has been mounting that implicates environmental stresses in the development of psychopathology. Thus, Steinberg and Durell (1968) have shown that entrance into military service is a significant precipitating factor of schizophrenia, and Brown and Birley (1968) were able to demonstrate that crises and life changes are associated with subsequent psychiatric hospitalization. Barthell and Holmes (1968) showed that social isolation during high school was associated with hospitalization for schizophrenia at least two years after high school graduation. Wechsler and Pugh (1967) demonstrated that psychiatric hospitalizations were significantly more common among people whose personal characteristics differed from the prevailing characteristics of the communities they lived in than among people who lived in homogeneous communities with which they shared important characteristics. All these studies suggest that environmental stresses play a significant role in the precipitation of psychiatric disorders, and they are presented as examples of a far wider literature.

These studies should not suggest, however, that psychopathology is a one-dimensional phenomenon. Social factors are implicated in the development of emotional disorders, but not everyone exposed to the social factors becomes disordered, and there are undoubtedly complex interactions between characteristics of the individual and characteristics of his or her social environment. Indeed, complex interactions most often characterize physical disease development as well. An example is breast cancer in mice:

> Apparently under natural conditions breast cancer occurs very rarely in this species. Special strains of mice can be bred, however, in which a high proportion of the offspring develop breast cancer spontaneously. Thus a genetic process is involved in the genesis of the disease. It has also been found that a particular virus is present in the milk of lactating mothers of these specially bred strains. If the offspring of such mothers are removed at birth from their mothers and suckled by mice who do not excrete this virus, no breast cancer develops. Thus, even though such baby mice possess the genetic characteristic, they do not develop breast cancer in the absence of the virus. Furthermore, if mice born from mothers who do not belong to this special strain, are removed from their mothers at birth, and are suckled by mice who do excrete the virus, they still do not develop breast

cancer. Thus exposure to the virus without the genetic predisposition is also without effect. In addition, not all mice born of and suckled by these specially bred mothers develop breast cancer; only female mice do, male mice being immune. Injection of female sex hormone, estrogen, into the male offspring, however, makes them as susceptible as the females. Thus the presence of the genetic factor plus the virus is without effect in the absence of the appropriate hormone. Finally, if mice in which all three factors are present are placed on a low caloric diet, the subsequent incidence of breast cancer is drastically reduced [Cassel, 1964, pp. 1483–1484].[3]

Efforts to discover relationships between sociocultural factors and psychopathology, and thus to identify groups of people at high risk of developing psychiatric disorders, have occupied the attention of social scientists for the last half century. This research interest, besides being of enormous theoretical importance, raises the hope of developing intervention programs that might reduce the magnitude of the problem of mental disorder. Until the early 1950s, most studies of social factors associated with psychiatric disability dealt with known psychiatric patients and sought to develop a greater understanding of them as a group and of how they differ from the general population. The increasing research funding in the early 1950s made possible a group of studies designed to extend the understanding of psychiatric disability into the population at large by identifying psychopathology in persons living in the community.

The pioneering effort to study social aspects of mental disorders in the United States was undertaken by Faris and Dunham (1939), using data assembled at state institutions and private hospitals in the Chicago area for the period 1922 to 1934 and from the County Psychopathic Hospital for the years 1930 and 1931. The authors showed that when all cases of mental disorder were plotted by residence at the time of admission, the resulting prevalence rates exhibited a regular increase from the more affluent and better-organized peripheral portions of the city to the central, poorer, more socially disorganized areas. After showing certain differences in this general spatial pattern for various diagnostic categories, the authors derived some hypotheses to account for their findings. The spatial pattern found for schizophrenic patients was quite similar to the pattern found for all patients combined.

First, the authors examined the possibility that people suffering mental disorders drift into the central slum areas of the city. If this hypothesis were true, argued the authors, the distribution of older cases would show a closer relationship to geographic area than the distribution of younger cases (since younger persons would presumably have had less time to drift). This hypothesis was rejected when older and younger cases were found in roughly the

---

[3]From "Social Science Theory as a Source of Hypotheses in Epidemiological Research," by J. Cassel, *American Journal of Public Health*, 1964, *54*, 1482–1488. Reprinted by permission of the American Public Health Association.

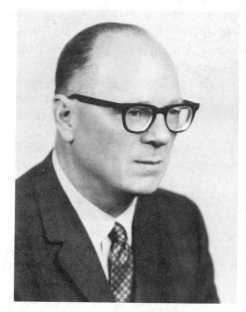 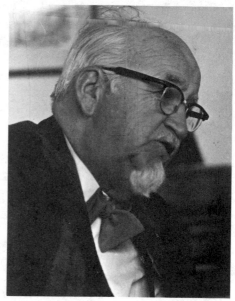

Robert Faris (left) and Warren Dunham, who pioneered the study of the social aspects of mental disorders. *(Photo of Faris courtesy of Mulholland Studios, and photo of Dunham courtesy of Warren Dunham.)*

same concentration in the central city. The alternative hypothesis—namely, that social conditions in central areas of the city were somehow a cause of the high rates of mental disorder found there—was then examined and found worthy of further study, particularly in light of the extensive social isolation found in the central city. In fact, Faris and Dunham concluded that "extended isolation of the person produces the abnormal traits of behavior and mentality" (1939, p. 173). In supporting the assertion that social causation seemed a more likely explanation for their findings than social selection, the authors noted, on the basis of other research, that conditions producing isolation are more frequent in disorganized communities and, from their own data, that admission rates for blacks, foreign-born persons, and native-born persons are all significantly higher in areas not populated primarily by their own members—that is, in areas where each group might be isolated by virtue of its minority status.

Nineteen years later, a study conducted in New Haven, Connecticut, that attempted to link social class to mental illness was published. In this study, Hollingshead and Redlich (1958) also dealt with identified psychiatric patients, considering as a patient any person who had been in treatment with a psychiatrist or under the care of a psychiatric clinic or mental hospital between May 31 and December 1, 1950, and who had been a resident of the greater New Haven area when treatment began. Data about these patients were taken from their clinical record. In addition, social and demographic data were collected by means of interviews with a 5% stratified sample of the New Haven community. The data collected from this sample were compared with the data collected from patients' records. Social class for patients and for the community sample was assessed using a formula that included area of residence, occupation, and education. Supplementary information was collected about the characteristics of psychiatric practice and about fee practices of agencies and private practitioners.

Hollingshead and Redlich were able to document that the poor are far more often coerced and compelled into entering treatment than the affluent, that identified mental disorder is generally more common among the lower socioeconomic classes and especially prevalent in the lowest class, and that while neurotic disorders are more common among the more affluent, psychotic disorders are more common in lower socioeconomic groups. They found significant differences in where, how, and for how long patients were treated—always favoring the highest social classes. Moreover, people in the higher classes spent more money on treatment. Hollingshead and Redlich examined their data in terms of the drift (social selection) hypothesis advanced by Faris and Dunham and came to the same conclusion as the earlier authors—namely, that psychotic patients from slum areas did not in fact drift into such areas as

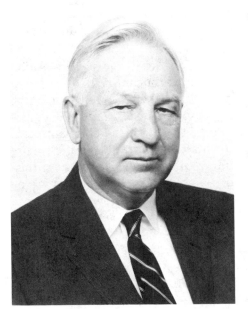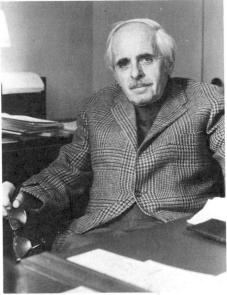

August Hollingshead (left) and Fredrick Redlich, who continued the study of the relationship of social factors—in particular, social class—to the rate of mental disorder. *(Photos courtesy of the Yale University News Bureau.)*

a consequence of their illnesses and that downward social mobility could not account for the unequal distribution of psychosis among social classes.

Two ambitious studies based on community surveys of mental disorder rather than on psychiatric patients known to treatment agencies were mounted in the early 1950s and reported in the 1960s. The first of these studies involved a sample of 1660 men and women aged 20–59 in an area of Manhattan, New York, and is known as the Midtown Manhattan study (Srole, Langner, Michael, Opler, & Rennie, 1962; Langner & Michael, 1963). The second project was undertaken in a rural area in Nova Scotia with a survey sample of about 1000 persons in both socially integrated and socially disintegrated communities by Leighton and his colleagues and was reported in three volumes (Leighton, 1959; Hughes, Trembly, Rapoport, & Leighton, 1960; Leighton, Harding, Macklin, MacMillan, & Leighton, 1963). This project is commonly referred to as the Stirling County study. Although the two studies differed somewhat in how they defined a psychiatric case, their estimates of the extent of psychiatric impairment in the general population were staggering. In the Stirling County study, it was concluded that "at least half of the adults . . . are currently suffering from some psychiatric disorder defined in the APA Diagnostic and Statistical Manual" (Leighton et al., 1963, p. 356). In the Midtown Manhattan study, which used a more limited definition of psychiatric impairment, nearly one-quarter of the sample was judged to be significantly psychiatrically impaired. These two studies reported prevalence at a particular moment in time rather than rates at which psychiatric disorders appeared to be generated in the communities studied, and both studies sought to identify factors related to the development of psychiatric disability.

The authors of the Stirling County study formulated a series of hypotheses, all of which related to the more general concept of social disintegration, within which they included such factors as lack of membership in associations, absence of strong leaders, few sanctions against deviant behavior, broken homes, frequent overt hostility, and poor communication among community members. They concluded that disintegrated social systems produce disintegrated personalities, but as to what aspects of a disorganized social system were specifically to blame, they could not be very specific. Their data led them to reject physical insecurity (inadequate food, shelter, clothing, sleep, or medical care), the frustration of sexual or aggressive impulses, and interference with one's sense of place in society or one's sense of membership in a particular human group as factors. The authors felt that the most harmful aspects of social disintegration were those that interfered with the achievement of love, recognition, spontaneity, and a sense of belonging to a moral order and of being right in what one does.

In the Midtown Manhattan study, ten stress factors were studied as possible causal factors in mental disorder in three socioeconomic-status groups. The authors found the effect of these stress factors to be additive and increasingly influential on subsequent mental disorder with decreasing socioeconomic status. Included were such factors as broken homes in childhood, poor health of parents or of self in childhood, economic deprivation, parental conflict, poor health as an adult, inadequate interpersonal affiliations, and socioeconomic, marital, and parental worries. As can be seen, these two major studies conceptualized the problem very differently and hence organized their hypotheses and presented their findings very differently. But neither had difficulty identifying social or demographic factors that might be related to the prevalence of psychiatric disorder.

In one of the very few studies of factors associated with the incidence of mental disorder, Hagnell (1966) examined the entire population of two villages (total population 2550) in southern Sweden ten years after they had been examined as part of another project (see Essen-Moller, 1956). In this reexamination, Hagnell was able to identify cases of mental disorder that had not been judged to be present ten years earlier and therefore to calculate incidence rates and to identify factors that appeared to be associated with the development of mental disorders. Using as the criterion of mental disorder his own clinical diagnosis plus evidence that the subject had consulted a physician (not necessarily a psychiatrist) for the condition, Hagnell found the average annual incidence of mental disorder per 100 population to be 0.88 in men between ages 15 and 59 and 2.27 among women in the same age range. Approximately 15% of these identified cases had at some time been admitted to a psychiatric hospital, and about 50% had at some time consulted a psychiatrist. Thus, about half of the cases Hagnell identified had never consulted a mental health specialist.

As to demographic factors that appeared to predispose persons to develop mental disorders, Hagnell identified as a particularly vulnerable group the wives of skilled workers and craftsmen. Persons who complained of symptoms of physical weakness and low energy at the start of the ten-year period (specifically, sleep disturbances and headaches) were significantly more likely to develop mental disorders, as well as persons who had complained of fatigue, nervousness, strain, and the feeling of being harassed. Finally, those persons judged ten years earlier as "listless" or "torpid" or otherwise possibly disturbed or abnormal were found upon reexamination to be overrepresented among persons judged to have some form of mental disorder. The worth of these findings rests on the *reliability and validity* of the diagnosis of mental illness as made by the author—that is, the consistency with which the same diagnosis was given to the same set of symptoms (reliability) and the extent to which the assigned diagnosis was correct (validity). Not only is validity an imponderable, but also no provision was made for assessing reliability of the diagnosis. I bring this overview full circle by noting that, in commenting on Hagnell's work, Dunham was moved to say "Perhaps it might be more desirable in future epidemiological studies to depend primarily on such operational definitions of a case as going to a psychiatrist, entering an outpatient clinic, or entering a mental hospital. The definition of a case by the 'author's diagnosis' as used by Dr. Hagnell in his study may present more difficulties than utilizing the social process as the selective agent" (1970, p. 226).

Low socioeconomic level and high social disorganization have repeatedly been shown to be associated with mental disorder. This association has been found in studies of the incidence and prevalence of treated cases, in studies of the general population, and in studies contrasting the environments of patients with the environments of some type of nonpatient comparison group.

Low social class as a stressor variable

In a review of the literature linking social class to psychopathology (in particular, to schizophrenia), Kohn (1968) has outlined and evaluated six hypotheses that have been advanced to account for the relationship found between the two. I have already commented on three of these hypotheses—low social integration, minority status, and high social isolation. Genetic differences associated with social class have been suggested, but no convincing data have yet been presented. Differences in parent/child relationships associated with social class have been suggested, but "there has not been a single well-controlled study that demonstrates any substantial difference between the family relationships of schizophrenics and those of normal persons from lower and working class backgrounds" (p. 167). Finally, excess stress in lower social classes has been postulated, and this theory is currently being evaluated by the Dohrenwends and their colleagues (see B. P. Dohrenwend & B. S. Dohrenwend, 1969; B. P. Dohrenwend, 1969; B. S. Dohrenwend & B. P. Dohrenwend, 1974). They suggest that field studies of mental disorder may overestimate the extent of psychopathology in lower classes by their failure to distinguish between relatively enduring symptomatology and short-lived symptomatology. The research question is thus "In lower status groups, to what extent is the excess of symptomatology generated by personality defects, of whatever origin (for example, genetic, childhood deprivation), and to what extent does such symptomatology consist of normal reactions to unusually harsh and numerous stressors in the contemporary situations?" (B. P. Dohrenwend, 1969, p. 147).

More research effort has gone into the study of low social class, or poverty, as a stressor than into the study of any other single social phenomenon. Research findings are persuasive in their consistency. A recent review of studies linking social class to psychopathology (B. P. Dohrenwend & B. S. Dohrenwend, 1974) found that, of 13 studies conducted in rural areas, 9 found the rates of all psychopathology to be highest in the lowest social class. Of 18 studies conducted in urban areas, 17 found the rates of all psychopathology highest in the lowest class. And the 2 studies conducted in geographic areas neither predominantly rural nor predominantly urban both found the highest rates of all psychopathology in the lowest class. Those studies that examined the relationship of social class to specific diagnoses found that rates of personality disorders such as alcoholism, drug abuse, and antisocial behavior show a consistent inverse relationship with social class; rates for neurosis and psychosis do not.

Although research studies show that the rate of psychopathology is consistently highest in the lowest social class, the actual rate differences are not great, averaging on the order of 3:1 (Dohrenwend & Dohrenwend, 1969, pp. 28–30). This difference is probably not of sufficient magnitude to warrant the establishment of a preventive intervention program, particularly since there is so little understanding of how poverty is linked to psychopathology. Mechanic (1972) has identified some of the complexities in understanding the relationship between social class and psychopathology by noting that

> the psychological impact of stress, of course, depends not alone on the occurrence of events but rather on the relationship between the demands an event makes and the individual's capacity to cope. . . . It has been too readily assumed by many writers in this field that the poor are always at a disadvantage, but it seems reasonable to anticipate that the poor are equally capable or superior to higher-status persons in dealing with some kinds of misfortunes. The development of coping capacities comes frequently through experience and practice, and in some areas of living, persons of lower economic status get greater opportunity to develop skills. Moreover, successful mastery builds confidence and a sense of effectiveness, and many persons of lower socioeconomic status, despite their low income, develop a strong sense of self. To talk of lower-status persons as a monolithic group on the basis of modest statistical differences among the social classes is conducive to asking the wrong research questions [p. 307].[4]

Contrast the differences in psychopathology rates among social classes with the difference in the incidence of lung cancer between nonsmokers and smokers. Lung cancer is 24 times as prevalent among heavy smokers as among nonsmokers (MacMahon, Pugh, & Ipsen, 1960, pp. 229–230), and a prevention program based on this very large differential not only could be quite inexpensive but could result in a dramatic decrease in the incidence of lung cancer. Psychopathology is only two or three times as common among socially isolated persons and among persons who are minorities in their own neighborhoods (whites in a predominantly black neighborhood or vice versa) as among other persons. These differences, like the differences among social classes, are not large enough to justify the establishment, even on a trial basis, of a preventive intervention program (see Bloom, 1975, pp. 305–316; Klee, Spiro, Bahn, & Gorwitz, 1967; Levy & Rowitz, 1972; Wechsler & Pugh, 1967).

The question then arises whether any social variable has been found that is so powerfully associated with some measure of psychopathology that the establishment of a preventive intervention program is justified; that is, has

---

[4]From "Social Class and Schizophrenia: Some Requirements for a Plausible Theory of Social Influence," by D. Mechanic, *Social Forces*, 1972, *50*, 305–309. Reprinted by permission.

any unequivocally high-risk group been identified? A review of the literature suggests that one high-risk group does exist—namely, people undergoing marital disruption.

Marital disruption as a stressor variable

In 1981 there were more than a million divorces in the United States, and each divorce affected an average of 1.22 children. Thus, more than 2 million adults and 1 million children were directly affected by divorce in a single year, representing 1½% of the total U.S. population (Bureau of the Census, 1974; National Center for Health Statistics, 1974, 1982; U.S. Department of Health, Education and Welfare, 1976; U.S. Department of Health and Human Services, 1980a). These figures might have little interest to any group other than demographers were there not a growing body of evidence that marital disruption constitutes a severe stress and that the consequences of that stress can be seen in a surprisingly wide variety of physical and emotional disorders.

Of all the social variables whose relationships to the distribution of psychopathology in the population have been studied, none has been more consistently and powerfully associated with this distribution than marital status. Persons who are divorced or separated have repeatedly been found to be overrepresented among psychiatric patients, while persons who are married and living with their spouses have been found to be underrepresented. In a recent review of 11 studies of marital status and the incidence of mental disorder reported during the past 35 years, Crago (1972) found that, without a single exception, admission rates into psychiatric facilities were lowest among the married, intermediate among the widowed and never married, and highest among the divorced and separated. This differential appears to be stable across different age groups (Adler, 1953), reasonably stable for each sex separately considered (Thomas & Locke, 1963; Malzberg, 1964), and as true for blacks as for whites (Malzberg, 1956). The same assertion was made even more recently by Bachrach, who noted that "utilization studies have generally shown that married people have substantially lower utilization rates than non-married people and that the highest utilization rates occur among persons whose marriages have been disrupted by separation or divorce" (1975, p. 3).

Not only are highest admission rates reported for persons with disrupted marriages, but the differential between these rates and similarly calculated rates among the married is substantial (see Table 5–5). Less extensive information is available nationally for private services (Bachrach, 1973), but the data indicate that admission rates into psychiatric inpatient units in private general hospitals are lowest among the married and highest among the separated and divorced, and that whereas admission rates for married men and married women are about equal, the rates for separated and divorced patients tend to be about twice as high among males as among females.

In examining the data in Table 5–5, it is worth noting that, first, regardless of sex, admission rates are highest for those with disrupted marriages. Second, the differential in admission rates between separated/divorced persons and married persons is far greater for men than women.

Analyzing data collected in Pueblo, Colorado, between 1969 and 1971, I found that admission rates into public and private psychiatric inpatient facilities were substantially higher for persons with disrupted marriages (divorced and separated combined) than for persons married and living with their spouses (Bloom, 1975, pp. 298–305), especially for males. Specifically, first-admission rates for males with disrupted marriages were 9 times those for males with nondisrupted marriages (30.0 per 1000 versus 3.3 per 1000). For first-admission females, the difference was in the order of 3:1 (10.7 per 1000 for disrupted marriages versus 3.2 per 1000 for nondisrupted marriages). Among patients with histories of prior psychiatric care, the differentials by marital status were greater for both sexes. For males, the ratio was about 16:1 (46.3 per 1000 for disrupted marriages versus 2.8 per 1000 for nondisrupted marriages), and for females, the ratio was about 6:1 (12.9 versus 2.2). Another way of viewing the data is to note that although divorced and separated males constitute only 6.5% of males age 14 and over who have ever been married, they constitute 46% of male patients in the same age span who have ever been married. Similarly, divorced and separated females constitute only 8% of ever-married females age 14 and over but 32% of ever-married female patients in the same age span. Finally, the data showed that each year more than 7% of males with disrupted marriages are admitted or readmitted to a hospital because of a psychiatric condition.

Equivalent results are generally reported from household survey studies. Srole and his associates (1962), in their Midtown Manhattan survey, found that "the midtown divorced of both sexes have the highest mental morbidity rates of all four marital status categories" (p. 185). Similar findings were reported by Blumenthal (1967) in Michigan, by Tauss (1967), based on data collected in Perth, Australia, and by Briscoe, Smith, Robins, Marten, and Gaskin (1973), from data collected in St. Louis. This last research group administered a structured interview to a representative sample of divorced and never-divorced men and women in St. Louis and found evidence of psychiatric illness in three-quarters of the divorced women and two-thirds of the divorced men (significantly greater proportions than they found with never-divorced subjects).

Two important sources of data link marital disruption to suicidal behavior. First, Shneidman and Farberow (1961) have examined some personal characteristics of attempted and committed suicides from the year 1957 in Los Angeles County. Data on committed suicides were obtained from the Los Angeles coroner's office; data on attempted suicides were obtained from Los Angeles physicians and from records of the county general hospital and the 16 Los Angeles municipal emergency hospitals. Of the persons who committed suicide, 13% were divorced and 8% separated. These figures are more than double the proportions of divorced and separated persons in the general population of the county. In a related study, Litman and Farberow (1961), in proposing a strategy for emergency evaluation of self-destructive potentiality, noted that "many suicide attempts, especially in young persons, occur after the separation from a spouse or loved one. . . . When there has been a definite loss of a loved person, such as a spouse, parent, child, lover, or mistress, within the previous year (by death, divorce, or separation), the potentiality for self-destruction is increased" (p. 51).

The second source of data linking suicide to marital status is the continuing reports of the National Center of Health Statistics. The most recent report (National Center for Health Statistics, 1970) covers the period 1959–1961 and is based on an analysis of total U.S. mortality data. According to these statistics, for white females, the suicide rate is higher among the divorced than in any other marital-status category, and the rate of the divorced is more than three times the rate of the married. For white men, the suicide rate is highest among the divorced, and the rate of the divorced is more than four times the rate of the married. The suicide rate of non-white females is highest among the widowed and second-highest among the divorced, for whom the rate is twice that of the married. Finally, among non-white males, the suicide rate is highest for the divorced, and the rate of the divorced is nearly two and a half times as great as the rate of the married.

Figures for deaths from homicide are even more striking. For both sexes and for both whites and non-whites, the risk of death by homicide is far higher for the divorced than for any other marital-status group. For white women, the risk is more than four times as high for the divorced as for the married. For white men, the risk is more than seven times as high for the divorced. Among non-whites, the risk is twice as high among women and three times as high among men.

Two studies demonstrate excess vulnerability to motor-vehicle accidents among the divorced. First, analysis of total U.S. mortality data published by the National Center for Health Statistics (1970) reveals that, for both sexes and for whites and non-whites alike, automobile fatality rates are higher among the divorced than among the members of any other marital-status group— about three times as high. Second, a study by McMurray (1970) showed that the accident rate of persons undergoing divorce doubled during the six months before and the six months after the divorce date.

A variety of studies have sought to link stress experiences to vulnerability to disease. Indeed, such linkages form the empirical basis of hypotheses about the etiology of psychophysiological disease. Holmes and Rahe (1967; also Rahe, McKean, & Arthur, 1967; Rahe, 1968; Theorell & Rahe, 1970) have developed a measure of stressful life events based on the amount of readjustment required by each such event and have shown that this measure distinguishes persons likely to become ill from those not likely to become ill (see also Cline & Chosy, 1972). Marital disruption figures heavily in this measure, which is discussed further in Chapter 6: the three most stressful life events—death of a spouse, divorce, and separation—all involve marital disruption.

Two recent studies suggest that alcoholism (both acute and chronic) is more prevalent among the divorced than among the married—a finding that corroborates conclusions drawn in much earlier literature. Wechsler, Thum, Demone, and Dwinnell (1972) studied the blood alcohol level of over 6000 consecutive admissions to the emergency service of Massachusetts General Hospital, excluding children under age 16, persons dead on arrival, persons admitted with psychiatric problems, including alcoholics not requiring medical services, attempted suicides, those receiving postoperative or continuing care, and those with dental problems not caused by injury. The authors found that "in both sexes, the divorced or separated had the highest proportion with positive Breathalyzer readings. . . . Divorced or separated men included 42 percent with positive alcohol readings" (p. 138). Widowers had the lowest proportion with positive readings (10%), and single (24%) and married men (19%) were intermediate. Rosenblatt, Gross, Malenowski, Broman, and Lewis (1971) contrasted first admissions with readmissions for alcoholism and concluded that their results "reveal a significant relationship between disrupted marriage and multiple hospitalizations for the acute alcoholic psychoses at ages below 45" (p. 1094).

Finally, with regard to death from disease, we can return to the special studies of the National Center for Health Statistics (1970). Both the widowed and the divorced have higher death rates for all diseases combined than married persons of the same age, sex, and race. Death rates from tuberculosis and from cirrhosis of the liver are consistently higher among the divorced than among the married. For white men and non-whites of both sexes, the death rate is higher among the divorced than among the married from cancer of the respiratory system, and for non-white males the death rate is higher among the divorced for diabetes and arteriosclerotic heart disease.

Three interrelated explanations of the relationship between marital disruption and mental disorder have been advanced. First, it has frequently been asserted that previously existing pathology reduces the likelihood that single persons will marry or stay married. In Turner's words, psychopathology "makes marriage less likely and, given marriage, is likely to speed divorce or separation" (1972, p. 365). Srole and his colleagues make a similar point:

> Unlike age and sex, marital status in our view cannot qualify as an independent demographic variable relative to mental health. On the contrary, elements of mental health may be crucially involved in determining whether or not individuals choose to marry; if they do so choose, whether or not they are successful in finding a spouse; and, if they are successful in this respect, whether or not the marriage is subsequently broken by divorce [1962, p. 175].

Briscoe and his colleagues (1973), in interpreting findings in their research already referred to, suggest that "one of the implications of finding such a significant amount of psychiatric illness in a divorced population is that psychiatric illness is probably a significant cause of marital breakdown" (p. 125). Crago, in her review of research studies linking marital disruption to psycho-pathology, also suggests this possibility: "Studies of hospitalization rates and marital status are sometimes criticized because the differences in rates may be due to effects of mental disorders on the marital status of individuals before they are admitted to a mental hospital. For example, if mental disorders tend to lead to divorce, this would boost the rate of mental disorders among the divorced and at the same time decrease the rate for married persons" (1972, p. 115).

The second hypothesis that has been advanced is that being married reduces one's vulnerability to a wide variety of illnesses. Turner, for example, suggests that different marital statuses may place individuals in different social systems that vary in supportiveness; thus the "marriage state [may be] protective against hospitalization" (1972, p. 365). Syme has recently reviewed the statistics linking mortality from disease to marital status and has concluded that "if the marital state provides an environment which reduces the risk of death from this long list of conditions, it may just be that a very profound and important influence is at work which is certainly worthy of prompt and careful study" (1974, p. 1045).

The third hypothesis is that marital disruption itself constitutes a significant stressor. This hypothesis falls under the rubric "crisis theory" (see Caplan, 1964; Parad, 1965; and Chapter 3 of this book). The national psychiatric admission rate statistics already cited, which show a substantially higher admission rate for separated than for divorced persons, support this hypothesis.

Even though marital disruption affects so many people and is more closely associated with psychiatric disorders than any other social variable, knowledge of the specific stresses triggered by marital disruption is relatively limited. A review of the U.S. literature suggests six specific stresses. First, the psychological and emotional problems associated with the breakup of a marriage appear to be intense. The termination of a marriage represents the death of a relationship and thus requires constructive mourning and a coming to grips with the resulting sense of failure, shame, and low self-worth. Second, particularly for women, there may be stresses associated with the need to do some thinking about employment, career planning, or additional education preparatory to establishing an independent economic existence. Third, legal and financial problems often occur. Separated women often find it impossible to get loans or to establish charge accounts. Parental rights are often poorly understood. Fourth, following the change from a two-parent to a one-parent family setting, child-rearing problems frequently emerge. Fifth, particularly for men, problems regarding housing and homemaking appear. And, sixth, for both men and women, particularly if they are beyond the early adult years, there are often serious difficulties in finding suitable social groups and satisfying social experiences.

DESIGN OF PREVENTIVE INTERVENTION PROGRAMS

Before a primary prevention program can be effectively instituted, a comprehensive analysis of the problem needs to be undertaken. Such an analysis must determine the frequency with which the problem occurs, its distribution and severity, those factors that set the stage for its appearance, those that cause the problem to appear once predisposing factors are present, and those that cause the problem to persist once it has appeared. It is this analysis that forms the rationale for the specific preventive intervention program and for its evaluation.

A number of such analyses have appeared in recent years, and it will be useful to examine a sample of them. Catalano and Dooley (1980) have inaugurated an analysis of the role of the economy (defined as those activities involved in the production and distribution of goods and services) in the development of psychopathology. In particular, Catalano and Dooley believe that "the status of an economy affects the psychological well-being of the population it supports" (1980, p. 27) and that regional or local economic changes can be forecast and controlled far more easily than national ones. Decisions affecting the economy, such as proposed changes in land use, can be influenced by urging the preparation and discussion of a social-impact statement analogous to the well-known environmental-impact statement. Similarly, corporations can be urged to undertake social audits of their performance analogous to their fiscal audits. Social audits would weigh the gains and losses to human resources within the corporation and within the communities it serves. Such audits could include consideration, for example, of the social costs of proposed changes in employment opportunities, such as opening a new plant, mass geographic transfer of employees, or modifications of working hours, and of the changing level of alcohol or other drug abuse among corporation employees.

At the reactive level, when specific economic changes are unavoidable, individual-level interventions can provide employees with early warning of impending changes and the time for anticipatory coping. Such coping can be facilitated by educational approaches designed to provide information on common reactions to job loss, for example, and behavioral-skill acquisition, such as stress-management techniques, new job-skill development, and strategies for obtaining new employment.

Carlson and Davis (1980) have undertaken an analysis of the literature on domestic violence as the first step toward developing preventive intervention programs in that area. Domestic violence appears to take place in more than one-quarter of American families, and about as many husbands as wives report being physically abused. Reported injuries and potential dangers are more severe among wives than among husbands, however, and accordingly far more attention is directed toward wife abuse than husband abuse (Carlson & Davis, 1980, pp. 42–43). The family can serve as a training ground for violence both by direct reinforcement and by observational modeling. Low self-esteem appears to predispose people to family violence. Physical violence within the family has a long and powerful historical tradition, and the right to use physical punishment is still given to parents and, under some circumstances, to spouses. Physical violence serves as a primary means of asserting superiority, particularly in families undergoing considerable social and economic stress. Any preventive program that hopes to succeed in reducing the incidence of family violence must keep these facts in mind.

At the level of the family and individual family member, Carlson and Davis propose changes in our ways of socializing children and training for improved family problem-solving skills, including education that distinguishes between assertiveness and aggressiveness. At the societal level, Carlson and Davis suggest the general reduction of violence by means of strict gun control, reduced TV displays of violence (particularly violence directed against women), a change in social norms so that behavior that is not tolerated outside the family will not be tolerated within the family, a ban on physical punishment of children, the elimination of sex discrimination in employment, reduction in sex-typing of family-related roles and responsibilities, opportunities for full employment, reduction of the stigma associated with receipt of public assistance, and constant monitoring of the state of family health and welfare.

The next two chapters present descriptions of primary prevention programs organized around the concept of stressful life events and programs focusing on mental health education strategies. Here I describe a sample of primary prevention programs that are organized around the identification of high-risk groups or high-risk situations—that is, groups that on the basis of epidemiological studies appear to be vulnerable or situations that appear to create special vulnerability (Gruenberg, 1981).

Each of these programs has been subjected to some form of evaluation. The importance of evaluation has been generally accepted by persons instituting experimental preventive intervention programs (Heller, Price, & Sher, 1980). In addition, the first issue of the new journal *Prevention in Human Services*, published in 1981, is devoted to the evaluation theme.

Preventing behavior symptoms in elementary school children

Starting in 1953, Glidewell and his associates undertook a 30-month evaluation of a school mental health program designed to have both a preventive and therapeutic effect on a group of elementary school children who were in the third grade when the project began (Gildea, Glidewell, & Kantor, 1967; Glidewell, 1968; Glidewell, Gildea, & Kaufman, 1973; Kantor, Gildea, & Glidewell, 1969). It has been found (see Glidewell & Swallow, 1969) that about 30% of American schoolchildren experience some form of school maladjustment. Accordingly, it seems quite appropriate to consider schoolchildren a high-risk group. The primary dependent variable under study was reports of behavior symptoms by mothers of children in the program. The mental health program had two component parts—an educational program for parents, led by persons who were not mental health professionals, and a school-based consultation program for teachers and administrators combined with a counseling program for parents and children led by specially trained psychiatric social workers.

Symptom reports were contrasted over time in three groups of children—those in control-group classrooms, those in classrooms in which the parent-education program was available, and those in classrooms in which the parent-education program *and* the school-based consultation and counseling program were available. Mothers were interviewed three times—initially, after 12 months, and after 30 months. Complete data were obtained from 426 mothers about their children. In addition to behavior-symptom reports, information was obtained on social class and sex of the child. The effectiveness of the program in meeting its preventive objectives was to be assessed by reduction in the appearance of new behavior symptoms in the experimental groups when contrasted with the children in the control classrooms.

The experimental programs were found to result in a significant reduction in reported symptoms for boys but not for girls. In addition, the programs appeared to have a more immediate effect on middle-class children. Lower-class children showed fewer new symptoms, but only during the second year of their participation. There was no persuasive evidence that the two program components combined were more effective than the parent-education program alone. The directors of this experimental program concluded that "probably the most significant aspect of the findings is that professional intervention into social systems such as schools can effectively *prevent* behavior symptoms" (Glidewell, Gildea, & Kaufman, 1973, p. 326).

Improving self-esteem in high school students

Hartman (1979a, 1979b) developed a preventive intervention program for a group of high-risk ninth- and tenth-graders in a Montreal high school. Risk was ascertained by tests that assessed self-esteem, psychological discomfort, and assertiveness and by additional assessment of stressful life events, availability of compensating positive experiences, and social relationships. The first set of three measurements identified the vulnerable population; the second set identified the degree of environmental pressure (sometimes called *press*) operative for each student. Students were randomly assigned to a preventive intervention program or to an assessment-only control group matched for sex and grade level.

Students assigned to the prevention program met for an hour weekly for eight weeks in groups of ten. The meetings were designed to teach a wide range of self-management skills and emphasized the acquisition of coping and social performance skills.

Hartman describes the results of this study as follows:

The measures of psychological risk showing the greatest amount of change following preventive skills training were the three vulnerability variables (self-esteem,
psychological discomfort, assertiveness) and peer-ratings from the press factor.
. . . A measure of situational social skills developed specifically for this study
showed clearly significant main effects for the intervention and vulnerability factors. Multiple comparisons revealed that the effect of preventive skills training
was most obvious for subjects exhibiting high vulnerability and low press. . . .
At the time of follow-up, three months later, the main effects of vulnerability and
the preventive program were still evident. . . . In summary, students undergoing
the intervention program revealed greater gains on self-report, peer, and teacher
rating measures than controls. These improvements in risk profiles were also
found to be evident at the time of follow-up [1979b, pp. 264–265].

Preventing delinquency

Bry (1982) described two efforts to prevent juvenile delinquency and substance abuse in seventh-graders at high risk for those behaviors. Risk was
assessed on the basis of low academic achievement motivation, a disregard
for rules, and a feeling of distance from their families. One study involved a
low-income urban school system; the other took place in a middle-class suburban school system. The two-year preventive intervention program consisted
of repeated exposures to a school environment in which it was clear that
desired consequences were gained through the student's own actions. Outcome measures included school grades and attendance records, since decreases
in these measures were known to follow delinquency and substance abuse.

Initial evaluation of the program yielded positive results: while attendance
and achievement decreased in the control group, they remained stable in the
intervention group. Results in the low-income and middle-income communities were identical.

One year later, a follow-up study found that there were fewer school-
related problems in the intervention group, significantly fewer students in the
intervention group than in the control group had never been employed, and
somewhat fewer members of the intervention group had reported substance
abuse and other forms of criminal behavior. A final follow-up study was
undertaken five years later. No differences in drug-related arrests were found
between the two groups, but delinquency measures (from county court records) were significantly less common in the intervention group than in the
control group.

Competency building for women receiving public assistance

Tableman, Marciniak, Johnson, and Rodgers (1982) developed a ten-week
life-coping-skills training package for women being supported by public assistance. The program was designed to teach life-planning and stress-manage-

ment skills and to enhance self-esteem. Sixty-five women participated in the experimental training program; 51 women served as controls.

Women in the training program attended weekly three-hour sessions. Transportation and child care were provided to facilitate attendance. The program objectives included efforts to help women feel better about themselves, accept responsibility for their own behavior, take control of their lives, and handle stress more effectively. Most meetings consisted of group discussions led by experienced group leaders, although specially developed written and visual aids were used as appropriate. The training program resulted in significant decreases in measures of psychological distress, depression, anxiety, and inadequacy and significant increases in measures of self-confidence and ego strength.

Reducing school maladaptation

The Primary Mental Health Project (PMHP) in Rochester, New York, has been in continuous operation since 1958 and has been unusually fully researched and reported by Cowen and his colleagues. This is a secondary prevention program aimed at early detection and correction of school maladaptation and emotional disorder; it is derivative in its philosophy from earlier work by Klein and Lindemann (1964).

In describing the rationale for the Primary Mental Health Project, Cowen wrote:

> The day-to-day activities of school mental health professionals have long been guided by prevailing conceptions of pathological behavior and by a *reactive* orientation to deficit. Psychologists and social workers in the schools have been cast in the role of "experts" or "trouble-shooters," called on to do their magic in the face of significant educational or interpersonal failure. Striking and understandable parallels exist between the specific problems of school mental health today and the broader ones confronting society in this area: Professionals are in woefully short supply. Demand for assistance, and certainly latent need, far exceeds resources. Established helping techniques are limited in value and their distribution across social strata is inequitable. Thus, the meager firepower generated from scarce mental health resources is directed to a relatively small percent of florid, rooted dysfunctions, which, unfortunately, are precisely the ones with the poorest prognoses [pp. 723–724].[5]

Cowen and his colleagues determined that about 30% of all children have problems adapting to school settings, that half of teachers' time during school hours is taken up with a very small number of maladapting children—a situation stressful for those children, for the many other children in the classroom, and for the teacher—and that school maladjustment is unusually visible

---

[5]From "Emergent Directions in School Mental Health," by E. L. Cowen, *American Scientist*, 1971, 59, 723–733. Reprinted by permission, *American Scientist*, journal of Sigma Xi, the Scientific Research Society of North America.

around the time of transition from elementary school to junior high or middle schools. In addition, they learned that these maladjusted children show evidence in their school records of having had difficulties during the very earliest elementary-school years, and on this basis they decided on the early-detection and -intervention program. Their hope was that this emphasis might "sharply reduce the incidence of chronic school maladaptation and, with it, heavy later service demands" (Cowen, 1971, p. 724).

The initial phase of the project (1958–1963) was directed primarily at the problem of early detection of school maladjustment and only secondarily at prevention of further maladjustment. One elementary school was selected as the site for the detection and intervention program, and two comparable neighboring schools provided control cases. A school psychologist and school social worker collected information on all new first-grade children in the experimental school by means of classroom observation, psychological testing, interviews with mothers, and analysis of teacher reports. On the basis of these combined data, children were divided into two groups—those who gave evidence of manifest or incipient maladaptation and those who did not. About one-third of each year's first-grade class was categorized as maladapting (Cowen, Izzo, Miles, Telschow, Trost, & Zax, 1963; Cowen, Pederson, Babigian, Izzo, & Trost, 1973; Cowen, Zax, Izzo, & Trost, 1966; Cowen, Dorr, Izzo, Madonia, & Trost, 1971; Zax & Cowen, 1967; Zax, Cowen, Rappaport, Beach, & Laird, 1968).

The intervention during the project's first phase was very modest. The two mental health professionals identified with the project steered the project away from traditional one-to-one clinical services and toward educative and consultative services for teachers, school administrators, and parents. Conferences were scheduled with teachers, the school principal, the school nurse, and other interested personnel. Special meetings were held for parents and teachers with experts in such topics as child development, human motivation, and the emotional and psychological needs of the young child. Direct service to children was provided in an after-school program. Children met in groups of no larger than ten for one hour a week for 20 weeks. During these meetings, activities ranged from woodworking to baking, and the intent was to provide a meaningful interpersonal experience in a relatively informal setting.

Cowen and his colleagues chose to evaluate the intervention program by contrasting all first-grade children in the experimental school with first-grade children in the two control schools. This comparison, undertaken when the children were in third grade and again when they were in seventh grade, suggested that the intervention program had been only partly successful. In the seventh-grade study, for example, the researchers contrasted the control and experimental children on 46 measures. They found that

> fourteen of the 46 comparisons between E [experimental] and C [control] school students reflected significant differences, although the pattern of differences is not clear-cut. The E school children were found to have lower grades, were more

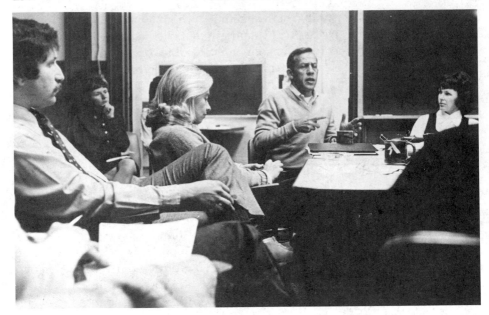

Emory Cowen explains the organization of the Primary Mental Health Project to workers in the project. *(Photo by Chris Quillen.)*

likely to be underachievers, and had poorer attendance records than C schoolers. On the other hand, they were less anxious . . . and scored higher than C school children on several standard achievement tests. It was not possible to do an adequate follow-up . . . because of the high degree of attrition. . . . Thus the results of this fairly long-term follow-up did not lead to definitive conclusions. The relatively weak follow-up findings may be the result of program inadequacies or the high attrition rates. Whatever the reasons, the positive effects of the preventive program were not demonstrated to be enduring with respect to the measures used [Zax & Specter, 1974, p. 191].

The second phase of the Primary Mental Health Project (starting in 1963) was inaugurated in part as a consequence of these ambiguous evaluation results and represented a major shift in the character of the intervention program. Now the program included far more direct service to the vulnerable children. First, six teacher aides were recruited and trained. These aides were all successful mothers with interest in and positive attitudes toward children. None of the aides had a college degree, and one had not finished high school. The aides were first assigned to teachers to assist in the classroom with children who required more attention than the teacher could provide. This procedure was later changed so that the aides provided supplementary experiences for certain children outside the classroom, usually in individual contacts. Second, an after-school day-care program was started, staffed by volunteer college undergraduates. Referrals to the after-school program were generally made because of acting out, apparent undersocialization, or poor achievement.

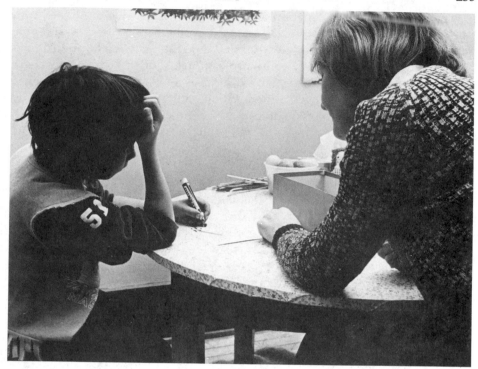

As part of the Primary Mental Health Project, a teacher aide gives special attention to this student. *(Photo by Chris Quillen.)*

Evaluations of the second phase were very encouraging. There was very little turnover of teacher aides, and referrals increased. Additional teacher aides were employed in several inner-city schools. Judgments of program effectiveness by teachers suggested that both the teacher-aide program and the volunteer-college-student program resulted in significant improvement in the children's behavior.

Since 1969, school mental health professionals have been trained to adapt the program to their own settings. Programs are currently underway in 30 schools in the area where the program originated and similar programs have been introduced in 300 schools in 40 school districts around the country (Cowen, Gesten, & Wilson, 1979). During the past decade important changes have continued to be made in program goals and in assessment procedures. Cowen, Gesten, and Wilson note that "discovering that the project had been more effective with shy-anxious children than with acting-out children or those with learning problems . . . gave rise to several new training programs to equip aides to work more effectively with the latter. . . . Growing interest in children's competencies and how to strengthen them led to the development of a measure of school-related competencies [which] was incorporated into the project's assessment and evaluation mainstreams" (1979, p. 295).

In the most recent evaluation of the Primary Mental Health Project, conducted in 1975–1976, outcome was assessed on the basis of teacher and aide ratings of children's problems, teacher and aide ratings of children's competencies, and school mental health professionals' judgments of children's improvement during the school year. Cowen, Gesten, and Wilson (1979) found that children in the experimental intervention program improved significantly on all dependent measures. In addition, in contrasting 176 experimental children with 72 matched control children who had not been referred to the program, the authors found that the experimental children exceeded the control children on all dependent measures. On 5 of the 11 dependent measures used in this part of the study, those differences were statistically significant.

The authors concluded their evaluation study by commenting that its findings "support the . . . view that PMHP serves young children with school adaptation problems, effectively. These new data strengthen the base of justification for programs in systematic early identification and prevention of school adjustment problems. Such programs are further supported by common sense. Prompt identification and effective intervention seem to be one important pathway to the essential goal of cutting down the enormous human and social costs of early school maladaptation" (1979, p. 302).

CURRENT STATUS OF PRIMARY PREVENTION

The great repositories of mortality and morbidity are no longer the infectious and nutritional diseases, as they once were. Today, the major currently unpreventable disorders are those that often have long-lasting consequences—heart disease, cancer, accidents, cerebrovascular disease, respiratory diseases, and mental disorders.

For the mental disorders, use of the traditional specific-disease-prevention paradigm suffers because of our continuing inability to find diseases—that is, psychiatric disorders with known biological markers. Weissman and Klerman (1978) have reviewed the substantial recent progress in psychopharmacology, genetics, and neurobiology and say that new psychiatric diseases may soon be found, particularly among what are now labeled schizophrenia, primary affective disorders, and mental retardation. If such new diseases were found, our diagnostic system would be quickly modified, of course, and a new series of studies could be inaugurated by invoking the traditional specific-disease-prevention paradigm, in the hope that ways of preventing these diseases might be found.

Weissman and Klerman note, however, that

the classical medical approach to causal explanation was to search for a single factor that would provide necessary and sufficient explanation. . . . This mode of causal explanation has proved highly useful for infectious disease, disorders due to nutritional deficiency, and for many, but not all, hereditary disorders. However, it has not been successful with the chronic diseases or psychiatric disorders and there has been a shift to a multifactorial mode of explanation [1978, p. 710].

Weissman and Klerman suggest that these potential factors are "multiple and include biological (genetic, biochemical, nutritional) and psychosocial factors (social stress, social class, migration, urbanization, economic change)" (p. 709).

With increasingly rare exceptions, it has been impossible to control illnesses without construing them in their biological, psychological, and socio-cultural contexts. For example, Sameroff and Chandler (1975) have shown that developmental defects associated with damage occurring around the time of birth, including anoxia (oxygen deprivation), occur primarily in high-risk social environments. Bates (1980) has shown that temperamental variables in childhood are predictive of later psychopathology only when social factors are taken into account. Cassel has shown that susceptibility to disease is likely to increase when people are new to an unfamiliar environment or when there is considerable social disorganization and that susceptibility to disease is greater in persons who are subordinate rather than dominant in a society or who are deprived of meaningful social contacts and social supports. He concludes that a high level of disease in general might be expected under conditions of social change and social disorganization and that "preventive action in the future should focus more directly on attempts at modifying these psychosocial factors, on improving and strengthening social supports, and reducing the circumstances which produce ambiguities between actions and their consequences" (1973, p. 547).

Eisenberg has recently noted that there is strong evidence that drug therapy for psychoses is insufficient without concurrent psychotherapy and social support and that, as a further indication of the important influence of social and cultural factors on the course and outcome of psychosis, the World Health Organization nine-nation study has shown that "patients from 'less developed' countries have considerably better prognosis than those in the 'developed' world. This observation stresses the importance of continuing to attend to the psychosocial environment rather than being dazzled by the illusory promise of combating illness by technical means alone" (1981, p. 15).

In that same paper, Eisenberg reviewed the recent work of Berkman and Syme, whose nine-year study with nearly 5000 adults in Alameda County, California (1979), found a significant relationship between social supports and lower mortality. Mortality was negatively associated with marriage, contacts with close friends and relatives, church membership, and informal and formal group associations, even after taking into account differences in social class, health, and health practices.

Prevention of mental disorders will succeed to the extent that basic and applied research maintains this multidimensional approach in its orientation. Health scientists are increasingly aware of the importance of psychological and social factors in the predisposition, precipitation, and perpetuation of most forms of illness (Engel, 1977, 1980). Thus, it is ironic that while there is increasing emphasis on biologizing the mental health field by expanding the search for organic factors in mental illness, primary care physicians are accelerating their attempts to psychologize and sociologize general medicine. The hope that control of the major, currently unpreventable disorders lies exclusively in our biology seems not only illusory but in defiance of an overwhelming amount of evidence. Culture invades physiology, and psychiatric symptoms are an exquisite final common pathway of a complex interaction of biological, psychological, and sociocultural forces.

Evaluation of the status of primary prevention programs in a typical community will generally show that preventable disorders continue to occur, that only a small proportion of the population is thriving, and that insufficient resources are allocated toward extending the frontiers of knowledge to diminish the incidence of emotional disorders. Because those disorders are rarely fatal and express their impact mainly in high morbidity rather than mortality, communities face unmet needs in their efforts to treat the already ill and are often reluctant to divert scarce resources away from that important humanitarian task (Lamb & Zusman, 1979). Yet, the public is not unwilling to seek preventive services. It is estimated (Cypress, 1981) that 17% of physicians' office visits during 1977–1978 took place primarily in the interest of preventive care. Clearly, a number of barriers exist that make it difficult to expand primary prevention activities in the field of the emotional disorders.

First, no national policy on the enhancement of mental health exists, although the President's Commission on Mental Health (1978) has proposed steps toward such a policy. This lack of national policy is reflected in a wide variety of phenomena. No one seems to be in charge of health maintenance or promotion. Responsibilities are fragmented even when assigned, and coordination among agencies is often impossible to achieve.

A second barrier is the difficulty in extending our knowledge about effective approaches to primary prevention. Continuing to extend our knowledge base will require increased numbers of skilled and dedicated scientists and expanded research support. Eisenberg has noted that "when one considers that the entire investment in the basic and applied research and the field trials that made the poliomyelitis vaccine possible was less than the cost of the illness burden from a single epidemic year of the disease, pursuit of the same strategy for other disorders is immensely appealing" (1981, p. 4). It may require a decade or longer to determine the extent to which preventive services have been effective. These longitudinal studies need not be prohibitively expensive in any one year, but there needs to be a stable and predictable support base over a relatively long period.

Gruenberg has recently commented about the need for better research in the field of primary prevention by noting that

> a special group of prevention advocates share three critical assumptions about the interventions they advocate. They assume that the interventions are harmless; socially acceptable and not frightening to the subjects; and able to prevent some

disorders on some reasonable basis. Whether or not they actually prevent a disorder is best found out by starting with a planned preventive trial. It is extraordinary that many of the fashionable mental health prevention programs have these characteristics, yet none of them have produced a preventive trial. Such programs as widow-to-widow counseling, to prevent extended depression; correction of low self-esteem in pregnant women to prevent neurotic symptom formation in their daughters; and enhancing the coping skills of mentally retarded parents and of their children to prevent mental retardation in the children are excellent examples of hypotheses that are best tested in the first instance by a carefully prepared preventive trial. If such educational and counseling methods actually have large effects, they deserve to become more widespread. If they do not, other preventable causes must be found to lower the incidence of these disorders [1980, pp. 1323–1324].[6]

A third barrier is our failure to accept the consequences of the growing realization that single-factor causal theories do not adequately explain the development of most forms of psychiatric disorders and that the concept of health is itself multidimensional. Effective preventive efforts will require the active collaboration of many professions, many agencies, and many social systems. These efforts will demand the active involvement of teachers, parents, the clergy, nutritionists, economists, architects, and so on. Although this sentiment is often subscribed to in theory, it is rarely adopted in practice.

Most activities in the field of primary prevention appear to equate health with the absence of disease and thus see their goal as the enhancement of health by reducing disease incidence. For more than 2000 years, however, an alternative view of health has had its adherents—a view that equates health with those "natural laws which will ensure . . . a healthy mind in a healthy body" (Dubos, 1959, p. 111). From this point of view, health is not a state; it is a process, a way of life. It is from this point of view that Williamson and Pearse described health as "intrinsically and distinctively a positive process not definable in terms of 'absence' of disease and/or disorder; hence not attainable through a 'preventive' approach necessarily directed to securing the absence of disease and disorder" (1966, pp. 293–294). This broad continuum in the concept of health brings with it an equally broad array of appropriate objectives, ranging from primary prevention activities that are designed to maintain a disease-free status quo to those activities that are designed to promote growth and wholeness and to help people make maximum use of their potential, independently of whether a disease process might be present.

Some preventive interventions can be effective if made available to individuals singly or in groups. Other interventions must be directed at social systems in order to have an ultimate effect on individuals. Reiff (1977) makes

---

[6]From "Mental Disorders," by E. M. Gruenberg. In J. M. Last (Ed.), *Maxcy-Rosenau Public Health and Preventive Medicine*, 11th Ed. Copyright © 1980 by Appleton-Century-Crofts. Reprinted by permission.

use of this distinction when contrasting the instability of individual marriage—a personal trouble—with the phenomenon in which 50% of marriages end in divorce. In this latter case, Reiff suggests, "there is something beyond the intrapsychic and interpersonal, something beyond the situation, and something in the social structure that accounts for these personal troubles" (p. 49). The clear implication of this line of reasoning is that any intervention that stops short of a thoroughgoing examination of societal conditions that are producing this much disruption may very well fail.

A final barrier lies within the mental health establishment itself and is reflected in contemporary practices and in the underlying societal values (see Perlmutter & Vayda, 1978). First, as Albee (1979) has noted, our society is oriented toward quick solutions to current problems, and mental health professionals are rarely enthusiastic about long-term planning aimed at long-term goals. Second, most members of the mental health establishment have been socialized into believing that treatment is a far more valued activity than prevention. Third, the mental health establishment is unprepared, either by training or by ideology, to advocate for needed social change to prevent mental disorders. Finally, members of the mental health establishment are part of a larger third-party reimbursement procedure that legitimizes little more than the provision of treatment for diagnosed disease (Albee, 1981). In such a fiscal environment, there is little motivation to develop preventive programs that are neither fundable nor reimbursable.

It may be necessary to develop an agency concerned solely with primary prevention, an agency that would serve the healthy for the purpose of maintaining and enhancing health and robustness. At one time, the public health agency played that role. Perhaps local health departments need to be encouraged to resume that responsibility in a late-20th-century version of an older, esteemed community service. Such an agency must deal with the entire spectrum of preventive services. It must recognize that health is a social as well as a biological phenomenon and that there are healthy ways of being sick, just as there are unhealthy ways of being well. It must legitimize and encourage holistic as well as specialized views of the process of health and of a healthy life and must attend to the entire range of contemporary stress, from the biological to the psychological to the sociological and cultural. It must take a broad view of health as not only the absence of disease but also the presence of joy in living and hope in the ultimate resolution of life's conflicts (Hoke, 1968).

CONCLUSIONS AND OVERVIEW

When the history of 20th-century efforts to control mental disorders is written, the great contribution of the last third of the century may well be seen in the movement away from consideration of predisposing factors in mental illnesses toward concern with precipitating factors. This movement away from a concern with the past and toward a concern with the present has come about, in part, from frustration with our efforts at remediation. But, in addition, a growing accumulation of empirical evidence has turned our attention away from the past. Kohlberg, LaCrosse, and Ricks (1972), for example, reviewing the literature linking childhood behavior and adult mental health, comment:

> To conscious experience, moods change, anxieties disappear, loves and hates fade, the emotion of yesterday is weak, and the emotion of today does not clearly build on the emotion of yesterday. The trauma theory of neurosis is dead; the evidence for irreversible effects of early-childhood trauma is extremely slight. Early-childhood maternal deprivation, parental mistreatment, separation, incest—all seem to have much slighter effects upon adult adjustment (unless supported by continuing deprivation and trauma throughout childhood) than anyone seemed to anticipate [p. 1233].

More recently, after reviewing the literature bearing on resilience and continuity in psychological development, Kagan (1976) has come to a similar conclusion:

> The total corpus of information implies that the young animal retains an enormous capacity for change in early patterns of behavior and cognitive competence, especially if the initial environment is seriously altered. The data offer no firm support for the popular belief that certain events during the first year can produce irreversible consequences in either human or infrahuman infants. If one limits the discussion to universal cognitive competences, in contrast to culturally specific skills, it appears that a slower rate of mastery of the universal abilities during the first two years places no serious constraints on the eventual attainment of many of the competences of pre-adolescence. . . . The first messages written on the *tabula rasa* may not necessarily be the most difficult to erase [p. 121].

But in a larger measure, the growing concern with current reality, with those factors that precipitate significant psychopathology, is an act of great affirmation. It recognizes what John F. Kennedy (1963) called the "harsh environmental conditions" that often are associated with mental illness. It legitimizes the search for effective primary preventions. And it draws us inexorably to the simple dictum of Moore (1970), "Human society ought to be organized in such a way as to eliminate useless suffering" (p. 5).

In reviewing the field of prevention, particularly primary prevention, one cannot help being impressed by both its complexity and its potential benefits. Two addresses by presidents of the American Orthopsychiatric Association to the association's members, delivered ten years apart, were devoted to urging the expansion of primary prevention activities. In 1962 Eisenberg called for a rededication by mental health professionals—both as professionals and as citizens—to the cause of prevention.

Ten years later, on the same platform, Bower (1972) focused his attention on children and on the key integrative social systems that exist in every society—those primary institutions that give pattern and meaning to the basic personality of the individual and to the society in which the individual lives.

These include the family, schools, and preventive health services. Bower suggested that prevention is difficult but that it is possible; the need for alternative social institutions (such as hospitals, jails, courts, and special schools) can be reduced or eliminated through the strengthening or rebuilding of the more fundamental integrative social systems.

In a review of the literature on primary prevention, Kessler and Albee (1975) suggest that a major source of resistance to the development of preventive intervention programs is that they require major social system changes. They suggest that many writers believe that

> patchwork solutions will not do, and that the whole structure of our polluted, industrialized, overpopulated, overenergized, overcrowded sexist and racist society breeds such massive human injustice and distress that the only hope for prevention is for major social reorganization. To prevent mental and emotional disorders, it is argued, we must abolish such injustices as unemployment, bad housing, social discrimination, personal insecurity, and poverty. As a consequence of the threat all of this holds to the status quo, the Establishment does little to encourage or support efforts at primary prevention in the social sphere because it believes, with some justification, that it would be funding programs aimed at a major redistribution of its power [p. 576].[7]

In spite of the general reluctance of the powerful to give up power, social systems can be and have been changed. Cowen and his colleagues have effected system changes in a set of public-school districts, and, to move to another arena, the prodigious efforts of Ralph Nader and his colleagues have resulted in major changes in the automobile industry's attention to the public interest and to public safety—that is, major changes in the automobile industry as a social system. With these changes have come substantial reductions in automobile fatalities (Whiteside, 1973).

In the context of these observations, the recommendations of the President's Commission on Mental Health (1978) regarding prevention seem prudent, appropriate, and timely. These recommendations—for establishment of a Center for Prevention within the National Institute of Mental Health, development of special programs directed toward children at risk, and development and evaluation of services and programs designed specifically for times of significant life stress—deserve the active support of all mental health professionals and professions. If we insist on waiting until all direct-treatment needs are met before allocating resources to prevention, we will doom our professions to the continuation of the hopeless spiral described at the beginning of this chapter. Of course, we may have to divert some money from direct treatment to undertake a significant effort in the field of primary prevention. Yet, when we consider the total cost of mental illness to our society, estimated to

---

[7]From "Primary Prevention," by M. Kessler and G. W. Albee, *Annual Review of Psychology*, 1975, *26*, 557–591. This and all other quotations from this source are reprinted by permission of Annual Reviews, Inc.

have been $17 billion in 1976 (President's Commission on Mental Health, 1978), that resource diversion not only is trivial but in fact represents one of the few hopes we have for ultimately controlling a major source of human suffering (Bloom, 1981b).

The potential of preventive intervention is almost boundless, although successful primary prevention of psychological disorders is undoubtedly more complex than most would care to admit. But history urges the continuation of preventive efforts. It is a fitting conclusion to this chapter to quote from the writings of C. E. A. Winslow, formerly of the School of Public Health at the Yale School of Medicine. Although these remarks were made 60 years ago, they have lost none of their urgency and none of their sense of hope.

> To state that the death rate of New York City has been reduced from 25 per 1000 in 1890 to 13 per 1000 in 1920 may perhaps leave one unmoved; but think for a moment what such statistics mean in terms of human life and human happiness. Today in that great city there are 201 death beds every twenty-four hours. If the death rate of thirty years ago were still in force there would be 384,—a saving of 183 lives with each revolution of the earth. If death be the wage of sanitary sin, nearly one half of the debt has been remitted in a period of thirty years.
>
> Or take a larger field. In the Registration Area[8] of the United States, the reduction in the death rate from four diseases only, typhoid fever, tuberculosis, diphtheria, and the diarrheal diseases of infancy between 1900 and 1920 amounts to a saving of 230,000 lives a year, 230,000 men, women, and children for the year 1920 alive and well who would be in their graves under the dispensation of a brief twenty years ago; more than 230,000 more for 1921, and still more for 1922, and on so far forward as our civilization shall endure. If we had but the gift of second sight to transmute abstract figures into flesh and blood, so that as we walk along the street we could say "That man would be dead of typhoid fever," "That woman would have succumbed to tuberculosis," "That rosy infant would be in its coffin,"—then only should we have a faint conception of the meaning of the silent victories of public health. For such achievements we may thank God and take courage for the future, bearing on our banners that eternal phrase of Cicero; "In no single thing do men approach the Gods more nearly, than in the giving of safety to mankind" [pp. 64–65].[9]

[8]The Registration Area includes those states participating in a coordinated vital-statistics reporting system.

[9]From *The Evolution and Significance of the Modern Public Health Campaign,* by C. E. A. Winslow. Copyright 1923 by Yale University Press. Reprinted by permission.

CHAPTER

6

Stressful-Life-Event Theory

T his chapter reviews and analyzes the recent research in the field of stressful life events. Stress has been defined as a "process in which environmental events or forces, called stressors, threaten an organism's existence and well-being" (Baum, Singer, & Baum, 1981, p. 4; Hefferin, 1980). Stress has also been defined as a condition in which there is a marked discrepancy between the demands made on an organism and the organism's capability to respond; the consequences can be detrimental to the organism's future in respect to conditions essential to its well-being (Caplan, 1981; McGrath, 1970). Stressful life events, then, are those external events that make adaptive demands on a person. These demands may be successfully met or may inaugurate a process of internal psychological or physiological straining that can culminate in some form of illness. Identification of stressful life events in a community combined with development of appropriate intervention programs may be one of the keys to the effective prevention of much emotional disorder.

By definition, stressful life events are contemporary. B. S. and B. P. Dohrenwend distinguish between stressful life events and personal dispositions. Stressful life events are

> those that are proximate to, rather than remote from, the onset of a disorder. For example, this category includes the recent death of a friend or relative but not the fact that an adult's father died when he or she was a child. The latter event is not irrelevant to life stress but is subsumed under personal dispositions, since we assume that the early death of a parent can affect an adult's behavior only insofar as its impact was internalized [1981a, p. 131].

Included among stressful life events but somewhat more removed in time from the more proximate events identified by the Dohrenwends are those episodes that produce what have been called *delayed stress responses*. These syndromes, according to Horowitz and Solomon, "often begin only after termination of real environmental stress events and after a latency period of apparent relief" (1978, p. 268). Interest in delayed stress reactions has intensified within the last several years as a consequence of the growing realization that Vietnam veterans appear to be surprisingly vulnerable to such reactions (see Figley, 1978; Williams, 1980).

Stressful-life-event research and its associated theory building represent a major effort to understand the role of psychological and sociocultural factors in the development of mental disorders. In the most recent report of the Surgeon General (U.S. Department of Health and Human Services, 1980b), a major goal articulated for promoting health and preventing disease is the more effective control of stress.

Inquiry into the role of stressful life events in human welfare is based on a very different paradigm from the one used in the analysis of specific psychiatric disorders. It is a paradigm that does not begin with the assumption that every specific disorder has a single or even a multiple necessary precondition. Rather, this paradigm is based on the clearly established association of stress with increased risk of illness. It assumes that we are all vulnerable to stressful life experiences and that "almost any disease or disability may be associated with these events" (B. S. Dohrenwend & B. P. Dohrenwend, 1974, p. 314).

Caplan has commented that "years ago we used to think that particular sets of such events in association with certain personality patterns would cause specific bodily or mental illnesses. Nowadays many of us believe that individuals exposed to such circumstances may suffer an increase in nonspecific vulnerability to a wide range of bodily and mental illnesses" (1981, p. 413). Cassel made a similar case when he wrote that "it is most unlikely that any given psychosocial process or stressor will be etiologically specific for any disease, at least as currently classified" (1976, p. 109; see also Cassel, 1973, 1974a, 1974b). Cassel's own research as well as his reviews of others' led him to conclude that although psychosocial processes enhance susceptibility to disease, the clinical manifestations of this enhanced susceptibility would not depend on the particular psychosocial stressor.

Four vulnerable persons can face a stressful life experience, perhaps the collapse of their marriage or the loss of their job. One person may become severely depressed; the second may have an automobile accident; the third may become alcoholic; and the fourth may develop a psychotic thought disorder—or coronary artery disease.

On the basis of the stress paradigm, preventive intervention programs can be organized to reduce the incidence of particular stressful life events, whenever possible, or to facilitate their mastery once they occur. In either case, one need not have undue regard for the prediction of the specific disorders that will be prevented, because this new paradigm abandons at the outset the search for a unique cause or set of causes for each disorder. Rather, the paradigm far more commonly examines the precursors of what Frank (1973) has called *demoralization* and what Dohrenwend and his colleagues (Dohrenwend, Shrout, Egri, & Mendelsohn, 1980) have more recently called *nonspecific psychological distress*. In contrast to the classic paradigm already described, the new paradigm has the following sequence of steps:

1. Identify a stressful life event, or set of such events, that appears to have undesirable consequences. Develop procedures for reliably identifying persons who have undergone or are undergoing those stressful experiences.
2. By traditional epidemiological and laboratory methods, study the consequences of those events and develop hypotheses related to how one might go about reducing or eliminating these negative consequences.
3. Mount and evaluate experimental preventive intervention programs based on these hypotheses.

This new stressful-life-event paradigm has turned our attention from long-standing predisposing factors in psychopathology to far more recent precipitating factors and is part of an even broader phenomenon. It has long been known that biological, psychological, and sociological factors differentially predispose persons to emotional disorders. With few exceptions, however, efforts to develop effective preventive services based on attempts to modify these early predisposing factors have been unsuccessful. Eisenberg has recently commented that "measurement of distant outcome places a terrible burden of proof on childhood interventions; they must be powerful indeed to be able to show a clear effect despite the vicissitudes of subsequent life experience" (1981, p. 4).

There is every reason to believe that prevention programs aimed at more successful management of stressful life events can be effective, particularly when we set about to build on what is already known about crisis theory and crisis intervention (Caplan, 1964, pp. 34–54; Mann, 1978; Parad, 1965; Parad, Resnik, & Parad, 1976). Many stressful life events, such as school entrance, new parenting, separation and divorce, retirement, and widowhood, are common; many are becoming more common; and few sustained and comprehensive services exist within our communities to assist people in mastering any of them.

If we keep in mind these two developments—the growing interest in contemporary stressful life events as well as in more distant predisposing developmental variables, and the growing acceptance of general as well as disorder-specific preventive interventions—we can better appreciate much of the recent research literature.

THE STUDY OF STRESSFUL LIFE EVENTS

Early clinical interest in the role of stressful life events is associated with the work of Cannon, Wolff, Meyer, and Selye. Cannon (1929) held that external stressors could invade the body through their effects on emotion. Wolff (1950) believed that external stressors produced protective reactions that had physiological as well as psychological components. Meyer (1951) taught that ordinary life events, if they were stressful, could play a role in the etiology of disease and urged that practitioners undertake systematic inquiry into such life events as part of their clinical assessments. Selye (1946, 1956) introduced the concept of the General Adaptation Syndrome to characterize what he believed to be a complex but nonspecific bodily reaction to stress and was instrumental in the beginning investigation of the biochemical nature of that reaction. Hinkle (1974) has summarized the implications of stress-related clinical research as of the post–World War II period by noting that "it seemed evident that there would probably be no aspect of human growth, development, or disease that would in theory be immune to the influence of the effect of a man's relation to his social and interpersonal environment" (p. 10).

An important early paper reviewing the evidence linking recent traumatic events to the occurrence of mental disorders was prepared by Reid (1961). Although that paper never used the phrase *stressful life event*, it is clear that Reid was dealing with exactly that concept. The field of stressful-life-event research came into its own and was virtually transformed by the development of the Social Readjustment Rating Scale (see Table 6–1) by Holmes and Rahe (1967; see also Holmes & Masuda, 1974; Rahe, 1979). Holmes had worked in Wolff's laboratory and followed Meyer's admonition to search for stressful events in the recent life of patients. He and his colleagues were persuaded that stressful life events, by evoking psychophysiological reactions, could play a precipitating role in many diseases.

Beginning in 1949, Holmes and his colleagues studied life stressors that over 5000 patients reported as occurring shortly before the onset of their illnesses. From this data pool, they assembled a list of 43 representative life events and proceeded to scale them in terms of stressfulness. In this process, they made two critical decisions. First, although most of the items in their list could be considered undesirable events, the concept of a stressful life event was not limited to such items but included desirable events as well. Stressfulness was defined in terms of the need for readjustment by the person undergoing the event, and desirable events (an outstanding personal achievement, for example) were thought to require a measure of readjustment just as undesirable events do (being fired at work, for example). Second, Holmes and his colleagues believed it was desirable to develop a rating scale of stressfulness derived from expert outside judgment rather than from judgments by the persons themselves. They sought to develop a scale in which each stressful event was given a single, universal weight. The methodological details of the development of the scale are described by Holmes and Masuda (1974).

TABLE 6–1. **The Holmes and Rahe Social Readjustment Rating Scale**

Rank	Life event	Mean value
1	Death of spouse	100
2	Divorce	73
3	Marital separation	65
4	Jail term	63
5	Death of close family member	63
6	Personal injury or illness	53
7	Marriage	50
8	Fired at work	47
9	Marital reconciliation	45
10	Retirement	45
11	Change in health of family member	44
12	Pregnancy	40
13	Sex difficulties	39
14	Gain of new family member	39
15	Business readjustment	39
16	Change in financial state	38
17	Death of close friend	37
18	Change to different line of work	36
19	Change in number of arguments with spouse	35
20	Mortgage over $10,000	31
21	Foreclosure of mortgage or loan	30
22	Change in responsibilities at work	29
23	Son or daughter leaving home	29
24	Trouble with in-laws	29
25	Outstanding personal achievement	28
26	Wife begin or stop work	26
27	Begin or end school	26
28	Change in living conditions	25
29	Revision of personal habits	24
30	Trouble with boss	23
31	Change in work hours or conditions	20
32	Change in residence	20
33	Change in schools	20
34	Change in recreation	19
35	Change in church activities	19
36	Change in social activities	18
37	Mortgage or loan less than $10,000	17
38	Change in sleeping habits	16
39	Change in number of family get-togethers	15
40	Change in eating habits	15
41	Vacation	13
42	Christmas	12
43	Minor violations of the law	11

Reprinted with permission from *Journal of Psychosomatic Research*, Vol. 11, pp. 213–218, T. H. Holmes and R. H. Rahe, "The Social Readjustment Rating Scale," copyright 1967, Pergamon Press, Ltd.

While research was continuing to explore the physiological concomitants of stressful life events, there was a remarkably rapid growth in the study of such events themselves, stimulated in large measure by the availability of the Holmes and Rahe scale. That scale made it possible to assign weights to events, total these weights across a broad array of such events, and then examine how the resulting total scores were related to subsequent illness. Research activity grew at such a pace that only six years after publication of the Social Readjustment Rating Scale, Barbara and Bruce Dohrenwend organized an international conference to bring many of the prominent stressful-life-event researchers together. The report of that conference (B. S. Dohrenwend & B. P. Dohrenwend, 1974) provides an eloquent summary of the state of stressful-life-event research as of that time.

The major thrust of that report for future research was to underline the complexity of the relations between stressful life events and subsequent disorder. In particular, the report urged the development of better measurement procedures and research designs, greater attention to conceptualization, and examination of factors that might moderate or intensify the effects of stressful life events. The field has been extremely responsive to these recommendations.

Recent stressful-life-event literature suggests that the role of stressful life events in precipitating illnesses is not as simple as investigators had initially envisioned (Aakster, 1974; Antonovsky, 1979; Barrett, 1979; Bunn, 1979; Crook & Eliot, 1980; B. P. Dohrenwend, 1979; B. S. Dohrenwend, 1978; Dooley & Catalano, 1980; Gersten, Langner, Eisenberg, & Simcha-Fagan, 1977; Jenkins, Tuthill, Tannenbaum, & Kirby, 1979; Mueller, Edwards, & Yarvis, 1978; Rabkin & Struening, 1976; Syme & Torfs, 1978; Tennant & Andrews, 1976; Wildman & Johnson, 1977; Zautra & Beier, 1978). These studies often, but not invariably, find that physical illnesses or psychological disorders are preceded by an excess number and intensity of stressful life events, but not enough is known that can help predict which specific persons are at unusually high risk.

The pathway between a stressful life event and subsequent illness is a complex one involving a number of important components. Rahe (1974) has proposed a series of steps that must be taken into account in understanding how a stressful life event may precipitate an illness: (1) past experience—that is, how the person has traditionally managed stressful life events so that they are more or less stressful than they would generally be, (2) psychological defenses—a person's abilities to deal with stressful life events so that they have no negative consequences, (3) physiological reactions—the nature of the physiological impact of those stressful life events that are not dealt with by successful psychological defenses, (4) coping—the ability to attenuate or compensate for physiological reactions, and (5) illness behavior—how individuals come to interpret the remaining physiological reactions as symptoms or as illness and how they decide to seek medical care.

Cobb (1974) has advanced a similar view. His scheme calls attention to (1) the objective and subjective stress associated with the stressful life event, (2) the physiological and behavioral straining that takes place in response to that stress, and (3) the subsequent development of illness and illness-related behavior. Cobb thinks of personal characteristics in much the same way as Rahe views past experience but also suggests that to understand the role of stressful life events in precipitating illness and illness behavior, we must appreciate the social situation within which the stressful life event is embedded. In particular, Cobb mentions the need to understand the current life situation, the nature of social supports available to the person, and the attitudes of peers and of medical care gatekeepers. Personal characteristics and the nature of the social situation are important mediating factors and can provide virtual immunity or excess susceptibility to illness in the face of stressful life events.

B. S. Dohrenwend (1978) has, like Cobb, conceptualized the process whereby psychosocial stress induces psychopathology. A stressful life event, usually undesirable and always requiring change or readjustment, leads to a stress reaction that is inherently transient, or self-limiting. Situational and psychological factors serve as mediators in determining whether this transient stress reaction will result in psychological growth, in the development of psychopathology, or in a lack of any substantial psychological change.

Chan (1977; see also Baum, Singer, & Baum, 1981; Lazarus, 1976) identified the process of appraisal, that process by which persons choose a particular pattern of reaction to a stressful life event, as one that might help account for the wide individual differences in reactions to stress so commonly reported in the literature. Chan identifies locus of control, sense of helplessness, chronic anxiety, and low self-esteem as central personality determinants of stress reactions. At the environmental level, strength of social supports appears to be most important as a stress-reaction determinant. On the basis of an analysis of these personality and environmental dimensions, Chan believes it should be possible to develop and validate a "vulnerability index"—a predictive measure of risk.

Sarason's theoretical framework for stress research views stress as following "a call for action when one's capabilities are perceived as falling short of the needed personal resources" (1980, p. 74). Stress can be handled by appropriate orientation to the task or, conversely, by such responses as unproductive preoccupation, anxiety, anger, depression, denial, or retreat into fantasy. Mediating factors can be classified as person or situational variables. Examples of person variables are such characteristics as the ability to anticipate danger, feel safe, or feel confident and history of stress-arousing experiences. Situational variables include such factors as available social supports.

The stress-response paradigm developed by B. P. Dohrenwend (1979) is based on Selye's (1956) formulations. This paradigm identifies four main elements: (1) an antecedent stressor, (2) mediating factors, (3) nonspecific physical and chemical changes, and (4) consequent adaptive or maladaptive responses. Conceptualizations generally similar to those just reviewed have also been advanced by Caplan (1981), Paykel (1979, pp. 82–85), and Warheit (1979, pp. 502–503).

Conceptual models linking stressful life events to illness have some common features. First, in the process of describing the links between stressful life events and subsequent disorders, life stressors need to be viewed within a social and psychological context. That context may contain factors that moderate the effects of stressful life events, such as a strong social support network or personal robustness, or factors that strengthen the effects of stressful life events, such as a history of poor crisis management, characteristic physiological overreaction, or a sense of external locus of control. Second, the long-term consequences of stressful life events are not necessarily deleterious—they may have no measurable consequences at all or may have adaptive and positive components. Finally, in evaluating the consequences of stressful life events, help-seeking patterns must be taken into account along with an understanding of the medical and psychological care system accessible to the person.

Albee (1979) has proposed a similar analysis in his formula stating that the risk of developing an emotional disorder is directly related to organic vulnerabilities and stress and inversely related to coping skills, competence, and the adequacy of social supports.

Keeping in mind the social context or situation, personal dispositions, and the stressful life event, we can examine the various hypotheses advanced to account for that chain of events. B. S. and B. P. Dohrenwend (1981b) have identified six competing hypotheses, shown in Figure 6–1.

Model A suggests that cumulations of stressful life events cause adverse health changes. The Dohrenwends call this model the *victimization* hypothesis. They believe that this model is appropriate to account for studies of extreme situations such as combat, incarceration in a concentration camp, or certain severe stresses, such as the death of a loved one, over which a person has no control. Model B suggests that psychophysiological strain mediates the impact of life events on subsequent illness—the *stress-strain* hypothesis. Support for this hypothesis comes from studies that show, for example, that if the effects of symptoms of psychophysiological straining are eliminated, correlations of stressful-life-event scores with measures of illness are significantly reduced.

Model C, the *vulnerability* hypothesis, supposes that preexisting personal dispositions and social conditions moderate the causal relation between stressful life events and psychopathology. This model forms the basis for the examination of the effects of mediating factors such as the strength of social supports, optimism, or locus of control on the relation between stress and illness. Model D, the *additive burden* hypothesis, suggests that personal dispositions and social conditions make an independent causal contribution to the occurrence of psychopathology. This model provides an alternative to the vulnerability hypothesis in explaining the role of personality variables or social resources in the precipitation of illness.

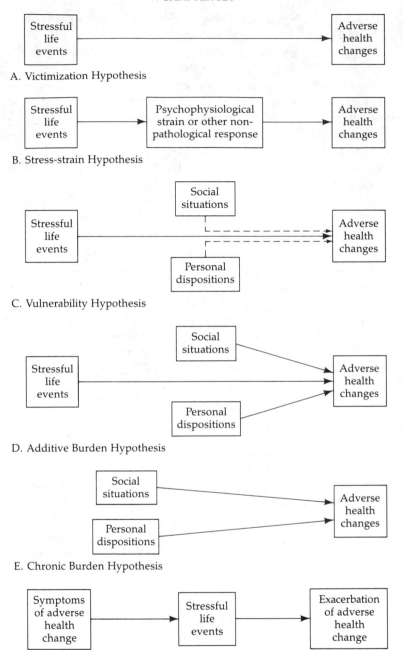

FIGURE 6.1 Six hypotheses about the life-stress process. From *Stressful Life Events and Their Contexts,* edited by B. S. Dohrenwend and B. P. Dohren-wend. *(Copyright © 1981 by Prodist. Reprinted by permission.)*

Model E, the *chronic burden* hypothesis, proposes that transitory stressful life events have no role in precipitating illness but, rather, that more stable personal dispositions and social conditions alone cause the adverse health changes. Finally, Model F proposes that the presence of a disorder leads to stressful life events, which, in turn, exacerbate the disorder. This model is called the *event proneness* hypothesis because proneness to stressful life events is thought to characterize persons who are already ill.

The principal activities in the field of stressful-life-event research can be grouped within these conceptual models. The psychological or physiological consequences of a particular stressful life event or of cumulative stressful life events are continuing to be examined in a very large number of studies. A growing number of studies are assessing the effects of mediating factors, including both personal and social-environmental characteristics. Fewer studies are seeking to identify positive consequences of stressful life events or are contrasting specific stressful life events in terms of their actual consequences. Finally, papers making general contributions to the methodology of stressful-life-event research have been quite numerous in recent years.

It is perhaps an indication of the continuing progress in the field of stressful-life-event research that Holmes has identified ten preventive measures that derive from the recent research using the Social Readjustment Rating Scale (see Table 6–1). These measures include the following:

> Become familiar with the life events and the amount of change they require. . . . Put the Scale where you and the family can see it easily several times a day. . . . With practice you can recognize when a life event happens. . . . Think about the meaning of the event for you and try to identify some of the feelings you experience. . . . Think about the different ways you might best adjust to the event. . . . Take your time in arriving at decisions. . . . Anticipate life changes and plan for them well in advance, if possible [1979, p. 51].

STRESSFUL LIFE EVENTS AND PSYCHOPATHOLOGY

Schizophrenia

In one of the earliest studies of the temporal relationship between the occurrence of life events and the onset of schizophrenia, Brown and Birley (1968) conducted in-depth interviews with 50 psychiatric patients who had had an acute onset of schizophrenia and, separately, with their relatives. Brown and Birley were interested in obtaining accurate data on the frequency of certain kinds of crises and life changes during the 13 weeks prior to onset of the disorder. The authors conducted essentially identical interviews with a general-population sample of 325 persons for comparison purposes. (These control subjects were asked about stressful events during the 13 weeks prior to the date of interview.) The authors determined the occurrence of events that "on common sense grounds are likely to produce emotional disturbance in many people" (p. 204). They also judged each event reported as either clearly independent or possibly independent of the disorder (that is, how completely the event was outside the patient's control).

Brown and Birley found that the patient group experienced substantially more stressful life events overall and, most important, this difference occurred in the three weeks immediately prior to onset. The rate of events for the patient group during this period was three times that in the general population—60% and 20%, respectively, experiencing at least one stressful life event. Outside these three weeks, the rates in the two groups were virtually the same. These results were obtained whether independent events were considered together with possibly independent events or separately. The authors concluded:

> There is reasonably sound evidence that environmental factors can precipitate a schizophrenic attack and that such events tend to cluster in the three weeks before onset. We do not regard the events as sufficient causes. We believe that a number of factors must contribute and perhaps coincide to produce the conditions necessary for an acute schizophrenic attack, and that we have demonstrated one of these—some sort of crisis or life change [p. 211].

In another early study, Steinberg and Durell (1968) reviewed the military records of every noncommissioned soldier in the U.S. Army who was hospitalized with a diagnosis of schizophrenia during 1956–1960. They found that the hospitalization rate during the early months of military service was markedly greater than during the second year. Steinberg and Durell found that only a very small proportion of the early hospitalizations was due to detection of chronic cases and therefore concluded that there was "a genuine increase in the rate of onset of acute schizophrenic symptoms during the early months of service" (p. 1104). These authors believed that their findings were consistent with the hypothesis that "a situation producing an intense need for social adaptation is an effective precipitant of acute schizophrenic symptoms in individuals predisposed to develop the schizophrenic syndrome" (p. 1104).

Several similar studies have since been reported, and Rabkin (1980) examined a number of them to determine whether stressful life events were related to the onset of schizophrenia. These studies fall into three types according to what comparison group is used: some studies contrast the frequency of stressful life events in schizophrenics and normals, others in schizophrenics and other types of psychiatric patients, and others in relapsing and nonrelapsing schizophrenics.

The two studies contrasting schizophrenics with normal controls found some support for the prediction that patients would report more recent stressful life events than controls. The five studies contrasting schizophrenics with other psychiatric patients did not find stressful life events to be more frequent for schizophrenics. If anything, such events appeared to occur more commonly for depressed patients. Finally, in the four studies contrasting schizophrenics who relapsed with those who did not, the relapsing patients reported more stressful life events. Rabkin concluded from her critical review that "life events may contribute incrementally to an already inflated stress level and so may influence the timing, if not the probability, of illness onset" (p. 424).

Affective disorders

To discover whether depressed patients attribute the same degree of required readjustment to stressful life events as do randomly chosen members of the general population, Schless, Schwartz, Goetz, and Mendels (1974) administered the Holmes and Rahe Social Readjustment Rating Scale to a sample of 76 hospitalized depressives along with a scale that measured the severity of depression. Depressed patients, both at the time of admission and at the time of discharge from the hospital, tended to rate the items in the stressful-life-event inventory as requiring more readjustment than normals did, although the ratings given by depressives and normals correlated very highly. Readjustment weights assigned by patients were found to be unrelated to the patient's age, sex, severity of depression, whether the patient had experienced the event or not, and degree of symptomatic improvement.

Paykel (1979) believes that life events are implicated in the genesis of most depressions except for a small minority that appear endogenous (physiological) in character. Although the vast majority of persons who undergo stressful life events do not become depressed, people who undergo these events are clearly at excess risk. Furthermore, the risk is particularly high immediately after the event and tends to diminish with passing time.

Dunner, Patrick, and Fieve (1979), similarly, found a high incidence of reported stressful life events during the three months prior to the episode among 79 patients in treatment for bipolar manic-depressive disorder. For patients whose first episode was manic, more men than women reported stressful life events prior to onset. For patients whose first episode was depressive, more women than men reported stressful life events. Among these events, the most common was childbirth.

Jacobs, Prusoff, and Paykel (1974) contrasted matched samples of 50 schizophrenics and 50 depressives all admitted for the first time for inpatient care. Depressives reported significantly more stressful life events than schizophrenics during the six months prior to onset of illness, particularly increases in the number of arguments with family members not living in the house and with closely related members of the other sex, such as steady girlfriends or boyfriends. An excess number of undesirable stressful life events was found for the depressives, but no such difference was found in the number of desirable events. Similarly, an excess number of events referring to exits from the social field (for example, death, divorce, leaving home) was found for the depressives, while no such excess of events representing entrances into the social field (for example, marriage, birth of a child, a new person moving into the home) was found. Depressives reported significantly more stressful life events in the area of finances and health than schizophrenics. The authors view their findings as consistent with the position that "life events are involved in the genesis of depression and schizophrenia" (p. 452). The relationship appears to be stronger for depressives than for schizophrenics and appears to involve more undesirable events (see also Rahe, 1979).

Neurotic disorders

Stressful life events appear to be implicated in the development of neurotic disorders. Cooper and Sylph (1973) found an excess number of stressful life events during the preceding three months in a sample of 34 patients with new cases of neurotic illness seeking medical care in London, contrasted with a matched nonneurotic sample. Serious threatening events (such as unexpected crises and news of failure) were particularly common among the new neurotics and uncommon among the controls. Cooper and Sylph calculated the proportion of neurotic illness attributable to stressful events and the average time by which the stressful life events advanced the onset of the neuroses (see Brown, Harris, and Peto, 1973). They concluded that "major events act as aetiological agents in the strict sense of provoking illnesses which otherwise, in terms of probability, would not occur until years later" (p. 427).

Tennant and Andrews (1978) surveyed a representative suburban sample of 863 persons in Sydney, Australia, and examined the relationship between a self-report measure of neurotic impairment (Goldberg, 1972) and three measures of stressful life events incurred during the previous year—total number of events, events weighted for emotional distress, and cumulated score weighted for life change. Although the three measures of stressful life events were highly correlated (correlation coefficients ranged from .79 to .89) and all three measures were modestly but significantly correlated with the measure of neurotic impairment, partial correlations suggested that only the measure of stressful life events weighted for distress was independently related to neurotic impairment. Tennant and Andrews concluded that "life events are pathogenic in neurosis because of the emotionally distressing impact and not simply because they produce life change" (p. 863).

Barrett (1979) studied stressful life events in the six months prior to onset in a group of 203 outpatients with neurotic disorders. His concern was mainly with neurotic depressives and with patients whose primary symptom was anxiety. In contrasting the depressed patients with those whose primary symptom was anxiety, Barrett found significant differences in the frequency of reports of undesirable events and events that represented a change in life setting. Such events not only occurred more frequently but were generally rated as more distressing among neurotically depressed patients than among those with anxiety, particularly when the event involved losses or changes in interpersonal relationships. By contrast, events that involved the need to carry out some instrumental behavior (for example, taking an examination, changing to a different line of work, financial difficulties, arguments) were seen as more stressful by patients with anxiety neuroses than by depressives.

Childhood disorders

Findings linking stressful life events in childhood with subsequent emotional difficulties are more mixed. Sandler and Block (1979) examined the relationship between life stress and maladjustment in a group of 99 maladjusting children and 44 matched nonmaladjusting children in four inner-city schools. The children were generally poor and of minority status. Most were from families on welfare. Life stress during the preceding year was assessed using a modification of the stressful-life-event scale developed for elementary-school children (Coddington, 1972a). The scale was completed by parents, and items selected for inclusion in the study were all judged to be events beyond the child's control—that is, events thought not to be confounded with the behavioral adjustment of the child. In addition, all items were independently rated as desirable, undesirable, or ambiguous. The nature of maladjustment was assessed by teachers and by parents.

Maladapting children were found to have suffered significantly more stressful life events, particularly undesirable ones, in the preceding year than adapting children, but the difference was found only for children not on welfare. That is, maladapting children on welfare and adapting children on welfare showed no differences in the frequency of stressful life events.

The authors suggest that some factors associated with being on welfare (perhaps including the availability of stronger social support systems) appear to moderate the effects of stressful life events. The fact that the stressful life events studied were not under the children's control "strengthens the implication of stress as a contributory cause of the children's adjustment problems" (p. 436).

Childhood stress and adult disorder

Robins (1979) has provided a recent review of her research linking childhood behavior and events to the development of antisocial personalities as adults and has found that replications of her work have supported the original findings—namely, that adult antisocial personality rarely occurs in the absence of serious antisocial behavior in childhood. Robins believes antisocial children undergo a long series of stressful life events over which they have very little control. She indicates that if scientists are to make progress in implicating stressful life events as causal factors in psychopathology, they will have to show, first, that the risk of such psychopathology is significantly greater among those persons who have undergone the event than among those who have not and, second, that there is a general consistency in the time interval between the event and its presumed consequences.

Crook and Eliot (1980) reviewed the research literature examining the consequences of parental death during childhood for adult behavior, specifically focusing on the development of depression. Most of the more than 20 studies they examined were case-control studies in which histories of parental death in a group of depressed patients and in some type of contrasting group were compared. These reviewers identified a series of complexities in this topic of study. First, the probability of parental death during childhood is related to age of parents, age of child, and social class. Second, there are severe problems in finding an agreed-on procedure for diagnosing adult depression or any of its subtypes. Third, highly varied comparison groups have been studied in order to determine the incidence of parental death in nondepressed persons. Such groups have included other psychiatric patients, normal controls, and persons with medical illnesses. Finally, numerous studies that seem quite comparable in design have yielded very inconsistent results. On the basis of their analysis of these published studies, Crook and Eliot concluded that "there is no sound base of empirical data to support the theorized relationship between parental death during childhood and adult depression or any subtype of adult depression" (p. 258). Similar conclusions have been reached by Tennant, Smith, Bebbington, and Hurry (1981).

STRESSFUL LIFE EVENTS AND PHYSICAL HEALTH

Fully as much interest has been expressed in the possible role of stressful life events in precipitating physical illness as in the precipitation of emotional disorders (see Cohen, 1979). Evidence linking stressful life events with subsequent physical disorder seems very persuasive. Hinkle (1974) has been examining the effects of changes in interpersonal relationships and of changes in the social and cultural milieu on health in a series of studies over the past 30 years. In a study of more than 500 telephone operators who were part of a comprehensive sickness-benefit program and who had worked for 20 years or more, Hinkle found a strong connection between stressful interpersonal and environmental difficulties and illness. He concluded that

> the longitudinal and retrospective life histories obtained from the frequently ill and moderately ill usually suggested that a cluster of illness coincided with a period when the individual was experiencing many demands and frustrations arising from his social environment or his interpersonal relations. These histories suggested that significant changes in the relations of ill people to their social group and in their relations to other important people in their lives were significantly associated with changes in their health [p. 21].

In Hinkle's studies of Chinese who immigrated to the United States soon after World War II, of Hungarian refugees who came to the United States in 1956, and of American prisoners of war in North Korea, excess illness was generally found. Among the Hungarian refugees, Hinkle wrote, "individuals differed markedly in their general susceptibility to illness. . . . The frequently ill people . . . had experienced a greater number of disturbances of mood, thought, and behavior" (1974, p. 29).

Aakster's (1974) survey of more than 1500 adults in Holland examined the interrelations of psychosocial stresses and health disturbances. Aakster's analysis indicates that although most of the variation in health disturbances is accounted for by generalized psychological dysfunction, specific disorders seem to be associated, in addition, with certain specific psychological difficulties. "Illness," Aakster has concluded, "is the more or less automatic result of a failure to adjust to stress. Stress was defined as a discrepancy between the ideal state of the individual in relation to his desired goals and the actual position in which he finds himself. We therefore infer that there is a close relationship between all kinds of failures of the individual in realizing his existential goals, and the development of illness" (pp. 88–89).

Gallin (1980) examined the use of medical services in a group of 124 relatively healthy women aged 20–40 in an ambulatory health care center. She found that those women who were poor, less well educated, and separated or divorced were likely to define the physician's authority very broadly and to feel that "their social resources were only nominally effective in mediating between them and the pressures of life-strains" (1980, p. 262). Gallin found that "these women visited the health center more frequently for vague, unorganized symptoms than women whose situations were less burdened" and that "the disadvantaged women's high use of medical services was an attempt to deal with their distress—social, psychic, and somatic—and consistent with and an adjustment to their deleterious life situations" (1980, p. 262).

Cooke and Greene (1981) examined the relationship between stressful life events and the report of both psychological and physical symptoms in a group of 131 premenopausal and menopausal women. They found that their subjects who developed psychological symptoms were reacting to general stress. These women appeared to be less able to cope with general stresses than formerly.

Totman (1979) has examined the responses to stressful life events in a sample of 25 males who were admitted to a coronary care unit because of a first myocardial infarction and a comparison group of males attending the ear, nose, and throat clinic at the same hospital. Totman found support for his hypothesis that, during the year prior to seeking medical care, the heart patients would have shown a significant decrease in involvement in goal-directed activities and in social interaction when contrasted with the ear, nose, and throat patients. The two groups had had about the same number and variety of stressful life events during the preceding year, but their reactions appeared to be quite different. Totman's conclusion is that "being cut off from customary pursuits and from familiar social contacts is potentially harmful to health—especially when no substitutes are formed" (p. 198). With regard to the specificity issue in the link between stressful life events and various disease responses, Totman concludes that "growing evidence that a similar class of life event is to be found in the pre-morbid histories of patients who develop psychiatric symptoms *and* patients who develop physical symptoms . . . brings to the forefront the possibility that physical and psychiatric illness are alternative responses to the same underlying 'problem' " (p. 198).

In another study, Totman, Kiff, Reed, and Craig (1980) examined the relationship of stressful life events to vulnerability to the common cold in a sample of 52 persons who were given experimental colds by nasal inoculation with a virus. These subjects ranged in age from 18 to 49 and came from many walks of life. Before inoculation with the virus, they were assessed on a variety of measures of recent life stress and given a number of personality inventories. The severity of the cold was measured by the amount of virus present in nasal washings. The authors obtained "clear evidence of a psychosomatic component in colds" (p. 155). Introverts developed significantly more severe colds than extraverts. Perhaps more important, these authors found that certain stressful life events, particularly those associated with changes in general activity level, were significantly related to the magnitude of the subsequent infection.

An interesting, if somewhat controversial, literature links stressful life events with the development of some cancers and with relapses following treatment for cancer (Achterberg, Simonton, and Matthews-Simonton, 1976). Schmale and Iker (1971) found a significant relationship between interviewer judgments of hopelessness or hopelessness potential in a sample of 68 women admitted for biopsy and subsequent laboratory reports of positive cervical cancer. Correct predictions were made in 50 of the 68 cases. These authors believe that "a high hopelessness potential provides a special somatic vulnerability through a loss of ego control for women who are already biologically predisposed to cancer of the cervix" (p. 98). Simonton and Simonton assert specifically that the most important predisposing factor in the development of cancer is "the loss of a serious love object, occurring six to eighteen months prior to the diagnosis. . . . The loss, whether real or imagined, has to be very significant; and even more important is . . . that it engenders the feeling of helplessness and hopelessness" (1975, p. 30; see also Schmale, 1972).

These authors present some data suggesting that there is a strong correlation between patients' positive attitudes and their clinical response to cancer treatment. The authors assume, however, not only that this correlation is a sign of a cause-and-effect relationship but that the direction of causality is that the positive attitude causes the good response to treatment. Even though the correlation of attitude and treatment response might hold in other studies as well, it would be critically important to distinguish among three equally plausible hypotheses: (1) attitudes cause treatment outcome, (2) treatment outcome causes attitudes; and (3) no cause/effect relation is involved in the correlation of these two variables, in that both may be related to a third variable, such as the severity of the condition for which treatment is being obtained (see also Cohen, 1979).

In a subsequent paper, Simonton, Matthews-Simonton, and Sparks (1980) examined the effects of psychological intervention (brief individual and group psychotherapy, relaxation and imagery enhancement, and health education) in the treatment of advanced cancers by contrasting survival duration in a group of 225 treated patients with nationally reported median survival durations for persons with the same disorders. National survival duration reports are in the range of 6–16 months; survival duration in the psychologically treated sample was about twice as long. The authors are circumspect in the interpretation of their findings and implicitly acknowledge the need for a stronger research design, but they do believe that "addressing the emotional issues presented by the patients in this study played a role in lengthening their survival" (p. 232).

Selzer and Vinokur (1974) studied a sample of 274 automobile drivers (selected to include a large number who had been in an automobile accident within the past year) and 258 automobile drivers who were in inpatient or outpatient treatment for alcoholism (of whom about 20% had been in an automobile accident within the past year). Demographic and personality variables were very modestly associated with accident history in both groups of drivers. Frequency of reported stressful life events during the past year and measures of current physical and subjective stress in a variety of life contexts (for example, marital and family life, working conditions, financial status, and health concerns) were substantially more highly related to accident history. Selzer and Vinokur concluded that life change and subjective stress measures "appear to be statistically more important than the demographic, personality, and social maladjustment variables that have previously been the focus of behavioral scientists. . . . relatively transitory life events, subjective stress phenomena, and the resultant changes they impose are an important factor in the traffic accident process" (p. 906).

Cassel (1974a) has concluded that one of the psychosocial factors that may play a role in reducing vulnerability to disease is the presence of other members of the same species. His conclusion derives from a review of animal studies as well as studies with human subjects, and he has proposed four hypotheses for consideration. First, the social process linking high population density to enhanced susceptibility to disease is not the crowding itself but the "disordered relationships that, in animals, are inevitable consequences of such crowding. . . . In human populations the circumstances in which increased susceptibility to disease would occur would be those in which there is some evidence of social disorganization" (p. 1041). Second, persons who occupy subordinate positions in the hierarchy of power or prestige will be particularly vulnerable to disease. Third, biological and social buffers exist (for example, coping capacities and social supports) that can cushion the individual from the physiological or psychological consequences of social disorganization. Finally, under conditions of social change and social disorganization, susceptibility to disease is in general increased.

Rowland (1977) examined a number of these hypotheses, reviewing the literature linking death among the elderly with three stressful life events— death of a significant other, relocation, and retirement. These three events have been identified as being particularly stressful under certain circumstances, particularly for the elderly. Rowland concludes that the evidence would argue that death of a spouse is detrimental, particularly for men and particularly within the first year of bereavement. Relocation, specifically from a private home to some type of group home for the aged or from one group setting to another, appears to predict death for those elderly persons who are already in poor health. Retirement appears to be a much more equivocal stressful life event, and it has not yet been possible to design a study in which the fact of retirement has been independent of prior health status.

Rowland has also examined the principal theories advanced to link these three stressful life events to premature death, including crisis theory, reinforcement theory, and learned-helplessness theory. Each model appears to generate important and researchable propositions. Crisis theory would suggest, for example, that prior coping styles and coping skills might play a role in determining whether relocation will lead to premature death. Reinforcement theory would lead one to examine patterns of reinforcement before and after relocation and changes in these patterns as a function of the event. Learned-helplessness theory would postulate, for example, a differential effect of forced versus voluntary relocation. In addition, each theory would emphasize somewhat different approaches to reducing the impact of relocation.

COMMUNITYWIDE STRESSFUL LIFE EVENTS

Some types of stressful life events, such as economic recession, may have an impact on an entire community and may be assessed without surveying individuals. Viewing economic downturns as stressful life events, however, does run the risk of committing the *ecological fallacy*—that is, the risk of assuming that an event that affects a community at large affects each community resident equally. The ecological fallacy would be committed by showing a relationship between economic downturns and communitywide well-being without showing that any particular individual suffered after experiencing economic stress. Another example of the ecological fallacy would be to discover that psychiatric-hospital admission rates are highest in those parts of the city in which there is a good deal of marital disruption and to conclude, as a consequence, that patients who are admitted are more often divorced than people in the community who are not psychiatric-hospital patients.

In spite of these problems in interpreting the findings of studies examining stressful life events that affect entire communities, a number of researchers have felt it to be useful to assess the extent to which such communitywide stressful events are associated with increases in various disorders. For example, Brenner (1973) found that increasing unemployment rates were highly associated with subsequent increases in mental-hospitalization rates. Catalano and Dooley (1977), in examining field-survey data collected in Kansas City, found that economic change was followed in one to three months by significant increases in self-reported life change and depressed mood.

In a more detailed subsequent analysis of the Kansas City data, Dooley and Catalano (1979) were able to examine the relationship between both economic and noneconomic life events and reported psychiatric symptoms in groups disaggregated by age, sex, and socioeconomic status. Data for the Kansas City study were obtained by interviewing one adult in each of 28 households chosen weekly for a period of 16 months. Economic life events included such phenomena as graduating from school, starting work, getting laid off, and acquiring property. Noneconomic life events included, for example, marriage or divorce, pregnancy, being arrested, and taking a vacation. Both types of events were also rated for whether they were generally seen as desirable or undesirable. Economic indicators at the community level included such variables as monthly unemployment rate and monthly inflation rate. Psychiatric symptoms were assessed by means of a standard short self-report measure (Langner, 1962).

Individually reported stressful life events were not found to be predictive of subsequent self-reported psychiatric symptoms. Economic indicators at the community level were significantly related to subsequent economic-life-event variables at the individual level, however, and to subsequent reports of psychiatric symptoms. Relationships tended to be stronger for men than women. There were no remarkable differences in the obtained relationships as a function of age, but the low-socioeconomic-status group was more responsive to economic change than the middle-income group. Dooley and Catalano concluded that "changes in a community's economy are associated with later changes in noneconomic . . . and economic events" (1979, p. 392). Furthermore, they concluded that "increases in unemployment and absolute economic indicators precede, by 4 to 8 weeks, increases in psychophysiological symptoms reported by samples of a metropolitan population" (p. 393).

In their recent review of the literature linking economic change and subsequent behavior disorder, Dooley and Catalano (1980) have conceptualized the links between economic change and treated disorder rates in a series of discrete steps. First, they postulate a link between environmental economic change (for example, increasing unemployment rate) and reported increased stressful life events, both economic and noneconomic, at an individual level. Second, these individual stressful life events may be linked to subsequent symptomatology. Third, this increased symptomatology may be linked to subsequent increases in demand for health-related services, resulting in an increased treated incidence rate.

Brenner (1979) has reviewed his own work linking economic characteristics of the social environment with physical and psychological disability. He has concluded that "major economic life changes . . . are associated with severe pathology in the areas of mental and physical health and criminal aggression" (p. 174). In addition, further analyses of his data have suggested that whereas "abrupt economic changes . . . are stress provoking . . . undesirable changes, such as unemployment and income loss, are substantially more generative of pathology" (p. 175).

Further work examining communitywide stressful life events was done by Bunn in Australia (1979, 1980), linking deaths from ischemic heart disease (IHD) to fluctuations in the business cycle. Australia suffered a severe economic depression during the five or six years before World War II and a smaller recession in 1961. Bunn used the national unemployment rate as an index of the business cycle. Rates of pharmaceutical prescribing by primary care physicians served as a measure of "national stress or morbidity" (1979, p. 773). Bunn found significant relationships between the unemployment rate and subsequent mortality rates from IHD, as well as subsequent drug prescribing. These associations appeared stronger for older groups. Time-lag variations in the IHD death rate and in the measure of national stress followed the fluctuations in the business cycle fairly closely (see also Jenkins, Tuthill, Tannenbaum, & Kirby, 1979).

Some studies, however, have found very weak relationships between communitywide stress and illness. Kasl and Harburg (1975) examined the extent to which high environmental stress (living in neighborhoods that were low on measures of socioeconomic characteristics and high on measures of crime, family disruption, and residential instability) could be shown to have consequences for perceived mental health and well-being. They surveyed 1000 married adults in four geographic areas in Detroit. Two areas were defined as high stress; the other two were low stress. One area in each stress group was populated mainly by whites, the other mainly by blacks.

Residents of high- and low-stress areas reported substantially different perceptions of their neighborhoods in the direction that would be predicted. That is, residents of high-stress areas saw their neighborhoods as far more unsafe and unsatisfying than did residents of low-stress areas, generally regardless of race or sex. Yet, these perceived environmental characteristics were unrelated to measures of mental health. Kasl and Harburg conclude that there is "very modest and spotty support for the general notion that variations in the nature of the urban environment, and in perceptions of it, play a role in the level of mental health and well-being" (p. 276).

The ecological approach to the study of stressful life events has undergone considerable criticism. Bunn's study, illustrative of this ecological approach, has been criticized by Kasl (1979, 1980) and by Lew (1979, 1980). Their critiques include pointing out the dramatic changes that have taken place in diagnostic practices regarding heart diseases (making the study of factors related to IHD mortality rates over time suspect); the lack of any a priori theoretical rationale for selecting any particular time-lag length (thus permitting chance findings to exert an undue influence); the discontinuity of ecologically based research and theory with clinical epidemiological research and theory focused on the individual; problems in much of the statistical manipulation of time-trend data;

and the prematurity of cause/effect assertions even when statistical and methodological problems are set aside.

One study (Bloom, 1975) has examined the relationship of both individual
and ecological measures of social disequilibrium to rates of treatment for psychiatric disorders. Social disequilibrium as a census-tract measure (for example, proportion of adult males who are divorced) was found to be highly
associated with treatment rates, but individual measures of social disequilibrium (for example, marital status of patients contrasted with marital status
of the total population) were found to be far more powerfully related to such
rates. Kasl (1979) is likely correct when he asserts that "when facing the results
of a macro-social or ecologic analysis, the safest attitude for the reader to adopt
is one of profound skepticism" (p. 784).

EFFECTS OF SPECIFIC STRESSFUL LIFE EVENTS

According to B. P. Dohrenwend's (1979) recent assessment of the literature
linking specific stressful life events to subsequent psychopathology,

> With respect to . . . whether stressful life events are important in the causation
> of . . . psychopathology in the general population, the best evidence is indirect.
> The reason is that this evidence comes not from epidemiological studies of com-
> munity populations under ordinary conditions but rather from studies of individ-
> uals and groups under extraordinary conditions imposed by natural and man-
> made disasters, especially the disaster of war. . . . Studies of such extreme situ-
> ations have provided compelling evidence that the stressful events involved can
> produce psychopathology in previously normal persons. . . . Certainly at the
> extreme of exposure to the brutalities of Nazi concentration camps, there is strong
> evidence that not only does severe stress-induced psychopathology persist in the
> survivors . . . but also that the survivors are more prone to physical illness and
> early death [pp. 3–4; see also Kinston & Rosser, 1974].[1]

Ursano and his colleagues (Ursano, 1981; Ursano, Boydstun, & Wheatley,
1981) have been monitoring the long-term consequences of one particular
stressful life event—being a prisoner during the Vietnam war. Their research
leaves no doubt that repatriated prisoners of war had to face a significant
degree of psychological stress and that there is an increased incidence of psychiatric illness in their sample.

This section will examine studies that have attempted to ascertain the
effects of other specific life stresses.

---

[1]From "Stressful Life Events and Psychopathology: Some Issues of Theory and Method," by B.
P. Dohrenwend. In J. E. Barrett, R. M. Rose and G. L. Klerman (Eds.), *Stress and Mental Disorder*.
Copyright © 1979 by Raven Press. This and all other quotations from the same source are reprinted
by permission.

High-rise housing

Gillis (1977) has examined the extent to which living in high-rise housing can constitute a chronic stressful life event. Previous research has tended to show that such settings create more strain for women than for men. In his study of 442 residents in a variety of public housing settings in two Canadian cities, Gillis found that women are more likely to experience psychological strain if they live in upper floors of high-rise units or on the ground floor. Men show the opposite pattern: those living on the ground floor or on the upper floors of high-rise units express least strain. Gillis believes that women feel unusually vulnerable on ground floors in public housing, which is often characterized by a high crime rate. Men, Gillis speculates, may be attracted to high-level living, which is often symbolic of successful upward mobility.

Loss of employment

Kasl (1979) has examined job loss and retirement as stressful life events and has reviewed studies linking these events to changes in mental health status. Job loss and retirement must be understood within a context that takes into account the meaning of work to the individual and the social, psychological, and physical setting in which the work takes place—that is, the work environment.

Kasl concludes that there is little evidence that the transition from work to retirement has a generally adverse impact on physical or mental health. Variations in postretirement adjustment seem to reflect continuities with preretirement status and adjustment, particularly in the areas of health, social and leisure-time activities, and general well-being. In contrast, loss of a job, particularly involuntarily, does cause stress, but of relatively short duration. Persons who become unemployed appear to adapt to that state and its consequences rather quickly, whether or not they find new employment, except for the stresses associated with economic deprivation.

Oliver and Pomicter (1981) examined the effects of unemployment on depression in 182 automotive assembly-line workers following an economic recession responsible for extended layoffs. They hypothesized that employment insecurity would be significantly and positively correlated with depression. Employment insecurity was measured objectively (by whether the employee had been laid off and by the employee's seniority) and subjectively (by perceived job instability).

Among employees who had not been laid off, depression scores were correlated with variables previously found to be related to depression—race, marital status, and education. In addition, optimism about the future of the economy was found to be related to level of depression. Among the group that had been laid off, depression scores were significantly related to judgments about the employee's future job and financial security rather than to any demographic variables such as marital status. While there were no significant differences in depression scores between workers who had and had not been laid off, the stressful character of being laid off could be seen in the high depression scores of workers who had little optimism that they would soon be rehired.

Husband absence

Another atypical stressful life event that has been studied is separation from husbands sent overseas during wartime. Representative of these studies is the clinical investigation by Bey and Lange (1974), who interviewed 40 wives of noncareer Army men sent to Vietnam. These wives described the stresses occurring before, during, and after the separation. Bey and Lange suggest a number of potentially effective preventive programs that could be inaugurated for these high-risk wives and indicate that similar programs could be introduced into civilian settings where husbands must be away from home periodically, sometimes for long periods.

Marital disruption

In investigations such as those by Holmes and Rahe (1967), separation and divorce are consistently judged by samples of professionals or community residents as among the most stressful events of adult life. Furthermore, in the stressful-life-event scales developed by Coddington and his colleagues (1972a, 1972b; Heisel, Ream, Raitz, Rappaport, & Coddington, 1973) for use with children, only death in the family ranks higher than separation and divorce of the parents in judged stressfulness (see also Gersten, Langner, Eisenberg, & Orzeck, 1974).

Two other types of studies underline the stressfulness of marital disruption. First, studies assessing morbidity and mortality rates as a function of marital status consistently show that separated and divorced persons are at substantially higher risk than persons in intact marriages (Bloom, Asher, & White, 1978). This statement holds true for psychopathology, many physical disorders, motor-vehicle accidents, alcoholism, suicide, and homicide. Second, as described in Chapter 5, admission rates into both inpatient and outpatient psychiatric facilities are far higher for separated and divorced persons than for persons in intact marriages, particularly among males (Bloom, 1975; Bloom et al., 1978; Crago, 1972; Grad & Sainsbury, 1966; Redick & Johnson, 1974; Robertson, 1974; Thomas & Locke, 1963). Community surveys have found that mental status is substantially poorer among persons from disrupted marriages than among persons in intact marriages (Blumenthal, 1967; Briscoe et al., 1973; Pearlin & Johnson, 1977; Radloff, 1975; Srole et al., 1962; Tauss, 1967). Related studies yielding similar findings have been reported by Belfer, Mulliken, and Cochran (1979), Kessler (1979b), Leff, Roatch, and Bunney (1970), Paykel, Myers, Dienelt, Klerman, Lindenthal, and Pepper (1969), Smith (1971), Udell and Hornstra (1975), and Zautra and Beier (1978).

Epidemiological studies.   In an analysis of presenting complaints of persons applying for mental health services, Udell and Hornstra (1975) collected information on all persons aged 18 or older who applied for care over a one-year period in a highly populated seven-county Midwestern area—nearly 7000 persons. Marital problems were consistently conspicuous, constituting more than 10% of chief complaints of public-sector inpatients, 20% of public-sector outpatients, 8% of private-sector inpatients, and 26% of private-sector outpatients.

Some stressful-life-event research data have been analyzed in terms of specific events, rather than total scores reflecting the accumulated impact of all events identified during a particular time period. Such studies often show separation and divorce to be significantly associated with subsequent psychological difficulties.

For example, Zautra and Beier (1978) sampled 454 adults in Salt Lake City to learn more about the relationship between stressful life events during the previous year, reported quality of life, psychological adjustment, and religious participation. Reported stressful life events were found to be significantly related to psychological adjustment even after the relationship of psychological adjustment to demographic factors and quality of life was taken into account. Reported stressful life events were also significantly related to the incidence of requests for mental health services. A number of variables interacted with life stress in relation to psychological adjustment. Zautra and Beier noted that "people with lower income, education, age, less religious participation, who were divorced or separated, reported more psychological problems chiefly when they were also undergoing life crises" (p. 130).

Smith (1971) attempted to delineate the temporal relationship between critical life events and onset of mental disorder in order to identify "risk-markers" that could serve as foci for a preventive mental health program. The initial study sample of 880 persons comprised all adult admissions to a regional mental health center during 1967–1968. This patient population and a general-population sample of 2414 persons were compared for the occurrence of certain critical life events within one year prior to contact. Of 19 such events, 5 emerged as significantly positive population risk-markers for mental disturbance requiring hospitalization—being in trouble with the police; development of problem drinking; divorce or separation; loss of employment; and having a member of the immediate family develop a problem with alcoholism.

Information was subsequently gathered from a second, smaller patient sample to "determine whether the risk-marker, if it occurred, occurred before or after a distinctly recognized change in psychological or social behavior" (p. 105). In most cases, the events occurred after the onset of psychosocial deterioration, including getting in trouble with the police and becoming unemployed. Divorce or separation preceded the onset of the disorder about as often as it followed it. The author concluded that divorce or separation as a risk-marker may "provide an opportunity to intervene with a healthy person prior to the onset of behavior and emotional decline" (p. 108).

The most common psychiatric disorder associated with marital disruption appears to be depression. Indeed, as already indicated, depression is probably the most common consequence of any significant stressful life event. To compare life-event rates of depressives and normals, Paykel and colleagues (1969) obtained information from 185 inpatients and outpatients on 33 stressful life events occurring during the six months preceding the onset of their depressive symptoms. Information on the same life events during the six months immediately preceding the interview was also obtained from an equally large control group of residents from the same community matched on sociodemographic variables. Overall, depressed patients reported three times as many events as controls. Of eight events that significantly distinguished between the two samples, all were more common in the depressed group. The events that most significantly distinguished between the two groups were increased arguments with spouse and marital separation. Twenty-three patients (12%) had experienced separation in the six months under study, compared with only two controls (1%).

Leff and colleagues (1970) undertook a retrospective study of environmental and behavioral events preceding breakdown in functioning in 40 hospitalized depressed patients. All stressful events occurring within one year prior to the breakdown were recorded. The average number of stressors was four, and many were clustered in the month immediately preceding the point of breakdown. The two most frequent stressful life events reported were sexual-identity threats (occurring in 30 out of 40 patients) and changes in the marital relationship (occurring in 19 of the 34 married patients).

Kessler (1979b) has attempted to determine the relative importance of differential exposure to stresses and differential tolerance of comparable stresses in understanding the relationship of stressful life events to psychological distress in a broad community sample. Information was available on social class, race, sex, and marital status. Psychological distress was assessed by means of a commonly used short self-report measure (Gurin, Veroff, & Feld, 1960). Subjects were interviewed twice, two years apart, making it possible to assess the interaction of the frequency and severity of stressful life events during the two-year period between interviews and the measure of psychological distress obtained at the first interview.

In contrasting married persons with separated and divorced persons, Kessler found that the maritally disrupted were more disadvantaged in functioning under both average and extreme levels of stress. Not only are separated and divorced persons more exposed to stress, they are also consistently more affected by those stressors than are persons in intact marriages.

An interesting sidelight on the role a person can play in his or her own marital disruption comes from a study by Belfer and colleagues (1979) of a sample of 42 persons who had undergone cosmetic surgery. Of these persons, four obtained a legal separation or divorce within six months after surgery without any prior indication that the separation was being planned or any evidence of an intervening family crisis. These authors suggest that it might be far better to help patients deal directly with their contemplated life change rather than deal with it indirectly by means of the symbolism of cosmetic surgery.

Clinical studies.   Another type of study that provides evidence on the stressful nature of marital disruption is based on self-reports by persons undergoing marital disruption. These studies serve to identify the specific nature of the perceived stress. Two studies are of special historical interest— the work of Goode (1949, 1956), who studied a sample of divorced mothers in Detroit, and of Locke (1951), who compared samples of divorced and happily married persons in one county in Indiana.

Goode interviewed 425 divorced mothers aged 20–38 at the time of divorce to explore factors influencing the trauma associated with divorce. The degree of trauma was measured by difficulties in sleeping, poor health, loneliness, low work efficiency, memory difficulties, and increased smoking and drinking. The women reported that the point of greatest disturbance occurred around the time of separation. Goode found that the trauma was greatest for women who were older, who had been married longer, who had two or more children, whose husbands had initiated the divorce, and who still had positive feelings for their husbands or wanted to punish them.

Locke interviewed 525 divorced persons and 404 persons judged by friends to be happily married in order to identify factors associated with marital adjustment and maladjustment. Items that were successful in differentiating the married from the divorced were incorporated into a measure of marital adjustment and included assessments of compatibility, sexual desirability, degree of communication, and amount of conflict over finances, religion, in-laws, friends, philosophy of life, and means of conflict resolution.

Several researchers have attempted to identify the specific problems faced by separated and divorced persons. Schlesinger (1969), noting that more than 90% of one-parent families are headed by the mother, listed the following as problems faced by single mothers: difficulties with children, needing to go to work, social and sexual problems, financial difficulties, and the problems associated with feelings of failure and shame. Schwartz (1968), commenting on the difficulties faced by divorced and remarried persons seen at a family agency, noted that "divorced persons . . . continue to be bound together . . . in ways that are destructive to themselves, the children, and their new family units" (p. 214).

Ilgenfritz (1961) reported on a group educational program for 12 single mothers and found that the major issues that were discussed were fear of being alone, concern with the loss of self-esteem as a woman, hostility toward men, practical problems of living, specific concerns regarding child rearing, and development of self-help strategies.

The economic problems faced by divorced persons, women in particular, have been extensively documented. In March 1970, there were 3,400,000 families with children that were headed by women. Three fifths of these families were on welfare (Stein, 1970). Only 38% of these families had incomes over $5000, and only 9% had incomes over $19,000. By contrast, 55% of intact families had incomes over $10,000. In 1974, families in which no husband was present had a median family income of $6413, while families in which a husband was present and in which the wife was not in the paid labor force had a median family income of $12,082 (Bureau of the Census, 1976). Brandwein, Brown, and Fox (1974) cite economic discrimination against women as a major reason for the financial difficulties of divorced mothers. Because few women are the recipients of job training, many have low-paying service jobs or semi-skilled factory jobs. Furthermore, the median earnings of full-time, full-year-employed women average about 55% of men's earnings, even for men and women in the same occupational categories. Child care and household responsibilities make it difficult for women to work full-time. Men complain about the economic strain involved in supporting two households, but Brandwein and colleagues note that only one-third of husbands contributed to the financial support of their former wives and children. Rheinstein (1972) has noted that the divorce rates in countries having family allowances and other forms of family support are all lower than that of the United States, even in quite industrialized countries, and has suggested that research should be undertaken to determine whether alleviating economic tensions within families might reduce the incidence of marital disruption.

Maritally disrupted persons, both men and women, are faced with maintaining a household, and some must provide child care as well. Hetherington, Cox, and Cox (1976) found that the households of divorced mothers and fathers were more disorganized than those of intact families. The irregular eating habits and erratic sleep patterns found in some of these families had the potential for exacerbating or precipitating mental health problems. Both Hetherington and colleagues and Brandwein and colleagues found that more men than women are likely to be helped with these problems by female friends or by hiring a housekeeper. Brandwein and colleagues noted that in Washington, D.C., the welfare department provided free homemaking services to single fathers but provided such services to single mothers only if they were mentally incompetent, chronically ill, or disabled.

Ferri (1973) noted that similar patterns of child care exist in Great Britain. Her work on single-parent families is an outgrowth of Great Britain's longitudinal National Developmental Child Study of all children born in England and Wales during a single week in 1958. At the time of her study, 1.7% of these children were living in families without their biological mother and 7.7% without their biological father. Single fathers had an easier time finding substitute mothering for their children than mothers had finding substitute fathering. Ferri stated "These findings may reflect differences in social attitudes toward men and women as sole parents" (p. 93). Such attitudes may act to isolate women, make it difficult for working mothers to find adequate child care, and place the entire responsibility for raising the children on the mother.

Marital disruption can precipitate intense and complex emotional reactions. Hetherington and colleagues (1976), Weiss (1976), and Hetherington, Cox, and Cox (1977) have examined such reactions. Hetherington and colleagues (1977) found that divorced parents felt more anxious, depressed, angry, rejected, and incompetent than married persons. Divorced men and women both experienced changes in self-concept. Men seemed to undergo greater initial changes because they were usually the ones to leave familiar surroundings. Fathers felt a lack of identity and a rootlessness and complained of a lack of structure in their lives. Men often engaged in a flurry of social activities as a way of resolving some of their identity problems. Familiar surroundings and the continued presence of their children provided the divorced mothers with a sense of security. Their changes in self-concept evolved more slowly than those of their former husbands, but the effects were longer-lasting. Divorced women complained of feeling unattractive and helpless and of having lost their identity as married women. The most important factor leading back toward a positive self-concept for men and women was the establishment of a satisfying heterosexual relationship.

Weiss (1976) has discussed the nature of stresses associated with marital disruption with about 150 men and women, usually in a small-group situation. Both sexes found marital separation distressing, and being the spouse who had initiated the separation minimized the distress only slightly. Weiss's most persistent finding was that even when the love and other positive feelings between the separated couple faded, a strong attachment remained. They felt drawn toward each other even when alternative relationships had been established. Weiss compared this marital bond to the attachment of children to parents described by Bowlby (1969). Both the maritally separated and children separated from parents had reactions that included rage, anxiety, maintenance of strong fantasy relationships with the lost person, and persistent efforts at reunion.

The findings of these studies converge on identifying a small but important number of problems faced by persons undergoing marital disruption. Such a list would include a generally weakened social support system; the need to work through the variety of psychological reactions to the disruption; problems with child rearing, resocialization, finances, education and employment planning, housing, and homemaking; and protection of legal rights. There is some consistent evidence that the most critical period in the marital disruption process is around the time of separation.

Within the past three years, an additional group of studies has been published continuing the identification of problems faced by persons undergoing marital disruption (Bane, 1979; Chiriboga, Coho, Stein, & Roberts, 1979; Chiriboga & Cutler, 1977; Chiriboga, Roberts, & Stein, 1978; Granvold, Pedler, & Schellie, 1979; Herman, 1977; Hetherington et al., 1976, 1977; Kelly, in press; Kitson, Lopata, Holmes, & Meyering, 1980; Kitson & Sussman, 1977; Raschke,

1977; Spanier & Casto, 1979; Wallerstein & Kelly, 1980; Weiss, 1976, 1979). Kelly (1982) has summarized these findings: stress associated with marital disruption is reported in terms of anger, depression, loneliness, economic difficulties, disequilibrium, regression, and ambivalent but persistent attachment to the spouse. These stress responses are invariably multifaceted and surprisingly long-lasting.

MEDIATING FACTORS IN REACTIONS TO STRESSFUL LIFE EVENTS

Interest in both personal and social resources that can serve to moderate reactions to stressful life events has been increasing over the past several years. Procedures for assessing the presence and extent of these mediating factors are not yet fully articulated, although there is considerable agreement on what are the most important mediating factors to be assessed.

In a recent review paper, Rahe (1979) describes the study of stressful life events as analogous to the identification of risk factors, such as high serum cholesterol levels for the development of coronary heart disease. Rahe notes that knowledge of such risk factors is useful in identifying a subpopulation more vulnerable to a particular disease than those people without the risk factor but cautions that risk factors are often very nonspecific and yield a large number of false positives.

Even where the strongest relationships have been found, correlations between the number of stressful life events and onset of illness are quite modest. According to Rahe, improved understanding of the relationships of stressful life events to illness onset will require closer examination of such mediating factors as the individual's perception of the event, social supports, psychological defenses, coping capabilities, and typical behavior during times of illness.

B. S. Dohrenwend and B. P. Dohrenwend (1974, 1978) comment on how little is known about the factors that mediate the impact of stressful life events. Such mediating factors may be physiological, psychological, or sociocultural. Dohrenwend and Dohrenwend indicate that further research on stressful life events must investigate the role of mediating situational factors—in particular, past experiences with the same event, the availability of social supports, the predictability of the event, and the amount of control a person has over whether the event takes place. Rabkin and Struening (1976) also note the need to analyze both internal and external mediating variables, such as personality characteristics or the availability of social support systems, in developing a more complete understanding of the relationship of stressful life events to illness.

Johnson and Sarason (1979), in their review of moderators of life stress, discuss social support, locus of control and perceived control, and level of arousability. They believe that high levels of social support may play a stress-buffering role and to some degree protect the individual from the effects of cumulative life changes. In addition, they suggest that people are more adversely affected by life stress if they perceive themselves as having little control over their environment. These authors conclude that level of arousability—that is, stimulation seeking—may determine the extent to which people are affected by life changes: the higher the level of arousability, the greater the reaction to life stress. Other moderating variables that they have identified include previous history of dealing with stressors; coping skills (often higher in persons who have previously experienced stress); certain behavioral styles, such as the Type A and Type B behavior identified by Friedman and Rosenman (1974); habitual use of certain defense mechanisms, such as repression or denial; and strategies for the appraisal of life events (Lazarus, 1966).

In an important test of some of these moderator-variable hypotheses, Warheit (1979) examined the role of loss-related stressful life events in depressive symptomatology by surveying a sample of 517 persons in the Southeastern United States twice, with three years between interviews. Warheit assessed the extent of depression at the time of both interviews and evidence of stressful life events associated with losses (particularly important in theories of the development of depression) occurring between the two interviews; help-seeking behaviors; personal, familial, and social resources; and a number of demographic variables, including socioeconomic status. The single most powerful predictor of depression scores at the second interview was depression scores at the first interview, but extent of loss-related stressful life events and availability of social resources were also important. Warheit described these relationships as follows: "In every instance those in the high-loss category, regardless of the presence or absence of personal resources, had significantly higher depression scores than those in the low/moderate-loss group. The data also suggest that the presence of resources significantly mitigates the impact of losses associated with life events" (p. 504).

Personal resources

At the level of personal resources, the most commonly studied mediating factors are coping ability, vulnerability, social competence, and locus of control (Crandall & Lehman, 1977).

Locus of Control.   Rotter (1966) introduced the concept of locus of control, postulating that individuals differ in the degree to which they perceive events in their lives as being under their personal control. Persons characterized by internal locus of control perceive events as being under their control; persons characterized by external locus of control perceive events as being the result of luck or fate or as due to powerful others. Johnson and Sarason (1978) examined the hypothesis that stressful life events would have their most adverse effects on persons with a sense of external locus of control. Results of their study, conducted with a sample of 121 university students, supported their hypothesis specifically in the case of undesirable life events. Only among persons who tended to externalize locus of control were significant correlations found between reported impact of undesirable life events during the previous year and dependent measures of depression and trait anxiety.

Coping ability.   Coping is defined as "efforts, both action-oriented and intrapsychic, to manage (that is, master, tolerate, reduce, minimize) environmental and internal demands, and conflicts among them, which tax or exceed a person's resources" (Cohen & Lazarus, 1979, p. 219). Pearlin and Schooler (1978) have made a very useful conceptual and empirical analysis of coping behavior—a response that serves to "prevent, avoid, or control emotional distress" (p. 3). These authors distinguish among social resources, psychological resources, and coping responses. Resources are what people *have* or *are;* responses are what people *do.* Social resources "are represented in the interpersonal networks of which people are a part and which are a potential source of crucial supports—family, friends, fellow workers, neighbors, and voluntary associations" (p. 5). Psychological resources "are the personality characteristics that people draw upon to help them withstand threats posed by events and objects in their environment" (p. 5). Coping responses are the "behaviors, cognitions, and perceptions in which people engage when actually contending with their life-problems" (p. 5).

In open-ended interviews, Pearlin and Schooler asked over 100 adults in Chicago to describe the problems they face and how they deal with them. Standardized questions that were developed after analyzing the interview responses were administered to a sample of 2300 Chicago residents. Statistical analysis of the coping-style questions revealed 17 coping factors, distinguished not only by problem area (marriage, parenting, household economics, and occupation) but also by their apparent functions or strategies.

One type of coping, for example, seeks to modify the situation that is the source of stress—negotiation in marital stress, punishment in dealing with parenting stress, seeking of advice, and so on. A second type of coping seeks to modify the meaning or significance of the stressful situation—making comparisons with the stresses endured by others, ignoring or minimizing the significance of the stressor, and so on. A third type of coping seeks to minimize the straining that constitutes the response to the external stress—acceptance, avoidance, trying not to worry, relaxing, and so on.

Pearlin and Schooler have assessed the relative efficacy of various coping strategies in various settings and contrasted the relative importance of coping strategies and psychological resources in moderating the relation between external stress and internal straining. They have also examined the relation of demographic factors to coping-strategy preferences and to the strength of various psychological resources. Although their specific findings will require replication and further elaboration, their work constitutes a highly significant beginning to the study of coping behaviors.

Cohen and Lazarus (1979) have identified five forms of coping—information seeking, direct action, inhibition of action, intrapsychic processes, and turning to others—and have applied this analysis to the examination of how people cope with the stresses of illness. In information seeking, the person tries to find out what problems exist and what, if anything, must be done. Direct action includes anything that is done about the problem. Since the skillful coper does not engage in action impulsively or ill-advisedly, inhibition of action is a mode of coping. Intrapsychic processes include all forms of defense—denial, avoidance, or intellectualization, for example. These defenses are particularly useful when the patient can do little about the problem except to allow therapeutic procedures to be applied. Finally, turning to others constitutes a form of coping, in that there is evidence that persons who are ill do better if they can maintain and use supportive social relationships. Cohen and Lazarus suggest that "the more helpless the person is, the more he or she must depend on cognitive or intrapsychic modes of coping" (1979, p. 221).

Cohen and Lazarus are in agreement with Pearlin and Schooler that our ability to assess coping behaviors is far from adequate. They have identified some of the major issues in such assessment. First, they suggest we must distinguish between thinking of coping as a generalized personality trait or disposition and thinking of coping as a process, perhaps unique to the particular stressful situation. In addition, they have identified a number of problems in assessing coping, such as (1) the realization that coping is not a single act but a complex constellation of many thoughts and acts, (2) choosing among a variety of ways to obtain information about coping, (3) difficulty in distinguishing among various modes of coping, and (4) difficulties in evaluating coping effectiveness.

Cohen and Lazarus conclude their review by noting:

> It is important for researchers in the field to plan future studies more carefully in order to . . . allow us to gain greater clarity about how coping affects recovery. First, we need a wider range and more consistency in the types of outcome variables examined. . . . Second, we must begin to try to specify which coping strategies are most effective across many illnesses and which are valuable in dealing only with certain specific illnesses. . . . Third, it may be useful to use both trait and process measures of emotional state in studying outcomes of illness, since each of these kinds of measures shows significant relationships with some medical outcomes but not with others. . . . Fourth, one must be careful about generalizing from results of non-intervention studies in the desire to make interventions to aid patients' coping. If those who seek information about a forthcoming surgery have more complicated recovery from surgery, that does not mean that withholding information will aid recovery efforts. . . . Fifth, we must consider seriously the outcome measures to be examined. There is a sense in which it is arbitrary to say that the course of recovery is better or worse insofar as the patient goes home sooner, takes less pain medications, has fewer complications, and fewer psycho-

logical complaints. . . . Sixth, . . . we need to broaden our assessment of coping over a longer time span so that we can determine how coping changes over time and situation [pp. 252–253].[2]

In spite of these difficulties, Cohen and Lazarus are convinced that we are in an early stage in the study of powerful forces that contribute either to health or to illness and that some of these forces can be manipulated in order to shorten the duration of illness and improve recovery rate.

Personality variables.   Kobasa (1979) examined the mediating effects of a number of personality variables on the consequences of stressful life events. In a sample of 837 executives who, as a group, had undergone considerable stress during the preceding three years, she isolated two groups of high-stress executives who differed on their reported illnesses—126 subjects above the median for total stress and below the median for total illness, and a second group of 200 subjects above the median for total stress and above the median for total illness. These two samples were then reduced to 100 subjects in each group. All were males, and most were between ages 40 and 59, married, parents, and college-educated.

Kobasa studied three personality variables related to coping style—degree to which participants felt they could control life events, involvement in or commitment to life activities, and extent to which they viewed change as an exciting challenge to further development. As expected, in the total group (including those executives below the median in stress) there was a significant but modest correlation between total stress and total illness scores.

Kobasa found numerous personality differences between the two groups of high-stress executives. She writes:

> This study provides a basis for understanding how persons can encounter great stress and remain healthy nonetheless. In order to do so, one must have a clear sense of one's values, goals, and capabilities, and a belief in their importance . . . ; a strong tendency toward active involvement in one's environment . . . ; an ability to evaluate the impact of any life event in terms of a general life plan with its established priorities . . . ; a belief that one can control and transform the events of one's experience . . . ; and finally, an ability to deal with external life stresses without their becoming threats to one's private sphere and causes of subjective strain [p. 420].

Zubin and Spring (1977) propose that the most important single concept underlying the various models advanced to understand schizophrenia is the concept of vulnerability. They postulate two major components of vulnerabil-

---

[2]From "Coping with the Stresses of Illness," by F. Cohen and R. S. Lazarus. In G. C. Stone, F. Cohen and N. E. Adler (Eds.), *Health Psychology—A Handbook.* Copyright © 1979 by Jossey-Bass. Reprinted by permission.

ity—inborn and acquired—and suggest that vulnerability is an enduring, relatively permanent trait. Inborn vulnerability is that which is "laid down in the genes and reflected in the internal environment and neurophysiology of the organism" (p. 109). Acquired vulnerability is due to the "influence of traumas, specific diseases, perinatal complications, family experiences, adolescent peer interactions, and other life events that either enhance or inhibit the development of subsequent disorder" (p. 109). Life-event stressors form a major component of acquired vulnerability in that they tax the organism's adaptive capacities.

Among the variables that should be taken into account in predicting a person's response to a stressful life event, Zubin and Spring include normatively perceived severity of the event, individually judged severity of the event, general competence, motivation to cope, and vulnerability. Zubin and Spring's review of the literature does not lead them to conclude that persuasive evidence of a link between preepisode competence and vulnerability exists. They do speculate, however, that reduced coping ability, characterized by frequent disequilibrium (particularly in the face of relatively mild threats), combined with high vulnerability, may significantly increase the risk of psychiatric disorder.

Antonovsky (1979) refers to those personal assets that increase resistance to disease or disorder as *generalized resistance resources*. Generalized resistance resources are characteristics of persons, groups, or social environments that are effective in avoiding and combating a wide variety of stressors so that tension (the straining that is the organismic response to an external stressor) is not converted into subjective stress, which is, in turn, a contributing factor in the development of disease. Antonovsky acknowledges the existence of specific resistance resources—that is, personal or social resources linked to reduced vulnerability to specific diseases—but he believes that generalized resistance resources are far more important, in part because their presence creates the possibility that people can locate disease-specific resources.

Perhaps the most fundamental generalized resistance resource, according to Antonovsky, is the sense of coherence—"a global orientation that expresses the extent to which one has a pervasive, enduring though dynamic feeling of confidence that one's internal and external environments are predictable and that there is a high probability that things will work out as well as can reasonably be expected" (1979, p. 123).

Kessler (1979a) has developed a model that postulates that "psychological distress . . . is the result of varying exposure to environmental stress events or situations . . . acting on individuals who possess varying vulnerabilities to stress" (p. 101). Unfortunately, no method is presently available to assess vulnerability (either constitutional or environmental) directly. But Kessler has been able to derive an indirect statistical measure of vulnerability. Reanalyzing data reported by Myers, Lindenthal, and Pepper (1975), Kessler was able to establish that higher scores by women than by men on a symptom checklist were due primarily to greater vulnerabilities to stress and only secondarily to being exposed to more stressful life events, Kessler's conclusion was that "the greater distress exhibited by women is due to the fact that they are more highly affected psychologically by stressful events and situations to which they and men are equally exposed" (p. 103).

Jenkins (1979) has identified a number of variables that might modify the relationships between stressful life events and subsequent disorder and has shown how one can view the interaction between stress and the organism at biological, psychological, interpersonal, and sociocultural levels. In using this model in the analysis of a study of health change in a sample of more than 400 air traffic controllers conducted by Rose, Hurst, and Herd (1979), Jenkins has been able to show, for example, that while life stress is generally associated with subsequent impulse-control problems, that association is particularly powerful only among those air traffic controllers whose educational level is no higher than their fathers'. That is, educational level of the participant, relative to educational level of the father, is a type of internalized status incongruity that makes it an important mediator between stressful life events and subsequent psychological or physical disorder. Similarly, the relationship between stressful life events and subsequent psychological disorder is found to be significant only among air traffic controllers below average in social coping resources.

Social competence. A final important factor that can moderate the effects of stressful life events is personal competence, particularly in social situations. Much human misery appears to be the result of a lack of competence—that is, a lack of control over one's life, a lack of effective coping strategies, and the lowered self-esteem that accompanies these deficiencies. This opinion is emerging out of an analysis of a substantial body of research from a variety of domains that appears to converge on competence building as one of the most persuasive preventive strategies for dealing with individual and social issues in many communities.

According to Iscoe, the development of competence involves obtaining and using information and other resources "so that the members of the community may make reasoned decisions about issues confronting them, leading to the most competent coping with these problems" (1974, pp. 607–609). As to the components of individual and community competence, Iscoe suggests, first, a repertoire of possibilities and alternatives; second, the knowledge of where and how to acquire resources; third, clout; and finally, as a consequence, hope, self-esteem, and power—not power in the sense of the ability to control others, but rather in the sense used by the Spanish author Salvador de Madariaga: "He is free who knows how to keep in his own hands the power to decide at each step the course of his life and who lives in a society which does not block the exercise of that power" (quoted in Bradley, Daniels, & Jones, 1969).

Ryan (1967) used the term *power* in the same sense when he wrote that

> self-esteem is to some extent an essential requirement to the very survival of the
> human organism . . . and is partially dependent on the inclusion of a sense of
> power within the self-concept. . . . A mentally healthy person must be able to
> perceive himself as at least minimally powerful, capable of influencing his envi-
> ronment to his own benefit, and further . . . this sense of minimal power has to
> be based on the actual experience and exercise of power [p. 50].

These authors contend that competence, power, and self-esteem are inextricably linked and that their loss may constitute a powerful stressor.

Masterpasqua (1981) has suggested that the interest in social competency
and in competency enhancement forms the basis for a natural linking between
the fields of developmental and community psychology. His rationale is based
on three premises that both fields appear to consider central in their thinking:
(1) that the drive toward competence is inherent, (2) that we need to study
the development of competence as it occurs in natural settings, and (3) that
the elucidation of real-life developmental needs can lead to the advocacy of
developmental rights in community settings. With regard to these developmental rights, Masterpasqua writes:

> My colleagues and I conceive of four broad categories of ecological contexts (levels)
> that need to be addressed in the advocacy of developmental rights: caregivers
> (e.g., parents, teachers, nurses, doctors), neighborhoods and communities, orga-
> nizations and agencies, and policymakers. Clearly, developmental needs change
> throughout the life cycle, and a corollary of this fact is that the ecological contexts
> that interface with the individual change in their salience depending on the devel-
> opmental period. So, for mother and newborn the ecological level of primary
> focus for advocacy of developmental rights is the hospital (organization) and its
> caregivers (physicians and nurses). For midlife adults the focus might be the work
> world (organizations), and for the elderly the focus might be nursing homes,
> retirement communities, family caregivers, and so on. The recognition that eco-
> logical levels are of varying significance for individuals at different developmental
> points not only helps clarify foci for advocacy of developmental rights but also
> helps identify the settings in which applied developmental research needs to
> occur [1981, p. 784].

Masterpasqua argues that an "ecology of human development can and should
become a basic science upon which community psychologists base their proactive plans for advocacy and change. Conversely, community psychologists can
pose ecologically meaningful questions (e.g., Is infant day care harmful?) for
applied developmentalists and sensitize developmentalists to the complexities
of the real-life settings in which ontogeny is embedded" (p. 785).

Empirical study of the roles of coping skills, social competency, and vulnerability in moderating the effects of stressful life events has only recently
begun. The concepts of vulnerability and of coping styles and strengths have
not yet been satisfactorily operationalized, but considerable progress can be
expected in the next several years. There is no question about the shared belief

in the importance of the study of this set of personal characteristics for the more complete understanding of stressful life events and their consequences.

Social resources

At the level of social or environmental resources, enormous activity is taking place around the concept of social support systems and social networks (Caplan, 1981; Dean & Lin, 1977). Cobb (1976) has recently reviewed the role of social support as a moderator of stressful life events. Cobb views social support as falling into one of three classes. Persons can be said to have social support, first, when they believe they are cared for and loved; second, when they believe they are esteemed and valued; and, third, when they believe they belong to a network of communication and mutual obligation. Cobb has shown that the presence of adequate social support is associated with the lack of complications of pregnancy, particularly among women high in life stress, with recovery from a variety of illnesses and response to a variety of medical procedures, with success in alcoholism recovery programs, with favorable management of the stress of involuntary unemployment, with successful coping with bereavement, and with better management of the illnesses and infirmities associated with aging.

Cobb comments that what is new about these studies is the accumulation of evidence that "adequate social support can protect people in crisis from a wide variety of pathological states: from low birth weight to death, from arthritis through tuberculosis to depression, alcoholism, and other psychiatric illness. Furthermore, social support can reduce the amount of medication required and accelerate recovery and facilitate compliance with prescribed medical regimens" (1976, p. 310). As for the processes by which social supports enhance health, Cobb believes that social support encourages coping (manipulation of the environment in the service of the self) and adaptation (change in the self in order to enhance person/environment fit).

Social relationships among the elderly. Lowenthal and Haven (1968) examined the role of strong personal relationships in the maintenance of health and psychological well-being during middle age and senescence. They postulated that having an intimate relationship—having a confidant—can serve as a buffer against age-linked social losses. Their sample consisted of 280 persons in San Francisco, aged 60 or above, interviewed yearly on three occasions. Assessments were made of number of social roles, level of social interaction, morale, and psychiatric impairment.

Low social interaction was found to be associated with poor morale; reported social losses in the past year were generally associated with poor morale as well. The presence or absence of a confidant had a dramatic attenuating effect on these relationships. Lowenthal and Haven found, for example, that "if you have a confidant, you can decrease your social interaction and run no greater risk of becoming depressed than if you had increased it. Further, if you have no confidant and retrench in your social life, the odds for depression become overwhelming" (p. 26). An additional finding was that "an individual who has been widowed within seven years, and who has a confidant, has even higher morale than a person who remains married, but lacks a confidant. . . . Among those having confidants, only 10 percent more of the widowed than of the married are depressed, but nearly three-fourths of the widowed who have no confidant are depressed, compared with only about half among the married who have no confidant" (p. 27).

The authors provide some very informative data on demographic characteristics of persons who do have confidants (for example, women are more likely than men to have confidants) and on the characteristics of these confidants (for example, most often spouses, friends, or children; rarely siblings or other relatives). These authors clearly view having a confidant as perhaps the most important type of social support that might be available to an aging person. They speculate that one reason for the greater life expectancy of women than men is their greater capacity and willingness to develop and sustain intimate relationships.

In another study that focused on the role of social supports in an elderly population, viewing aging as a stressful life event, Abrahams and Patterson (1978–1979) surveyed a sample of 445 persons aged 65 and above in a New England town. Their survey was based on a structured interview conducted in the respondent's home. They sought to assess the prevalence of various forms of psychological impairment and to contrast psychologically healthy and impaired persons in terms of demographic characteristics and social interactions. On the basis of these analyses, the authors sought to identify some of the factors that result in excess vulnerability to the stresses of aging.

A total of 8% of the study population reported being severely depressed; 17% of the sample had one or more symptoms of impairment. Impairment was not found to be associated with age or sex, but it was found more commonly among persons living in deteriorated neighborhoods and among less well educated persons. Healthy aged persons were found to have significantly stronger social relationships outside the household, to be significantly higher on social initiative, and to have significantly more varied daily lives.

As for the factors that appeared to make some persons more vulnerable to the stress of aging, the authors identified loss of significant others, reduced physical vitality, and unhappiness about retirement from work. Both impaired and healthy persons in this study tended to make very little use of community services and did not differ in their help-seeking behavior. The authors suggest that preventive measures such as increasing community support systems and increasing knowledge about the need for neighborhood or peer support groups could be helpful in reducing vulnerability to the aging process.

Social support and psychological well-being. Andrews, Tennant, Hewson, and Vaillant (1978) provided information on a very brief measure of coping style (immature versus mature) and social support (including availability of support in times of emergency, neighborhood interaction, and community participation). Neurotic impairment was significantly more common among immature copers than mature copers and among persons with few social supports available in times of emergency. Of the 226 persons low in stressful life events, high in coping, and high in social support, only 12.8% were found to be at risk of being psychologically impaired. Of the 67 persons high in stress, low in coping, and low in social support, 43.3% were found to be at risk of psychological impairment. In this study, which the authors think of as only a first step, coping style and social support did not serve to moderate the effect of stressful life events on psychological impairment; rather, each appeared to have an independent and additive effect on impairment.

Burke and Weir (1977) studied 189 couples in Ontario, measuring life stresses, satisfaction with the spouse's helping efforts, job and marital satisfaction, and mental and physical well-being. In both husbands and wives, measures of well-being were significantly positively correlated with satisfaction with spouse's helping efforts and negatively correlated with level of stress. The significance of the relationship between well-being and satisfaction with spouse's helping efforts persisted even when the authors controlled for level of stress. But at the same time, the reported helpfulness of spouses was found to be significantly greater under conditions of high experienced stress. The authors concluded that "marital helping can be viewed as a moderator of the relationship between stress and well-being, influencing the degree to which stress will be translated into psychophysical symptomatology" (p. 129).

Eaton (1978) reanalyzed some of the data previously collected by Myers et al. (1975) in New Haven, Connecticut, particularly regarding the relationship between the availability of social supports and psychiatric symptoms. He identified several indexes of the extent of social support available to each respondent (currently married, club membership, church membership, having friends or relatives visit often, going out to visit others often, having a very close friend, and not living alone). These eight items did not constitute a coherent scale, however, and Eaton therefore examined their individual relationships to the psychiatric-symptom measure. Two variables, being married and living with others, were found to be associated with the relationship between reported stressful life events and psychiatric symptoms. Among persons who were unmarried or who lived alone (the variables are, of course, not independent of each other), that relationship was significantly stronger than among persons who were married or who lived with others. That is, stressful life events appeared to have a greater impact on subsequent psychiatric symptoms among persons with weaker social supports.

Lin, Simeone, Ensel, and Kuo (1979) examined the independent contributions of stressful life events and social-support strength to self-reports of psychiatric symptoms in a sample of 170 Chinese Americans in the District of Columbia. These authors viewed social support as support available through one's social ties to other persons, to groups, and to the larger community. The authors used a measure of weighted stressful life events, a self-report psychiatric-symptom checklist, and a short scale assessing the availability of various forms of social support. In addition, they recorded occupational level and marital status of each respondent.

Psychiatric symptoms were more commonly reported among unmarried people, people of lower occupational prestige, those with more reported stressful life events, and those with poorer social supports. The social-support measure was the most powerful predictor of psychiatric symptoms. "Marital status, occupational prestige, and stressful life events combined to explain about 8% of the variance. . . . The variance explained in the dependent variable increases to 21% when social support is incorporated into the model" (p. 113). Availability of social supports and incidence of stressful life events were independent of each other, and hence each could, in theory, be examined for its potential for control or enhancement as part of a preventive intervention program.

Sarason (1980) has examined the nature of social supports as a moderating factor in understanding stress responses in an innovative laboratory setting where the nature of social supports was manipulated experimentally. During a 20-minute period before a difficult anagram task, members of the experimental group participated in a discussion designed to create a social support network and a sense of sharing. Among subjects who were high in test anxiety, those who had participated in the group-building discussion scored significantly higher on the anagram task than those who had not. In a second experiment in which social support was generated by a brief empathic comment regarding a subject's inability to solve the anagrams, similar findings were obtained. Sarason has concluded that "under certain conditions social supports function as a moderator by counteracting undesirable consequences of high anxiety" (p. 26).

Social support and physical illness.   Medalie and Goldbourt (1976) examined the role played by anxiety and psychosocial problems in the development of angina pectoris (a chronic but not life-threatening heart disorder) in a longitudinal five-year study of 10,000 male Israeli civil servants aged 40 and above. The incidence of angina pectoris was found to vary by age, by area of birth, and by a number of physiological variables but at the same time was found to be higher among persons reporting high anxiety, a high level of family problems, and psychosocial difficulties. Anxiety, psychosocial problems, and family problems appear to strengthen the relationships between physiological factors (such as electrocardiographic changes, cholesterol levels, systolic blood pressure) and angina. The risk of developing angina pectoris was found to be about 20 times as high among persons with all risk factors present as among those with none present.

One additional variable was assessed—the perceived love and support of one's wife. The authors found that, with high levels of anxiety, the incidence of angina was significantly reduced in men who reported having a loving and supportive wife. Medalie and Goldbourt concluded that

> preventive measures, like antismoking, reducing cholesterol and blood pressure levels and weight, will probably help to reduce the incidence of . . . angina pectoris. But . . . no matter how well this is done, the major sources of risk for angina pectoris will be missed, unless it is accompanied by a detailed investigation of the subject's personal, family, and occupational life situations. The latter will allow the physician to assess the strengths and stresses in order to help the patient solve or adjust in a more satisfactory way to recurrent problems and thus reduce his anxiety [p. 918].

Lynch (1977) has gathered an impressive array of both statistical and clinical data to support his assertion that the lack of social support systems can lead to a variety of disorders, particularly coronary artery disease. In his words, "The lack of human companionship or the loss of a loved-one can have serious effects on our physical and mental well-being. In terms of cardiovascular disease, the evidence is remarkably consistent . . . human companionship appears to play a vital role in the healthy functioning of the heart" (p. 87).

Gore (1978) examined the role of the availability of social supports in mediating physical illness in 100 married men who were involuntarily unemployed as a consequence of two industrial-plant shutdowns. Gore suggests that "support increases coping ability, which is the etiological gate to health and well-being" (p. 157). Participants were interviewed by public health nurses on five occasions ranging from six weeks before the scheduled shutdowns to two years after the shutdowns. The dependent measures of health included, in addition to self-report scales, assessment of serum cholesterol levels. Social support was measured by a 13-item index, with participants subsequently divided into a high-support and a low-support group.

Some changes in serum cholesterol level were found over time in the two level-of-support groups, but Gore was not sure about the validity of the findings and was unable to interpret these changes as indicative of increased illness in the lower-support group. With respect to the self-report measures, however, the results seemed clearer and, according to Gore, suggested that the loss of employment, "in the absence of a continuing sense of self-worth maintained through supportive relationships, contributes to negative health responses" (p. 164).

Implications for program and policy development

Research in the field of social networks and social support has become so voluminous that one can now examine it in order to identify its implications for program development and social policy. One such overview has been provided by Mitchell and Trickett (1980), who have concluded that "although it seems clear that social networks are important aspects of one's life . . . how they operate and whom they affect in what way are questions still largely unanswered. The promising nature of the research literature is a hopeful sign of further clarifying work in this area" (pp. 37–38).[3]

As to the implications of the research and theory thus far, Mitchell and Trickett suggest that, first, social network concepts will need to be tied more closely to the specific settings and populations where these concepts are being developed, and, second, "even if social network analysis demonstrates unquestionably that a particular group is at risk because of deficiency in networks, the intervention strategy adopted would depend on a number of variables, such as the resources available to implement an intervention, the way one assesses the nature of the environment in which the intervention is to occur, and the theoretical and ideological perspective of the change agent" (p. 38).

With these cautions in mind, Mitchell and Trickett suggest that, first, social network analysis will help in the development of intervention programs because it will focus attention on the social context of behavior; second, concern with social networks will have an impact on the training of mental health personnel because they will need to develop skills in understanding and working with community resources; third, assessment of social networks can be used as a tool for evaluating the community adjustment of previously hospitalized psychiatric patients; fourth, evaluation of social networks in different neighborhoods and within different demographic groups can help in the identification of community problem areas and needs and general quality of life; and, fifth, interest in social network analysis can lead to an improved understanding of the functioning of natural support systems and possible ways of improving them.

Mitchell and Trickett note, in concluding their review, that

> there are also implications that shifting to a social network orientation may require some reorientations in the thinking and practice of mental health professionals. These include an increased emphasis on understanding the social systems in which individuals are embedded, a decrease in emphasizing intrapsychic explanations in favor of an interpersonal, skill-development orientation, and a rethinking of the available intervention strategies that include increased contact and collaboration with nonprofessional community resources. The concept of social network as a mediator of social support provides a conceptual orientation for a reemphasis on the community component of community mental health centers [pp. 41–42].

METHODOLOGICAL ISSUES IN THE STUDY OF STRESSFUL LIFE EVENTS

As should be clear, identifying the role of stressful life events in precipitating emotional disorders is more complex than one might think. Rabkin (1980) has reviewed some of the major methodological difficulties. Among these, she mentions (1) the use of retrospective study designs, (2) insufficient attention paid to the selection of subjects and control groups, (3) lists of stressful life events that are inadequately defined or conceptualized or are insufficient in scope, (4) inability to distinguish the onset of illness from help-seeking behavior, and (5) inadequate statistical procedures. Rabkin notes that not only may stressful life events vary in perceived severity, but they may be expected or unexpected, familiar or novel, desirable or undesirable, sudden or gradual, discrete or prolonged, variously under the control of the person being studied, and part of or separated from the advance signs of impending illness (see also Miller & Ingham, 1979, pp. 318–324).

In a parallel paper, Cleary (1980) has identified nine methodological problems in the design and reporting of stressful-life-event research and has proposed suggestions for dealing with them. These problems are (1) failure to describe important characteristics of the sample being studied so that replications will be possible, (2) failure to use a carefully enough chosen list of items so that no major events are missed and so that the events can be disentangled from their presumed consequences, (3) failure to standardize the conditions for the collection of stressful-life-event data, in order to increase reliability, (4) failure to check on the validity of stressful-life-event reports, (5) failure to specify how scale values have been calculated, (6) failure to specify time intervals within which stressful life events are to be identified and time intervals between those events and the subsequent dependent measures of adjustment, (7) failure to use an identified and appropriate rationale in the selection of dependent measures, (8) failure to use an undistorted base rate for life events or for undesired outcomes in the study of stressful-life-event predictors of maladjustment, and (9) failure to use appropriate statistical procedures in describing and analyzing data.

Dohrenwend, Krasnoff, Askenasy, and Dohrenwend (1978) examine some of the criticisms of the Holmes and Rahe Social Readjustment Rating Scale that have been raised and describe their proposed solutions. Regarding the issue of weighting stressful life events versus simply counting them, Dohrenwend et al. believe that the preponderance of research to date has found more significant results using weighted rather than unweighted measures. A second issue is the practice of assigning each stressful life event a fixed rating of importance rather than soliciting judgments of importance by the person being studied. Dohrenwend et al. believe the former to be an appropriate methodology in view of the research interest in assessing the importance of stressful life events as environmental inputs unconfounded by predispositions or outcomes.

To improve the study of the effects of stressful life events, Dohrenwend et al. have enlarged the list of such events, defined each of them less ambiguously, and classified them according to whether they may or may not be among early signs of illness, according to their desirability, and according to how often they might be expected to occur throughout a variety of sociocultural settings. They have also developed what they believe to be an improved procedure for scaling such events in terms of required readjustment or change. Although their results are admittedly imperfect, Dohrenwend et al. hope their proposed procedure will lead to a "general and permanent methodological gain in studies of stressful life events" (1978, p. 228).

Stressful life events in children

Coddington (1972a) has undertaken a series of studies to examine the clinical belief that children's illnesses often follow stressful life events. To evaluate this hypothesis, it was first necessary to develop a children's version of the life-events inventory. Coddington chose to model his version after the methodology developed for adults by Holmes and Rahe (1967). Coddington prepared separate versions of the questionnaire for preschool-age children, elementary-school-age children, junior-high-school-age children, and those in senior high school. Ratings of each item in terms of the judged amount and duration of change that would result were made by a sample of teachers, pediatricians, and mental health workers. Coddington found very high agreement among the three groups of judges, with rank-order correlations never lower than .85, and he was able to construct four age-specific stressful-life-events inventories, in which each event was weighted in terms of life-change units (see Table 6–2).

In a subsequent study, Coddington (1972b) applied the scales to a representative sample of 3620 children in Columbus, Ohio, to establish expected norms and to examine questionnaire responses in relation to sex, race, and socioeconomic class. Coddington found no difference in life-change-unit scores by sex or by socioeconomic class. However, life-change-unit scores were significantly related to age. A regular increase in life-change-unit scores with increasing age was found in every demographic subgroup.

In a third study (Heisel, Ream, Raitz, Rappaport, & Coddington, 1973), the life-events inventory was applied to a sample of 34 children with juvenile rheumatoid arthritis, 35 hemophiliac children, 32 general pediatric inpatients, 31 children undergoing surgery for hernias or appendicitis, and 88 children seen at a child psychiatric outpatient clinic. In comparison with age-matched normal controls, these children, with the exception of the hemophiliacs, had had two or three times as many and as severe stressful life events during the year prior to the onset of their medical conditions. There was no difference among the various patient groups. These authors concluded that stressful life

TABLE 6–2. Life-event scores (in life-change units) by age group

Life events	Pre-school	Ele-mentary	Junior high	Senior high
Beginning nursery school, first grade, seventh grade, or high school	42	46	45	42
Change to a different school	33	46	52	56
Birth or adoption of a brother or sister	50	50	50	50
Brother or sister leaving home	39	36	33	37
Hospitalization of brother or sister	37	41	44	41
Death of brother or sister	59	68	71	68
Change of father's occupation requiring increased absence from home	36	45	42	38
Loss of job by a parent	23	38	48	46
Marital separation of parents	74	78	77	69
Divorce of parents	78	84	84	77
Hospitalization of parent (serious illness)	51	55	54	55
Death of a parent	89	91	94	87
Death of a grandparent	30	38	35	36
Marriage of parent to stepparent	62	65	63	63
Jail sentence of parent for 30 days or less	34	44	50	53
Jail sentence of parent for 1 year or more	67	67	76	75
Addition of third adult to family (e.g., grandparent)	39	41	34	34
Change in parents' financial status	21	29	40	45
Mother beginning to work	47	44	36	26
Decrease in number of arguments between parents	21	25	29	27
Increase in number of arguments between parents	44	51	48	46
Decrease in number of arguments with parents	22	27	29	26
Increase in number of arguments with parents	39	47	46	47
Discovery of being an adopted child	33	52	70	64
Acquiring a visible deformity	52	69	83	81
Having a visible congenital deformity	39	60	70	62
Hospitalization of yourself (child)	59	62	59	58
Change in acceptance by peers	38	51	68	67
Outstanding personal achievement	23	39	45	46
Death of a close friend (child's friend)	38	53	65	63
Failure of a year in school		57	62	56
Suspension from school		46	54	50
Pregnancy in unwed teen-age sister		36	60	64
Becoming involved with drugs or alcohol		61	70	76
Becoming a full-fledged member of a church/synagogue		25	28	31
Not making an extracurricular activity you wanted to be involved in (i.e., athletic team, band)			49	55

TABLE 6–2 (continued)

Life events	Pre-school	Ele-mentary	Junior high	Senior high
Breaking up with a boyfriend or girlfriend			47	53
Beginning to date			55	51
Fathering an unwed pregnancy			76	77
Unwed pregnancy			95	92
Being accepted to a college of your choice				43
Getting married				101

From "The Significance of Life Events as Contributing Factors in the Diseases of Children, III: A Study of Pediatric Patients," by J. S. Heisel, S. Ream, R. Raitz, M. Rappaport, and R. D. Coddington. In *Journal of Pediatrics*, 1973, *83*, 119–123. Copyright 1973 by The C. V. Mosby Company. Reprinted by permission.

events are diagnostically nonspecific and that "the child required to face major changes in his environment must adjust his internal milieu both psychologically and physiologically, or, more likely, both" (1973, p. 122).

Sandler and Ramsay (1980) factor-analyzed the responses of a group of ten clinical child psychologists who had been asked to judge the degree of similarity between pairs of stressful-life-event items in a list of 32 such items. From this factor analysis, Sandler and Ramsay were able to identify seven sets of items that appeared to tap different content categories—losses (for example, death, divorce, or hospitalization of parent or friend), entrances (for example, addition to the family, moving to a new house), family troubles (for example, worsening of parents' mood, loss of job by parent, arguments between parents), positive events, primary environment change, sibling problem, and physical harm. Study of the relation between scores on each of these categories of stressful life events and adjustment ratings as assessed by parents revealed that the items in the entrance and family-troubles clusters were significantly related to adjustment ratings in a sample of 104 inner-city children attending kindergarten through third grade. Maladapting children scored significantly higher than control children on those two stressful-life-event clusters.

Desirable and undesirable stressful life events

A number of studies have addressed the question of desirability or undesirability of stressful life events as an approach to determining what type of event is most closely related to negative consequences. Klassen, Roth, and Hornstra (1974) determined that there was generally good agreement in a community sample regarding the desirability or undesirability of various stressful life events. A probability sample of 190 adults in Kansas City judged whether each of 40 events in a stressful-life-event inventory was "a good thing or a bad thing for most people." A total of 70% or more of the participants judged 19 of the items to be desirable events; 70% or more judged 16 of the items to be undesirable. Thus, according to the authors' definition of 70% as the cutoff criterion of unambiguity of judgment, only five items were viewed as ambiguous in terms of their desirability: retiring from work; being released from prison or acquitted of other than a minor traffic offense; entering the armed services; having a new person move into the house, other than a newborn child; and having a family member leave home.

Very few differences in judged desirability were found as a function of sex, age, marital status, or education. Seven items were judged significantly more desirable by white than by black participants. Particularly significant were three items—improvement in job, new love relationship, and acquisition of property. These items all involve changes in responsibility, and the authors speculate that the limited nature of the opportunity structure for blacks may cause them to perceive such events as relatively undesirable.

Mueller, Edwards, and Yarvis (1977) examined their own survey data collected in Sacramento to determine whether all stressful life events or just undesirable ones are related to self-reported measures of well-being. Their analysis suggested that the frequency of undesirable stressful life events was substantially more highly correlated with well-being than were measures that combined desirable and undesirable stressful life events. In addition, the authors noted that "regardless of whether desirability is defined by respondents or independently, the relationship of desirable events to psychological status appears to be weak or negligible. Undesirable events, by comparison, are strongly linked with measures of psychological impairment" (pp. 314–315). Finally, the reported relationships appeared very similar whether stressful life events were summated in weighted or unweighted form.

Vinokur and Selzer (1975) examined the question whether undesirable stressful life events have greater effects than desirable events on physical and psychological well-being. The original concept of a stressful life event was one that required significant readjustment or change regardless of its desirability. Vinokur and Selzer argued, however, that desirable events might actually reduce stress. Furthermore, since the perceived desirability of many events (for example, moving to another city) may vary among people, it is necessary to determine the degree of desirability for each stressful life event on an individual basis.

These authors studied a sample of over 1000 male automobile and truck drivers in order to learn more about the effects of stress and personality variables on traffic accidents. A traditional stressful-life-events scale was modified so that desirable and undesirable events could be distinguished from each other. For example, the original item *Changes in working conditions* was modified into two items: *Improvement in working conditions* and *Deterioration in working conditions*. Furthermore, respondents were asked to rate the degree of stress or pressure evoked by each event and to indicate whether the event was desirable or undesirable. Dependent measures included assessments of aggression, paranoid thinking, depression, suicidal proclivity, physical anxiety and tension responses, amount of drinking, and involvement in traffic accidents. Finally, subjects completed a scale designed to determine the extent to which perceived social desirability of answers influenced their responses.

Vinokur and Selzer calculated the number of events checked by each participant as having occurred during the preceding year, the weighted total of these events based on the traditional stressful-life-events scale, and the perceived impact of these events as judged by each participant. These totals were calculated separately for the events judged desirable and for those judged undesirable. Finally, a series of difference scores was calculated for each subject by subtracting the total score for desirable events from the same score for undesirable events.

The three types of scores (number, weighted total, and perceived impact) turned out to be so highly correlated (all correlations were above .90) that there were no differences among them in terms of their relationships with the dependent variables. The authors found that the scores based only on undesirable events were consistently more closely related to their dependent measures than were the scores based on desirable events or the difference scores. The measure of social desirability had no effect on the relationships obtained. Weighted scores that reflect the amount of change or readjustment judged to be required by each stressful life event were insensitive to the judged undesirability of the event. Since the undesirability of stressful life events is a crucial component in assessing them, self-ratings of readjustment appeared to be more suitable than fixed measures of readjustment derived by others.

The authors believe that these relationships are genuine and of a causal nature—undesirable life events "contribute to physical illness and psychological impairment" (p. 333). In the authors' words, "the contribution of life events to psychological impairment is mediated by stress that is evoked by some undesirable aspect of the events rather than by change per se" (pp. 333–334). Similarly, Crandall and Lehman (1977) found in a sample of 81 undergraduates that reported undesirable-stressful-life-event ratings were significantly correlated with reported psychiatric symptoms.

In a multidimensional analysis of the concept of life change, Ruch (1977) identified three aspects of life change—degree of change, desirability of change, and the life area in which the change occurs. Her work has added to the original concept of life change, which was unidimensional, being defined solely in terms of necessary social adjustment. A sample of 211 undergraduate students were asked to estimate the intensity and duration of social readjustment required for each of the Holmes and Rahe stressful-life-event items. Results of this analysis were almost identical to those obtained in the original standardization study. Factor analysis of the data, however, yielded the three aspects of life change mentioned above. Ruch concluded that although the concept of life change involves both quantitative and qualitative dimensions, the quantitative dimension (degree of change) seems more primary, in that persons making judgments of degree of change appear to consider desirability and life sphere as well as magnitude.

Zautra and Simons (1979) surveyed 454 adults who represented a stratified sample of the 26 census tracts in the catchment area of one community mental health center in Salt Lake City. Both desirable and undesirable life events were assessed at the individual and census-tract levels. Dependent variables at the individual level included self-report measures and reports of help-seeking behavior. Census-tract dependent variables included measures of mental health service utilization and a number of indicators of socioeconomic status and social disequilibrium, such as percentage divorced, median family income, occupational level, and education.

With regard to undesirable life events at the individual level of analysis, the results of the analysis were as expected—the incidence of undesirable life events was positively correlated with measures of psychological distress and negatively correlated with measures of psychological adjustment. The incidence of positive life events was far less powerfully related to the dependent measures, but in general it was positively correlated with measures of psychological adjustment.

At the community level of analysis, both desirable and undesirable life events were related to measures of service utilization and to measures of socioeconomic status and disequilibrium. Undesirable life events were highly associated with low socioeconomic status; desirable life events were highly associated with high socioeconomic status and low divorce rate. Mental health service utilization rates were significantly associated with the absence of desirable life events and were not associated with the presence of undesirable life events. "Individuals who required services tended to report a high number of recent negative life events . . . areas with high rates of service utilization, however, appeared to be best characterized by the relative absence of positive life events. It appeared that negative events were the immediate life stressors, but that positive life events may have served an important preventive function for areas within the community" (p. 448). These authors believe that it may be as useful to identify the frequency of desirable as of undesirable events in people's lives, and they suggest that "investigations of positive life events may complement epidemiological studies of mental illness by providing evidence of events which may promote well-being in addition to identifying stressful events which increase the risk of pathology in a community" (p. 450).

Subjective judgments of stress

Another issue of concern has been how to weigh the severity of individual stressful-life-event items. Specifically, researchers differ on whether each such item should be assigned a universal weight, as originally proposed by Holmes and Rahe (1967), or whether respondents should be asked to judge the impact the event had on them.

B. P. Dohrenwend (1979) takes an unequivocal position on the need to measure the impact of stressful life events independently of self-reports. He writes that it is

> incredible that some researchers have advocated scoring the magnitude of life events . . . in terms of subjective ratings by the individuals whose stress experiences in relation to their psychopathology are being studied. . . . This procedure is virtually guaranteed to confound the relationship between stress and psychopathology. Typically, for example, psychiatric patients rate such events as more stressful than nonpatients . . . just as persons who have experienced heart attacks after a particular life event or series of life events are likely to rate such events as more stressful than a person who has survived the events without a heart attack [p. 8].

Mueller et al. (1978) contrasted 187 newly admitted mental health center patients and a randomly selected nonpatient sample of 321 persons drawn from the same geographic area, looking at the incidence of reported stressful life events during the preceding 30 days. The life events in the questionnaire were categorized according to their judged desirability and their judged independence of psychological status.

Patients reported a significantly greater number of events at the time of entry into treatment than the nonpatient control group. This difference was due mainly to the reports of undesirable events and was not found for events judged to be independent of psychological status. The authors also found that, in both groups, the frequency of reported stressful life events was significantly associated with less positive general well-being as gauged by a brief self-report measure. The authors concluded that "the difference between patients at admission and nonpatients appears to result from patients reporting more undesirable events of the kind that could well be confounded with their current psychological state" (pp. 21–22). It is this very confounding that B. P. Dohrenwend is seeking to avoid.

Schless, Teichman, Mendels, and DiGiacomo (1977) contrasted reported stressful life events during the previous year among 56 newly admitted psychiatric inpatients with those reported by a matched group of 56 medical and surgical patients and a larger community sample of persons interviewed as part of a general-population epidemiological study. Psychiatric patients reported significantly more events than the medical and surgical patients, who, in turn, reported significantly more events than the community sample. Eight events were reported significantly more commonly among the psychiatric patients than among the medical and surgical group. Of these, the largest differences were in increased arguments with spouse, increased arguments with family, and a child leaving home. The authors are, however, cautious in proposing a cause/effect relationship, since the first two of those three events may in fact have been symptoms, rather than causes, of the psychiatric disorder—again a confounding of stressful life events and psychopathology.

By way of contrast, Sarason, Johnson, and Siegel (1979) have developed the Life Experiences Survey—a measure that asks respondents to rate a series of potentially stressful life events as either desirable or undesirable and according to the degree of personal impact the event had—and Horowitz, Wilner, and Alvarez (1979) have developed a scale to make possible a detailed study of the subjective impact of stressful life events. These latter authors proceeded from the belief that what was needed was an instrument "that measures the current degree of subjective impact experienced as a result of a specific event. With such an instrument investigators can observe individuals over periods of time following the occurrence of an event, compare subgroups for degree of subjective distress after a particular life event, or contrast life events in terms of their relative impact on different populations" (p. 209).

The scale Horowitz et al. developed is used to report the impact of any particular stressful event. The items refer to the subject's feelings during the past week regarding the event. Factor analysis of the 20 items in the scale revealed two clusters of seven and eight items, one measuring intrusion ("Images related to it popped into my mind") and the other measuring avoidance ("I stayed away from things or situations that might remind me of it"). The scale has been found useful in assessing the effectiveness of brief psychotherapy undertaken to treat stress-response syndromes and has been found to differentiate such patients from medical students reporting on their reactions to the first cadaver dissection; medical students scored substantially lower on both the intrusion and avoidance scales.

Grant, Gerst, and Yager (1975) administered the same stressful-life-event scale to a sample of 171 psychiatric patients, 181 controls, and 165 relatives of the patients and controls. All participants were asked to assign a weight to each event, just as had been done in the original research by Holmes and Rahe (1967). Rank-order correlations of judged severity of each of the 43 items across the three groups were very high, but psychiatric patients consistently attached a greater magnitude to the events than controls did. While both patients and controls ranked marital separation as the fourth most stressful event, for example, patients weighted the event as nearly 35% more stressful than did controls.

Askenasy, Dohrenwend, and Dohrenwend (1977) have shown that subjective judgments of the severity of stressful life events vary substantially with the educational level and cultural background of the judges. The authors suspect that "the near universal consensus inferred from previous research . . . is in point of fact a middle-class consensus . . . shared by social circles with values and interests in common in many different parts of the world" (p. 438).

In addition to the assessment of stressful life events by using standard-weighted event items or by relying on self-reported measures of undesirability and impact, Brown (1974) has proposed a third procedure, involving judgments of impact made by independent raters who follow a carefully designed interview format and who do not have information about outcome or perceived stress. Brown, agreeing with Dohrenwend, argues that it is crucial to be able to assess the importance of a stressful life event independently of knowing subsequent outcome if one is ever to develop a sound theory of how stressful life events may be causally related to illness. In the absence of that careful rating, three sources of invalidating contamination exist:

> In direct contamination . . . the respondent may report more disturbing life events to make sense of his illness; in indirect contamination, anxiety of the person or some other such trait may lead both to a greater reporting of life events and subsequent illness. And in spuriousness the account of life events may be accurate, but the association of events with illness may be due to another factor such as general anxiety, which leads both to a greater tendency to experience distress in response to life events and also a greater illness rate [p. 237].

Brown suggests, however, that, in assigning a standard index of importance to each event, an enormous amount of individual information is sacrificed. Furthermore, unless a stressful life event is carefully described, each subject can interpret the item differently. Brown believes that a stressful life event can be understood only in its social context and that careful interviewing is necessary to appreciate that context.

Tennant, Smith, Bebbington, and Hurry (1979) have reported that raters can reliably judge severity of stressful life events on an individual basis, as Brown has proposed, by determining the unique social context in which the event took place. These ratings are made on the basis of a wide-ranging semi-structured interview, and the severity of reported life events is judged independently of knowing the subject's response or the outcome of the event. This procedure of individually assessing the contextual threat of stressful life events stands in contrast to the more traditional procedure of assigning a fixed weight to each event in a finite list.

The need for prospective studies

Starting in 1974, researchers examining the state of stressful-life-event research have been unanimous in asserting that the field now needs to inaugurate a series of prospective cohort studies. Epidemiologists have developed two general research strategies for finding connections between certain events and subsequent disorders. One research design, called the *case control* method, contrasts a group of persons having a particular disorder (the cases) with a matched group of persons without the disorder (the controls) to determine whether a suspected antecedent event has occurred significantly more often in the group of cases than in the control group. The other research design, called the *cohort* method, contrasts a group of persons who have undergone a particular event with a matched group of persons who have not, to determine whether a suspected outcome has occurred significantly more often in the first group than in the second. MacMahon and Pugh (1970) write: "A case-control is usually less costly than a cohort study—in terms of both time and resources—and is therefore frequently undertaken as a first step to determine whether or not an association exists between the suspected cause and effect. . . . Cohort studies may then be undertaken to gain added confidence in the existence of a relationship and to measure more accurately its strength" (p. 43).

B. S. Dohrenwend and B. P. Dohrenwend (1974) have suggested that one of the central questions yet to be answered is "What is the risk that some form of disability will follow the occurrence of stressful life events?" They state: "Only studies of cohorts who differ with respect to stressful life events provide any information about the magnitude of the risk that illness or disability will actually follow these events, information without which the practical implications of research on stressful life events [are] far from clear" (p. 315).

In a later publication, B. S. Dohrenwend and B. P. Dohrenwend (1978) have reviewed the direct and indirect evidence relating life stress to illness. They conclude that "the correlates of stressful life events are not limited to any particular types of disorder. On the contrary, life events have been shown to be related to many somatic disorders including heart disease . . . fractures, and childhood leukemia . . . , to performance deficits among teachers and college students . . . , and to psychological disorders including acute schizophrenia . . . depression . . . and suicide attempts" (p. 8). They point out, however, that current research findings "do not provide a clear picture of the nature and strength of this relationship" (p. 9; see also Rahe, 1979, p. 3). B. S. Dohrenwend and B. P. Dohrenwend (1978) indicate that typical case-control studies do not provide "the information that we need to estimate the magnitude of the risk that disorder will follow as a consequence of experiencing stressful life events. To get this information we need cohort studies based on samples of the population of persons who have experienced whatever life events are of interest rather than case-control studies based on samples of persons who have become ill" (p. 12).

Rabkin and Struening (1976), in their critical analysis of the studies of life events, stress, and subsequent illness, note that "the purpose of life events research is to demonstrate a temporal association between the onset of illness and a recent increase in the number of events that require socially adaptive responses on the part of the individual. The impact of such events is presumed to be additive; more events are expected to have greater effect. The underlying assumption is that such events serve as precipitating factors, influencing the timing but not the type of illness episodes" (p. 1014).

Although the notion that socially induced stress can serve as a precipitating factor in chronic diseases is gaining acceptance among many scientists, Rabkin and Struening (1976) caution that the actual magnitude of the relationship is quite small. In addition, these authors note the often-reported low reliability and validity of measures of stressful life events, the evidence that certain life events may be advance signs of subsequent illness rather than independent of it, and the fact that correlations do not prove the directionality

or existence of cause/effect relationships. These authors believe that any significant increase in our understanding of stressful life events as illness precip-
itants will require prospective studies.

Eastwood (1975) examined the relationship between psychiatric and physical disorder in 124 London psychiatric patients and 124 psychiatrically normal
persons carefully assessed and matched for age, sex, marital status, and social
class. Both male and female psychiatric patients had significantly more major
physical disorders and psychosomatic conditions than were found among the
normals. Cardiovascular and respiratory diseases were particularly prevalent
in the psychiatric group. Eastwood concluded that "the concept of . . . a generalized psychophysical propensity of disease appears to be a useful and alternative model to the one which seeks only specific cause-and-effect relationships. The notion of multiple aetiology in disease, and multiple responses . . .
to agents threatening . . . health, is a greater acceptance of the realities of the
ecology of ill health" (p. 87). Eastwood suggests that prospective studies be
undertaken to clarify the etiological role of stressful situations in precipitating
both psychological and biological disorders.

In considering what directions further research should take, Goldberg
and Comstock (1976) suggest that "further retrospective studies seem imprac-
tical both because of biased recall and because of possible interaction between
events and diseases, particularly mental illnesses. More in order are well
designed prospective studies using random samples of the population, a range
of outcome illnesses, outcome variables clearly distinguishable from independent variables, and an account of the effects of mediating factors" (p. 156).

Dean and Lin (1977), who have examined the mediating role of social
support in the connection between stressful life events and both physical and
psychiatric illness, believe future research should be prospective and should
involve annual measurement of stressful life events, social supports, and health.
Three central hypotheses need to be tested: (1) social support moderates the
impact of stressful life events, (2) the moderating effect of social support will
hold true for healthy as well as ill persons, and (3) the availability of social
support is itself a dynamic variable—that is, it not only influences the effects
of stressful life events but also can be influenced by stressful life events.

Finally, Paykel (1978) recently reviewed much of the research linking stressful
life events with the onset of psychiatric illness and calculated a measure of
relative risk based on an analysis of a series of studies contrasting psychiatric
patients with general-population controls. Paykel estimated that the risk of
psychiatric illness following major stressful life events was on the order of 2–
7 times greater than when no significant life events were reported. Risks
appeared greater following life events judged to be more stressful and greater
for subsequent depression and suicide attempts than for schizophrenia. Perhaps as important as this summary statement, was Paykel's observation that
the vast majority of persons undergoing stressful life events do not become
ill, and that to understand how background factors play a role in determining
who does become ill, we will have to move away from retrospective studies

and toward prospective studies in which persons undergoing some stressful life event are matched with persons not undergoing the event. In this way we will be able to identify the actual excess risk of illness associated with the event.

Syme and Torfs (1978) have examined the relation between stressful life events and hypertension and, in that context, comment on the specificity issue. They believe that social, psychological, and physiological factors undoubtedly interrelate in bringing about hypertension. Different stress-related factors may be implicated in the predisposition, precipitation, and perpetuation of hypertension. It may also be that there are both disease-specific and more-general factors involved—some stress-related factors may be specific to hypertension; others may be associated with generalized increased susceptibility to illness.

Because there appear to be no stressful-life-event-specific diseases or disorders, any case-control study, in which persons with a particular disorder are contrasted with suitably matched controls without the disorder, runs the risk of significantly underestimating the deleterious consequences of any particular stressful life event or group of such events. Only cohort studies can identify all such consequences.

Very few prospective cohort studies have been reported in the literature. In addition to Warheit's study (1979), already described, it will be useful to report on one additional study examining the relation of changes in social support over time and changes in psychological adjustment. In this study, Holahan and Moos (1981) administered two surveys, one year apart, to the husbands and wives in a randomly selected sample of 267 families in the San Francisco Bay area. The scales included a number of measures of social supports, recorded negative life-change events during the year between the two surveys, and assessed depression and psychosomatic symptoms. Although the relationship between social support and psychological maladjustment was low in an absolute sense, the study did find that decreases in social support in the family and work environments were significantly related to increases in psychological maladjustment one year later.

EXAMPLES OF STRESS-RELATED PRIMARY PREVENTION PROGRAMS

Some primary prevention programs focus on particular stressful life events. Examining these programs will give the concepts presented in the previous pages some reality in terms of their implications for preventive intervention program development and evaluation.

College entrance

One such program took place on a college campus and involved helping a group of 200 freshman students master the stresses associated with the transition from being a high school senior living at home to being a college

student living away from home (Bloom, 1971b). The unusual vulnerability of
college freshmen to stresses during the early months in college is well known.
While about 5% of the student body in the average university seeks psychiatric
help each year, the incidence of help seeking is unusually high among freshmen. The dropout rate is twice as high for freshmen as for seniors. It has been
suggested that freshmen constitute a specific high-risk group, and this project
developed, carried out, and evaluated a strategy designed to provide meaningful interventions to assist freshmen in this role transition.

The theoretical constructs that were most useful in conceptualizing the
project and in planning its specific objectives and activities were related to the
developmental tasks of adolescence. Review of the literature suggested that
students could be helped toward the completion of five major tasks: (1) developing independence as well as appropriate interdependence, (2) developing
the ability to recognize and deal with uncertainty, (3) developing a personal
set of values and standards that may or may not reflect those of peers or
parents, (4) developing a sense of sexual identity and of satisfaction with one's
own masculinity or femininity, and (5) developing mature interpersonal relationships and social skills.

The project had three interrelated objectives. The first was to learn something about the personality changes that take place during a young person's
college career. The second was to learn how the college student views the
university. The third was to develop an ongoing process with a defined group
of college students so that these research findings could be fed back to the
participating students in a manner they would find growth-inducing and stress-
reducing. It was hoped that this feedback would help the student achieve
emotional maturity, adapt successfully to the college community, avoid psychological disability, and stay in school.

The project was designed to accomplish its third objective by (1) providing
a sense of membership in a group and thus reducing feelings of isolation, (2)
giving group members some reference facts with which to compare themselves, thus reducing feelings of uniqueness, (3) giving group members the
opportunity to express their reactions to the university, (4) giving group members some intellectual tools by which to better understand the stresses acting
on them and their reactions to these stresses, (5) providing formalized opportunities (in the form of questionnaires) for group members to think through
their own beliefs, and (6) providing a resource person for students to talk with
in the event of some crisis.

Information was collected by means of questionnaires. The timing of the
questionnaires, their general themes, and specific items had been derived
partly from an exploratory project, carried out during the preceding year, in
which two graduate students and I met with three groups of freshmen weekly
during the fall semester to learn about the lives of these 36 students and how
and when crises occurred. On the basis of these meetings and a review of
much of the published literature on the subject of college-student mental health,

a series of questionnaires were designed. They were administered to the entire freshman class during orientation week and at key times during the year—after one month in college, after Christmas vacation, shortly after the start of the second semester, and just before final examinations in the second semester. Progress reports based on analyses of these questionnaire responses were prepared by me at irregular times and distributed to all participating students.

The process of preventive intervention was based on a number of principles fundamental to the project. First, data collection and dissemination techniques had to be inexpensive. This principle was invoked primarily because of the conviction that the project, should it successfully achieve its objectives, ought to be suitable, wholly or in part, for use at other universities, regardless of their resources. The second principle was that the participating students had as much to give to the project as to get from it. The communication between students and project director was clearly two-way. Some data-collection forms and many individual items were suggested by students. Students were asked to evaluate the forms and the feedback, and changes were made on the basis of these evaluations. In general, the intervention aspect of the project was an ongoing process between this group of students and one faculty member. Students were invited to visit with me, and a few did—often because of some crisis in their lives.

The third principle was that students, accustomed to learning by reading, could profit from the opportunity to read selected articles on topics relevant to project objectives. Students were asked what topics interested them. When articles were found that it was thought might be informative and interesting, authors' and publishers' permission was sought to reproduce and distribute these articles free of charge to the 200 students in the project. In all, six articles were distributed during the year, dealing with such topics as mental health on the college campus, campus unrest, and sexuality in college-aged persons. The fourth principle was that the type of feedback the students would receive should be appropriate to the means of disseminating the feedback. Since reports to participating students were in the form of statements sent by mail, it was decided that they should not be individualized. The reports gave information about the entire cohort, typically in terms of percentages of males and females responding to items in a certain manner. Another type of report quoted back to cohort members comments they had made about their experiences during Christmas vacation. In this report, students were identified only by sex and by in-state or out-of-state residential status.

The fifth principle was that I would not establish a continuing, regular therapeutic relationship with any student member of the project. An adequate array of therapeutically oriented facilities existed on the campus, and the strategy of the project—preventive intervention by anticipatory guidance—was incompatible with the establishment of long-term therapeutic relationships. When information obtained from a student suggested it, I scheduled a single appointment with that student. Finally, as a sixth general principle, for purposes of program evaluation, an effort was made to follow all members of the project, regardless of whether they remained on the campus as students in good standing. It became clear, as students left the university, that follow-up was going to be time-consuming. Two facts became apparent quite soon after the follow-up of students was begun. First, students welcomed this contact with the project, and, second, contact by letter was virtually useless in obtaining information from students. Students are apparently poor letter writers, however interested they are in maintaining contact. The telephone became the technique of choice for establishing and maintaining periodic contact with students who left the campus.

Evaluations of the pilot project were generally favorable. In contrast to a comparison group of freshmen, the experimental group had a somewhat higher survival rate, and of those no longer on the campus, a significantly larger portion of experimental-group students continued their academic involvement in other settings. In addition, of students who left the university, a majority of the members of the experimental group continued to live away from home, while a majority of the comparison group returned to their parental home.

Widowhood

Another example of an area in which preventively oriented programs have been established is in the development of intervention services for the widowed (Clayton, 1975; Parkes, 1981; Raphael, 1977; Silverman, 1967, 1972; Silverman et al., 1975; van Rooijen, 1979; Walker, MacBride, & Vachon, 1977). Silverman's program was designed to facilitate the transition from the role of wife to that of widow in new widows under age 65, using as helping agents other widows who had themselves already made the transition successfully.

In her review of the literature and in her own studies, Silverman found that newly widowed persons rarely considered using traditional mental-health-related agencies unless they had used them before widowhood. In fact, Silverman suggests that there may not be an appropriate role for the psychiatric clinic in the lives of widows, particularly during the early stages of mourning. Rather, what is required is a service that is available immediately after the death occurs, can reach every new widow, has legitimate access to the newly widowed population, and can provide a range of services, including all existing community resources. On the basis of this analysis, Silverman concluded that "the most effective caregiver . . . is another widowed person who has recovered" (1967, p. 44).

The "Widow-to-Widow" program was developed on the assumptions that the caregiving widow aide would be able to use her own experience and special empathy to help newly bereaved widows and that she would be able to provide acceptable and extended support. Silverman notes that the "findings of the Widow-to-Widow program indicate that widows and widowers often develop emotional disturbance when they cannot give up their role of wife or husband, i.e., when they continue to live as they had when their spouse was alive" (1972, p. 96). The widow aides must help the new widow give up the role of wife, return to earlier roles—for example, as paid workers— or establish new roles, deal with the secondary mourning that often emerges six months or a year after the spouse's death, and resume a socializing life-style. The widow aide can talk about her own grief and become a role model and a bridge back to the real world.

During the first year and a half of the program, efforts were made to reach 300 new widows. A total of 67 women could not be reached. Of the 233 who were reached, 142 (61%) accepted at least some of the widow-aide services. Younger widows (particularly those with children and those who were not working) were most receptive. Widows needed to talk and to experience the friendship of the widow aide. The problems discussed included housing, child rearing, finances, difficulties with relatives, and job training. Widows needed assurance that they could successfully weather the difficulties they faced, and talking with someone who had coped with the same problem was clearly valued.

This project has not yet been quantitatively evaluated, but qualitative observations suggest that large numbers of newly widowed persons find the widow caregivers enormously helpful to them in the crisis that follows the death of the spouse.

A second major approach to reducing the negative consequences of wid-owhood as a major life stressor is the self-help group. In a recent evaluation of such a group, THEOS, Lieberman and Borman (1981) have analyzed data from a large follow-up study of a group of widows and widowers who were current members of the self-help group, were former members, or had been invited to join but had chosen not to. Several hundred persons were involved in the follow-up study, which included two questionnaires administered one year apart.

Respondents were asked to describe their most pressing widowhood-related problems. Role problems—that is, problems of establishing a role as a single person—were mentioned by 61% of the respondents. Nearly one-third of the sample mentioned problems of depression. In evaluating the effective-ness of the self-help group, the authors divided the sample according to how actively participants had been involved in the program. Their analysis sug-gested that active participation positively affected the mental health status of the participants, particularly in reducing depression and in increasing self-esteem.

Finally, in a two-year study of postbereavement adaptation of a group of 162 widows, Vachon, Lyall, Rogers, Freedman-Letofsky, and Freeman (1980) contrasted adaptation in two groups, one of which consisted of widows who were paired with another widow to provide emotional support and practical assistance. These helper-widows had previously participated in a training seminar that examined issues related to widowhood, and the widow-to-widow program consisted of supportive telephone calls and both individual and small-group meetings.

These authors found that the intervention subjects and the control subjects (those who were not part of the widow-to-widow program) were equally disturbed one month after bereavement but that widows in the intervention program were less depressed and less preoccupied with the past. One year after widowhood, the control group had caught up with the intervention group in personal adjustment, but the intervention group was superior in terms of resocialization. At two years, health was substantially better in the intervention group than in the control group. The authors concluded that those widows who received the intervention services followed the same general course of adaptation as the control subjects, but their rate of achieving a satisfactory level of adaptation was accelerated.

Multiple stresses

Roskin (1982) developed a preventive intervention program for persons who had sustained two or more significant stressful life events within the previous year. Intervention consisted of six weekly meetings involving didactic presentations and group discussions in the context of a supportive orientation. Fifty-five persons were involved in the program.

Roskin found that the program appeared to have positive consequences for depression, anxiety, and interpersonal oversensitivity and that the program was most helpful for those participants who had experienced greater numbers of stressful life events. In particular, those participants who had experienced the death of a family member or close friend appeared to improve most.

High school entrance

Felner, Ginter, and Primavera (1982) examined the effectiveness of a preventive intervention program designed to facilitate the transition from junior to senior high school—a common and predictable stressful life event. Moves from one school to another have often been found to result in decreases in academic achievement, increased classroom behavior problems, and heightened anxiety, particularly in interpersonal situations. The project took place during the summer before high school entry and involved 65 students. A control group of 120 matched nonproject students was also identified.

The project was designed to increase teacher and student support during the transition to high school and to reduce the difficulties of mastering the tasks associated with the transition. All project students were assigned to one of four designated home-room teachers, and during the summer these teachers contacted the parents of their students in order to increase the amount of perceived social support available from teachers, to decrease the students' sense of anonymity, and to help students gain access to important information about school expectations and regulations.

In addition, the school schedule and organization were revised so that students in the experimental project would take their four primary academic subjects only with other project students. Thus, it was hoped, a stable peer-support system could be established.

Both project and control students were evaluated at midyear and again at the end of the school year. Students were evaluated in terms of their self-concepts, their perceptions of the social climate of the school, and their grades and attendance records during both the previous and the current school years.

Control students were found to be absent from school significantly more often during the first school year than students in the intervention project and to have earned significantly poorer grades. While the self-concepts of students in the experimental program generally remained stable during their first year in high school, self-concepts of control-group students showed marked declines. Finally, students in the experimental program reported significantly more positive feelings about the social climate in the school than did control-group students. In particular, experimental students reported higher levels of teacher support, affiliation, and involvement; significantly more favorable impressions of the personal-growth-enhancing aspects of the school environment; and significantly more favorable judgments of how well organized the school was. Virtually all the differences between experimental and control groups over time were due to declines in the ratings by control students rather than to increases in ratings by experimental students.

The authors conclude by noting that "overall, these findings support the arguments that attempts to understand and modify social environments . . . can be fruitfully adapted to preventive programs designed to increase people's ability to cope with the adaptive tasks of life transitions" (Felner, Ginter, & Primavera, 1982, p. 288).

Separation and divorce

Finally, it will be useful to present some of the details of a six-month program that we established to assist people who were undergoing a marital separation and divorce in Boulder County, Colorado (Bloom, Hodges, & Caldwell, 1982).[4] Since marital separation is not a legally reportable event, there is no certain way of identifying all persons potentially eligible to participate in such an intervention program. The procedure we followed was to use the mass media (newspapers and radio, as well as posters in supermarkets, laundromats, and so on) and direct mailing to human service agencies and to appropriate practitioners (attorneys, physicians, clergymen, mental health professionals) to publicize the "Separation and Divorce Program." The pro-

[4]This program was undertaken with the support of a research grant from the National Institute of Mental Health (Grant number MH26373), and we are pleased to acknowledge that support on this occasion.

gram was described in deliberately ambiguous terms, with no mention of the availability of services to participants.

Requirements for eligibility were as follows: (1) the person had to be legally married at the time of the inquiry but living apart from the spouse because of marital discord, (2) it had to be the first marriage for the person making the inquiry, (3) the length of separation could not have exceeded six months, and (4) the person had to reside in Boulder County, Colorado. Both husband and wife in a separated couple were eligible to be in the study, but in fact only three couples participated.

After eligibility was established, assignments to the experimental intervention and to a no-treatment control group were systematically alternated at the ratio of two persons in the intervention program for each one person in the control condition. All persons assigned to the intervention group were contacted by an intervention-program staff member, who administered the initial interview before indicating the availability of intervention services. Persons assigned to the control condition were interviewed by research assistants (advanced graduate students in clinical psychology). Referrals to community agencies were made in this group as seemed appropriate. A total of 101 persons were assigned to the intervention program and 52 to the no-treatment condition.

Interviews were conducted at the time of entrance into the study and again six months later (by which time participation in the preventive intervention program was completed). Additional interviews will be conducted 18 and 30 months after entrance into the program. The evaluation reported here is based on an analysis of initial and six-month data for all subjects interviewed on both occasions. Six-month data were obtained from 100 of the 101 members of the intervention group and from 50 of the 52 members of the control group.

Data collection took place by means of in-person interviews that required between 90 minutes and 2 hours to complete. The initial interview consisted of a number of component parts, including (1) a participant consent form, (2) residential tracing information to facilitate locating the participant when the time arrived for the next interview, (3) demographic information, (4) information on the events surrounding the separation, prior and current histories of help-seeking behavior, current life problems, and characteristics of the support network, (5) information about socialization patterns and practices, (6) information about income and expenses, (7) housing and homemaking information, (8) career and employment information, (9) a symptom checklist covering the six months prior to separation, (10) information about parenting, and (11) a stressful-life-events inventory covering the six months prior to separation. The six-month interview was designed to obtain information about the six months since entrance into the program and generally paralleled the initial interview.

The intervention program. Each program participant was assigned to one of three full-time supervised program representatives, who were paraprofessionals with extensive volunteer counseling experience. Twenty program participants constituted a full caseload, and there were never more than 60 participants in the program at any one time. The program representatives provided emotional support and crisis intervention and served as the link between the participants and the rest of the program. Program representatives played an active outreach role, contacting the participants regularly, developing opportunities for group and individual social interaction, making referrals to other parts of the program and to community agencies, and following up throughout the period of participation in the intervention program.

In addition to the program representatives, five specialized study groups were available, each led by a subject-matter expert who was associated with the project a maximum of four hours a week. Both group and individual contacts were made available, depending on the demand for services as well as the nature of the issues under consideration.

One study group focused on the career-planning and employment problems common to the newly separated—developing marketable skills, finding employment, changing jobs, and long-range occupational and career planning. The leader of this group was a psychologist experienced in career and educational counseling. The second study group focused on legal and financial issues—establishment of credit, eligibility for loans, child custody, visitation rights, maintenance and child support, and the process of divorce litigation. This group was led by an attorney experienced with clients seeking divorce. The third group dealt with child-rearing and single-parenting problems—children's reactions to the separation of their parents, visitation issues, behavior problems, and enhancing personal adjustment. The group leader was a psychiatric social worker who specialized in working with children. The fourth group, led by a home economist, dealt with housing and homemaking issues—finding a place to live, home repairs, money management, consumerism, food purchase and preparation, and time management. The fifth study group dealt with issues associated with socialization and personal self-esteem—enhancing the self-concept, loneliness, resocialization in the world of the single, and feelings of social and personal inadequacy. The leader was a psychiatric social worker with extensive clinical experience.

Outcome measures.   Since the intervention program was designed to provide services in five areas, five area-specific problem scores were calculated from questionnaire items. The same items appeared on the initial and the six-month interviews, permitting analysis of changes in problem scores over time. In addition to obtaining estimates of problem severity related to each program area, problem scales included such questions as the frequency of work-related symptoms and the severity of problems in the areas of sexual satisfaction, loneliness, the establishment of new relationships, and child rearing.

In addition to these five area-specific problem scores, two other groups of items were selected to assess the frequency and intensity of psychological problems. First, nine items were combined into a measure of psychological distress and maladjustment. These items included current attitude toward the separation; severity of problems in the area of mental and physical health, guilt, self-blame, and competence; and estimates of the magnitude of the perceived benefits of the separation. The second group of items was based on the Symptom Checklist (Bloom & Caldwell, 1981). This scale has two sub-scales—Neurasthenia and Anxiety—and also yields a total score.

Results. Participants in the study appeared to be demographically sim-ilar to the overall Boulder County adult population (Bloom, Hodges, Caldwell, Systra, & Cedrone, 1977). No significant demographic differences were found between the intervention and control groups. An analysis of the demographic characteristics of Boulder city residents (the city contains about half of the total county population) who filed for divorce in 1977 was conducted by the Human Resources Department of the City of Boulder (Conger, Shepard, & Szot, 1978). This analysis indicated that about half of all divorces were obtained by persons aged 30 or younger, length of marriage at the time of divorce averaged about three years for childless couples and eight years for couples with children, 43% of divorcing couples were parents, and divorcing parents had an average of 1.89 children.

Contrasting the 59 participants who chose to make use of any of the study groups with the 41 who did not revealed that initial problem scores on each of the five study-group topics were not significantly different, although non-users had lower problem scores in each of the five areas than eventual users. In contrast, initial general psychological problem measures tended to favor the users of study groups. Users of study groups scored significantly lower on the Symptom Checklist Anxiety Scale than nonusers.

Program participants were given the opportunity to evaluate their con-tacts with intervention-program components monthly. Most returned only one evaluation during the six-month program. All participants completed at least one evaluation; the average number of completed evaluations was 1.4 per participant. The program was judged very favorably. Study-group expe-riences were thought to be good; program representatives were judged to be skillful and easily available when needed.

Six-month program evaluation. To evaluate the impact of the interven-tion program, nine statistical analyses (one for each dependent measure based on data obtained at the six-month interview) were performed. Of the nine analyses, five indicated that there were significant differences between the intervention and control groups. In all cases where significant differences were found, intervention-group participants reported fewer problems and better psychological adjustment than members of the control group.

Members of the intervention group also showed a significant decrease in general-psychological-problem scores across time. The intervention group sig-nificantly reduced its psychological distress and maladjustment score from pre- to posttest. On the Anxiety and Neurasthenia subscales of the Symptom Checklist, equally significant improvements from pre- to posttest were found. No equivalent improvement was found in the control group. On the total Symptom Checklist score, the intervention group reported significantly fewer problems than the control group at the six-month interview. In this case, however, control-group members reported more symptoms than they had initially, while intervention-group members remained at about their initial level.

Two sources of information attested to the usefulness of the intervention program—reports by program participants and statistical comparisons of the six-month adjustment scores of participants and control-group members. Although the intervention program had planned thematic components, and although program participants found the study groups helpful, most of the improvement was general rather than specific. Participation in problem-focused study groups did not result in any appreciable reduction in the severity of those problems. Knowledge that special services were available may have had a more powerful general effect than actually making use of those services.

The importance of the general improvement should not be minimized, however. Decreases in the Neurasthenia and Anxiety scores represent reductions in fatigue, nervousness, tenseness, weakness, and ill health; increases in the ability to cope and to carry out important life tasks; and decreases in anxiety-related physiological responses to stress. Findings in the present study suggest that high Neurasthenia scores are specifically associated with difficulties in child rearing and single parenting. In a recent paper, Berger has suggested that there has been a revival of interest in the concept of neurasthenia and that "periods of heightened interest in neurasthenia in the psychiatric literature coincide with periods and locales of decreased cohesion of the larger group" (1973, p. 562; see also Bloom & Caldwell, 1981). There can hardly be a better example of decreased group cohesion than the dissolution of a marriage.

Even more important, the nature of the general improvement lends considerable support to the primary prevention goals of the program. Reductions in anxiety and in general fatigue, along with improved coping skills and physical well-being, are exactly the results one would hope to obtain in a program that seeks to reduce the incidence of diagnosable psychopathology in a vulnerable high-risk group such as the newly separated.

CONCLUSIONS AND OVERVIEW

Activities in the field of primary prevention that draw on stressful-life-event theory are very vigorous. Although much remains to be learned, there is a sense that significant advances in preventive intervention are taking place. These advances appear to be due mainly to the high level of interest in stress and its consequences for both general health and psychological well-being. Many common stressful life events have been identified, and a significant beginning has been made in understanding under what circumstances these events can impair health. Furthermore, as has been seen, a number of preventive intervention programs based on these theories and conceptualizations have been mounted and evaluated. We are only at the beginning of this line of inquiry, but there is every reason to be optimistic about its long-term effectiveness in reducing both incidence and prevalence of a broad array of disorders.

CHAPTER

7

Mental
Health
Education

In the spring of 1964, the regulations governing the administration of Title II of Public Law 88-164 (the Community Mental Health Centers Act) provided the definition of a community mental health center in terms of services such centers were required to offer. Among those services were consultation and education, available to community agencies and professional personnel. A subsequent federal publication designed to clarify this requirement defined mental health education as follows: "The primary goal of mental health education is to promote positive mental health by helping people acquire knowledge, attitudes, and behavior patterns that will foster and maintain their mental well-being" (National Institute of Mental Health, 1966, p. 4).

Thus, mental health education appeared to have two major components: one directed toward mental health professionals and their colleagues throughout the community human service delivery system (often called "staff development," "continuing education," or "in-service training") and the other directed toward the public (Mazade, 1974, p. 674). This latter emphasis on prevention by education of the public, or, as it is sometimes called, "consumer education," emerged as the more important of the two from the point of view of community mental health, and it will be the chief focus of this chapter.

In his discussion of the role of the mental health educator in the community mental health center, Goldston has observed: "The mandated inclusion of consultation and education services represents a new approach in community mental health programming and a distinct challenge to the responsible staff of a community mental health center. The challenge calls for pioneering

311

efforts in an area which heretofore appears to have been relatively neglected and in which limited opportunities have existed for professional training and practice" (1968, p. 693).

RECENT HISTORY OF MENTAL HEALTH EDUCATION

The reputation of mental health education, at least so far as education of the public is concerned, was already tainted in 1964 owing to the widely publicized experiences of Elaine and John Cumming (1957) some years earlier, who attempted to mount and evaluate a six-month intensive mental health education program in a small community in Canada. Defining mental health education as "education about the nature of those already ill" (1957, p. 159), the Cummings found not only that their program (a mixture of films, group discussions, and media exposure) had no measurable effect on attitudes toward the mentally ill but also that their conscientious efforts at both education and evaluation met with hostility, anxiety, and rejection. The culmination of these reactions was an invitation to the mental health education project staff by the mayor of the community to leave town (1957, p. 44).

The report of their work somehow cast its shadow on the entire mental health education enterprise, even though the Cummings were the first to be critical of their own efforts. They had entered the community without invitation, had very little sense of the context of currently held attitudes toward the mentally ill, had only a small and unstable constituency, and in retrospect considered the assumptions that were fundamental in planning their program to be "naively conceived" (1957, p. 91).

In 1965 the field sustained a second blow—this time from an evaluation of a carefully chosen group of published studies pertinent to mental health education, or, as the author called it, education for positive mental health (Davis, 1965). Davis's findings—perhaps overstated, to be sure—were anything but reassuring:

> A mental health education program may be thought to consist of four major parts: (1) substantive content, (2) medium or vehicle; (3) audience; and (4) goal. . . . Our original assumption was that the major obstacles to success in conducting programs would turn up in the bottom three rows, specifically: (1) dependent variables would be difficult to measure; (2) audiences might be resistant to the information; (3) the delicacy of the content might require special techniques, such as discussions led by a psychiatrist. On the whole, this assumption was not borne out by our review of the literature. . . . Rather, the major problem appears to be this: *mental health educators have little or nothing specific and practical to tell the public* [Davis, 1965, p. 138].

In addition to these historical developments, few formal professional training programs have ever been available for persons interested in becoming mental health educators. As a consequence, mental health education has been the runt of the community mental health center's required-services litter. In

Beisser and Green's book *Mental Health Consultation and Education* (1972), the subject of mental health education occupies about 10 pages out of a total of 145. In Vacher and Stratas's book *Consultation-Education: Development and Evaluation* (1976), their program is consistently described as a consultation program in their text, and the word *education* does not even appear in the subject index. A similar imbalance between consultation and education can be found in Mannino and MacLennan (1978). In a survey of consultation and education activities conducted in community mental health centers during a representative month in 1973 (Bass, 1974), staff hours devoted to public information are not included in the total, with the result that "consultation and education" is in effect a euphemism for what is overwhelmingly mental health consultation.

More recently, however, Ketterer (1981) has systematically identified the educational components of consultation and education services. In his classification of the methods used by consultation and education staff, he specifically includes (1) competency training for community populations and (2) public information methods.

With regard to competency training, Ketterer indicates that the most widespread application of education and training methods has been carried out by specialists interested in "improving the coping skills and competencies of normal and at-risk groups. The premise is that by improving the competencies and coping skills of populations at risk, individuals and groups will be better able to manage predictable and unpredictable life crises and events" (p. 133). Ketterer describes public information methods as involving the "dissemination of mental health information to relevant caregivers and populations in the community" (p. 137) and says that whereas consultation involves face-to-face reciprocal interactions between the consultant and the consultee, the distribution of public information is more unilateral, the direction of action being from the public information specialist to the target group. Public information strategies are used to

> inform the public about mental health problems and about available treatment and prevention services. . . . provide general information to the community that promotes positive mental health, individual growth, and a more enriched life. . . . ease client transitions back into community life and to increase a community's acceptance of formerly institutionalized individuals returning to the community. . . . provide important information to people in the community who are in key positions to affect the lives of others. . . . [and] influence public policies that affect the mental health and well-being of individuals and groups in the community [pp. 138–139].

CURRENT STATUS OF MENTAL HEALTH EDUCATION

Within the last few years, the field of mental health education has clearly revived, and although it is a field characterized as much by promise as by accomplishment, it is vigorous and active (see, for example, Marshall, 1977, especially Chapter 1; Mico & Ross, 1975; Ridenour, 1969; Sauber, 1973; Somers, 1976; U.S. Department of Health, Education and Welfare, 1977a).

In a recent paper prepared for the Michigan Mental Health Association, Williams (1979), a strong advocate of mental health education, wrote as follows:

> How can we explain the high cost and ineffectiveness of the system in addressing mental health needs? No simple answer can be put forth at this time. Yet I would submit that the problem stems largely from the basic—and faulty—assumption that undergirds our current mental health system: that in order to benefit from mental health services, one must be willing to (1) accept client or patient status, and (2) seek out clinical or treatment services. What other options do we have? I believe mental health education is the strongest approach available to us. There are at least three reasons for this: (1) education affects larger groups or populations than traditional service delivery approaches, (2) education does not require that people take on client or patient status, and (3) education builds on the strengths and competencies of people rather than focusing on illness and pathology. Expressed in its most basic form, education is more acceptable to people than clinical or treatment approaches and therefore is capable of affecting a larger number of people who are motivated by the principle of growth and development. The key lies in the word 'motivated.' There is an essential difference between the motives of one entering therapy and the motives of one entering an educational experience. And it is this difference which makes education a largely untapped resource within the mental health field. The primary motive of the person entering therapy is that of reducing the amount of pain being experienced in his or her life. The primary motive of the person entering an educational experience, on the other hand, is that of learning and growth. He or she may be experiencing pain, but it is desire to grow and develop that propels one into an educational experience [pp. 4–5].[1]

Goldston (1968) has proposed that mental health education includes two broad areas of functioning: general educational services—"activities and tasks which every community mental health worker might assume in order to increase his effectiveness as a community agent" (p. 694)—and specific educational functions, "which require the skills of a professionally trained community mental health educator" (p. 694). Among the general educational activities, Goldston mentions (1) community organization and interagency collaboration, (2) community assessment, particularly regarding knowledge of and attitudes toward mental illness and health, mental health services, and mental-health-related needs, (3) identifying foci of stress and mental illness, (4) establishment and provision of mental health consultation programs, and (5) educational programs for prospective and current patients and their families. Among the specific educational activities, Goldston identifies (1) professional training for other caretaking groups, (2) general educational and mental health educational programs for the public, (3) consultation to mental

---

[1]From "Mental Health Education: The Untapped Resource," by R. T. Williams. Paper developed for the Mental Health Association, Michigan, December, 1979. Reprinted by permission of Roger T. Williams.

health center staff, (4) staff in-service education, (5) rehabilitative education for former patients and their families, and (6) development of specific educational materials and programs.

A very useful approach to domain definition has been inaugurated by the National Committee for Mental Health Education, a national organization of mental health educators founded in 1967. The group has proposed the following definition of mental health education:

> Mental health education is a distinct group of interventions designed to assist people in acquiring knowledge, skills and attitudes that directly contribute to their mental health and to their effect on the mental health of others. Such interventions enable people to cope with and act on their environment and seek to create environments which are more supportive of human life. Mental health education is applicable to a wide variety of purposes and target groups, and has unique potential for preventing emotional disability and for promoting growth in people and community groups [McMillen & Williams, 1977, p. 2].[2]

According to the National Committee for Mental Health Education, mental health education has six distinguishing characteristics:

1. It is a method or group of methods intended to advance mental health through learning.
2. Its methods are derived from the fields of mental health, psychology, sociology, education, and mass communication.
3. Although sometimes used in conjunction with clinical services, it is uniquely different from clinical interventions.
4. It can be used to help a variety of populations and is not limited to clients or to those seeking clinical assistance.
5. It can serve a variety of purposes ranging from improving the adjustment of institutionalized patients, to creating an informed and caring community, to helping people lead happier, more mentally healthy lives.
6. Its potential is greatest in the realm of prevention and in promoting positive mental health, as a consequence of its ability to reach large numbers of people who might not want or need clinical services and its ability to create a more supportive environment in which people can live.

The National Committee for Mental Health Education has outlined the major target groups and purposes of mental health education: (1) Education of the general public, particularly regarding mental health problems and resources and to promote positive mental health. (2) Education of at-risk non-client populations, to assist people in coping with predictable life-stage transitions, in living under stressful conditions more effectively, and in gaining

---

[2]From *Ideas*, March, 1977, R. McMillen and R. T. Williams (Eds.), National Committee for Mental Health Education.

skills to deal with symptoms of distress. (3) Education of clients and their significant others, to assist the client in becoming a skilled and knowledgeable consumer of mental health services, to enhance the therapeutic program of a client or patient, and to facilitate the transition of a client back into community life. (4) Education of those in the community who are in a key position to affect the lives of others, such as persons affiliated with human service agencies, school systems, and law enforcement agencies, attorneys, physicians, and public health nurses. Objectives in these educational efforts for caregivers include improving such persons' ability to be effective mental health resources, to accept increasing responsibility for the general level of the mental health of the community, and to recognize emotional problems and to make appropriate referrals to other community agencies. (5) Education of those who are in a position to influence public policy, such as elected officials, board members, and government authorities. Objectives in these educational efforts include developing greater understanding of the impact of all public policies on mental health and greater support for public policies that promote mental health.

Adelson and Lurie provide a similar set of emphases in their definition of mental health education:

> Mental health education may be conceived as having two broad goals: (a) Increasing the understanding, knowledge, and capacity of the individual to effectively cope with problems and crises as these arise in daily life and also special times in the life span. (b) Increasing the knowledge, understanding, and capacity of the community and its subsystems—governmental bodies, public and voluntary agencies, such as school, welfare, police, church, hospital—to cope responsibly and effectively with 'social problems' through programs of prevention, treatment, rehabilitation, and change [1972, pp. 520–521].[3]

CONSUMER HEALTH EDUCATION

Fortunately for the active advocates of mental health education, a larger, older, and better-established field—consumer health education—is in existence, from which much can be learned. Most of the issues that are of concern to mental health educators (for example, basic definition of domain, strategies for the evaluation of effectiveness, reaching particular high-risk groups, or developing persuasive educational materials) are of concern to consumer health educators as well. Furthermore, since physical well-being is so powerfully associated with psychological well-being, the work of consumer health educators and of mental health educators is interdependent. Duncan states that although the fields of health education and mental health education have areas of uniqueness, there does appear to be a substantial confluence between them and that "both fields have much to gain from this emerging relationship" (1979, p. 13).

---

[3]From "Mental Health Education: Research and Practice," by D. Adelson and L. Lurie. In S. E. Golann and C. Eisdorfer (Eds.), *Handbook of Community Mental Health.* Copyright 1972 by Goodyear Publishing Co., Inc.

In fact, Swisher (1976) has developed an approach to health education that places individual emotional development at the core of the curriculum. Swisher's assumption is that "enriched emotional development will prevent a variety of health problems" (1976, p. 387). Thus, Swisher contends that school health curricula should expose students to a set of systematically planned emotionally enriching experiences. These experiences should, according to Swisher, deal with four major dimensions: (1) personal skill building around such issues as self-concept and decision making that are necessary for personal satisfaction with life, (2) interpersonal skill building around such issues as listening, acceptance, and relationship establishment that are necessary for successfully functioning as an individual within a society, (3) extrapersonal skill building in areas related to a more comprehensive understanding of the environment and its impact on the individual, and (4) health-problem skill building that allows the individual to cope effectively with health maintenance and illness management.

The field of consumer health education is expanding rapidly, mainly as a consequence of (1) the increasing prevalence of chronic disease and the growing necessity for people to take responsibility for their own health, (2) the development of new technologies for mass communication (the most noteworthy being the computer and a variety of innovative mass-media approaches such as public television channels with the capability for two-way communication between broadcaster and audience), and (3) the growth of the consumer movement (Marshall, 1977).

Definition and goals of consumer health education

In the report of the President's Committee on Health Education, established by President Nixon in 1971, the field of health education is defined as follows: "People tend to confuse health 'information' with health 'education.' 'Health information' is simply facts. And facts are widely available. . . . Health education motivates the person to take the information and do something with it—to keep himself healthier by avoiding actions that are harmful and by forming habits that are beneficial" (President's Committee on Health Education, 1973, p. 17).

Another definition, developed at about the same time, is somewhat broader in character but also emphasizes action: Health education is a "process with intellectual, psychological, and social dimensions relating to activities which increase the abilities of people to make informed decisions affecting their personal, family, and community well being. This process, based on scientific principles, facilitates learning and behavioral change in both health personnel and consumers, including children and youth" ("New Definitions," 1974, p. 34).

More recently, a more comprehensive definition of the term *consumer health education* was adopted by the Task Force on Consumer Health Education, jointly sponsored by the National Institutes of Health, the American College of Preventive Medicine, and the John E. Fogarty International Center for Advanced Studies in the Health Sciences:

> The term 'consumer health education' subsumes a set of six activities that—(1) inform people about health, illness, disability, and ways in which they can improve and protect their own health, including more efficient use of the delivery system; (2) motivate people to want to change to more healthful practices; (3) help them to learn the necessary skills to adopt and maintain healthful practices and life styles; (4) foster teaching and communication skills in all those engaged in educating consumers about health; (5) advocate changes in the environment that will facilitate healthful conditions and healthful behaviors; and (6) add to knowledge through research and evaluation concerning the most effective ways of achieving these objectives [Somers, 1976, p. xv; see also p. 15].[4]

Consumer health education: An overview

Marc Lalonde, the former Minister of National Health and Welfare in Canada, has urged that one must look beyond the traditional view that levels of health in any society can be improved only by improving the delivery of health services. Lalonde argued that future improvements in level of health lie mainly in "improving the environment, moderating self-imposed risks and adding to our knowledge of human biology" (1974, p. 18). He suggested that there are two broad objectives in the health field—to reduce mental and physical health hazards and to improve the accessibility of high-quality mental and physical health care. To achieve these two objectives, Lalonde proposed a number of strategies, including health promotion.

Of the nearly two dozen possible courses of action proposed by Lalonde that could be followed in undertaking a health-promotion strategy, many dealt directly with health education. Included were the development of educational programs on nutrition; increasing the awareness of the gravity and underlying causes of traffic accidents, deaths, and injuries; promoting a more widespread understanding of coronary artery disease; creating a more realistic sense of urgency about the problem of mental illness; increasing awareness of the hazards of self-medication and of problems due to abuse of alcohol, drugs, and tobacco and to venereal disease; and promoting and coordinating school and adult health education programs (Lalonde, 1974, pp. 67–68).

Two major studies have recently suggested that educational campaigns can have demonstrable effects on behavior and attitudes but that the effects take far more time than was originally thought. A new poll conducted by Louis Harris and Associates for the National Conference of Christians and Jews, dealing with attitudes toward black persons ("A New Racial Poll," 1979), indicates that between 1963 and 1978 attitudes have become slowly but consistently and often dramatically more favorable. In the area of smoking and health, the

---

[4]Reprinted from *Promoting Health: Consumer Education and National Policy,* by Anne R. Somers (Ed.), by permission of Aspen Systems Corporation, © 1976.

recent Surgeon General's report (U.S. Department of Health, Education and Welfare, 1979c, Appendix, Table 2) indicates within recent years the start of a slow but consistent decrease in the prevalence of smoking among adults. In 1964, for example, 52.9% of adult males were current smokers and 22.2% were former smokers. In 1975 the same measures were 39.3% and 29.2%. For women, the 1964 figures were 31.5% current smokers and 7.4% former smokers. In contrast, in 1975, 28.9% of women were current smokers and 14.5% were former smokers.

Levy, Iverson, and Walberg (1980) reviewed a series of 22 studies that examined the effectiveness of school nutrition education programs published between 1968 and 1978, examining their impact on nutrition knowledge, behavior, and attitudes. Although classical nutritional diseases are rare in the United States, subclinical signs of malnutrition are far more common, particularly among people who exist at or near the poverty level. The 22 studies varied in their theoretical emphases and in their methodological strengths, as well as in their effectiveness. The authors found that studies that used media in effective ways "appear to have untapped potential for influencing nutrition behavior and may need to be the focus of future nutrition education research" (p. 123).

In a recent review of studies using the mass media for health promotion, Flay, DiTecco, and Schlegel (1980) organized their evaluation in terms of both the dependent (outcome) and independent variables in such studies. As for dependent variables, these authors noted that it is important to distinguish between the impact of mass-media approaches on (1) exposure to the message, (2) awareness of the message, (3) comprehension of the message, (4) belief in the message content, (5) persistence of any change in attitude caused by the message, and (6) changes in behavior. As for the independent variables (characteristics of the media approaches), these authors indicate that it is important to consider (1) characteristics of the message source, (2) message content, structure, and style, (3) the medium and how it is used, (4) characteristics of the audience, and (5) the specific objectives of the mass-media approach.

Flay et al. found that some conditions seem to be conducive to causing change in beliefs and attitudes—particularly the following:

> (1) arousing involvement in the issue and/or motivation to change; (2) much repetition by several sources, via multi-media, over long periods of time (i.e., years, not weeks or months); (3) novelty in the way the message is presented (in order to maintain attention and increase the chance of arousing involvement); (4) targeting very specific issues and providing consistent alternative attitudinal structures; and (5) high quality production of materials (equal to that of commercial mass media production) to ensure attention [p. 135].[5]

[5]From "Mass Media in Health Promotion: An Analysis Using an Extended Information-Processing Model," by B. R. Flay, D. DiTecco, and R. P. Schlegel. In Health Education Quarterly, 1980 7, 127–147. Copyright 1980 by Human Sciences Press, Inc. This and all other quotations from the same source are reprinted by permission.

Four other program attributes are needed in order to increase the likelihood that there will be behavior change as well: "(1) incorporation of information pertaining to behavioral alternatives and skills development within the communication message itself; (2) promotion of interaction with the audience (e.g., via telephone or written materials); (3) supplementation with face-to-face clinics; and (4) mobilization or restructuring of community resources" (p. 136).

In summarizing their analysis, Flay and colleagues say:

> The first requirement is to reach the target audience. Many programs have probably proved ineffective because not enough people were exposed to [them]. . . . Once exposure is achieved, it is no use reaching people's living rooms if they do not attend to the message. Appeals to multiple motives . . . in novel ways; with repetition across sources, channels, and times; will help get attention. An expert . . . who presents a clearly targeted concise, easily understood message will also increase attention, as well as ensure comprehension. . . . Acceptance of . . . the message is also more likely if the source is credible . . . and presents the message in an arousing and involving (i.e., motivating) way. Changes in attitudes and intentions are more likely if that source also offers social support, and asks for (and gets) active participation (answer a questionnaire, keep a diary, etc.). Repetition in many ways, involvement, active participation, and social support, all together, also increase the likelihood of persistent changes in attitudes and intentions. . . . The chances of behavior change are maximized only when explicit ways to change are provided [p. 142].

Flay, DiTecco, and Schlegel believe that "the earlier pessimism about the effectiveness of mass media in health promotion should now give way to a cautious optimism and more sophisticated development" (pp. 142–143).

Recent health education programs

Some recent health education efforts will now be reviewed for two reasons. First, as already indicated, the fields of consumer health education and mental health education, just like physical and psychological well-being, are interdependent. Second, since the field of consumer health education is older and better established, it provides examples of approaches to prevention that have methodological and conceptual applicability to the newer field of mental health education.

This review cannot be comprehensive, of course. If you would like to know more about the methods and effectiveness of health education, you might examine *Health Education and Behavioral Science,* by Paul R. Mico and Helen S. Ross (1975); *Promoting Health: Consumer Education and National Policy,* edited by Anne R. Somers (1976); and *Toward an Educated Health Consumer: Mass Communication and Quality in Medical Care,* edited by Carter L. Marshall (1977); as well as recent issues of the *Health Education Quarterly.*

The sharp reduction in cigarette smoking in recent years has already been mentioned. This reduction has come about largely as a consequence of a persistent health education campaign. The vast majority of Americans are now aware of the harmful effects of cigarettes, and many smokers have reduced or stopped smoking or are trying to (see also Tuomilehto, Koskela, Puska, Björkqvist, & Salonen, 1978).

Heart disease prevention.   One of the largest and most important programs undertaken in the United States to reduce the incidence of heart disease is taking place in California (Maccoby & Alexander, 1979; Maccoby & Farquhar, 1975; Maccoby, Farquhar, Wood, & Alexander, 1977; Meyer, Nash, McAlister, Maccoby, & Farquhar, 1980; see also Leventhal, Safer, Cleary, & Gutmann, 1980, for a critical analysis of this project). These scientists successfully used health education instructional and mass-media techniques to help effect behavioral change in the areas of diet, exercise, and smoking.

Maccoby, a specialist in communication research, and Farquhar, a professor of medicine and specialist in the prevention of heart disease, were drawn to the study of the role of health education in the prevention of heart disease because of the very high incidence of the disorder, particularly in Westernized countries. They noted that heart disease in the United States alone causes 180,000 deaths and 550,000 nonfatal illnesses annually and costs an estimated $10 billion a year in medical expenses (Maccoby & Farquhar, 1975). As for the preventability of heart disease, these scientists have noted that

> while the rate of incidence of heart disease differs for inhabitants of different countries, it also changes for the same people migrating to different environments. The Japanese have the lowest rate among the Westernized countries. But this is true only for the Japanese living in Japan. When they migrate to Hawaii, their rate of coronary heart diseases increases; when they move to California, their risk increases further still. In other words, the Japanese have no built-in protection against the disease. When their diet and exercise patterns become more like those of Americans, so does their coronary heart disease rate [Maccoby & Farquhar, 1975, p. 115].

Because of the persuasive research linking faulty diet, lack of exercise, and smoking to increased risk of heart disease, these scientists launched an effort to reduce the prevalence of these risk-producing behavior patterns.

These authors were very aware of the difficulties involved in attempting to change behavior. They were also aware that not all attempts at changing behavior by means of health education have been successful. They concluded from their reviews of the literature that "people who hold erroneous views on such matters as diet, drugs, or smoking would be more likely to be influenced by communications advocating positions not too different from their own" (Maccoby & Farquhar, 1975, p. 116). In addition, they concluded that they wanted to work at the community level—that is, that they should attempt to have a measurable impact on behavior in an entire community of persons at risk of developing heart disease, using mass media alone in their health education program.

Accordingly, the authors located three semirural communities in northern California. They performed an initial survey of random samples of persons aged 35–59, ascertaining the level of information and the nature of attitudes and behaviors with respect to diet, exercise, and smoking. They then conducted physical examinations in specially established clinics. The authors obtained a very high response rate: more than 80% of their randomly drawn samples were both interviewed and examined.

One of the three communities served as a control. Four surveys of all study participants were conducted one year apart in the three communities, including the "no treatment" control community. A media campaign was conducted in the second community over the next three years. In the third community that same media campaign was supplemented by an intensive instructional program for selected members of the group determined to be at high risk of developing heart disease. The media campaign was designed and pretested by professional media experts not only to inform and motivate people but also to stimulate behavior changes that would reduce the risk of heart disease. Because nearly 20% of the population in the three communities was Spanish-speaking, the entire media campaign was bilingual. The health education campaign included TV spot announcements and radio spot announcements and minidramas. Local newspapers carried specially prepared columns dealing with diet and with pertinent health issues. Other printed items were prepared, including a basic information booklet, a cookbook, and a heart health calendar. Additional messages were prepared using billboards and business cards.

The special additional intensive program in the third community was aimed at two-thirds of the highest 25% of the people at risk (as assessed with a number of scales that measure risk of heart disease). The remaining third of the high-risk population served as the control group for this special intensive program. Participants in the special program received instruction in groups of 15 or, if unable to attend group meetings, individually in their homes. Again, the emphasis of this special program was on effecting changes in diet, exercise, and smoking behaviors.

In information, attitudes, and behavior, people changed more in the two towns where the media program took place than in the control town. In addition, people in the high-risk group who received intensive instruction changed more than people who were only exposed to the general mass-media information program.

Risk-reduction effects were found after two years in both communities where the health education program had been inaugurated. The level of risk of coronary heart disease decreased by 17% in those two communities. In contrast, the risk increased more than 6% in the control community. During the first year of the program, changes in behavior were seen most clearly in the community with the two-phase health education program. By the end of the second year, however, significant further decreases in risk had taken place in the community with the mass-media health education program alone. That is, the mass-media program plus intensive instruction had more rapid effects, but similar reductions in risk were achieved through mass media alone after one additional year.

The experimental communities showed significant reductions in smoking, systolic blood pressure, and plasma cholesterol, as well as overall risk of coronary heart disease. Significant reductions in saturated-fat consumption were also found.

Results of the five-year evaluation of a comprehensive Finnish program to reduce the incidence of cardiovascular disease have recently been reported (Klos & Rosenstock, 1982; McAlister, Puska, Salonen, Tuomilehto, & Koskela, 1982; Wagner, 1982). This program, established in 1972, initially attempted to achieve a number of intermediate objectives—improvement in the detection and control of hypertension, reduction in smoking, and promotion of diets lower in saturated fat and higher in vegetables and low-fat products.

The program was comprehensive in that it used six procedures for attaining its objectives: (1) improved preventive services through identification of persons at high risk and provision of medical attention, (2) dissemination of information on health maintenance, (3) efforts to persuade people to change their behavior on the basis of this information, (4) competency building in the area of self-control, environmental management, and social action, (5) social support building and community organizational development to facilitate social action, and (6) environmental change.

The initial effects of the program were studied by contrasting the experimental community with a neighboring county in which the experimental program did not exist. No significant changes in the measured characteristics were found in the control community during the five-year period. In contrast, a number of significant changes were found in the experimental community, including reduced cholesterol level in men and reduced smoking and blood pressure in both men and women. Although the eventual reduction in mortality rate has yet to be shown, the authors believe their health-promotion goals are being met.

Medical care cost and quality.　　The Blue Cross Association (see Somers, 1976, pp. 145–149) has reviewed its experiences with health education, looking at effects on medical costs and quality of care. With regard to cost, its review concludes:

> While not presenting conclusive evidence of reduced *total* costs for care for specific groups, some studies do suggest large cost savings as a result of changes in the pattern of utilization. . . . These findings suggest that certain types of patient education do promote the substitution of self-care and information-seeking for acute care services. On balance, organized patient education has demonstrated

its effectiveness in reducing the unnecessary utilization of certain health care services and in encouraging the use of the most appropriate, least-cost settings for care [Somers, 1976, pp. 146–147].

With regard to quality of care, the report concludes:

> Several studies have demonstrated the beneficial impact of patient education on the *process* of patient care. The use of an interdisciplinary team to provide educationally oriented support to patients with congestive heart failure has resulted in increased knowledge among study patients in one sample regarding diet, medications, disease process, and even more importantly, increased adherence to the treatment regimen. Other research suggests that patient education enhances patient understanding of and compliance with the process of care. With respect to health care *outcomes*, studies have shown the quality-increasing effects of patient education. At the University of Southern California Medical Center . . . the initiation of a multifaceted program of patient education was associated with a reduction of approximately two-thirds in the incidence of diabetic coma from 1968 to 1970. Similarly, in another study, a significantly higher percentage of congestive heart failure patients receiving educational support improved in their ability to function, as measured by the American Heart Association classification. Also, recent work at Massachusetts General Hospital has shown that the provision of intensive preoperative and postoperative information and guidance contributed to reduced pain among surgery patients. These studies point to the potential of patient education in enhancing health status [p. 147].

Recovery from elective pediatric surgery.   In a related study, 80 children scheduled for various types of elective minor surgery were divided randomly into two groups, along with their parents. Wolfer and Visintainer (1975) tested the hypothesis that the group of children and parents who received systematic psychological preparation and continued supportive care would fare better than the group who received normal nursing care. The experimental surgical preparation included information about events, experiences, role expectations, and appropriate responses, as well as previews of procedures by means of play techniques. The hypothesis was consistently supported by significant differences in ratings of upset behavior, cooperation with procedures, pulse rates, resistance to induction of anesthesia, posthospital adjustment, and parental anxiety and satisfaction.

Geriatric medical care.   Health education approaches appear to be particularly appropriate for the elderly. With regard to this group, Lombana has said that "although counseling for remedial purposes can have a vast impact on the life of an individual, the implications of preventive guidance are even more far-reaching. If it were possible to help our citizens more thoughtfully to direct the course of their lives, prepare in advance for retirement, maintain appropriate health habits, develop satisfying avocational interests, and maintain a healthy self-esteem, the despair of millions of Americans could be drastically reduced" (1976, p. 144). Lombana includes in her list of preventive approaches (1) preretirement counseling, (2) lifelong health education, (3) avocational opportunities and leisure activities, (4) programs of information on available services, (5) educational and recreational opportunities, (6) education of the general public, (7) counseling of families of senior citizens, and (8) adequate training and employment of professional and paraprofessional counselors. These approaches all represent the field of health education in action.

A similar position has been taken by Poindexter, who suggests that "it should be clear that the public health efforts toward the elderly should be not merely to prolong a life but to prolong the usefulness of life and reduce the preventable infirmities of old age" (1976, p. 133).

Dalzell-Ward, writing in Great Britain, approaches the definition of health education by contrasting it with other forms of preventive medicine. He writes:

> The classical methods of preventive medicine are universally applicable to all members of a community. A vaccine works in exactly the same way in everyone and is independent of individual vagaries, save in the rare cases of hyper-sensitivity. . . . Environmental control of water and food supplies, atmospheric pollution and the abolition or containment of toxic processes in industry benefit all irrespective of their personal circumstances. Similarly, ante-natal care and the surveillance of the health of small children operates in the same way biologically, although it may be facilitated by social circumstances and personal intelligence. Health education, on the other hand, depends for its effect on the voluntary change of behaviour of individuals. Briefly, personal and group behaviour can influence health and disease in the following ways. (1) Giving up a dangerous behaviour pattern; (2) Adopting a new and positive behaviour pattern; (3) The voluntary use of services of a primary preventive character—like immunization, or of a secondary preventive character—like cervical cytology; (4) Taking decisions about personal health in the light of knowledge and perception of problems [1976, p. 101].[6]

As for the potential of health education, Dalzell-Ward writes:

> We stand on the frontier of a new type of preventive medicine which will be advanced by health education. In the general community, mass communication undoubtedly will be developed and will be increasingly used, but with more refinements of analysis of effectiveness. However, this is only part of the process, and person-to-person health education, either by individual counselling or in groups is one of the gains in the last 25 years which must be consolidated. . . . Much of the future potential will lie in the field of mental health in terms of personality development and suggestions to people as to how they can organize their personal lives, relationships with families and groups, and so control their reactions to challenge to minimize aggression, pathological anxiety, and faulty decision taking [1976, p. 109].

[6]From "The New Frontier of Preventive Medicine," by A. J. Dalzell-Ward. In *Public Health*, 1976, *90*, 101–109. Copyright 1976 by The Society of Community Medicine. Reprinted by permission.

Consumer health education problems and prospects

In spite of the persuasive evidence that health education can improve health status, there are numerous problems in fully implementing a health education program. Marshall describes some of these problems as follows:

> If . . . cervical cancer can be detected through a simple Pap smear, why is it that only 5 percent of women over 20 years of age undergo annual Pap smears, as recommended? If recurrence of rheumatic fever can be prevented, why is it that only 5 percent of those who have had rheumatic fever are under appropriate preventive treatment? If hypertension is susceptible to control, why is it that only half the people with hypertension are even as much as aware of their condition? While behavioral research provides clues to the individual's resistance to appropriate preventive and medical behavior, there are as yet no programs to transform this data into the required positive motivational and educational approaches for the public as a whole or for target audiences at particular risk to specific chronic diseases. Despite continued assertions of the benefits of prevention, the low level of financial support for the health education of the American public suggests its low actual priority in the health care system. Of $83 billion spent for health care in the United States in 1973, according to the President's Committee on Health Education, 92 to 93 percent was spent on medical care for the sick; 4 to 4.5 percent on biomedical research; 2 percent on such public health measures as rodent control; and less than one-half of 1 percent for health education [1977, p. 10].[7]

It should be clear, however, that with proper information and guidance, consumers of health services can do much on their own to improve their health. Furthermore, there is considerable evidence that levels of health among the healthy can be more successfully maintained by becoming better informed about health-related facts of life. Consumer health educators are developing increasing effectiveness in having an impact on the total population as well as on specified subgroups at special risk, and there is reason to be optimistic about the expanding role of consumer health education in the development of healthier communities.

THE PRACTICE OF MENTAL HEALTH EDUCATION

Mental health education programs can be described along three major axes: (1) the target group, (2) the program content, and (3) the techniques used in delivering the program content to the target group. Adelson and Lurie (1972) have observed that mental health educators concentrate their efforts on three main target groups. First of all, there are persons who are themselves at special risk of developing emotional disorders—for example, persons undergoing developmental crises such as school entrance, marriage, beginning parenthood, or retirement; persons undergoing stressful life events; and persons who exist under chronically stressful conditions, such as those who

---

[7]From *Toward an Educated Health Consumer: Mass Communication and Quality in Medical Care*, by C. L. Marshall. U.S. Public Health Service Publication No. (NIH) 77–881. Washington, D.C.: U.S. Government Printing Office, 1977.

are chronically unemployed or ill-housed. Second, there are persons who vary in terms of their degree of power in the community—that is, persons who are in positions of power in the local community and in a position to influence social policy and funding as well as persons who are relatively powerless and who can be helped to develop increased control of their own destinies. Finally, there are persons who have responsibilities to care for others, such as teachers, public health nurses, ministers, and the police.

In some ways, the most difficult aspect of the work of the mental health educator concerns the decisions that must be made about the content of a program, once the target group has been identified. In planning the content, mental health educators must develop a comprehensive and accurate understanding of the target population and also of mental health educational techniques. At the same time, mental health educators need to be aware of their own goals in working with a particular target population. Adelson and Lurie write: "If the goal is that of encouraging the improvement of mental health facilities and services, the content may be statistics on mental illness and the lack of current resources. . . . If the goal is encouraging employers to hire the 'recovered patient,' a meeting may be arranged to demonstrate that former patients are articulate and normal in appearance" (1972, p. 522). Korchin, in discussing mental health education, says that "with a parents' group, the focus is . . . likely to be on matters of child development and their import for later mental health. . . . to be effective, an educator must not only have a broad knowledge of psychopathology, development, intervention methods, social problems, and understanding of the organization and facilities of mental health, but also have the knowledge and skills of communication and group processes, required of a fine teacher or consultant" (1976, p. 538).

Mental health educators use three main techniques: (1) lectures, demonstrations, and films, typically used in group settings; (2) the mass media—newspapers, radio, television; and (3) small face-to-face discussion groups. Mental health educators have long provided mental health information through talks to organized groups. Sometimes commercial movies or television programs are shown, followed by a discussion. Mental health associations and many mental health agencies provide a speakers' bureau and furnish professional mental health staff members as speakers to groups. The National Institute of Mental Health has prepared a comprehensive list of materials such as films and pamphlets that are available for use by mental health educators (U.S. Department of Health, Education and Welfare, 1977a).

Probably the most commonly used vehicle for the provision of mental health education to the public or to important segments of the public is the mass media. Many of the programs reported in this chapter use the mass media. Joslyn-Scherer has recently prepared a volume that describes the field of therapeutic journalism. She writes:

Certainly communication is necessary for every system's maintenance and growth. Journalism is a method of choice when we can use this medium to plan, organize, carefully produce, structure, and distribute at will a variety of messages directed toward the advancement of the individual system, the community system, the network of helpers, and these three systems in interaction. . . . When messages of this type are being used toward the goals of systemic augmentation, restoration, and rehabilitation, we call them *therapeutic* [1980, p. 69].

Small-group discussions can communicate information and can effect both attitude and behavior change. Adelson and Lurie write:

> The increasing emphasis on small groups in mental health education is coordinate with the increasing use of small groups in other settings and with other purposes such as psychotherapy groups. . . . It might be said that with the use of groups there is a movement away from a recipient to a participant model. The mental health educator who recognizes that education is a participative process acts primarily as a facilitator of the group process and secondarily as a resource person with special knowledge [1972, p. 521].

There is considerable evidence that where people participate actively in the educational process, change is likely to take place more rapidly and be longer-lasting.

A number of imaginative mental health information projects have appeared in the past several years that have yet to be evaluated. Among those that seem unusually promising are publications for and about health and mental health service consumers (for example, Marshall, 1977; Mishara & Patterson, 1977); curriculum materials for dealing with particular life stressors such as divorce (for example, Fisher, 1978) or with specific skill-building needs (North Carolina Department of Public Instruction, 1974; Sirbu, Cotler, & Jason, 1978); the printing and distribution to catchment-area restaurants of place mats bearing mental health information in celebration of Mental Health Month (Prairie View Mental Health Center, Newton, Kansas) or information about local mental health services (Tri-City Community Mental Health Center, East Chicago, Indiana); the description of the local mental health and mental retardation program, in a format that resembles the game of Monopoly, that was prepared by the Columbus, Ohio, Mental Health and Mental Retardation Board (see also Morrison & Libow, 1977); and the "Peace Yourself Together" mass-media campaign developed by the Northside Community Mental Health Center in Tampa, Florida (Ehrlich, 1981). Abernathy (1979) has described a mental health information program that is implemented by means of a small, portable computer and display terminal.

The staff mental health educator at Prairie View Mental Health Center assists professional staff members in writing columns that appear frequently in catchment-area newspapers. These columns (all headlined "Let's Talk about It . . . ") begin with a problem statement presented in personal terms—"I think my husband has a drinking problem," "My 7-year-old son is failing in second grade," "I am terribly worried because my husband periodically talks about suicide," "I have an elderly neighbor whom I almost never see"—and then discuss the issue from a variety of points of view (see Dibnor, 1974). A newspaper called *TODAY* . . . *Your Mental Health in Your Community,* prepared by and for mental health professionals, clients, and ex-clients, is published by the Mental Health Association of Erie County, Inc., in Buffalo, New York, and is distributed free of charge throughout the county. Finally, a number of simulation games have been developed for use in health and mental health education (Clark, 1976; Sleet, 1975; Sleet & Stadsklev, 1977).

Recent mental health education programs

The Alternatives Project. The Alternatives Project (Sundel & Schanie, 1978; U.S. Department of Health, Education and Welfare, 1977b), a mental health preventive education and public information program using mass media (both TV and radio), was conducted in Louisville, Kentucky, during a 60-week period in 1973–1974. Its ultimate objective was to reduce both incidence and prevalence of mental disorders. The project staff undertook to assess three intermediate goals: improvement in public attitudes toward personal mental health issues, increased awareness of community mental health resources, and increased use of community mental health resources.

A total of 21 brief messages were aired. Each message was either 30 or 60 seconds long and included the telephone number of the local crisis and information center. Evaluation procedures included examining the pattern of telephone calls to the center and conducting structured telephone interviews with a representative sample of 500 Louisville households before the mass-media program began and with a different sample of 500 households each 20 weeks during the 60-week program.

Here are two examples of the radio spot announcements, followed by two examples of the television spot announcements.

Radio Spot 1. *Questions about sex.*

Sound effects of boys talking and then laughing.

Male Voice: "The story was funny to the rest of the guys . . . but you didn't get it. You're eleven . . . and they're a couple of years older. You thought you knew about sex. Could there be more to it? That might explain those feelings you've had lately. It's scary. And it really needn't be. Your drives . . . your feelings . . . are perfectly normal. Sex is not a dirty word. Get someone you trust to fill you in."

Announcer: "An idea from River Region Services. Helping you build a life you can live with . . . through ALTERNATIVES. 589-4470."

Radio Spot 2. *Same old thing.*

Man: "Get up. Go to work. Come home. Eat. Watch TV. Same old thing all the time. That's living?"

Woman: "It's like being on a treadmill. Do the cooking, do the laundry, do this . . . do that . . ."

Teenage Male: "Exams and classes. The whole thing's a drag. That's all."

Announcer: "If this is your life, change is possible if you will change. An idea from River Region Services. Helping you build a life you can live with . . . through ALTERNATIVES. 589-4313."

TV Spot 1. This message argues that although alcohol and drugs may be used to solve problems, they do not offer a real solution. In fact, alcohol and pills generally fail to solve the basic cause of the pain or difficulty; they are often used as an avoidance mechanism. The spot aims at mobilizing people to deal with their real problems.

TV screen shows montage of pills and alcoholic beverages.

Man's Voice: "So they didn't give me a raise! Who needs that two-bit company? What I need is a drink."

Woman's Voice: "These arguments leave me a nervous wreck . . . fighting over every little thing. Where are my pills?"

Announcer: "Anyone who tells you that drinking or taking pills isn't a solution is a fool. But anyone who tells you that either is the best solution is a bigger fool. How many drinks does it take to get a raise? How many pills does it take to bring back love?"

TV screen shows the ALTERNATIVES slogan and telephone number.

TV Spot 2. A supportive message for older persons who feel their usefulness and effectiveness are gone.
TV screen shows older man walking through the park.

Man's Voice: "Just lately, I've discovered that some people have my life all worked out for me. It's called being a 'senior citizen.' I feel like it means I'm supposed to get out of the way. Not make any waves. I feel like I'm not as good as I used to be."

Announcer: "You might feel that way . . . but you're wrong, because the truth is—you've got more talent, more good ideas, and more experience than a lot of people. And a lot of people could be helped if you shared your knowledge and experience. You're not going to give up now, are you?"

Second Announcer: "An idea from River Region Services. Helping you build a life you can live with."

Findings indicated, first, a significant positive impact of TV messages on the number of adults calling the crisis and information center; second, a significant general increase in knowledge about local community mental health resources; and, third, a significant increase in the ability of interview respondents to make a cognitive assessment of the problem situation presented in the media message. With regard to knowledge of local community mental health resources, better-educated persons were found to have substantially more information than less well educated persons at every interview period. But less well educated persons showed the greatest proportional gain in knowledge during the 60-week program.

Sundel and Scharre concluded that "the results of the project offer a strong endorsement for utilization of mass media in prevention programs (1978, p. 304). They were able, in addition, to develop some persuasive suggestions for making such mental health education programs even more effective in the future.

Prevention of depression.   In a recent study of the effectiveness of a two-week-long television miniseries on behavior and mood, Muñoz, Glish, Soo-Hoo, and Robertson (1982) conducted a telephone survey the week before the series started and the week after it ended, in order to examine its effects on viewers. The series consisted of nine four-minute segments shown three times daily as part of the local news program. Ten segments were prepared, but one segment was preempted by a late-breaking news story. The segments were drawn from a recent volume that dealt with social-learning and self-control approaches to the prevention of depression. Each approach was described and then modeled using videotapes of everyday situations portrayed by students.

Telephone numbers were selected at random from the San Francisco telephone directory, and 162 persons aged 18 or older responded to both the pre- and postprogram interviews. The interviews included a set of behavioral questions, a measure of depression, and the determination of which segments were watched. The behavioral items paralleled the themes of the individual segments—for example, doing something pleasant, rewarding oneself, relaxing, trying to think positive thoughts. A 20-item depressive-mood scale was administered to assess respondents' mood during the past week. In the post-program interview, after the behavioral and mood scales were administered, the respondents were asked whether they remembered watching the segments of the program.

Two of the specific behavioral items increased significantly during the two-week period—telling oneself to stop thinking upsetting thoughts and taking time to relax. One general item also increased significantly—thinking about how to keep oneself from getting depressed. No significant changes in reported mood were found in the sample as a whole. But when the sample was subdivided according to initial level of depression, the sample with higher initial scores who had watched the segments showed a significant reduction in depressed mood when contrasted with those persons with higher initial scores who had not watched the program.

The authors are cautious in their interpretations of the findings, but they do suggest that the miniseries appeared to have a significant immediate effect on both depression-related behavior and mood.

Orientation to psychotherapy.   One well-controlled study examined the consequences of a brief educationally oriented preparation of clients for entry into treatment. Jacobs, Charles, Jacobs, Weinstein, and Mann (1972) oriented some patients and some psychiatric residents and then randomly assigned 120 low-socioeconomic-status psychiatric-clinic patients to one of four conditions: oriented patient to be seen by oriented psychiatric resident; oriented patient to be seen by nonoriented resident; nonoriented patient to be seen by nonoriented resident; and nonoriented patient to be seen by oriented resident. The 15-minute orientation of patients and of residents was undertaken by the chief resident. Psychiatric residents were told about the difficulties lower-class patients might have in exploring their feelings, in accepting the concept of psychological motivation, and in tolerating delay in receiving help. Patients were told about how discussing problems with a psychiatrist was different from discussing problems with a family doctor or surgeon, particularly as regards talking about personal feelings.

Nonoriented patients seen by nonoriented residents were judged to be significantly less likely to profit from insight therapy, were seen significantly more often only for evaluation (without offers for treatment), and reported significantly less improvement than all other groups.

Attitudes toward mental retardation.   Douglas, Westley, and Chaffee (1970) examined the effectiveness of a mass-media program designed to increase acceptance of a planned sheltered workshop for mental retardates. Two small rural communities in Wisconsin were selected. A six-month mental health education program using the mass media was inaugurated in one community; the second community served as a control setting.

The media campaign consisted of 20 news stories, five feature stories, and a Mental Retardation Week advertisement in the local newspaper; posters and a display of articles made by trainable retardates set up in a local barber shop; an uncounted number of news items broadcast over local radio; a well-publicized meeting in a church concerning what the community should do about mental retardation; items in church bulletins; special speakers at three service clubs and a 4-H club; and an announcement of the start of a year-long project on the subject of mental retardation undertaken by the Junior Chamber of Commerce.

Every tenth household in the two communities was chosen to be surveyed, yielding a total of 134 homes in the experimental community and 169 in the control community. For some reason, initial response rates were substantially lower in the control community than in the experimental community. After initial refusals to participate and later loss of some households that had participated initially, a total of 85 residents in the experimental community and 60 in the control community met all requirements of the study.

No significant pre-to-post changes were found in the informational items on the questionnaires, but attitudes toward community-based programs for the mentally retarded became significantly more favorable in the experimental community than in the control community. In addition, the authors found that the program was particularly effective with persons with relatively little education.

Family-life education programs

One of the target groups that have long had the attention of mental health educators is parents. Parents are often unusually receptive to information about parenting and to inaugurating behavior change when such change seems indicated. In addition, social scientists interested in preventive intervention are commonly drawn to working with children and with those persons who play a guiding role in their welfare—that is, their parents. The field of family-life education has emerged from this interest in the education of parents and children (see Goodwin, 1972), and an entire issue of the journal *Family Relations* (October 1981) was recently devoted to the topic of family-life education.

Ulrici, L'Abate, and Wagner (1981) have categorized family skill-training programs for couples and families on the basis of their theoretical orientations, particularly according to whether the emphasis is on building emotional skills, cognitive skills, or behavioral skills. Programs that focus on emotional skills have such goals as developing intrapersonal and interpersonal awareness and increasing interpersonal sensitivity. Programs that focus on cognitive skill building have such goals as learning new facts about family life or learning how the history of the family can influence present family functioning. Programs that focus on behavioral skills have such goals as solving behavioral problems through problem-analysis procedures, teaching effective behaviors and extinguishing inappropriate behaviors, or engaging in practice through some form of behavioral rehearsal, such as role playing or simulation exercises.

Pierre the Pelican. The family-life education program that has been in existence for the longest continuous period is undoubtedly the Pierre the Pelican series, originated in Louisiana in 1946 by the late Loyd W. Rowland. The pelican is the Louisiana state bird and, undoubtedly as a consequence of the French influence in Louisiana, has, since time immemorial, been named Pierre. The pamphlets were designed to be distributed to all parents of first-born children in Louisiana. There are 28 pamphlets in all, distributed one each month during the first year, every other month during the second year, every fourth month during the third and fourth years, and every six months during the fifth and sixth years. Rowland described the pamphlets as "especially designed to cover good principles of child rearing—beyond the area of physical care. . . . The pamphlets . . . are simple, are cast at the sixth grade reading level, are illustrated by sketches, have the continuity made possible by the character Pierre, comprise a series, make use of questions, are of optimal length, and make an effort to cover topics of principal interest to young parents" (quoted in Greenberg, Harris, MacKinnon, & Chipman, 1953, p. 1147).

Perhaps the best way to describe the early days of this pamphlet series is to use Rowland's words:

> I left a good professorship in psychology to work in programs of child development, and have had a very exciting experience in doing so. It was hard to get started, but the now defunct Woman's Foundation of New York in 1946 gave us

$5,000 to develop the first 12 pamphlets of the Pierre the Pelican program and send the materials to all parents of first-born children in Louisiana the first year of the operation. It was strictly a one-string affair, I can tell you. I used to write the material during the week, go down on Saturday and Sunday to my office and cut the stencils and run them off and mail the chapters to the critic readers, one at a time. When we had heard from them and read their suggestions we raced to the printer. We were always just one jump ahead of the deadline in the distribution of the materials. By October of 1947 we had finished the twelve pamphlets and were broke. We asked the Mental Health Authority of Louisiana to take over the program, and by that time there was enough interest that this was accomplished with ease [Rowland, 1975].

The titles of some of the 12 pamphlets distributed to new parents during the first year illustrate the topics covered in the series: "Is 'Bright Eyes' Watching You?," "Talking Starts by Listening," "Sitting Up Is Wonderful to Do," "Let's Think about Discipline," and "Even a Baby Needs Friends His Own Age."

An early evaluation of the Pierre the Pelican series was undertaken by Greenberg et al. (1953), who examined the effect of the pamphlets on the feeding behavior of parents. No such effect was found, but the authors acknowledged that the effectiveness of the pamphlets should not be judged solely on the basis of changes in feeding practices. In the concluding section of that evaluation study, Greenberg and his colleagues did indicate that Pierre was favorably received by parents. They wrote: "After the first three months of distribution, self-addressed return post cards were mailed to recipients. . . . 50.7 per cent were returned, and every answer was in favor of continuing the series. Of those returning the cards, about 90 per cent answered that they were saving the pamphlets, and without being asked, 82 per cent volunteered . . . that they had found Pierre helpful" (p. 1155).

Rowland has described that and other evaluation studies:

Twelve graduate students at the Tulane School of Social Work undertook to interview mothers (and fathers when they could) who had received the program. And as a control group, those parents whose children were born the month before the program started. . . . They got positive results, showing the program to be effective. . . . Then about the following year, Dr. Greenberg and his group made a study, and he was not able to find any measurable results from the program in terms of its effects on the eating habits of children—that was the only criterion reported on in his paper. . . . I knew he was going to read the paper before the Maternal and Child Health section of the American Public Health Association, and so was present when he read it. I invited him to lunch after he had finished the paper and he said, as accurately as I can quote him, "I'm sorry the results came out that way because my wife and I found the series very helpful in rearing our son." I laughed and told him I would quote that remark many times.

Next came a study by the Department of Mental Health of Michigan. . . . The conclusions of most interest to us were the ones numbered 1 and 4. "(1) There are significant differences in the child rearing knowledge expressed by parents who have used the Pierre letters and those who have not and this difference is in favor of the letter readers." and "(4) The Pierre and control parents were compared in relation to their answers to the concept questions (i.e., questions involving understanding of child rearing practices, but not dependent on economic or other environmental situations). The Pierre group was significantly better informed than the controls on these items. This result is the most striking evidence that the Pierre letters are an effective means of educating parents."

In spite of the good two-out-of-three record, I have come to relax confidence in evaluation studies of mental health education programs that rely upon statistical methods. Much better it is to adopt the supermarket approach worked out by the girls in my office when I was Director of the Louisiana Association of Mental Health. On their coffee break they would go across the street to the big supermarket, sidle up to a young mother who had a child about four years old, and find an excuse to talk—first ask the age of the child, and next, "Did you receive the Pierre the Pelican program?" Then watch for the big smile that would come onto their faces and hear their expressions of how helpful the program had been. Then they would want to talk and tell all about it . . . so much so that we had to set a limit to the coffee breaks! [Rowland, 1975].

Parent discussion groups.   One of the earliest efforts to conduct and evaluate a mental health education program with parents using the discussion-group method was reported by Hereford (1963), who was interested in helping parents become more effective. Hereford wrote:

Very few parents actually attend courses on parenthood offered in a regular educational program. Various organizations reach many parents through programs on parent-child relations, frequently consisting of a lecture by an expert, or a panel discussion, or perhaps a film, but these are usually sporadic attempts, with no continuity intended. . . . Unlike some other areas of education, that of parent-child relations is concerned primarily not with knowledge, information, and facts, but with concepts, ideas, and attitudes. Since the ultimate goal in any attempt at educating parents in the parental role is to change the parent's behavior in his relations with his child, merely providing the parent with factual information and knowledge is not enough [1963, pp. 4–5].[8]

The mental health education program that Hereford directed was conducted over a four-year period in Austin, Texas, and was designed to (1) develop and establish a way of helping parents with their parent/child relations and (2) evaluate the method in terms of the resulting attitudinal and behavioral changes.

Hereford looked for a method that would allow active parental participation and would be feasible, economical, acceptable, and testable. He selected the discussion-group method because it met all these criteria. According to Hereford, the discussion-group method would result in working with parents who not only would be active participants but also would be personally involved

[8]From *Changing Parental Attitude through Group Discussion,* by Carl F. Hereford. Copyright © 1963 by the Hogg Foundation for Mental Health. This and all other quotations from the same source are reprinted by permission.

in the process. To assure maximum involvement and participation by parents, Hereford selected group leaders who were not mental health professionals. In this way he hoped to place the responsibility for the success of the program on the shoulders of the participants rather than the leader. Hereford trained a total of 104 such group leaders and employed 22 of them in the study. The remaining leaders found employment elsewhere in the community.

The program consisted of six weekly two-hour meetings. Films on various aspects of parent/child relationships were frequently shown at the start of a meeting and stimulated the discussion that followed. Participating parents decided on the content of each meeting and on how that content was to be presented. No agenda was developed in advance, and no textbook was used.

Initial assessment of program participants took place during the week before the start of the program; final assessments, four to six weeks after the program ended. Seven such cycles (each lasting about three months) took place during the four years of the study. The effects of the program were evaluated by contrasting program participants with three other groups of parents: (1) parents who attended at least one of a series of lectures by professionals in the field of parent/child relationships, (2) parents who registered for a discussion group or a lecture series but did not attend; and (3) parents who did not register for or attend either the discussion group or the lecture series. Assessment consisted of parent attitude surveys, parent interviews, teacher ratings, and sociometric evaluation of the children.

Five parental attitudes were assessed: (1) confidence in parental role, (2) attitudes toward causation of child's behavior, (3) acceptance of child's behavior and feelings, (4) parent/child interaction and mutual understanding, and (5) mutual trust. Two areas of child behavior were assessed: (1) relationships with classmates and (2) classroom adjustment. Hereford hoped to show that parents who attended the discussion-group sessions would show positive changes in their attitudes and behavior; that children, though not directly involved in the program, would show positive changes in their behavior; that participants in the discussion-group program would show more change than members of each of the other experimental groups; and that the amount of change would be related to the degree of participation in the program.

A total of 903 persons in 775 families participated in all phases of the study. About 40% were in the experimental discussion-group program, 11% in the lecture-series control group, 18% in the nonattendant control group, and 30% in the random control group.

Hereford has provided a short summary of the program results:

1. Parents who attended the discussion-group series *did* show positive changes in their attitudes as measured by the Parent-Attitude Survey. These changes were significantly greater than those of parents in the three control groups. 2. Parents who attended the discussion groups also changed their attitudes and behavior as shown by responses to the Parent Interview, again significantly more than parents in the control groups. 3. Children of parents who attended the discussion meet-

improved in their classmate relations significantly more than did the children of parents in the control groups, but not in their ratings by teachers, even though none of the children participated in the program. The observed changes in the attitudes and behavior of discussion-group parents were apparently strong and pervasive enough to influence the social acceptance of their children by classmates. 4. The number of discussion meetings attended, the amount of verbal participation in the discussion, and the frequency of personal references generally proved to be unrelated to the quantity of attitudinal and behavioral change in the parents. Nor did the individual nonprofessional leader prove to be a factor of any importance, giving rise to the conclusion that the discussion group method *per se*, not the leader, is the crucial element involved [1963, pp. 136–137].

Hereford's final conclusion is worth quoting: "Group discussions led by a nonprofessional leader . . . proved to be a powerful method for changing attitudes and behavior in the area of parent-child relations. The low cost of this method, its ready acceptance by participants, and its flexibility make its use as limitless as the ingenuity of the organizer of educational programs" (p. 143).

Perhaps the best-known approach to family-life education is Thomas Gordon's Parent Effectiveness Training. Gordon (1977) has described the origin of that program in the early 1960s as his response to two beliefs—first, that building the profession of psychology on the foundation of the medical model was doomed to failure and, second, that the task of the psychologist was to give knowledge to the public. These two beliefs stressed prevention and education rather than therapy. Gordon wrote:

> In working with children and youth, I gradually began to comprehend that these young people were not "sick," nor did they need psychotherapy. Quite the contrary, when I got to know them well, most of them struck me as remarkably healthy and often creatively resourceful in their attempts at coping with the destructive and repressive behaviors of their parents and teachers. . . . The parents who brought their "problem children" to me, always with high hopes that I would bring about radical changes in their behavior, were not "sick" either. . . . Instead, most of them were trying hard to be effective parents. They were concerned, conscientious, and eager to raise responsible kids. Usually, they were worried about the youngster or disappointed in the way he was turning out, but they could not be accused of child neglect, nor of failure to discipline their children. Most were doing what they thought best for the child, usually being the kind of parents their own parents were with them [1977, p. 176].

Drawing on his experience in developing and teaching human-relations training programs for executives, Gordon designed an educational program for parents that had the following characteristics: (1) It was easily portable geographically and easily taught to a variety of professionals. (2) It was brief, requiring one three-hour session a week for eight weeks. (3) It was completely divorced from the medical model and the language of treatment. Rather, its metaphor came from the field of education, and it used such terms as *course*, *instructor, students, textbook, assignments,* and *tuition.* (4) It was far less expensive than therapy, averaging around $2 per instructional hour. (5) It attracted fathers as well as mothers, mainly by being scheduled at night. (6) It was geographically accessible to parents by being scheduled in churches, homes, and neighborhood conference centers. (7) It was self-supporting. There are now over 7500 trained instructors nationwide.

The orientation of Parent Effectiveness Training can be seen in the skills that parents develop in the program. Gordon mentions the ability to (1) talk about their children in terms of behaviors rather than in terms of personality characteristics—"Kathy left her clothes in the living room" rather than "Kathy is sloppy and inconsiderate," (2) respond consistently and with honesty to their children's behavior, (3) communicate with their children in ways that facilitate bilateral understanding, (4) confront children whose behavior is unacceptable to them by sending statements about their own feelings rather than blaming, preaching, warning, and so on—"I am too tired to play with you," not "You are being a pest," (5) learn the destructive effects that punishment and power can have on both children and the parent/child relationship, (6) understand the pitfalls of excessive permissiveness or excessive authoritarianism and the advantages of a problem-solving strategy in which both parent and child win, and (7) resolve differences between parents' and children's values without damaging the relationship.

Follow-up interviews with parents who have completed the program reveal numerous reported changes in behavior. Controlled studies have shown that parents who went through the program, contrasted with parents who did not, show greater confidence in themselves as parents, greater mutual understanding and trust between parent and child, better understanding of children, less inclination to use authority, improvements in parents' self-concepts, more distaste for punitive and rigid discipline, more willingness to listen to the child's problems and complaints and to accept the child's right to hold different views from the parents', and more democratic attitudes toward the family. In addition, some studies show that children improve their school performance and their self-esteem.

Sirbu et al. (1978) examined the utility and effectiveness of group parent training. Sixty mothers of preschool children participated in the study. The mothers were randomly assigned to four groups. Mothers in Group 1 were given a course of five weekly two-hour sessions based on a commonly used programmed textbook on child management. Mothers in Group 2 were given the same course but without access to the textbook. Mothers in Group 3 were given the textbook to read but did not meet in groups. Mothers in Group 4 did not use any materials and did not have a professional group leader. Rather, they met for five weekly two-hour sessions and informally discussed any problems they were having with their children.

The effectiveness of the mental health education programs was assessed by a questionnaire that tapped knowledge of child behavioral principles, a measure of the amount of stress and the amount of satisfaction parents were deriving from their children, and two measures of sensitivity to children that assessed how mothers would likely behave in a variety of situations with their children.

There were no significant differences in effectiveness among the three techniques used in the educational program, but on three of the outcome measures, mothers in Group 4 (the no-treatment control group) did significantly worse than all others. The authors concluded that "it is the clear and systematic presentation of behavior modification principles that is more important than the format (written, lecture, or both) in which the principles are presented" (Sirbu et al., 1978, p. 168). Mothers in all three training groups showed significant increases in knowledge of behavior principles and significantly reduced emotional reactions to children's behaviors. The authors summarize their conclusions by noting that "to the extent that parent training is preventive of child behavior problems . . . packaged programs similar to the one used in this project may be adequate. Just as parents are encouraged to participate in prenatal classes with each pregnancy, they could also be offered a prevention-oriented class in child management" (pp. 168–169).

Spoon and Southwick (1972) have described their family-life education program, developed as a service of the North Central Kansas Guidance Center in Manhattan, Kansas. The major goal of their program was the "promotion of mental health—defined as the ability to meet the demands of daily living on the basis of acceptance of self, and understanding and skill in interpersonal relations—in mentally healthy families" (1972, p. 279). Spoon and Southwick described the specific objectives of their program as follows: "(1) To promote mental health through increasing understanding of family life and modifying attitudes toward family life . . . (2) To provide a service appropriate to all persons who are supporting the sponsoring agency through taxes . . . and (3) To serve as a screening agent and referral service to the sponsoring agency's treatment staff" (pp. 279–280). Thus, this program served both a mental health education and a casefinding function.

Family-life education groups were established through the sponsorship of cooperating agencies—churches, clubs, nursery schools, school counseling programs, social service programs, and so on. Each program consisted of eight two-hour meetings held at a convenient time and place, with topics to be discussed selected by the participants. Topics most commonly chosen included discipline, parent/teenager relationships, and husband/wife communication. Although the family-life educator could make initial statements on these topics, much of the meeting time involved group discussion and the sharing of ideas.

The group leader helped in the initial establishment of rapport among group members, served as a discussion leader and resource to the group, and facilitated discussion so that anxiety was kept at an optimal level and important ideas and feelings were recognized. The aim of the discussion group was education, not therapy. The focus was as much on group process as on content. Attention was given to feelings just as much as to ideas. Emphasis was placed on ways group members were similar, rather than ways they were different.

During the first year of this program, 15 groups were conducted. About 200 people attended at least one session, and about half attended all the sessions of their group. Most of the dropping out occurred after the first session. An evaluation questionnaire was administered before and after the program. Participants not only rated the discussion-group experience very favorably but also reported changes in their behavior with their children and spouses. They indicated that they had gained "a greater objectivity about their lives along with the necessary flexibility, motivation, and openness to try to improve themselves" (p. 284).

Reducing child-abuse potential.   Thomasson, Berkovitz, Minor, Cassle, McCord, and Milner (1981) developed a 16-session family-life education program for poor rural parents who appeared to be at high risk for child abuse. Of the initial group of 79 participants, 49 attended 10 or more sessions. An inventory that had been shown to identify attitudes commonly associated with the potential for child abuse was administered at the first session, at the last session, and seven weeks later at a follow-up evaluation session.

The program was designed with the primary goal of preventing child abuse and secondarily to improve parenting skills. The goals were to offer information about child development and parenting, to provide a vehicle for parents to share their problems and concerns with one another, and to orient parents to community resources. Child care was available during the program, and a monetary stipend was provided for attendance. The 16 sessions generally alternated between large-group meetings with speakers and films and small discussion groups.

Results of this program appeared quite positive. Initial scores on the child-abuse-potential scale were significantly higher in this group than in the normative sample on which the scale had been developed. Scores decreased significantly from pretest to posttest. Interestingly, initial scores were significantly higher among persons who did not complete the program than among those who did. Scores at the seven-week follow-up evaluation were not significantly different than at the end of the program.

Scores on the child-abuse-potential scale decreased most in the group of parents with moderately elevated initial scores. Scores decreased far less among parents with the highest initial levels of child-abuse potential. Thus, it appears that the program was less successful with parents with the greatest potential risk for child abuse than with parents whose risk was high but not extreme.

Frank and Rowe (1981) have described their efforts to reduce the risk of child abuse or psychiatric disturbance in children by conducting weekly two-hour educational meetings with small groups of mothers and their children under age 4. Although some mothers were self-referred, most were referred by medical or social-work personnel because "a particular mother-child pair is considered 'at risk' to develop problems in their relationship" (p. 170). The educational program was designed to teach mothers about infant and child development and to discuss infant and child behavior as it related to developmental theory. The authors believe that when mothers increase their understanding of child development, they will have more appropriate expectations of their children's behavior and will be able to respond more usefully to their children's needs.

Evaluations thus far have been limited to self-reports by mothers, but these reports appear to be favorable and seem to stress the exact objectives that the authors have for the program—that is, that it is easier to be an effective mother as one understands more about why a child is behaving as he or she is.

Home-based mental health education. One of the challenges facing health educators interested in providing family-life education is how to make most efficient contact with their target population. This problem is particularly important for young families—people aged 19 to 34—who make up about 30% of the American population. An analysis of such families reveals that they are frequently not oriented toward group education but rather toward home-based education. Young families make most of their decisions at home in privacy, and they are influenced in these decisions by magazines, newsletters, or pamphlets they receive at home.

On the basis of these conclusions from previous research, Hennon and Peterson (1981), two Wisconsin specialists in family resources and consumer sciences, developed a series of ten single-theme learn-at-home packets, dealing with such topics as choosing parenthood, family management, consumer decision making, credit, and family nutrition. These packets were made available to university-extension-program faculty members in all Wisconsin counties, and an in-depth study of the effectiveness of this approach to family-life education was undertaken with a sample of 82 young families in nine Wisconsin counties. These families agreed to read the packets and participate in a telephone interview to help evaluate their quality and usefulness.

The interviews were conducted six months after the packets had been distributed. Fifty-nine families reported having read all ten packets. In general, families found the packets informative and useful. The packets filled some immediate needs and were judged to be practical, helpful, clear, and interesting. The authors also found that the packets that dealt with a particular need that the family had at a given time were evaluated most favorably. Virtually all families liked the idea of having the learn-at-home packets. Younger families living in rural areas found the packets most useful. About two-thirds of the families reported having used at least one of the ideas in the packets in the six months since they had received them.

Hennon and Peterson conclude that young families can be reached by learn-at-home packets and that their delivery system was effective and efficient regardless of the educational level, place of residence, or employment status of the adults in the families they reached.

Parents of problem children.   Gordon, Lerner, and Keefe (1979) developed a program for parents of problem children, oriented toward helping parents modify their children's problematic behavior by teaching parents techniques for behavior analysis and change. Twelve families were involved in the two groups that were described and evaluated in this study. Each family carried out a home project involving "observation of the problematic behavior, daily record keeping, and systematic intervention" (p. 48). One unusual aspect of this program was that the group leaders asked each family to make a cash deposit that could be earned back by attendance and completion of weekly assignments during the 8–10 weeks that the groups met.

One couple, for example, chose to develop a home project designed to decrease noncompliance with parental requests in their 9-year-old son. They collected data on noncompliance for an 18-day period and then began to use a system of praise for compliance along with additional reinforcement by means of family social activities. A substantial reduction in noncompliance was found.

Attendance was very high throughout the group sessions, and parents reported a high level of satisfaction. Significant reductions in maladaptive behavior were reported in the children, particularly regarding tense disposition, aggression, and conduct problems. The authors indicated that their program was educational in its focus and that because it emphasized learning a set of skills, participation seemed to diminish "the sense of guilt, shame, frustration, and hopelessness that most parents seeking professional help experience" (p. 54).

In another study dealing with problem children, Johnson and Breckenridge (1982) developed a two-year parent/child education program for 1–3-year-old children and their parents. The program took place in Houston, Texas, and was designed for low-income Mexican-American families. During the first year of the program, project staff made home visits and organized several weekend sessions for entire families. English classes, medical examinations of the children, and assistance in gaining access to other community agencies were also provided. During the second year, mothers and children participated in program activities four mornings each week. In addition, there were evening programs that involved the fathers. The entire program required about 500 hours of participant time. A total of 64 children were involved in the experimental program; another 64 served as no-treatment controls.

Because young boys typically have more behavior problems than young girls, in evaluating the effectiveness of this intensive program the authors chose to analyze their results separately by sex of the child. Over the next four years, the authors found that the program appeared to have its greatest impact on boys. Boys in the experimental group had significantly fewer behavior problems than boys in the control group: control boys were more destructive and overactive, were less emotionally sensitive, and engaged in more attention seeking. Girls in the control and experimental groups did not differ.

Social competency and social-skill building

Perhaps the most exciting single aspect of mental health education has been the growing effort over the past decade to improve mental health by increasing social competency and social skills (see, for example, Eisler & Frederiksen, 1980). This movement has emerged out of a body of research and an ideological position. The body of research focuses on the wish for competence as a motivating force. Interest in competence as a legitimate area of research dates from the work of White (1959), who suggested that "something important is left out when we make drives the operating forces in animal and human behavior" (p. 297). White felt that many kinds of behavior could not be successfully conceptualized simply in terms of primary drives:

> This behavior includes visual exploration, grasping, crawling and walking, attention and perception, language and thinking, exploring novel objects and places, manipulating the surroundings, and producing effective changes in the environment. The thesis is then proposed that all of these behaviors have a common biological significance: they all form part of the process whereby the animal or child learns to interact effectively with his environment. The word *competence* is chosen as suitable to indicate this common property. Further, it is maintained that competence cannot be fully acquired simply through behavior instigated by drives. It receives substantial contributions from activities which, though playful and exploratory in character, at the same time show direction, selectivity, and persistence in interacting with the environment. Such activities in the ultimate service of competence must therefore be conceived to be motivated in their own right. It is proposed to designate this motivation by the term *effectance*, and to characterize the experience produced as a *feeling of efficacy* [1959, p. 329].

White's ideas have recently been elaborated by Bandura (1977), and the literature that has been developing in the past two or three decades on how to assess personal competence was recently reviewed by Sundberg, Snowden, and Reynolds (1978). Some authors (Iscoe, 1974; Ryan, 1967) contend that competence, power, and self-esteem are inextricably linked. A. N. Schwartz has made a similar point in discussing quality of life for the aged. His response to the question of the essential ingredient in successful aging is unequivocal: "Without hesitation I would answer that the essential ingredient is positive self-regard, the maintenance of self-esteem. Without that gold, all else is dross. What is at stake for the aged is self-esteem which, I submit, is the linchpin that holds everything else in its appropriate place" (1975, p. 470).

Similarly, in reviewing her 15-year research program to identify the effects of various patterns of parental authority on the development of children's and adolescents' ability to master their environment, Baumrind said: "I have made the assumption that the qualities basic to instrumental competence are and will continue to be of benefit to the individual and the society. I believe that the abilities both to accommodate to social mores and laws and to take self-assertive and autonomous action in opposition to those mores and laws when their legitimacy cannot be defended are essential to healthful, successful functioning . . . in any society" (1975, p. 13).

Social-competency building in children. At least two recent major projects have shown that it is possible to increase self-esteem in young children by enhancing their social or interpersonal problem-solving skills. Spivack and Shure (1973; Shure, 1979; Shure & Spivack, 1982) worked with 4- and 5-year-old day-care and kindergarten participants to improve the children's interpersonal problem-solving skills, including the ability to understand causal factors in interpersonal problems, the ability to see alternative solutions to typical problems, and the ability to evaluate the likely consequences of these alternative solutions. Spivack and Shure contend that the quality of social adjustment is determined largely by these cognitive skills, and they have developed procedures for assessing them, for increasing them, and for training teachers and mothers how to improve them. They have found that these skills are easily taught, that teachers and mothers make equally good training agents, that the training effects last at least two years after training, and that when these social skills are enhanced, social adjustment improves.

Allen, Chinsky, Larcen, Lochman, and Selinger (1976) worked with third- and fourth-grade children in a comprehensive program in problem solving that included training in social-problem solving. Using the same rationale as Spivack and Shure, these authors trained teachers to improve children's problem-solving behaviors by improving problem formulation, the search for alternative solutions, the identification of obstacles to these solutions, and the assessment of consequences. Children receiving the training scored significantly higher than control children on a problem-solving measure and generated significantly more alternative solutions. Furthermore, the experimental group showed a significant increase in scores on a measure of internal locus of control, assessing the extent to which people believe they have the ability within themselves to control their own destiny rather than depending on powerful others, fate, or providence.

Competency building in adults. Although much of the work in competency building deals with children, there is some research examining the consequences of increased competency in adults. One such study, reported by Gatz, Barbarin, Tyler, Mitchell, Moran, Wirzbicki, Crawford, and Engelman (1982), dealt with efforts to enhance individual and community competence in adult community workers and in the community residents with whom they worked. A total of 22 community workers, all aged 50 or above and 97 comparably aged community residents participated in this study; another sample of 30 community residents served as a posttest control. The project was carried out in two suburban mental health catchment areas. Community workers were trained in a two-day workshop and then for the next two years worked part-time in project activities and attended weekly meetings to review cases, share information and support, and improve their skills.

The goal of the program was to increase adaptive strengths of both workers and residents, particularly the sense of self-efficacy, trust, and hope, and problem-solving skills in dealing with day-to-day issues that might arise in this group of older adults. Pre-to-post changes included increased knowledge of community services, increased number of community information channels, and increased life satisfaction. Residents developed a stronger internal locus of control, which was judged to be associated with their increased knowledge of available community services and agencies.

A related line of research is the one linking interpersonal competence and the availability of social support systems to the incidence of infectious and chronic disease—a body of research recently reviewed by Cassel (1973). Cassel showed that the most common infectious diseases are not caused by virulent microorganisms acquired through exposure to sources of infection outside the body but rather by the activities of microorganisms that are constantly in the environment and in the body, generally doing no harm unless the person is under stress (see also Dubos, 1965, pp. 164–165).

After reviewing a number of studies attempting to identify these stresses, Cassel concluded, first, that "in human populations, increased susceptibility to disease should occur when . . . individuals do not receive any evidence (feedback) that their actions are leading to desirable and anticipated consequences" (1973, p. 543). Cassel's review of the research suggested that this situation is likely when people find themselves in an unfamiliar environment. This may happen to migrants or to persons caught up in rapid social change or to persons living in an area undergoing considerable social disorganization. A second general conclusion was that susceptibility to disease is greater in persons who are subordinate than in those who are dominant in a society. Third, Cassel suggested as a general finding that susceptibility to disease is far lower in persons who have strong group social supports than in persons who are deprived of meaningful social contacts.

Cassel's conclusion was that a high level of disease in general might be expected under conditions of social change and social disorganization and that "preventive action in the future should focus more directly on attempts at modifying these psychosocial factors, on improving and strengthening social supports, and reducing the circumstances which produce ambiguities between actions and their consequences" (p. 547).

Another group of findings linking competence to adjustment and health is emerging from the study of a phenomenon called *learned helplessness* (Abramson, Seligman, & Teasdale, 1978; Depue & Monroe, 1978; Maier & Seligman, 1976). This research, like that reviewed by Cassel, includes studies of a variety of species, including human beings. The original learned-help-lessness research showed that animals exposed to inescapable and unavoid-able electrical shocks in one situation later failed to learn to escape shock in a situation in which escape was possible. Exposure to uncontrollable events appears to interfere with an animal's ability to see a causal relationship between its behavior and subsequent events. Exposure to uncontrollable aversive events appears to reduce the subsequent motivation to try to escape these events and seems to produce significant emotional disruption. In general, helplessness appears to be surprisingly easily learned by animals, including human beings, and its consequences are measurable in the animal's intellectual, motivational, and emotional life.

The concept of learned helplessness has been invoked as a means of understanding reactive depression (viewed as the consequence of experienc-ing an aversive event over which one had no control), number of children (greater when parents have learned helplessness), internal versus external locus of control (learned helplessness leads to a sense of external control), infant development (more rapid and healthier when the infant has control of the environment), and urban stress (lack of control of stresses such as noise leads to fatalism).

The converse of learned helplessness is learned competence, and as I have shown, learned helplessness can be successfully "treated" and replaced by a sense of mastery and competence. Sue and Zane (1980) have examined the links between learned helplessness and community psychology. They believe that "the application of helplessness theory has utility in viewing community phenomena" (p. 137). Specifically, they argue that, first, laboratory studies consistently demonstrate the importance of having control or a sense of control over one's life; second, where persons in a community lack control, psycho-logical well-being and the psychological sense of community may be dimin-ished; and, third, the theory of learned helplessness provides both a means for conceptualizing certain community processes and directions for intervention.

Social-skills training.   A number of studies of the efficacy of social-skills training have appeared in the past several years. Argyle, Bryant, and Trower (1974; see also Argyle, Trower, & Bryant, 1974) compared brief psychotherapy and social-skills training in a group of 16 psychiatric patients whose symptoms included complaints in interpersonal situations. Social-skills training tended to maintain its effectiveness longer than the brief therapy even though therapy patients had twice as many treatment hours as patients in the social-skills training group. Stone, Hinds, and Schmidt (1975) taught elementary-school children strategies for dealing with problems typical in their age group. Con-trasted with a matched group of children who had not received the three-day training, trained children were generally superior in all measures of problem solving. Levenson and Gottman (1978) developed a measure of social com-petence in the areas of dating and assertiveness and found that three different eight-week training programs for samples of college students with either one of these two problems resulted in significant improvement in both areas of interpersonal skill.

Walton and Russell (1978) developed a ten-day mental health teaching unit, focusing on affective education, to be used with high school health education classes, and evaluated its effectiveness with a sample of 248 students in four high schools in west-central Florida. They were interested in whether participants in the learning experience would show less alienation and more positive self-concepts and whether the psychological climate of the classroom would be perceived as positive. Two sets of materials were used—one consisting of commercially available filmstrips and the other consisting of a sight-and-sound show assembled by the authors.

Representative concepts that were presented and discussed during these ten class periods included the following:

- *Awareness.* "Knowing and consciously realizing what one is seeing, hearing, and feeling . . . tends to increase [one's] ability to perceive self as a worthy person in a complex, changing environment of people, places, things and events" (p. 663).
- *Love and Nature.* "To function competently as a human being, one needs to be able to work, to play, and to love. . . . When experiences have included a loving, accepting and understanding relationship with other people, chances of becoming an accepting, understanding and loving person are enhanced" (p. 663).
- *Between Two Worlds.* "Individuals have deep feelings of personal needs and wants. Early in life, these needs are met rather fully and quickly. But as one grows, personal needs and wants often differ from the needs and wants expected by others. At such times, individuals are caught between two worlds—normal conflicts in decision-making situations between one's inner world and one's outer social world" (pp. 663–664).

Measures of effectiveness were collected during the last class period. Significant decreases in alienation and increases in self-concept were found regardless of which set of materials was used. In addition, participants showed a reduction in dogmatic, inflexible classroom behavior and less tendency to feel they could not accomplish what was asked of them.

Elias (1979) examined the effectiveness of a videotaped ten-session training program to improve the socially related problem-solving skills of preadolescent and adolescent emotionally and academically handicapped boys. Two months after the program ended, 52 boys who had participated were found to have significant decreases in overall personality problems, emotional detachment, inability to delay gratification, and social isolation, as well as greater gains in self-reliant learning behaviors, compared with a control group of 57 boys from the same institution.

Lindsay, Symons, and Sweet (1979) instituted a training program for socially inept adolescents, emphasizing such competencies as initiating conversations, joining conversational groups, assertiveness, dealing with authority figures, interviewing skills, and heterosexual interaction. The program involved 33 adolescents and included free-play sessions, explanations of verbal and non-verbal social skills, role playing, group discussions, and review sessions. Evaluation indicated that the program produced improvements in rated social skill, self-reports of social behavior, and social aspects of personality. In addition, the adolescents themselves regarded the program as both practical and supportive.

Hartman (1979a), working with asymptomatic high school students, found that social-skill training was both economical and effective in dealing with behavior problems that constituted advance signs of maladjustment. The effectiveness of the eight-hour training program was maintained at a three-month follow-up assessment. Kirschenbaum, DeVoge, Marsh, and Steffen (1980) evaluated their multifaceted Social Skills Development Program, inaugurated in seven elementary schools in Cincinnati to help children who were exhibiting such behaviors as acting out, moodiness, general immaturity, and academic difficulty, and found their program to be generally effective on a number of dimensions.

Haynes and Avery (1979) found that a 16-hour training program, incorporated into a junior-level English class, increased self-disclosure and empathy skills in high school students. Monti, Curran, Corriveau, DeLancey, and Hagerman (1980) contrasted the effectiveness of social-skill training and sensitivity training in two groups of 23 psychiatric inpatients or day hospital patients in a Veterans Administration medical center. Each training program took 20 hours and was administered in 1-hour units four days per week for five consecutive weeks. Immediately after the program, the social-skills group showed significantly greater improvement in social skills and decreases in social anxiety, both on self-report measures and on a simulated social-interaction test, than the sensitivity training group. These differences were maintained at a six-month follow-up assessment. Monti et al. concluded that their results "very strongly support the efficacy of doing social skills training with psychiatric patients in a day hospital setting" (1980, p. 247).

S. D. Brown (1980) contrasted the results of a 30-hour psychoeducational program in coping skills and an equally long group counseling program in a sample of 40 clients in a community mental health center. The clients in the coping-skills program showed significant improvements in general anxiety, fear, and assertiveness in comparison with the counseling group, both immediately after the program and at a three-month follow-up assessment. In addition, significantly fewer psychoeducational-program clients were hospitalized within one year after participation in the program than clients in the counseling group.

Other reports of social-skill training have been published by Farris and Avery (1980), working with married couples, Filipczak, Archer, and Friedman (1980), with disruptive adolescents; Miller, Wilson, and Dumas (1979), with schizophrenics in remission; Wells, Hersen, Bellack, and Himmelhoch (1979), with unipolar nonpsychotic depressives; and Zilbergeld and Ellison (1979), regarding the use of social-skill training as an adjunct to sex therapy.

A number of reviews evaluating published studies of the effectiveness of social-skill training with a variety of special groups have recently appeared. As is often true of such critiques, they tend to be less favorable than individual studies, some of which may not be sufficiently rigorous in their design or analysis. For example, Wallace, Nelson, Liberman, Aitchison, Lukoff, Elder, and Ferris (1980), summarizing the published studies of social-skills training with schizophrenic patients, found that although self-reports of anxiety and discomfort can show improvement following social-skills training, the improvement does not occur for all patients and, perhaps more important, does not often generalize to new situations. These authors suggest that social-skills training for schizophrenics could be more effective if it were of longer duration and if opportunities for generalization were designed into the training program.

In another review of the literature on the treatment of schizophrenics through various forms of behavior modification, including social-skills building, Gomes-Schwartz came to a similar conclusion. She suggested that social-skills training is based on the premise that "schizophrenic withdrawal and isolation is a result of earlier failures to learn appropriate techniques for interacting with others" (1979, pp. 455–456) and that those techniques can be taught. But although generalization to new role-playing situations seems good, generalization to natural settings is quite limited. Furthermore, there is very little evidence that behaviors learned in social-skills training last very long after the training.

Twentyman and Zimering (1979) recently reviewed some 150 social-training experiments with particular regard for the relative effectiveness of such experiments contrasted with other forms of behavioral training, including various psychotherapies.

> When compared to waiting list or no-treatment control groups, behavioral training is clearly superior in teaching new social behaviors. Moreover, treatment efficacy is not restricted to certain types of patients but has been found with clients of widely differing demographic characteristics. Differences between therapies have been small or nonexistent when skills training has been compared with traditional psychotherapy or other treatments which provided subjects with information about handling problem situations. . . . To date, treatment programs have been based on methods merely considered effective rather than on empirically validated treatment procedures. This may be one reason for the paucity of evidence supporting skills methods over other forms of therapy. When empirically validated

treatment components are obtained, the therapeutic efficacy may substantially increase and gains relative to other forms of therapy may be produced. . . . The evidence in support of generalization of treatment effects must be considered tentative at this time. Treatments which have extended the traditional clinic boundaries into naturalistic settings hold promise for producing greater treatment gain. . . . To be effective, behavior training must provide those skills which will enable clients to obtain the most reinforcement even in those situations where the contingencies are not favorable [pp. 389–390].[9]

Conger and Keane recently reviewed the literature on social-skills intervention with isolated or withdrawn children. They concluded that "although some of these techniques appear to hold promise, the conclusions are limited owing to methodological problems, such as small numbers of subjects, different assessment procedures across studies, and lack of extended follow-up" (1981, p. 478).

CONCLUSIONS AND OVERVIEW

Mental health education, as well as its parent, consumer health education, is in the midst of an enormous expansion. As the cost of health services increases, health economists are reexamining all kinds of programs that show promise of preventing either psychological or physical disorders. Among these programs are those that focus on health maintenance or disease management in large population groups. For psychological disorders, no approach to health maintenance or disease management holds more promise than mental health education.

Havik (1981) recently reviewed 25 published studies examining the effectiveness of providing patient information and education in reducing the duration or disability of physical disease. Most of the studies were done with surgical patients, and all used extremely brief interventions, averaging about 30 minutes.

Havik found that 96% of the measures of effect favored the group of patients who received the information and education over patients in a control group. Information and education appeared to have the greatest effect in reducing somatic complications and in improving psychosocial well-being. Havik summarizes his findings by noting:

Patient education and patient information do have an effect on psychological adjustment and physical recovery of patients with physical illness. The effects are observed over a broad spectrum, covering emotional, interpersonal, and physiological variables that are of importance for the total well-being of medical patients. In addition, the intervention programs are very brief, they can be administered to groups of patients, and they can be incorporated in standard treatment and

---

[9]From "Behavioral Training of Social Skills: A Critical Review," by C. T. Twentyman and R. T. Zimering. In *Progress in Behavior Modification*, 1979, *3*, 319–400. Copyright 1979 by Academic Press. Reprinted by permission.

care programs without a great need for additional professional expertise [1981, pp. 193–194].

It is encouraging to note that persons now most closely identified with the field of mental health education are undertaking the assessment of its impact. In each of the mental health education programs just described, some effort was made to evaluate its effectiveness.

Mental health education, like all education, is more than the presentation of information. Mental health education is a *process* that involves the sharing of information, but much more. Mental health educators hope to use that information to foster group and community discussion, and out of that discussion can come individual changes in attitudes, opinions, and behavior. The President's Committee on Health Education made this point when it stated "Health education is a process that bridges the gap between health information and health practices" (1973, p. 17).

Under the best of circumstances, the mental health education process can lead not only to individual modifications in behavior but to collective modifications in behavior—that is, to social action that can result in genuine community change.

4

Beyond Community Mental Health

The two chapters in this section address communitywide issues in mental health. The first chapter deals with various approaches that can be taken to understanding the community, its structure, its quality of life, and its needs. The second chapter introduces the field of community psychology by providing an orientation to its context, its values, and its approaches to improving community well-being. These two chapters illustrate ways in which the mental health professional can function in order to serve the entire community, not only those who are at high risk or who have already sought help for an emotional problem.

CHAPTER

8

Assessing Community Structure and Community Needs

Just as there are conceptual parallels between mental health consultation, a community mental health activity, and psychotherapy, a clinical activity, so there are parallels between the assessment of community characteristics and the assessment of individual characteristics. Both clinical assessment and community assessment involve, ideally, a quantitative and objective judgment of strengths as well as weaknesses and, where weaknesses are found, a set of prescriptions for remediation. Furthermore, for assessment to have any value, there must be a set of standards by which individual or community characteristics can be measured.

In an annual physical examination, for example, the physician checks for symptoms (the patient's complaints) and signs (laboratory or other objective data) and compares them with "normal" symptoms or signs. The physician may know that certain symptoms are normal for a patient of a particular age or may find that certain laboratory findings are abnormal and require additional study. A psychological assessment might contrast a person's intellectual behavior with normative intellectual behavior for people of that age and might conclude that the person's intellectual performance is advanced or retarded or within normal limits and, if advanced or retarded, by what amount. Other psychological examinations assess personality characteristics and, within the limitations of personality theories, offer a remarkably sophisticated view of the person as a functioning human being with certain strengths and weaknesses, feelings and needs, anxieties and coping style. Psychiatric examinations have objectives similar to those of psychological examinations, although assessment techniques are somewhat different. But in all these cases, there are assessment instruments (the stethoscope, the microscope, the set of Rorschach inkblot cards, the standardized interview) and some more or less clear definition of normal performance that allows abnormal performance to be identified.

The diagnostic examination is perhaps the most basic element of the mental health professional's work—that element on which the processes of prevention and remediation are based. Development of individual assessment procedures has been going on for a long time, and the procedures, in a very large proportion of cases, are of unquestionable value. The history of community assessment is far shorter, and its value is less clearly documented. The purpose of this chapter is to review the efforts to apply assessment procedures to communities—efforts to take the pulse, so to speak, of the community.

CONCEPTS OF COMMUNITY

Sociologists and social psychologists have long studied the community as an entity, and it is to them we must turn for a basic understanding of that social unit. It would be useful to review the concepts of community employed by some of the most influential writers in the field. According to Sanders (1966, p. 26), "A community is a territorially organized system coextensive with a settlement pattern in which (1) an effective communication network operates, (2) people share common facilities and services distributed within this settlement pattern, and (3) people develop a psychological identification with the 'locality symbol' (the name)." Sanders suggests that most people, inevitably, have a narrow view of a community and that, in contrast, social scientists try to get a broader view of the community and try to understand it with detachment and completeness. Since this task is exceedingly complex, social scientists have developed four somewhat different approaches to studying the community.

First, some social scientists think of the community as *a place to live* and study communities by collecting responses to such questions as: What kinds of people live in the area? What are the employment opportunities, the shopping facilities, the opportunities for recreation? What are the chief religious groupings, the general educational level, the housing pattern? What are the prevailing community attitudes and sentiments? What is family life like? How are newcomers received? As you can see, many of these questions can be answered only in qualitative terms.

A second approach to studying the community is to see it in *demographic, ecological,* or *spatial* terms. In using this approach, the social scientist studies the spatial distribution of people, of occupations, and of activities and commonly makes use of subarea analyses of communities. By contrasting subareas, the social scientist can define neighborhood characteristics and can study the interrelationships of these characteristics. Having determined the basic elements of the community, at least from a demographic point of view, the researcher can identify how these elements change over time and can determine, for example, that an increasing proportion of the population of the central city are members of minority groups, or that crimes against property are substantially more common in certain areas of the community, or that certain forms of disruptive behavior occur with unusually high frequency in those sections of the city in which certain demographic characteristics prevail. This second approach to the study of the community, in contrast to the first approach, is highly quantitative in character.

A third strategy for studying the community is to take the *ethnographic approach* and to try to understand the community as a way of life. This approach, often used by anthropologists, is highly subjective and usually requires extensive periods of residence in the community, fluency with the local language, and a high level of participation in community life. The spatial and demographic characteristics of the community are not separated out for study; rather, researchers using the ethnographic method seek to develop insight into the total culture. Because of the subjective nature of the approach, Sanders says it "is as much a creative as a scientific act" (1966, p. 18).

Finally, one can study a community by concentrating on its *social relationships*—the patterns of interactions through which daily activities are carried out. In other words, this approach involves considering the community as a social system. Using this approach, sociologists examine patterns of social relationships and their groupings into larger and more complex social units.

Warren is another important theorist in this field. His approach to defining the community is as follows: "It is the unescapable fact that people's clustering together in space has important influences on their daily activities which gives us perhaps our best clue to a definition of the community as a social entity. We shall consider a community to be *that combination of social units and systems which perform the major social functions having locality relevance*" (1972, p. 9). Warren divides these locality-relevant functions into five categories. First is *production-distribution-consumption*—that is, local participation in the process of producing, distributing, and consuming those goods and services which are a part of daily living and access to which is desirable in the locality. Second is *socialization*—a process by which society or one of its constituent social units transmits prevailing knowledge, social values, and behavior patterns to its individual members. Third is *social control*—a process through which a group influences its members to behave in conformity with its norms. Fourth is *social participation*, opportunities for which are provided by religious organizations, other voluntary organizations, the business community, the family, extended kinship relationships, and other, less formal associations. Fifth is *mutual support* in time of need, provided by family and friends as well as by institutionalized governmental public welfare and social service mechanisms. This view suggests that the community serves to provide the means of satisfying both individual and societal needs (see Warren, 1972, pp. 10–11, and Sanders, 1966, pp. 51–52). Warren proposes that certain characteristics of communities are crucial in determining how these five functions are carried out, and he specifies, as three special dimensions along which communities vary, *autonomy* (the extent to which a community is self-sufficient in carrying out its functions), *coincidence of service areas* (the extent to which residents in a community are served by institutions from the same community), and *identification* (the extent to which residents have a sense of belonging to the community).

Bernard (1973) makes a useful distinction between the term *community* and the term *the community*. After noting that most definitions of community include the concepts of locale, common ties, and social interaction, she proposes that the major component of the concept of *the community* is locale. In contrast, the major components of the concept of *community* are common ties and social interaction. The concept of community involves personal intimacy, emotional ties, moral commitment, social cohesion, and continuity in time (see Bernard, 1973, pp. 3–4; see also Rossi, 1972, pp. 90–97).

It is not difficult to identify the common elements in the concepts of community advanced by Sanders, Warren, and Bernard. All acknowledge that the community is multidimensional and that a variety of approaches can be used to study it. All see utility in qualitative as well as quantitative approaches to the task of community analysis. All view the community as having a geographically defined locality, and all acknowledge that there is, to use Sarason's (1974) felicitous term, a *psychological sense of community* as well. All see the residents of a community as interdependent and identify certain functions that must be performed in order for a community to be viable. Thus, the task of assessing community characteristics and community needs requires both objective and subjective measurements. In assessing the school system, for example, one might gather information about such variables as the number of students, the number of teachers and administrative staff, and the budget. At the same time, one would examine more subjective variables, such as public attitudes toward the school system or values and beliefs about education in general. A comprehensive analysis of the educational establishment in a community might well include studies of neighborhood differences in attitudes toward local elementary schools; factors associated with differing dropout rates in various sections of the community and during various time periods; morale, illness patterns, and turnover rate of teachers; objective academic test scores of a random sample of students and test-score changes over time; postsecondary-school educational plans and educational activities of new high school graduates; and voting patterns on school-bond referendums.

The various approaches to the study of the community identified in this section have become traditional, and many social scientists are identified with only one of these approaches. Thus, according to Bernard (1973), some scientists look at communities in terms of their ecology, others in terms of social-class structure, others in terms of distribution of power, and still others in terms of how human relationships are established and maintained. Bernard, for one, sees these traditions as having a certain inertia, which breeds conservatism and stultifies research and theory (1973, pp. 8–10).

COMMUNITY SUBAREA ANALYSES

With the possible exception of a few suburban communities which consist of street after street of almost identical houses and in which demographic characteristics show very little variation from one neighborhood to another, most communities in the United States are not homogeneous. Most communities have their rich and poor section and both white and non-white ghettos. Delinquency and crime are often more common in certain sections of the city than in others. There are neighborhoods inhabited largely by young families and other neighborhoods populated almost exclusively by adults. With the development of community mental health centers, mental health professionals have become increasingly interested in their communities and in the neighborhoods within their communities. This interest in community subareas, relatively recent in practicing mental health professionals, has actually been of central concern to demographers for more than two generations (see Burke, 1974; Shevky & Bell, 1955), and the Bureau of the Census of the United States Department of Commerce has, since the census of 1910, used the concept of the census tract in tabulating census information.

Census tracts are small areas into which large cities and adjacent areas have been divided. Census-tract boundaries are established by a local committee in collaboration with the Bureau of the Census so that the tracts are relatively uniform in size of population. The average census tract has 3500–4000 residents. It is the intention of the Bureau of the Census to maintain these boundaries intact over a long period so that comparisons may be made from census to census. In many communities, agencies tabulate locally collected data by census tract, further increasing the potential usefulness of census-tract divisions. Census tracts were created in 1910 and in 1920 were analyzed for 8 cities. The number of cities was increased to 18 in the 1930 census and in 1940 increased again to 60. By the 1970 census, 241 Standard Metropolitan Statistical Areas (towns, cities, counties, or groups of contiguous towns, cities, or counties that contain at least one city of 50,000 or more inhabitants) were identified, and each was divided into census tracts, which were separately analyzed. In the 1980 census that number had increased to 323.

Information for each census tract is available concerning general population characteristics (for example, age, sex, marital status, type of household, and number of own children), social characteristics of the population (for example, nativity, school enrollment, means of transportation to work), labor-force characteristics (for example, employment status, occupation, type of industry), income characteristics (for example, median family income, source of income, incomes below poverty level), and housing characteristics (for example, persons per room, value of owner-occupied units, housing units containing complete kitchen facilities, age of housing-unit structure). In census tracts where a certain number of blacks or of persons of Spanish language or Spanish surname live, similar information is separately tabulated for these two groups.

When one adds to this array of information other information locally collected and tabulated by census tract, it is immediately apparent that the characterization of neighborhoods in rather precise quantitative terms is possible. These neighborhood descriptions can be enormously useful to persons responsible for planning mental health or other human services and to others who need to understand how social factors are associated with phenomena of interest, such as rate of psychiatric hospitalization, number of school dropouts, or number of new cases of tuberculosis or venereal disease. The use of census statistics for community analyses is being strongly encouraged by the National Institute of Mental Health (1975a, 1975b).

One way in which the subareas of a community can be analyzed is illustrated by a study I did on data collected in Pueblo, Colorado (Bloom, 1975, and see Figure 8–1). Pueblo was divided in 1970 into 34 census tracts with an average population of 3500 each. One of these tracts is the Colorado State Hospital and does not figure in the data to be presented. This particular analysis had two fundamental purposes: first, to examine how individual census-tract characteristics interrelated and to develop broad dimensions along which census tracts could be compared and contrasted and, second, to examine the relations between these dimensions and measures of psychopathology in order to develop a greater understanding of the complex relations between community social characteristics and mental disorders.

From all the data available for census-tract analysis, I chose data on the 35 variables that seemed to have the most potential for contributing to an understanding of the sociocultural organization of the community. Of the 35 variables, 27 were taken from census-tract publications of the Bureau of the Census, and 8 were available from local sources. By means of statistical analyses developed by Tryon and Bailey (1970), it was possible to determine whether *clusters* of census-tract characteristics could be identified. A cluster was defined as a number of mathematically interrelated variables that, as a group, seemed to be representative of one clearly specifiable census-tract characteristic.

The 35 variables I selected are shown in Table 8–1. Each variable is defined, and the lowest, highest, and average census-tract scores are shown. One remarkable characteristic of Pueblo, and of cities in general, is the high degree of variability among census tracts on so many of the variables. There are 12 times as many Spanish-surnamed people in the census tract highest on this variable as in the census tract lowest on this variable. The ratio between highest and lowest census tracts is on the order of 16:1 for people living alone, 20:1

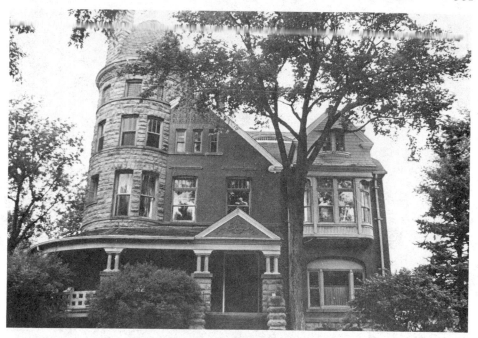

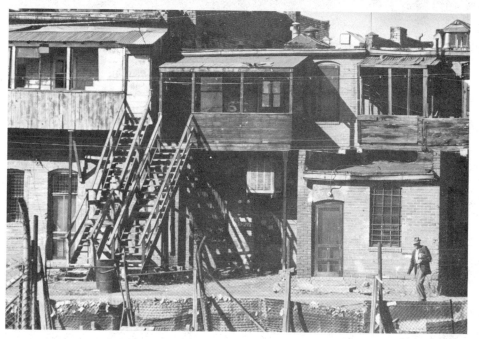

FIGURE 8.1   Homes in areas of high and low socioeconomic affluence in Pueblo, Colorado. *(Photos by John Suhay.)*

TABLE 8–1. Ranges, means, and definitions of selected census-tract variables for Pueblo, Colorado, 1970

Census-Tract Variable	Range		Mean	Definition
	Low	High		
Demographic characteristics				
1. Population	624	9280	3522.5	Total population
2. Median age	19.6	41.0	26.8	Male median age
3. Sex ratio	82.8	121.1	104.7	Females per 100 males
4. Foreign born	0.4	8.3	2.5	Percent foreign born
5. Spanish surname	6.6	84.5	35.1	Percent Spanish surname
6. Fertility ratio	27.3	51.5	40.7	Number of children under age 5 per 100 females age 15–44
7. Education	8.5	12.7	11.1	Median school years completed—persons age 25 and above
Community participation				
8. Library-card holders	113.6	452.9	259.4	Public-library-card holders per 1000 population—age 5 and above
9. YMCA members	0.0	25.8	6.6	YMCA members per 1000 population—age 3 and above
10. Golf-club members	0.0	27.8	5.0	Municipal-golf-club members per 1000 population—age 21 and above
11. Public health nursing visits	0.0	120.8	31.5	Public health nursing caseload per 10,000 population
Family characteristics				
12. Household population	1.9	4.1	3.2	Population per household
13. Young children	12.2	40.3	26.1	Percent married couples with own children under age 6
14. People living alone	3.5	57.1	18.0	Percent occupied housing units occupied by one person
15. Household population density	3.0	27.7	12.7	Percent occupied housing units occupied by more than one person per room
16. Residential stability	38.0	78.9	60.3	Percent of population age 5 or above in census year living in same house as 5 years earlier
17. Married women in labor force	16.1	48.4	32.4	Percent nonseparated women in labor force
18. Children living with both parents	58.5	93.5	80.1	Percent population 18 and under living with both parents

Census-Tract Variable	Range		Mean	Definition
	Low	High		
Housing characteristics				
19. Single homes	21.2	100.0	83.4	Percent of all structures containing one housing unit
20. Rooms per housing unit	2.8	5.5	4.6	Median number of rooms per housing unit
21. New housing	0.7	50.0	15.7	Percent of all housing units built in ten-year period prior to census year
22. Housing-unit value	$7000	$20,600	$11,538.60	Median value of owner-occupied housing units
23. Owner-occupied housing	18.0	92.8	71.4	Percent occupied housing units owner-occupied
24. Housing lacking plumbing	0.3	30.9	7.5	Percent year-round housing units lacking some or all plumbing facilities
25. Central heating	23.0	100.0	70.2	Percent year-round housing units with central heating
26. Vacant housing	0.6	8.3	3.2	Percent year-round housing units available and vacant
27. Household fires	0.0	2.2	0.6	Percent of all housing units that had a reported fire
Socioeconomic characteristics				
28. Family income	$5707	$12,112	$8060.00	Median family income
29. Unemployment	0.0	14.4	6.2	Percent of male civilian labor force unemployed
30. White-collar workers	1.7	29.2	10.4	Percent employed males in professional, technical, and kindred occupations
31. Families receiving ADC	0.0	25.8	10.2	Percent of families receiving Aid to Dependent Children federal assistance
Personal disruption				
32. Delinquency	0.0	8.7	4.4	Juvenile delinquents per 100 population age 18 and under
33. Suicide rate	0.0	3.2	0.6	Suicides (accumulated over six years) as proportion of total population
34. School dropouts	0.0	36.0	16.8	School dropouts per 100 population age 18 and under
35. Marital disruption	12.8	508.7	91.7	Number of divorced and separated males for every 1000 married nonseparated males

Adapted from *Changing Patterns of Psychiatric Care*, by B. L. Bloom. Copyright 1975 by Human Sciences Press. Reprinted by permission.

for proportion of foreign-born, 17:1 for proportion of white-collar workers, and 39:1 for marital disruption.

Analysis of the pattern of interrelationships among the 35 census-tract characteristics revealed that it was possible to group 26 of them into three clusters. The other 9 variables were not strongly enough related to any of these three clusters to be part of one. Two of the clusters will be examined.

I labeled the cluster accounting for the greatest proportion of the pattern of statistical relationships among the 35 variables *socioeconomic affluence*. The 12 variables making up this cluster, along with their intercorrelations, are shown in Table 8–2. The average correlation of any 2 of the 12 variables was .57, which is relatively high for analyses of this kind. The actual naming of the cluster took place after the statistical analyses were completed; the task in naming clusters is to try to capture the essential character of the variables that compose the cluster.

This cluster identifies census tracts along a dimension that includes direct measures of affluence and a variety of indexes highly associated with affluence. After identifying a group of variables that form a cluster, one can assign a cluster score to each census tract. Census tracts that get high socioeconomic-affluence-cluster scores are characterized by high median family income and high value and good condition of owner-occupied housing; high level of education and high proportion of employed males in professional, technical, and kindred occupations; large numbers of library-card holders and golf-club members; high proportion of married women in the labor force; low proportion of Spanish-surnamed people; low unemployment; low household population density; and a low percentage of families receiving Aid to Dependent Children. The correlation coefficients in Table 8–2 indicate, of course, that these 12 variables were found to be mathematically related. That is, if one knew the median family income in a census tract, for example, one would be able to predict the other 11 characteristics of the census quite accurately. Of the 12 variables, the one that might be the most surprising is the percentage of married women in the labor force. Contrary to what one might expect— namely, that it is in the poorer families that a second income is needed and that therefore it is in the poorer subareas that one would find wives gainfully employed—it is in fact in the more affluent census tracts that married women can be found in the labor force in greatest number. This one dimension, socio-economic affluence, accounted for nearly half of the entire pattern of relationships among the 35 variables.

The second cluster has been labeled *social disequilibrium* and consists of 10 variables, whose intercorrelations are shown in Table 8–3. Looking at Table 8–3, you can see that a census tract high in social disequilibrium was one that was characterized by housing units with few rooms, a high rate of marital and familial disruption, many people living alone, little owner-occupied housing, a high rate of delinquency, few single homes, many vacant housing units, frequent household fires, and a lot of school dropouts. In Pueblo, as in all

TABLE 8–2. Correlations between the variables making up the "socioeconomic affluence" cluster

Census-Tract Characteristic	Census-Tract Characteristic										
	1	2	3	4	5	6	7	8	9	10	11
1. Housing-unit value											
2. Family income	+.87										
3. White-collar workers	+.80	+.72									
4. Education	+.81	+.74	+.71								
5. Golf-club members	+.79	+.70	+.59	+.58							
6. Spanish surname	-.74	-.70	-.69	-.86	-.58						
7. Central heating	+.59	+.58	+.51	+.61	+.65	-.56					
8. Families receiving ADC	-.57	-.64	-.47	-.55	-.44	+.70	-.29				
9. Library-card holders	+.50	+.45	+.55	+.39	+.32	-.43	+.36	-.15			
10. Married women in labor force	+.65	+.62	+.55	+.72	+.35	-.70	+.42	-.43	+.47		
11. Unemployment	-.45	-.54	-.42	-.45	-.23	+.54	-.16	+.71	-.05	-.62	
12. Household population density	-.58	-.48	-.61	-.63	-.66	+.61	-.78	+.38	-.33	-.28	+.13

TABLE 8–3. Correlations between variables making up the "social disequilibrium" cluster

Census-Tract Characteristic	Census-Tract Characteristic								
	1	2	3	4	5	6	7	8	9
1. Rooms per housing unit									
2. Marital disruption	−.85								
3. People living alone	−.87	+.88							
4. Owner-occupied housing	+.87	−.85	−.92						
5. Delinquency	−.65	+.43	+.54	−.52					
6. Single homes	+.79	−.81	−.94	+.94	−.51				
7. Vacant housing	−.68	+.71	+.53	−.63	+.44	−.52			
8. Children living with both parents	+.83	−.70	−.83	+.87	−.79	+.83	−.52		
9. Household fires	−.65	+.74	+.62	−.57	+.57	−.56	+.59	−.61	
10. School dropouts	−.78	+.64	+.74	−.72	+.85	−.71	+.60	−.87	+.65

Adapted from *Changing Patterns of Psychiatric Care,* by B. L. Bloom. Copyright 1975 by Human Sciences Press. Reprinted by permission.

other U.S. cities studied, personal disruption was found to be highly associated with environmental disruption. The average correlation between variables in the social-disequilibrium cluster was .73. This second cluster accounts for an additional 32% of the pattern of relationships among the 35 variables. That is, between the two clusters just described, a total of nearly 80% of the entire pattern of correlations has been accounted for. Those census tracts high in socioeconomic affluence tend to be low in social disequilibrium, although the degree of this relationship is smaller than one might suppose. The correlation between the two cluster scores is − .60. Squaring this correlation, you get .36, which indicates that if you tried to predict census-tract social-disequilibrium scores from census-tract socioeconomic-affluence scores, the magnitude of your errors would be reduced by only 36% from what they would have been had you made the prediction without knowing the relationship between social disequilibrium and affluence.

A useful view of the city and county of Pueblo is afforded by an examination of the geographic distribution of census-tract cluster scores. In Figures 8–2 and 8–3, you can see the census tracts of Pueblo County. (The census tracts within the central city are drawn to scale, but all census tracts outside the central city have had to be significantly compressed in size.) The shadings indicate whether a tract falls in the upper, middle, or lowest third of scores on a cluster. The cluster scores that define each third are shown at the bottom of each figure.

Census-tract cluster scores were arbitrarily calculated so that the average census tract would have a score of 50, and the distribution of census-tract scores has a standard deviation of 10. As you can see in Figure 8–2, the most affluent tracts form two groupings—one in the north-central portion of the city and the other in the southwestern portion. Tracts with moderate scores on the index of socioeconomic affluence are located in the northeastern and southwestern quadrants of the city. Three of the southern rural tracts (bottom right in the figure) are included in the moderately affluent group. Those tracts with the lowest level of affluence are located in the central portion of the city and in the rural sections of the county to the north and east.

Census-tract scores on the social-disequilibrium index are shown in Figure 8–3. The concentration of high scores in the central area of the city is readily apparent.

As already indicated, the correlation between the census-tract measures of social disequilibrium and socioeconomic affluence is negative, but the two indexes are in no sense measuring the same neighborhood characteristic. Scores on the two measures are negatively correlated, but not perfectly so. Thus, from a statistical viewpoint, it is not surprising that two census tracts in the inner city are high on both measures and that the rural tracts surrounding the central city tend to be low on both measures.

In summary, then, in 1970, the inner portion of the central city could be characterized as low in affluence and high in social disequilibrium. Moving

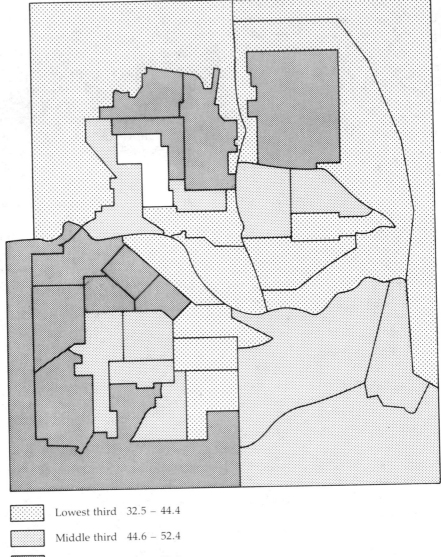

Lowest third   32.5 – 44.4

Middle third   44.6 – 52.4

Upper third   52.5 – 72.1

Figure 8.2   Socioeconomic-affluence-cluster scores for Pueblo County, Colorado, 1970. From *Changing Patterns of Psychiatric Care*, by B. L. Bloom. (*Copyright 1975 by Human Sciences Press. Reprinted by permission.*)

somewhat outside the inner city, one finds decreasing social disequilibrium and increasing affluence. In the rural areas surrounding the city, affluence generally decreases, as does social disequilibrium.

These tables and figures illustrate the use of census-tract data for characterization of community subareas. Each community presents its own special pattern of neighborhoods, and depending on one's purposes in preparing

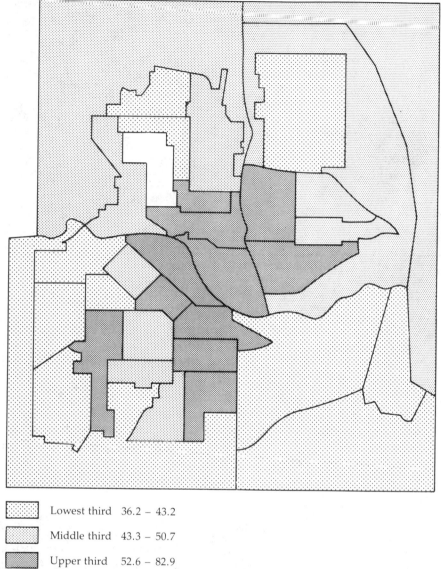

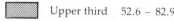 Lowest third   36.2 – 43.2

Middle third   43.3 – 50.7

Upper third   52.6 – 82.9

Figure 8.3 Social-disequilibrium-cluster scores for Pueblo County, Colorado, 1970. From *Changing Patterns of Psychiatric Care*, by B. L. Bloom. *(Copyright 1975 by Human Sciences Press. Reprinted by Permission.)*

subarea analyses, different variables can be selected. Just as one can make a social and demographic analysis of neighborhoods, one could analyze psychiatric-patient caseloads, delinquency rate, crime statistics, infectious-disease incidence, or voting behavior. All these analyses offer the potential of allowing one to see more deeply into the character of a community.

It is possible, for example, to examine the relationships between com-

TABLE 8-4.   Correlations of census-tract characteristics with age-adjusted admission rates to psychiatric facilities in Pueblo, Colorado, 1970

	Census-Tract Characteristic	
Type of Admission and Type of Facility	Socioeconomic Affluence	Social Disequilibrium
First inpatient admission		
Public facilities	− .56	+ .78
Private facilities		+ .49
Repeat inpatient admission		
Public facilities	− .44	+ .84
Private facilities		+ .45
First outpatient admission		
Public facilities		+ .79
Private facilities	+ .54	
Repeat outpatient admission		
Public facilities		+ .75
Private facilities		

Note: Correlation coefficients not shown were not significantly different from zero.

munity subarea characteristics and rates of psychopathology. Such an analysis, for the city of Pueblo, Colorado, is shown in Table 8-4. As you can see, the social-disequilibrium characteristic of census tracts is far more closely related to most admission rates than is the socioeconomic characteristic. Census tracts with high social-disequilibrium scores yield disproportionately large numbers of psychiatric inpatients and outpatients, particularly into publicly supported facilities. In contrast, census tracts high in socioeconomic affluence yield disproportionately *few* psychiatric inpatients into public inpatient facilities and disproportionately large numbers of patients into private outpatient facilities. It is this type of analysis, when combined with others—such as contrasting demographic characteristics of psychiatric patients with characteristics of the general population—that helps identify high-risk groups.

ASSESSMENT OF COMMUNITY NEEDS

The emergence of the field of community mental health has brought with it an interest in the assessment of mental-health-related needs, since such an assessment would need to be part of any rational planning effort. The field of need assessment has developed very rapidly, and a number of excellent comprehensive presentations of the state of the field are available (for example, Bell, Sundel, Aponte, Murrell, & Lin, 1982; Hagedorn, Beck, Neubert, & Werlin, 1976; Hargreaves, Attkisson, & Sorensen, 1977; Warheit, Bell, & Schwab, 1977).

Siegel, Attkisson, and Cohn define the field of need assessment in the following way:

Basically, assessment is an attempt to describe and understand the mental health needs in a geographic or social area. This involves two distinct steps: the application of a measuring tool or assortment of tools to a defined social area; and the application of judgment to assess the significance of the information gathered in order to determine priorities for program planning and service development. . . . Assessment is a part of mental health planning. It provides one important informational input to a much broader planning process that leads to: (a) a mental health plan; (b) the selection and operationalization of specific program activities; and (c) the evaluation of these program activities [1977, p. 46].

Warheit et al. (1977) have summarized and illustrated each of the major approaches to need assessment: (1) key informant, (2) community forum, (3) rates under treatment, (4) social indicators, and (5) survey. The key-informant approach assesses mental health needs on the basis of information secured from those in the area who are in a position to know the community's needs and patterns of use of mental-health-related services. The community-forum approach relies on individuals who are asked to assess the needs and service patterns of those in the community. In comparison with the key-informant approach, the community forum involves a wider circle of participants and is usually designed around a series of public meetings. The rates-under-treatment approach is based on an enumeration of persons who have used the services of pertinent health and welfare agencies and assumes that the needs of the population can be estimated on the basis of the number of persons who have received care. The social-indicators approach is based on inferences drawn from descriptive statistics found mainly in public records. Finally, the survey approach is based on collection of new data from samples of the population by means of interviews eliciting, for example, information about their health, social well-being, and patterns of service utilization.

The professional has long had the greatest power in the assessment of needs, and it is only in relatively recent years that mental health professionals have sought to discover what their clients or potential clients want. The private-practice model is one, after all, in which a service is offered and in which, as long as the practitioner makes enough money, there is very little need to identify needs that the service does not meet. For the past several decades, privately practicing mental health professionals have generally been able to attract a large enough clientele. The professional staff of many public mental health clinics and community mental health centers came out of this entrepreneurial heritage, and with very few exceptions, they saw themselves as the primary source of wisdom about community mental health needs. As a result, the most common sequence of events in the development of staffing patterns for mental health centers involved, first, a decision, on the basis of some explicit or implicit formula, that this center with this budget needed so many psychiatrists, psychologists, social workers, psychiatric nurses, paraprofessionals, administrative staff, and so on. Only later, if at all, were attempts made to identify community needs to which the staff might be responsive. Often, by the time those needs were identified, no funds remained with which to hire the appropriate personnel. Thus, by the time it was discovered that a significant proportion of the clients of a community mental health center had need for legal advice or homemaker services or transportation, for example, funds no longer existed to employ these kinds of staff.

Expert assessment of needs

Lemkau (1967) discusses three general strategies for developing expert assessment of needs. First, he suggests that it is possible to *compare the services offered by one community with those offered by others* and to "relate those of a community that we presume is excellently served to the needs of the population under study" (p. 65). This method requires that there be some standards by which adequacy of community mental health services can be judged and that the community under study be measured by those standards. But, as Lemkau continues,

> convenient as such comparisons are, and useful as they may sometimes be for propaganda purposes, they are hardly to be taken seriously as scientific measures of actual need. . . . The principal flaw in such evaluations of need is, of course, that they are actually evaluations of the kind and amount of service given. Thus they reveal only the needs that have been modified by public demand; this demand which influences public policy, is determined by the level of education of the community [pp. 65–66].

A second strategy is to *collect and interpret service statistics*, or data on patients in treatment—that is, to "use data from the study of discovered cases that, according to some already determined criterion, need service" (p. 66). Although this technique of estimating need for mental health services has been used since the early 1800s, it involves the assumption (usually incorrect) that "people who do not demand treatment or do not have treatment demanded for them are healthy and have no medical needs" (p. 66).

Regarding the use of treated rates as an index of the extent of psychiatric disorder in a community or in subpopulations within a community, Blum wrote "In the past, becoming a patient has been the primary case-finding method for psychiatry; it must not be overlooked in planning future community studies" (1962, p. 272). Yet, the defects of this method of case identification are readily apparent. From the large pool of potential patients, an unknown proportion elect to become or are selected to become actual patients. Not only is the proportion unknown, but it is likely that identified patients are not a random sample of the larger potential-patient pool. Becoming a patient is the end result of a complex chain of events dependent on the nature of the symptomatology, the alternative forms of support available, social class, community value systems, the availability of treatment facilities, economics, and willingness to accept the patient role.

One final objection commonly raised to the use of treated rates in epidemiologic investigations is that the act of hospitalization for a psychiatric disorder is less an indication of psychopathology on the part of the patient than it is an indication of society's reaction to what it labels deviant behavior. Although this hypothesis has been a popular one, it has, until recently received little systematic attention. But two papers by Gove (1970a, 1970b) have presented substantial empirical evidence that the primary determinant of hospitalization as well as of the consequences of hospitalization is the patient's psychiatric status.

It is conceivable that a person may be denied the patient role, having petitioned for it, but this is rare. It is reasonably safe to assume that identified psychiatric patients have some form of disability, although, as Goffman (1961) and Rosenhan (1973) have shown, once in the psychiatric care system, it is sometimes amazingly difficult to get out. The problem with using patient-care data as a measure of psychiatric disability in a population is not only the danger of systematic underestimation, however. In addition, one has to assume that although rates based on identified patients may be lower than rates based on population surveys, patient rates are sufficiently highly correlated with rates calculated on the basis of population surveys to serve as "true" psychiatric-disability rates. B. P. Dohrenwend and B. S. Dohrenwend noted, for example, that relations between treated rates and social class are "strongly affected by such factors as the greater availability of private psychiatrists to high-income groups . . . and the relatively favorable orientation to psychiatric treatment" of high-income groups and thus concluded that they could not assume that "an empirical relation between social status and rate of psychological disorder based on treated rates necessarily reflects the true relationship" (1969, p. 7).

Accordingly, Lemkau identifies a third strategy—a *survey of the general population* or of a sample of that population. But such surveys are expensive and suffer from severe problems of reliability and validity. Although an estimate of the proportion of the total population in need of mental health services would be a superb index of community need, studies deriving such estimates have yielded widely divergent results. An overview of the more than 40 population surveys conducted in the past 30 years in nearly that many communities was presented by B. P. Dohrenwend and B. S. Dohrenwend (1969), and the range in the reported prevalence rates of identifiable mental disorder was from less than 1% to over 60%—a range that defies credibility. Furthermore, except for social class, which has generally been found to vary inversely with obtained rates, few variables on which communities can be differentiated have been shown to be consistently related to disorder-rate variations. And social class is not strongly enough associated with obtained rates to account for the extraordinary variation in findings. The Dohrenwends have concluded that "there is no way to account for this great variability on substantive grounds. Rather, the differences are found to be related to differences in thoroughness of data collection procedures and, even more, to contrasting conceptions of what constitutes a 'case'" (1969, p. 170). Manis, Brewer, Hunt, and Kerchner, in their discussion of the problems in arriving at a valid measure of the prevalence of mental illness, come to a similar conclusion: "Our interpretation is that the differences in the reported rates of untreated illness arise *primarily* from lack of agreement, stated or implicit, in the criteria used to establish the cutting-point between the sick and the well" (1964, p. 89). Similar results were obtained in a study contrasting American and British procedures of diagnosing psychiatric patients (Cooper, Kendell, Gurland, Sartorius, & Farkas, 1969; Kramer, 1969; Zubin, 1969).

This variation in obtained rates led Pasamanick to note:

> It is the borderlines between the psychoses, on the one hand, and the neuroses, personality disorders and psychosomatic psychophysiologic disorders, on the other, and between them, that we encounter major difficulties. It is between the latter three and no illness, or with social maladjustment without psychiatric disorder, that we encounter our greatest unreliability. Since these are our most common disorders, surveyors, of course, have, as a consequence, arrived at the fantastically varying rates which create such hilarity in the literature [1968, p. 38].

In a related observation, the Expert Committee on Mental Health of the World Health Organization concluded that "in epidemiological studies, the definition of a 'case' is of crucial importance. The Committee has come to the conclusion, however, that there seems to be little prospect of producing a definition which would cover all the major and minor aberrations in social behavior or manifestations of disordered thought and would be applicable to all communities throughout the world, irrespective of their cultural background and social customs" (World Health Organization, 1960, p. 15). This is the issue of content validity, of course, and B. P. Dohrenwend and B. S. Dohrenwend comment that "it is doubtful whether content validity, in the strictest sense, can be achieved in the measurement of untreated psychological disorder, since there appears to be no universe of items which experts agree on as defining the variable" (1965, p. 56).

Even when used to assess a less equivocally defined disorder, household surveys have been shown to be inadequate. Consider the case of developing a survey instrument by which it might be possible to identify alcoholics. In an imaginative effort to assess the validity of such an instrument, Mulford and Wilson (1966) selected a sample of urban housing units "loaded" with addresses of households containing known alcoholics and concealed this fact from their otherwise carefully trained interviewers. The questionnaire the interviewers used was derived from a substantial body of previous research in the community—research that had shown the questionnaire to be of acceptable reliability and validity—yet, using this instrument, the interviewers missed half of the known alcoholics. Failure to identify known alcoholics was not random. The interview instrument was about twice as successful in identifying lower-socioeconomic-status alcoholics as it was in identifying alcoholics who had higher incomes and education.

There is no reason to believe that the problem of false negatives (failure to identify known cases) by means of household surveys is unique to surveys of alcoholics. In the Midtown Manhattan study (Srole et al., 1962), nearly half (19 out of 40) of the current psychiatric outpatients surveyed were judged not to have impaired states of mental health.

Even if the problem of false negatives did not exist, there would remain the distinct possibility that cases identified by means of community surveys (particularly persons never in psychiatric treatment) might differ in such significant ways from patients known to caretaking agencies as to constitute false positives. Major studies of psychiatric disability based on community surveys (for example, Srole et al., 1962, and Leighton et al., 1963) have concluded that substantial proportions of the general population are psychiatric cases and that the large majority of these cases have never been in treatment. Unfortunately, no studies to date have determined whether such persons are at higher risk of becoming patients at some future time than persons found reasonably free of psychiatric disability in the same surveys (see B. P. Dohrenwend & B. S. Dohrenwend, 1965, p. 57). These researchers assume that the psychiatric conditions of such untreated "cases" are similar to those of typical psychiatric patients. To test this assumption, B. P. Dohrenwend used two rating scales to rate samples of community leaders, heads of households, outpatients, and inpatients in northern Manhattan. In contrasting, for example, those heads of households judged to be almost certainly psychiatric cases with clinic outpatients judged similarly, a significant difference was found in degree of impairment. The outpatients were significantly more impaired. On the basis of this and other findings, Dohrenwend concluded that "typical 'cases' in the community, according to the Midtown Study and the Stirling County Study psychiatric ratings, are simply not the same as typical cases in either outpatient clinics or mental hospitals" (1970, p. 1061).

There are still other problems in assessing mental health in a general population, particularly if one is interested in evaluating social class or other sociocultural variables as possible etiological factors. It has been found that there are significant differences in symptom expression between members of different ethnic groups suffering from the same medical (Zola, 1966) or psychiatric (B. P. Dohrenwend, 1969) condition. Questionnaire replies are difficult to interpret across social classes and ethnic groups because of systematic differences in modes of symptom expression (Crandell & Dohrenwend, 1967), in acquiescence (B. P. Dohrenwend, 1969; Phillips & Clancy, 1970), and in perceived social desirability (Dohrenwend & Chin-Shong, 1967; Phillips & Clancy, 1970). Clear sex differences in symptom expression have been found (Phillips & Segal, 1969). It has been shown that respondents from the general population are less likely to be rated as cases on the basis of interviews conducted by psychiatrists than on the basis of interviews interpreted by psychiatrists but conducted by others (Dohrenwend, Egri, & Mendelsohn, 1971). Self-reports of stressful events are increasingly being used as part of the assessment of mental health, although one study has raised a question about the reliability of such self-reports (Hudgens, Robins, & Delong, 1970).

We are thus drawn to conclude that the best available population-survey instruments designed to assess psychiatric disability not only fail to identify known patients but succeed in designating as cases such a high proportion of people (the vast majority of whom have never sought treatment) that their validity has yet to be convincingly established.

Assessment of community opinion

According to Hargreaves, Attkisson, Siegal, and McIntyre (1974), "Identification of community views on mental health problems and service priorities is an important aspect of mental health needs assessment. . . . The majority of mental health programs either have ignored community input in planning or have considered their community advisory boards to be adequate reflectors of mental health priorities in the communities they serve" (pp. 55–56). Although, on occasion, the advisory board of a community mental health center may be representative of the community, and its members may have the skill to provide input into the program-planning process, this is relatively rare. As a consequence, if one wants to learn about the community's perception of mental-health-related needs, there is little alternative to asking the community directly. What one learns will be impressionistic or quite precise, depending on the methods used, but will often add quite significantly to what is learned from experts.

Two general procedures can be used to learn the views of local residents about mental-health-related issues—the survey method and the group-interaction method.

Surveys may be designed to be administered to a representative sample of community residents or of community agencies or of specified types of people—for example, psychiatric patients—but in all cases opinions are asked on such questions as: What are the most important problems the community is facing? What sources of help are available for these problems? How good are these services? What additional services are needed? How do community characteristics contribute to community problems? Surveys may be conducted door to door, by mail, by telephone, or in front of supermarkets. The questions can be open-ended (for example: What do you think are the most important mental health problems in the community?) or may be in a form that requires respondents to choose from among certain given answers (for example: Rank the following problems in terms of how severe they seem to be in this community: alcoholism, child abuse, divorce and separation, problems of old age, mental retardation, and suicide).

Representatives of social agencies (both public and private) can be asked to evaluate other agencies, to indicate to whom they make most of their referrals and from whom they get most of their referrals, to suggest whether, in their opinion, additional services are needed in the community or whether there is an oversupply of certain services, to describe the most commonly encountered problems in their agency and their theory of why these problems occur, and so on. There is no end to the questions that can be posed, and as long as samples of respondents are chosen carefully and the survey replies are skillfully analyzed, much can be learned.

The group-interaction method of assessing community needs encourages participants to exchange ideas about mental-health-related problems in a semi-public setting. Such procedures are quick and inexpensive, allow for diverse elements in the community to express their views, can start a problem-solving process, and can help locate persons who might be willing to play a role in subsequent problem solving. However, not everyone who should attend a forum or workshop will do so, some who attend will not speak, and it is not uncommon for unrealistic expectations to be generated (Hargreaves et al., 1974, pp. 57–83). Delbecq (1975) has recently reviewed a series of techniques that have been developed to facilitate group techniques for program planning and need assessment.

One way of assessing mental health needs using the method of the community survey was recently proposed by Pyszka and Hall (1975) for the Department of Social and Health Services of the state of Washington. The method proposed by these authors consists of personal interviews with a representative sample of community residents. The purpose of the interviews is to elicit information on which estimates of the need and demand for mental health services can be based. Their proposed data-collection method is fairly complex. First, a sample of households is selected, and an initial interview is conducted with the head of the household or the spouse. The person being interviewed is then asked to identify the other members of the household who are 13 years old and older. One of these other household members is randomly chosen, and the person being interviewed is asked to provide information about the mental health of that selected individual. Finally, that selected individual is interviewed. Note that the needs of young children are not assessed. All interviews are fairly structured, involving questions the responses to which can easily be coded for tabulation and analysis. The purpose of the interview with the household head is to obtain information on the *need* for mental health services, and accordingly the individual is asked what, in his or her opinion, the needs of the community, of the household, and of the selected household member are. The purpose of the interview with the selected household member is also to obtain information on the need for mental health services, but in this case the method is to directly assess the person's mental status. *Demand* for mental health services is measured by asking both the head of household and the selected household member questions about service-use patterns and awareness of service availability. Pyszka and Hall offer information on sampling, design of instruments, and recruitment and training of interviewers.

Sallis and Henggeler (1980) have examined the strengths and weaknesses of a variety of techniques for conducting community-needs assessments, including epidemiologic techniques, the use of social and health indicators, measuring utilization rates for various human service agencies, community-survey methods, and the community-forum approach. Their conclusions and recommendations are worth noting:

> Although the social and health indicators and the rates-under-treatment approaches . . . are frequently used, they provide little information about specific community mental health needs. . . . On the other hand community surveys and community forums are infrequently employed even though they . . . help specify community mental health needs. . . . However, despite the strengths of these latter methods there is little empirical support for the isolated use of any single needs assessment strategy. . . .
>
> Needs assessment techniques cannot be improved until they are evaluated systematically, hence it is important to empirically clarify their respective contributions and biases. To facilitate this process, techniques can be employed simultaneously and independently to provide multiple evaluations of community needs. These independent priority rankings can then be examined to determine areas of concordance and discordance. . . .
>
> Another approach to the evaluation of needs assessment techniques is the sequential use of multiple methods. . . . For example, hypotheses generated from the social and health indicators approach could be validated through surveys of community residents or professionals. Community forums could then be used to further validate, clarify, and generate increased support for intervention programs designed to meet identified needs [pp. 207–208].[1]

SOCIAL INDICATORS

Social indicators are statistics and other forms of information that enable a community (or nation) to assess its characteristics and to determine where it is in relation to where it wants to be. The act of collecting community information on some systematic and regular basis has a long tradition. The United States census has taken place every decade for nearly 200 years and now includes a large number of questions related to social conditions (questions about education, quality of housing, family composition, and so on). A hundred years ago, Herbert Spencer called for the collection and analysis of information on such variables as religion, culture, morals, styles of life, and use of leisure time and suggested that "these facts, given with as much brevity as consists with clearness and accuracy, should be so grouped and arranged that they may be comprehended in their ensemble, and contemplated as mutually dependent parts of one great whole. The aim should be so to present them that men may readily trace the consensus subsisting among them with the view of learning what social phenomena coexist with what others" (1882, p. v).

Although Spencer's interest appears to have been primarily theoretical, interest in applying the analysis of social variables came into being in the late

---

[1]From "Needs Assessment: A Critical Review," by J. Sallis and S. W. Henggeler. In *Administration in Mental Health*, 1980, 7, 200–209. Copyright 1980 by Human Sciences Press. Reprinted by permission.

1920s under the auspices of the federal government. It was hoped that once sources of social stress were identified, effective strategies for reducing them could be planned. Interrupted by the depression of the 1930s and by World War II, interest in the analysis of social variables reappeared after the war, first at the level of the United Nations and subsequently within the United States.

The term *social indicators* is generally attributed to Bauer, who in 1966 edited a book by that title. Since that year, the term has gained very wide usage. Indeed, in 1972, an annotated bibliography of more than 1000 works related to social indicators was published (Wilcox, Brooks, Beal, & Klonglan, 1972), and more than half of the listed works had been published since 1970. Sheldon and Parke say that such terms as *social indicators, social reporting,* and *social accounting*

> emerged from an awareness of rapid social change, from a sense of emerging problems with origins deep in the social structure, and from . . . a commitment to the idea that the benefits and costs of domestic social programs are subject to measurement and to the belief that each newly perceived, albeit ancient, inadequacy in the society should, and would, call forth a corrective response from a federal government whose efficacy would be assisted by social measurement, planning, and new management analytical techniques [1975, p. 693].

The most widely known definition of *social indicator* is found in a federal publication titled *Toward a Social Report.* According to this source, a social indicator is "a statistic . . . which facilitates concise, comprehensive and balanced judgments about the condition of major aspects of a society. It is in all cases a direct measure of welfare and is subject to the interpretation that, if it changes in the "right" direction, while other things remain equal, things have gotten better, or people are 'better off' " (U.S. Department of Health, Education and Welfare, 1969, p. 97). This definition includes three important components— the quantitative nature of the social indicator, its use in the assessment of both strengths and weaknesses of a community or a society, and its unambiguous interpretability. Social indicators are thus measures of social problems (or their absence) and, taken together, indicate the quality of life. By taking such measures from time to time, one should be able to see clearly whether social problems in a community are getting better or worse. Presumably, a problem could be identified that would be seen as so severe that there would be a call to action; subsequent measurements of the problem would serve to evaluate the effectiveness of the action program. Thus, social indicators, if properly chosen, can serve the same function at the community level that body temperature and IQ serve at the individual level. In a review of the social-indicator literature, Oborn says that "the two most important uses of social indicators stressed by writers at all levels are: (1) as guides in decision-making or policy making; and (2) as aids in evaluation of current programs" (1972, p. 10).

Rossi and Gilmartin (1980) have recently prepared a comprehensive handbook of social indicators in which they discuss the important characteristics and uses of social indicators, how to construct social indicators, both existing and new data sources for social indicators, and techniques for the analysis and reporting of findings that emerge from the study of such indicators.

Selection of social indicators

The idea of social indicators can be seen as an effort to develop an assessment procedure parallel to and complementary to the highly successful economic indicators, or economic index. Economic theory is relatively well developed, and the complex economic consequences of, for example, increasing unemployment are fairly well understood. Accordingly, the use of such an economic indicator as unemployment rate—or inflation rate, to cite another example—is well justified. Kahn proposes that the development of social indicators could, "to some degree, correct the incomplete or inaccurate picture of society derived from economic indicators alone and begin to remedy a tendency to underinvest in social data collection and analysis" (1969, p. 89). But there is considerable question about how one is to select from among the hundreds of pieces of social information one could collect in any community in the absence of any guiding theory or set of principles. Sheldon and Freeman (1970) suggest that

> evoking the economic analogy and proposing the development of social indicators that parallel economic indicators is confusing and in part fallacious. Despite its weaknesses and limited rigor, economic theory provides a definition and the specifications of an economic system, and the linkages are at least hypothesized, if not empirically demonstrated, between many variables in the system. . . . Although some social scientists have proposed similar usefulness for social indicators . . . this is not even a reasonable anticipation. There is no social theory, even of a tentative nature, which defines the variables of a social system and the relationships between them. . . . Yet, without the guidance of theoretical formulations concerning significant variables and their linkages, one can hardly suggest that there exists, even potentially, a set of measures that parallel the economic variables [pp. 102–103].[2]

Accordingly, most social indicators have been chosen by an inductive rather than a deductive procedure. Through analysis of the full spectrum of information available about any community, it has been possible to identify those specific variables that make major contributions to variations over time and to eliminate those variables that duplicate each other. As a consequence, social scientists have been able to select a small set of social indicators to apply to any community at periodic intervals. For example, the Urban Institute has proposed 14 aspects of the quality of life and for each aspect has selected one best indicator ("Measuring the Quality of Life," 1971). The 14 aspects are poverty, for which the indicator is the percentage of low-income households;

[2]From "Notes on Social Indicators: Promises and Potential," by E. B. Sheldon and H. E. Freeman, *Policy Sciences*, 1970, *1*, 97–111. This and all other quotations from this source are reprinted by permission of the authors and Elsevier Publishing Company, Amsterdam.

unemployment, for which the indicator is the percentage of unemployed; racial equality, indicated by the ratio of non-white unemployment to white unemployment; mental health, indicated by suicide rate; health, indicated by infant mortality rate; traffic safety, indicated by traffic-death rate; air pollution, indicated by the air-pollution index; income level, indicated by per-capita income; housing, indicated by the cost of housing; social disintegration, indicated by the narcotics-addiction rate; community concern, indicated by per-capita United Fund contributions; public order, indicated by reported-robbery rate; education, indicated by draft-rejection rate; and citizen participation, indicated by the presidential voting rate.

It is instructive to examine this list in some detail. First, the 14 aspects of quality of life were not deduced from any theory. They were simply thoughtfully selected. Other groups could well have chosen a somewhat different list. Second, each indicator is quantitative and readily available in most communities. Indeed, it might appear that one criterion used in the selection of the indicators was availability. Third, the indicators clearly differ in degree of closeness to the variables they purport to index. Thus, while the indicators of health, traffic safety, air pollution, and income level seem straightforward enough, using draft-rejection rate to index education, or suicide rate to index mental health, or narcotics-addiction rate to index social disintegration seems far more open to debate. Fourth, there is undoubtedly some redundancy in this list of indexes, and the list can probably be shortened. For example, it is likely that the indicators of poverty, income level, and housing are highly intercorrelated and that one of them could serve for all three. But until social indicators are derived from a theory of society or a theory of community, there is little alternative to being quite pragmatic in the initial selection of social indicators. After that, a variety of statistical procedures are available for determining independence and redundancy, and research studies can be undertaken for determining utility.

Other lists of social indicators have been proposed. A United Nations expert committee concerned with the measurement of "level of living" (United Nations, 1954) proposed 12 categories: health, food and nutrition, education, conditions of work, employment situations, aggregate consumption and savings, transportation, housing, clothing, recreation and entertainment, social security, and human freedoms. These 12 categories were subsequently collapsed into 7: nutrition, shelter, health, education, leisure, security, and environment (Drewnowski & Wolfe, 1966). In Denmark, the list includes the following categories: children and family, physically handicapped, social welfare, social gerontology, work force and labor conditions, agriculture, housing, youth and education, and leisure-time activities. In France, the list of categories for which data are currently being collected comprises: life expectancy, health protection, evolution of the family, participation of women in economic and social life, old people's place in society, behavior toward marginal populations, employment trends, role of education, cultural development, adaptation to change, social mobility, receptivity of society to the outside world, distribution of national wealth, utilization of income, pattern of assets, role of welfare, housing, organization of the countryside, urban development, and patterns of time utilization (U.S. Senate Committee on Labor and Public Welfare, 1970). In a recent U.S. government publication, the first to issue statistical data under the general heading of social indicators in such a way that they could be compared over time, information is organized around eight so-called social concerns: health, public safety, education, employment, income, housing, leisure and recreation, and population (U.S. Office of Management and Budget, 1973; see also Rossi, 1972, pp. 98–126).

As you can see, these lists have much in common; yet, each tends to emphasize certain aspects of the social condition and deemphasize others. In reviewing these various sets of social indicators, Oborn notes that "the various categorizations of social indicators according to subject area . . . are based on normatively selected areas of human needs, and while it is conceivable that one list of categories could be universally agreed upon, it is doubtful whether such agreement would ever take place or whether it is important that it should" (1972, p. 39).

Three socially relevant community characteristics appear to be of nearly universal interest—general health (sometimes including mental health and nutrition), education, and social welfare and public safety. Specific measures suggested for these general social-indicator areas include the following (U.S. Office of Management and Budget, 1973). For general health, specific measures of life expectancy, disability, and access to medical care have been proposed. Examples of measures of life expectancy are life expectancy at birth, life remaining at ages 30 and 50, and infant mortality rate. Examples of disability measures are days of disability per person per year, admission rates into mental hospitals and into nursing homes, rates at which persons are limited in their major activities because of chronic conditions, and injury rates. Examples of measures of access to medical care are extent of health-insurance coverage, proportion of expenditures for personal health care covered by private insurance, and personal confidence in ability to obtain good health care. For education, measures include high school graduation rate, school dropout rates, prekindergarten enrollment, reading achievement, rate of educational participation by the adult population, college-entrance rates, and number of degrees awarded. Measures of social welfare and public safety include percentage of persons below the poverty income level, number of substandard housing units, degree of satisfaction with neighborhood, rate of violent crimes, rate of crimes against property, and percentage of persons afraid to walk alone at night.

Two points should be made about these examples of social indicators. First, these indicators are both objective (life expectancy at birth) and subjective (personal confidence in ability to obtain good health care). Yet, whether the measures are objective or subjective, they are presented in quantitative terms. The point to be stressed is that there is no reason that attitudes or opinions cannot be assessed in reliable and quantified form. The second point is that in most cases, but not all, it is clear how changes in these indicators are to be interpreted. That is, one would like to see, over time, an increase in life expectancy, a decrease in infant mortality rate, a reduction in days of disability, an increase in reading achievement, and so on. But other indicators are more equivocal. Is a decrease in the admission rate into nursing homes or mental hospitals a good or a bad sign? Is a decrease in school dropout rate necessarily a good sign? Is it a good sign if there is no difference in reading comprehension or mathematical skill between high school graduates and those persons who drop out of high school before graduation?

Problems with social indicators

One general area of difficulty in the social-indicator approach to the analysis of community structure and community needs has already been mentioned—namely, the absence of a persuasive theory of community.

A related concern among persons who undertake critical reviews of the social-indicator literature has to do with the interpretation of changes in the magnitude of social indicators. If unemployment rises from 8% to 9%, few would see this increase as anything other than an indication of a growing problem. If body temperature goes up in a person already feverish, it is difficult to interpret that change as good news. But social-indicator changes are not that easily interpreted. An increase in the number of days lost from work because of illness or injury could signal a decrease in the health status of the employed population. But it could equally well indicate a liberalization of employment policies regarding sick leave (see Sheldon & Freeman, 1970, p. 98).

Fundamental in the development of social indicators, as in the development of any indirect measure, is the issue of validity—the degree of correspondence between an abstract concept (such as health or quality of life) and the procedure used to measure it. There is considerable criticism about the relation between certain social-indicator concepts and their measurement. In discussing measurement in the field of education, for example, Cohen says "When we survey the voluminous, yet unsuitable, data now available for assessing the products of education, we must conclude that practically none of it measures the output of our educational system in terms that really matter (that is, in terms of what students have learned)" (1967, p. 89). Although health-related expenditures are often used as an indicator of health status, Bell comments that "no one can say with any precision, what kind of correlation exists between various expenditures on health and the actual state of the nation's health" (1967, p. 80). The authors of *Toward a Social Report* (U.S. Department of Health, Education and Welfare, 1969) suggest that

> many of our statistics on social problems are merely a by-product of the informational requirements of routine management. This by-product process does not

usually produce the information that we most need for policy or scholarly purposes, and it means that our supply of statistics has an accidental and unbalanced character. . . . We have measures of death and illness, but no measures of physical vigor or mental health. We have measures of the level and distribution of income, but no measures of the satisfaction that income brings. We have measures of air and water pollution, but no way to tell whether our environment is, on balance, becoming uglier or more beautiful. We have some clues about the test performance of children, but no information about their creativity or attitude toward intellectual endeavor [pp. 96, xiv].

In a critical review of health-status indicators, Goldsmith (1972) asserts that definitions of health are ambiguous and imprecise (involving, as they do, such terms as *social well-being, fruitful creative living,* and *cheerful acceptance*), that the purposes of health-status indicators need to be clarified, and that most currently used measures are inadequate. In developed countries, general measures of mortality are no longer useful, because of the vastly decreased contribution of infectious disease to the overall mortality rate. Infant mortality rate (number of deaths of children under 1 year of age per 1000 live births), the most popular of all indexes of mortality, is of limited reliability and not particularly useful as a health indicator in developed countries. Measures of morbidity (illness) are even more difficult to interpret because of problems of definition (How sick is sick?), problems of reliability, and the extraordinary variation among cultural and ethnic groups in the reactions to the same apparent clinical condition (see Zola, 1966, for example).

Access to medical care, as already mentioned, is indexed by such measures as extent of health-insurance coverage, expenditures for health services, and degree of personal confidence in the ability to obtain good health care. Yet none of these indicators gets at the fundamental question—do people in need of medical care get it? A new approach to measuring access to medical care has been proposed by Taylor, Aday, and Andersen (1975). These authors asked a sample population, whose members had experienced 1 or more of 20 symptoms, how many times they had visited a physician for those symptoms. The authors then asked a panel of physicians the number of visits appropriate for these symptoms, and they noted the difference between the two sets of numbers. They found that "nonwhites, rural farm people, the poor, and those who have no usual place to go for medical care . . . have less access to care than would be judged appropriate . . . [and that there is] possible 'over-utilization' among certain groups such as children and people who see specialists as their regular source of care" (p. 39).

Another problem with social indicators is that their value for forecasting future social conditions and social issues is questionable. Predicting and explaining social phenomena are very different matters. Prediction is most precise under stable conditions; explanations are developed most validly under changing conditions. People in the business of social forecasting must assume that past trends can be extrapolated into the future. When the assumption is correct, the predictions seem magical. In those circumstances, however, predictions are likely to be trivial. Henry (1978) called the business of social fore-casting "the future hustle" and noted that econometric models built in the early 1960s functioned well during our stable economy of that decade but that forecasting errors in the economically unstable 1970s were so large as to make those models virtually useless.

Finally, although the literature suggests that social indicators are used mainly as guides to policy decisions and as aids in the evaluation of social programs, these two uses, according to Sheldon and Freeman (1970), are the ones least easily defended. With regard to the use of social indicators in form-ing policy decisions, they state:

> It would be foolish to argue against the use of indicators in program planning and development, or to expect their employment to disappear as a means of influencing politicians and their electorates. But it is naïve to hold that social indicators in themselves permit decisions on which programs to implement, espe-cially that they allow the setting of priorities. . . . Priorities do not depend on assembled data. Rather, they stem from national objectives and values and their hierarchical ordering.
>
> In short, when used for purposes of setting goals and priorities, indicators must be regarded as inputs into a complex political mosaic. That they are potentially powerful tools in the development of social policy is not to be denied. But they do not make social policy development any more objective. Advocates of policy can strengthen their position by citing hard data and so can critics of those policies. In a situation where all sides have equity of resources to gather, interpret, and communicate indicator information, it could be argued that social indicators can serve to develop a more rational decisionmaking process in social policy devel-opment. But this is unlikely to be the case very often and in instances of unfair competition indicators are essentially a lobbying device [pp. 99–100].

The notion that data are selectively used to support a point of view and that competing factions need to have equal access to sources of data is important. The same concept prevails in the legal profession—namely, that the adversary system works best when the two sides have access to equally qualified legal staff. In both instances, when the basic assumption of equal access fails, the process is corrupted.

With regard to the use of social indicators for program evaluation, Sheldon and Freeman say:

> Concurrent with the movement to promote social indicators, there has devel-oped a strenuous effort on the part of key individuals in and outside of govern-ment to estimate the gains that are derived from the initiation and expansion of different types of preventive and rehabilitative action programs. The terms "eval-uation research" and "cost benefits analysis" now are common jargon among a vast number of such practitioners, planners, and politicians. The rationality of being able to estimate the benefits of expenditures of money, time, and manpower is virtually incontestable, and the utility of knowing whether existing and inno-vative programs work clearly is desirable.
>
> The empirical situation however is that there have been but a handful of respect-able evaluation studies of social action programs: There simply are not very many

craftsmanlike evaluations of national programs, and there is increasing dissatisfaction with the failure to document by careful research the current massive programs now underway to improve the occupational, educational, mental and physical health status of community members. As a consequence, there is a temptation to argue for social indicators as a substitute for experimental evaluations. The fact . . . is, however, that social indicator analyses cannot approximate the necessary requirements of sound design in order to provide for program evaluation.

Investigators who have thought about the problems of evaluation generally agree that there is no substitute for experimental research that differentiates between the effects of treatments and programs . . . and of extraneous contaminating factors. . . . Experimentally designed evaluations often are not possible. . . .

The use of indicators to evaluate programs would require one to be able to demonstrate, via statistical manipulations, that programs determine the outcomes measured by the indicators rather than other factors "causing" the results. There is no possibility at the present time of meeting the requirements of controlling for contaminating variables with available statistics that may be regarded as indicators, at least ones that cover large groups of individuals. In order to locate and identify factors that may be contaminating, knowledge of the determinants and interrelationships between determinants is required. Information is not available in many fields of social concern to do such analyses well, either on an empirical basis or a theoretical one [pp. 100–101].

This is not to say that social indicators cannot be used for improved descriptive reporting, for analytical studies of social change, and for the prediction of future developments. But even these objectives, involving analyses of community characteristics and their changes, can be met only if measures are carefully chosen, reliably gathered, and skillfully analyzed.

ASSESSMENT OF LIFE QUALITY

Assessment of the quality of life is based on self-report measures, rather than on evaluation of objective measures such as annual income, value of owner-occupied housing, or crime rates. Campbell, who has been centrally involved in assessing life quality for 25 years, justifies the study of perceived life quality by noting:

We cannot understand the psychological quality of a person's life simply from a knowledge of the circumstances in which that person lives. There are many good reasons for knowing the context of people's lives—their environmental condition, their economic status, their work life—but none of this information gives us more than a partial explanation of why some people find their lives enjoyable and satisfying and some do not. The mind does indeed influence our perception of the world . . . [so] that the correspondence between our objective conditions and our subjective experience is very imperfect. If we try to explain the population's sense of well-being on the basis of objective circumstances, we will leave unaccounted for most of what we are trying to explain [1981, pp. 1–2].[3]

[3]From *The Sense of Well-Being in America: Recent Patterns and Trends*, by A. Campbell. Copyright © 1981 by McGraw-Hill Book Company. Used with the permission of McGraw-Hill Book Company.

Social scientists have been interested in the concept of quality of life for many years (for example, Andrews, 1974; Andrews & Withey, 1974, 1976; Flanagan, 1978; Zautra & Goodhart, 1979). According to Campbell, when people are asked the most important factors in determining their quality of life or sense of well-being, they mention, first, economic security, followed by family life, personal strengths, friendships, and the attractiveness of their physical environment. Few of these values can be measured in dollars. Rather, the sense of well-being is a private experience, and as Campbell notes, "we can only learn about it if the person is willing to tell us about it" (1981, p. 16).

Social scientists interested in salient community characteristics are increasingly realizing the importance of understanding quality-of-life judgments. In particular, they are interested in three general questions about life quality. First, what is happening to those judgments over time; second, do judgments of quality of life vary according to where people live; and third, do judgments of quality of life vary according to important demographic characteristics, such as sex, age, ethnic group, and socioeconomic status? Answering these questions requires that representative samples of community residents be located, that their opinions be skillfully solicited and analyzed, and that these opinion surveys be conducted more or less regularly.

The principal dependent measures used by Campbell and his associates in the assessment of well-being are (1) happiness, (2) positive and negative affect, or emotion, (3) life satisfaction, and (4) stress. The principal domains within which these questions of well-being are asked are marriage, family life, friendships, standard of living, work, neighborhood, place of residence, the nation, housing, education, health, and the self. Finally, the independent variables that Campbell and his colleagues have examined are these: (1) Status—for example, do people of high status (economic, educational, or occupational) enjoy more satisfying lives than people of low status? (2) Marriage—for example, are married people happier than unmarried people? (3) Social networks—for example, to what extent are people supported by a network of friends and family, and to what extent is this degree of support related to feelings of well-being? (4) Employment—for example, are people who work happier than people who are retired? (5) Neighborhoods and housing—for example, do the physical circumstances where people live have a significant relation to degree of happiness? (6) The nation—for example, is satisfaction with life in the United States associated with a sense of well-being? (7) Aging and the life span—for example, how is age associated with degree of happiness? (8) Health—for example, how do health and physical attractiveness relate to happiness, satisfaction with self, and sense of well-being?

Campbell's surveys took place in 1957, 1971, 1972, 1976, and 1978. In 1978 nearly 3700 persons were interviewed. Survey respondents were randomly selected from all over the continental United States, and the interviews, somewhat over one hour long, were conducted in the interviewees' homes.

As a sample of Campbell's findings on quality of life, two sets of data will be briefly described—information about community satisfaction and about satisfaction with the neighborhood. Campbell writes:

> The larger the community in which people live, the less likely they are to describe themselves as satisfied with it. . . . The public schools are the object of much criticism, much more than in the smaller communities. . . . The condition of the streets and roads, the collection of garbage, police protection, police-community relations, and adequacy of parks and playgrounds are all less well-regarded by people in the large cities than by people in the smaller towns. . . . Recent surveys have asked people living throughout the country where they would choose to live if they could have their preference. If these people all lived where they say they would like to live, the large cities would lose half their population and the rural areas would more than double. . . . The Great White Way which may have seemed attractive to small-town and rural people in earlier generations seems to have lost a good deal of its glitter. . . .
>
> In general people tend to express greater satisfaction with their neighborhood than they do with the larger community in which they live, although if they are satisfied with one, they are likely to be satisfied with the other. . . . It is clear that the poorer the condition of the buildings, the lower the satisfaction with the neighborhood. This is what one might expect; more surprising is the large number of people living in physically deteriorated areas who declare themselves entirely satisfied with their neighborhood. . . . Reasonably enough, people who do not know their neighbors are not as likely to express satisfaction with their neighborhood as people who do. . . . Satisfaction with neighborhood is most strongly determined by the individual's perception of the condition of neighborhood housing, of the friendliness of its residents, of its security from criminals, and of the convenience to work and shopping. Most Americans are generally satisfied with the neighborhood they live in. . . . But about 10 percent describe themselves as dissatisfied in some degree, and they are likely to perceive their neighborhoods as lacking in these important qualities [1981, pp. 153–157].

Zautra, Beier, and Cappel (1977) examined quality of life in a sample of 454 adult residents of a large suburban community who were interviewed in their homes. In addition to identifying the major dimensions in quality of life, these authors studied the extent to which these dimensions were influenced by six key demographic variables—age, sex, marital status, education, income, and religious participation.

In assessing quality of life, these authors measured the self-reported sense of contentment and pleasure, life changes, psychiatric symptoms, and major social-role performance in the areas of personal growth, family, work, household, economic, as well as church and community responsibilities. They also collected information on use of professional agencies in the community for dealing with personal problems. A factor analysis of the items making up the quality-of-life measure revealed three general dimensions—reports of happiness, community participation styles, and value preferences. The latter dimension seemed less important than the first two. The reports of happiness included happiness with family life, with personal life-style, with economic well-being,

and with the ability to manage life crises. The measure of community participation styles included such variables as family activities, work responsibilities, and social and religious participation and fellowship.

All six of the demographic variables were associated with the major quality-of-life factors. Of the six, age and marital status were the most important.
Many of the specific findings of the study can be noted in the following concluding comments provided by the authors:

> The demographic correlates of quality of life reflect major social inequities which
> a community creates for certain subgroups of community members. The results
> of this study show that life quality differs for males and females, and individuals
> with different education and income, and is even more variable for people of
> different ages and for single, married, and divorced individuals.
>
> The results suggest that the community resources available may short-change
> the younger groups who have higher Life Crises scores. . . . The older people, in
> contrast, appeared to have lesser needs for mental health services. They needed
> more activities of interest to them, more ways to participate in the community.
>
> The divorced respondents were also a troubled group, but not necessarily because
> of a marriage failure. . . . The results suggest that these people turn to community
> mental health centers for assistance. Different community services should be
> designed for the very different needs of these groups. . . .
>
> In summary, the findings suggest that the quality of life of members of a com-
> munity can be meaningfully, even though incompletely, assessed, and that such
> ratings can be usefully interpreted to compare communities and to understand
> better where a given community has its shortcomings [Zautra et al., 1977, p. 96].[4]

Shin (1980) compared two statistical procedures for measuring general
satisfaction with various aspects of community life in a study of nearly 1500
persons in seven Illinois cities who were interviewed by telephone and asked
to rate their satisfaction with the public schools, medical care, their housing,
government services, and neighborhood safety. Respondents, who were selected
by means of a random telephone dialing procedure, were asked to rate each
of these community aspects on a 4-point scale: very satisfied, somewhat satisfied, somewhat dissatisfied, or very dissatisfied.

The two procedures measured, first, average level of satisfaction with each
of the five community resources among the respondents in each city and,
second, variation of judgments of quality among citizens in each city for each
of the five community resources. That is, the first measure assesses average
level of judged quality, and the second assesses the distribution in those levels
of judged quality. It is Shin's argument that knowing the average level of
satisfaction of a group of citizens with a certain agency tells us very little about
the variation in those judgments of satisfaction and that both pieces of information are important in assessing community characteristics.

[4]From "The Dimensions of Life Quality in a Community," by A. Zautra, E. Beier, and L. Cappel.
In *American Journal of Community Psychology*, 1977, 5, 85–97. Copyright 1977 by Plenum Publishing
Corporation. Reprinted by permission.

Shin found that the two measures were quite independent of each other; that is, it was not possible to predict variability knowing average level of satisfaction. Accordingly, Shin concluded that "government officials and scholars should take into account both the levels and distributions of subjective indicators in order to assess and plan for the greatest amount of happiness among the greatest number of their citizens in the context of limited resources" (1980, pp. 533–534).

Handal, Barling, and Morrissy (1981) have developed a scale to assess characteristics of the residential environment. The scale taps both perceived and preferred social and physical characteristics of a neighborhood and also assesses level of satisfaction with the environment. Thus, in addition to the measure of satisfaction, it is possible to derive six measures that describe the environment—perceived social characteristics, perceived physical characteristics, preferred social characteristics, preferred physical characteristics, social-characteristics discrepancy score (the difference between perceived and preferred social characteristics), and physical-characteristics discrepancy score.

These authors first administered their test instrument to a sample of 120 residents in a single neighborhood. In this study, they tested three hypotheses, all of which were confirmed. First, they found that perceived physical characteristics played the greatest role in determining satisfaction. Second, measures of both perceived and preferred characteristics contributed significantly to neighborhood satisfaction. Third, the discrepancy scores between perceived and preferred measures were inversely related to satisfaction.

A second study (Morrissy & Handal, 1981) contrasted two differing neighborhoods. In addition, the test-retest reliability of the scale was examined. Morrissy and Handal found, first, that the scale had an acceptable level of reliability and, second, that the two neighborhoods differed on each of the six measures of neighborhood characteristics in predictable ways. They found, further, that the relationships between the six measures of neighborhood characteristics were related to the measure of satisfaction in a somewhat different pattern in the two neighborhoods, suggesting that satisfaction may have different meanings in different communities.

Cresswell, Corre, and Zautra (1981) assessed life stressors and perceived quality of life among the employees of a medical hospital for whom they were designing a counseling program. Using a measure of self-efficacy, obtained from a subset of items on the scale assessing perceived quality of life, as the major dependent variable, these authors found that the employees who were least satisfied in the various quality-of-life areas were those who were separated from their spouses, were over age 55, or had lower education levels, large families, and low incomes. These results were used in designing an employee counseling program.

> Because perceptions of self-efficacy were best predicted by family/support concerns, therapy programs which focus on these concerns could be most effective. Suggested interventions included workshops focusing on promoting more satis-

fying relationships among family members, managing parental responsibilities, and strengthening the marital bond. . . . Satisfaction with the quality of one's leisure activities was an unexpectedly strong predictor of perception of self-efficacy. . . . More attention to recreational concerns in treatment and planning programs was also recommended. . . .

Work concerns were also important to self-efficacy. . . . Because the employee-counseling program was affiliated with the work organization, it was in a unique position to assist both employees and their supervisors. A supervisory training program which focused on job design and effective superior-subordinate communications was suggested as a cost-effective way of improving employee job satisfaction. . . .

Our results indicated that positive perceptions of self-efficacy in general and job, family/support, and financial experiences were related to positive life events. Programs could thus be implemented to assist employees in identifying and enhancing specific positive experiences on-the-job and in family environments [Cresswell et al., 1981, pp. 159–160].[5]

CONCLUSIONS AND OVERVIEW

By the skillful combination of social-indicator data, subarea-characteristic analyses, and need assessments, it should be possible to develop a useful view of the community as a social system with its strengths and weaknesses. On the basis of such analyses, proposals for reducing or eliminating weaknesses and increasing strengths can be presented to the community and debated. Conflicting ideologies about the quality of life and about the role of human service agencies in improving the quality of life can be identified and debated as well. One special consequence of conducting an open assessment of community organization and needs is that the decision-making processes of community governments and human service agencies become more public and the decision makers more informed.

A number of years ago, Warren (1965) prepared a book called *Studying Your Community*, designed to help citizens and community workers take a systematic look at some important aspects of their communities. It is instructive to review the aspects of the community that Warren identifies as worthy of examination in order to make sure that, in our attention to the details of community assessment, we do not lose sight of the major overall dimensions of the task. These community aspects comprise (1) the background, history, traditions, and setting of the community, (2) its economic life, employment, and working conditions, (3) its governmental structure, politics, and criminal justice system, (4) its processes of community planning, especially zoning and land use, (5) housing conditions and urban redevelopment, (6) its educational system, libraries, and museums, (7) recreation, both commercial and publicly

---

[5]From "A Needs Assessment of Perceived Life Quality and Life Stressors among Medical Hospital Employees," by S. L. Cresswell, B. H. Corre, and A. Zautra. In *Journal of Community Psychology*, 1981, 9, 153–161. Reprinted by permission.

supported, (8) its religious traditions and activities, (9) its public assistance and welfare services, (10) community services for children and families, (11) health services, including provisions for special groups such as the aged or the handicapped, (12) communication media, (13) intergroup relations and tensions, (14) participation in voluntary organizations, and (15) the process whereby various community services and organizations are coordinated.

This chapter has touched on almost every one of these community attributes. An increased understanding of the community on the part of community leaders can be extremely helpful in their efforts to improve the quality of life of community citizens.

CHAPTER
9

Community Psychology

Most mental health professionals working in community mental health centers are clinically trained, and as we have seen, their primary concerns are with the emotional well-being of the persons they serve. For these professionals, the community mental health movement holds the hope that the mental health service delivery system can be reorganized so as to better meet community needs, that innovative mental health services and mental health resources can be developed that will reduce the prevalence of emotional disorders in the community, and that preventive services can be established that will reduce the incidence of emotional disorders. Some of these hopes have been realized, and others will surely be realized in the future.

Yet, all along, many mental health professionals have been uneasy about this effort to get more services more quickly to more people. There has been the fear that the additional psychotherapy, the early casefinding, the expanding consultation might allow professionals to deal more effectively with troubles but not with issues—a helpful distinction proposed by C. Wright Mills (1959). *Troubles* arise when an individual's values are perceived as being threatened; *issues* arise when a society's values are so perceived. Rappoport and Kren have said that "any matter involving controversy or uncertainty over the well-being of substantial numbers of people can be called a social issue" (1975, p. 838). Although the community mental health movement may be successfully addressing itself to the treatment of troubles, we must go beyond community mental health if we are to resolve the issues. The conceptual and scholarly field concerned with analyzing and modifying social systems and dealing with social issues from the point of view of psychology is called *community psychology*. A number of books have been published that concern themselves almost entirely with this new field (see, for example, Gibbs, Lache-meyer, & Sigal, 1980; Heller & Monahan, 1977; Iscoe, Bloom, & Spielberger, 1977; Mann, 1978; Rappaport, 1977; Sarason, 1974; Zax & Specter, 1974).

CONCERNS OF THE COMMUNITY PSYCHOLOGIST

Goodstein and Sandler (1978) have examined the field of psychology from the point of view of the promotion of human welfare. In this task, they identify four specialties of psychology—clinical psychology, community mental health, community psychology, and public-policy psychology. Each approach is examined in terms of the target population, the content and approach of the intervention, and the necessary knowledge base. In their analysis, they pay particular attention to the fields of community mental health and community psychology and suggest that since these two fields have such basic differences in philosophy, target, content, process, and knowledge base, they would do well to disengage from each other.

For example, whereas the field of community mental health looks toward troubled individuals and members of the helping professions within a given catchment area as its principal targets, the field of community psychology looks toward social systems—systems of deviance control and of socialization and support—as its principal targets. Community mental health is concerned with service delivery and its evaluation and with such indirect services as mental health consultation, training, mental health education, and program planning and coordination; community psychology is concerned with social-system analysis and social-system modification. As for the approach to inter-vention or the intervention process, Goodstein and Sandler write: "It is no longer enough for the professional psychologist to work competently and humanely with individuals needing help; professionals must work to change the norms, values, and structures of systems" (1978, p. 888).

Finally, whereas the knowledge base of the clinical psychologist comes from the clinical literature, and the knowledge base of the community mental health psychologist is supplemented to draw on program-evaluation literature as well as the literature on such techniques as mental health consultation and mental health education, the knowledge base of the community psychologist must include such fields as group process, decision making, planned social change, social-systems theory, the sociology of deviance, environmental and ecological psychology, and organizational development. It can therefore be argued that whereas the field of community mental health is concerned mainly with preventing emotional disorders and with finding innovative ways of helping individuals adjust to existing social systems, the field of community psychology is concerned mainly with changing social systems to better meet the needs of those individuals.

Rappaport (1977) says that a psychologist working in the community must be interested and involved in reshaping social structures to serve the people who live within them. Similarly, Muñoz, Snowden, and Kelly (1979) say that community psychologists need to function in natural settings, playing the roles of observer, participant, and change agent.

In a recent critical analysis of this postulated domain of community psychology, McClure, Cannon, Allen, Belton, Connor, D'Ascoli, Stone, Sullivan, and McClure (1980) suggest that although community psychology and community mental health can be distinguished in theory, these two fields are not yet distinguished in practice. They note that the commonly agreed-on defining characteristics of the community psychology orientation are "(a) a competency-prevention-oriented theoretical perspective, (b) a preference for organizational and community ecological levels of intervention, and (c) the need for an ecologically valid research base" (p. 1000), and that "community psychology's competence-enhancement or primary-prevention orientation and its organizational-community intervention level are believed to differentiate it from the deficit or repair orientation and the individual/small-group intervention level of community mental health and clinical psychology" (p. 1001).

These authors examined the contents of four major journals in the fields of community mental health, community psychology, and social psychology. They found that these conceptual distinctions are yet to be reflected in the nature of the published research. They concluded that "no evidence was found supporting the position that community psychologists are more likely than community mental health professionals to be oriented toward non-deficit, competence-building, primary-prevention, or organizational-community theoretical perspectives or interventions" (1980, p. 1007). In addition, they concluded that "the data indicate virtually no growth of an interpretable, empirical, intervention research base clarifying the relationships between individual functioning and higher ecological variables. The vast majority of well-designed empirical research studies reported in these four journals were at the traditional individual/small-group level" (p. 1007). McClure et al. believe, however, that the "failure to intervene and assess at community-organizational levels reflects more a failure to develop a technology distinctive from traditional mental health individual/small-group approaches than a failure to conceptualize on an ecological level" (p. 1008).

Dealing with societal issues rather than with individual troubles requires the examination of a new set of postulates and assumptions and a commitment to a new set of tasks. Reiff (1968) articulated the basic postulate when he affirmed that social forces play a significant role in determining human behavior. He suggested that, therefore, the primary task in community psychology is to intervene at the social-system level. The social environment does not have to be a source only of demands and constraints; it can also provide rewards that do not depend entirely on the satisfaction of inner impulses. The social environment can be a source of stimulation and challenge, and these attributes can lead to changes in behavior and to changes in ego structure that alter the balance of intrapsychic forces (see Fried, 1964).

While the clinician generally assumes that the locus of a problem lies within the individual, the community psychologist has the option of assuming that the locus may be within the social system—that human misery is created by the community. The clinician has traditionally made a commitment to the patient, believing that each patient is unique, accepting continuing responsibility for the care of that patient, and acknowledging ultimate accountability to that patient. To the community psychologist, it is the community that is unique and the community to which he or she is committed and accountable. Rather than having needs defined by other mental health professionals or by colleagues in the helping services, the community psychologist looks to the entire community for a definition of needs. And the needs that are of greatest interest are not restricted to traditional mental health problems. To the community psychologist, whatever aspects of the community act to limit quality of life are of concern.

The community psychologist is interested in determining how the community creates and perpetuates disability and in how it enhances development and growth. Even though the relationship between people and their social context can be enhanced by improved individual adaptation, the community psychologist's commitment is to improve this relationship by effecting changes in the social systems in which people live—by redesigning the host environment so that the symptom disappears (Kelly, 1970). Because of this commitment, the community psychologist must evaluate interventions by their social consequences, as well as by their clinical consequences. He or she must anticipate problems and help plan for the future of the community rather than respond only to the community crisis of the moment. And the community psychologist must take a broad view of community resources. For, in fact, resources—ideas, assistance, and support—are everywhere in the community. These sources of help must be located and linked together.

With this background, you can begin to anticipate what ideological, conceptual, and empirical issues are of central concern to the community psychologist: What makes for a healthy community? How is the community to be conceptualized? How can its subsystems be identified and their interdependencies documented? How is individual behavior affected, both for good and for bad, by these social systems and social processes? How can the nature of social support systems within the community be determined? What methods of social-system intervention can increase the satisfactions we attain in our communities? How are decisions made in the community, and how can the decision-making process be democratized? What methods and concepts will permit us to anticipate needs and to develop resources to meet these needs before they reach crisis proportions? And how can interdependence be fostered so that a true sense of community develops?

The task of understanding and changing community dynamics is not easy. It has been asserted that social factors influence behavior, that we need to change environments rather than people (Shatan, 1969), and that our goals should be to make communities sources of health (Kubie, 1968), but critics have pointed out that we have no theory of community intervention (Hersch, 1968), that we do not understand how the community works or how to change it, that we have no techniques for influencing social policy or treating the community, that the relation of community forces to the production of psychopathology is far from clear (Dunham, 1965), and that we have no evidence that social change will eradicate mental illness (Kolb, 1968a).

In spite of these assertions, which properly attest to our very limited understanding of what or who the community is, in the minds of many advocates of the newly emerging view of community mental health there is no alternative other than to learn more about the interactions between community dynamics and individual dynamics. The new community mental health professional should have, in the words of Kelly, "the spirit of a naturalist who dotes on his environment; of the journalist, who bird-dogs his story; and of the conservationist, who glows when he finds a new way to describe man's interdependence with his environment. The recommended way to prevent professional extinction is participation in the local community; the preferred antidote for arrogance is an ecological view of man" (1970, p. 524).

That this gradual transition from a primary interest in the individual to a primary interest in the society has been taking place in the thinking of theorists and practitioners is amply illustrated in a recent review of NIMH-sponsored research (Segal, 1975). Segal describes how this change was manifested in research in the field of race relations.

A quarter of a century ago, it was still widely believed that discriminatory behavior simply reflected prejudiced attitudes; the sole research emphasis was the psychodynamics of prejudice. But then it was learned that most discrimination results not from blatant bigotry but from the ordinary behavior of people who, at worst, are "the gentle people of prejudice," people who simply follow standard institutional practices, be they discriminatory or nondiscriminatory. The questions have more and more become: Why are institutional practices as they are? What forces make for continuity and for change in patterns of race relations?

With this broadening of research perspective has come a number of concomitant shifts in the nature of the research. From being almost entirely concerned with measuring prejudice and its place in personality dynamics, the research has shifted . . . to studying institutional practices and the complex interaction of individual personality, situational context, and larger institutional organization. From being preoccupied with assessments of personality, particularly with devising adequate tests of prejudice, the research has shifted . . . to studying behavior in its natural contexts, particularly the comparative study of how the same individuals behave in a variety of discriminatory and nondiscriminatory situational and institutional contexts. From being preoccupied with the individual, the research emphasis has shifted . . . to studying larger social and economic structures, including political-economic systems as a whole. And in what may be the most important shift of all, research that was once almost entirely preoccupied with static arrangements has come more and more to realize the strategic research value of studying the processes of social and individual change [p. 280].[1]

In the field of poverty research, Segal notes a similar trend.

In the recent past, the focus was on the psychology of the poor, an underlying and often explicit assumption being that a "culture of poverty," transmitted from generation to generation, kept the poor from rising in the stratification system. Out of a raging controversy over the validity of such an attribution of cause has come a recognition that the values and attitudes of the poor represent adaptation to a set of social and economic conditions. These values and attitudes are readily modified by changing conditions. Moreover, recent evidence on intergenerational mobility clearly demonstrates that the culture of poverty has little to do with determining who in any generation falls to the bottom of the social scale. The underlying factors are to be found more in the educational and occupational systems, in racial discrimination, in the treatment of the aged, and in our system of financing medical catastrophes [pp. 280–281].[1]

To cite one more example, research in the field of crime and delinquency has shown a similar transition in recent years.

At one time, research in this field was predicated on the assumption that one could neatly dichotomize the adult population into criminals and noncriminals, the juvenile population into delinquents and nondelinquents. The object of research was to characterize the personalities, life histories, or genetic endowments of the criminals or delinquents; the natural subjects of such research were those convicted of and incarcerated for criminal acts. The assumption that it makes sense to thus dichotomize the population has proved to be false; there are very few members of the population who have not committed some violation of law at some time in their lives. The genesis of criminality, though still not precisely known, is at least known to lie in the interaction of biological potential, life experience, personality, situational exigency, and social structural locus. And incarcerated criminals and delinquents have long since been shown to provide a very biased sample from which to generalize [pp. 281–282].

These interests in person/environment interaction, in ways of influencing human behavior through the analysis and modification of environments or societal values, and in issues far broader than mental health have emerged in all mental health professions. They have influenced the activity patterns of community nurses, community social workers, and community psychiatrists and have prompted the development of the field of community psychology (see Anderson, Cooper, Hassol, Klein, Rosenblum, & Bennett, 1966; Kelly, 1971).

The field of theory, research, and practice that is related to, but beyond the domain of, community mental health is almost limitless, and a full explo-

[1]This and the following two quotations are from *Research in the Service of Mental Health: Report of the Research Task Force of the National Institute of Mental Health*, by J. Segal (Ed.). Department of Health, Education and Welfare, Publication No. (ADM) 75–236. Washington, D.C.: U.S. Government Printing Office, 1975.

ration of it is well beyond the scope of this volume. It includes concern for patient rights, child advocacy, rape prevention, race relations, poverty, crime and delinquency, environmental protection, housing improvement, population control and family planning, sexual orientation, desegregation, drug use and abuse, and self-destructive behaviors, to mention but a few topics. Accordingly, two major areas of activity from this large field—social ecology and environmental assessment, and population research—have been selected to illustrate important recent developments in community-relevant social-science concern. Discussion of these two areas can serve only to suggest the nature of a far greater body of knowledge.

SOCIAL ECOLOGY AND ENVIRONMENTAL ASSESSMENT

Freeman (1978) has reviewed some of the recent research on mental health and the environment. He notes that "scientific investigation of the relationship between the environment and mental health involves mainly ecology and epidemiology; the first discipline is concerned with studying living organisms in relation to their environment and the second with variations in rates of illness related to the strengths of environmental factors in different populations" (p. 117).

Insel (1980) has recently summarized the status of the field of social ecology as it relates to mental health. Since, from the social-ecological perspective, mental health is intimately linked to the social environment, "the sine qua non of preventing mental illness involves understanding and assessing the social environment" (p. 63).[2] According to Insel, the field of social ecology is at present concerned mainly with the preliminary steps of conceptualizing and classifying social environments.

The social and physical components of any environment give it its unique character. Assessing environmental characteristics appears to be just as difficult as measuring individual personality, but important first steps have been taken. Approaches to environmental assessment fall into two general categories: (1) self-report measures collected from persons who live in the environment or act as observers of it and (2) objective measures that assess such variables as noise level, population density, temperature, lighting, humidity, and color. Self-report measures include scales assessing a wide variety of social characteristics, such as conflict, cohesion, expressiveness, leadership styles, and adaptability.

Studies have shown relations between rates of emotional illness and both physical and social characteristics of the environment. Before effective environmental interventions can be undertaken, though, it will be necessary to make significant progress in four areas. First, we must develop an adequate

[2]From "Task Force Report: The Social Climate of Mental Health," by P. M. Insel. In *Community Mental Health Journal*, 1980, 16, 62–78. Copyright 1980 by Human Sciences Press. This and all other quotations from the same source are reprinted by permission.

concept of how the environment affects mental health. Insel proposes that "environmental variables account for more variance in behavior than measures of either personality traits or biographic or demographic background data. . . . The way people perceive their surroundings influences the way they behave in that environment" (1980, pp. 75–76).

Second, we need a classification scheme for measuring and comparing widely different environments along similar dimensions. "Although there are a variety of approaches to classifying social environments, the conceptual consistency of the typologies developed to date argues for a limited number of underlying dimensions. Relationship, personal development, and system maintenance and system change variables are constants in the analyses of social environments" (Insel, 1980, p. 76).

Third, we need to investigate the relations between environmental variables and behavioral or psychological outcomes. Again, Insel comments: "This area of study requires research under controlled conditions. Once particular environments are identified as harmful to mental health, interventions can be designed to change destructive conditions. The relevant questions here are what are the most effective means of changing social environments? what are the problems or obstacles obstructing change? and what are the side effects of changing social environments? (1980, p. 76).

Finally, it will be important to undertake those studies necessary to determine what the most effective interventions are. Insel points out that although development of this area must wait until the interventions are available, it is clear that "participatory planning and continual monitoring of environments by those who must function within them increase the probability of achieving an optimum environment" (1980, p. 76).

Brogan and James (1980) undertook a factor analysis of a very large number of both physical and sociocultural environmental indexes in a random sample of 100 of the 743 city blocks forming one community mental health center catchment area in Atlanta, Georgia, and related them to 29 indexes of deviant psychosocial behaviors. This analysis made it possible to contrast physical with sociocultural indexes in terms of their relations to deviant behavior. Deviant behavior was gauged by such measures as arrest rates, homicides, fires, known drug problems, number of patients in psychiatric inpatient and outpatient facilities, and high school dropouts.

The more than 100 indexes of the physical environment and the more than 100 indexes of the sociocultural environment were reduced to 25 and 18 indexes, respectively, by means of a series of data-reduction analyses. The final physical-environment indexes included such variables as percentage of front yards that are dirt, percentage of block area covered in trees, percentage of front yards with cars in them, percentage of yards that are fenced, and average morning noise in decibels. Sociocultural indexes included such variables as percentage of families with income below poverty level, average number of persons per room, percentage of structures with ten or more family units, and percentage of population in professional or managerial occupations.

The results of this analysis yielded a list of physical and sociocultural variables that were significantly associated with each of the psychosocial-deviance measures. Physical variables and sociocultural variables contributed about equally to each of these associations. Studies of this type need to be repeated in order to determine whether any of these relationships are stable either across time or across communities. Results of such studies, in the words of the authors,

> could be used to estimate probable levels of various . . . problems and facility needs for dealing with them. A very important additional point is that the physical environment in urban areas is largely shaped by decisions being made by the urban-planning profession, and these decisions are now being made in ignorance of whatever effects, for better or for worse, they may have on the psychosocial health of the people who live in the environments created [Brogan & James, 1980, p. 520].

A similar study conducted earlier (Bloom, 1966) examined the relations of census-tract characteristics in Pueblo, Colorado, to nine measures of social disequilibrium—familial disruption (proportion of persons under age 18 not living with both parents), marital disruption, unemployment rate, proportion of households in which there was a fire, proportion of students who dropped out of school, juvenile delinquency rate, public and private first-admission rates for psychiatric disability, and suicide rate. Environmental measures included assessments of community participation, family characteristics, socioeconomic measures, housing characteristics, general-health measures, and several demographic variables.

Social disequilibrium was generally highest in census tracts with relatively few single-family homes, higher proportions of persons with Spanish surnames, less community participation, lower educational level, and lower median family income. Familial and marital disruption, juvenile delinquency, and public-psychiatric-hospital admission rates were high in census tracts characterized by a high proportion of foreign-born persons, high female median age, low community participation, low population per household, low educational level, low socioeconomic level, relatively few single-family homes and homes that were new, many vacant housing units, and high incidence of tuberculosis. The relation of social disequilibrium and low socioeconomic status and high social isolation seems clear from these findings, although the cause-and-effect relationship is undoubtedly more complex than simply a matter of financial status.

Theories of social causation will gain credibility, however, only when correlation findings such as these are extended to prospective studies that show that changes in environmental characteristics can result in subsequent reduction of social disequilibrium. Monahan and Vaux (1980) illustrate the growing interest in the relations between characteristics of the environment and mental health by examining two particular environmental domains—the physical and the economic. They examined two physical characteristics in detail—noise and population density. In the economic environment, Monahan and Vaux examined economic status, unemployment, and economic change.

As for the effects of noise on mental health, Monahan and Vaux summarize the literature by noting that "under certain circumstances noise may decrease attention and affiliative behavior between people, increase aggressive behavior, decrease the probability that people will come to one another's aid, and contribute to tension-related illness" (p. 17). As for population density, Monahan and Vaux conclude that although results of investigations are not always in agreement, "density may clearly impair performance, depress mood, obstruct social affiliation, generate social withdrawal, and contribute to helplessness, decrease helping behavior, and contribute to health problems" (p. 18). As for the relation between socioeconomic variables and mental health, Monahan and Vaux conclude that "socioeconomic status, unemployment, and societal economic change seem to have an effect on a wide variety of physical, behavioral, and affective problems, although these effects are heavily mediated by individual difference variables such as social support" (p. 21).

The final conclusions of Monahan and Vaux warrant quoting:

> We believe that whenever environmental stressors may be prevented or diminished, as in the case of noise, the mental health professional should make every effort to do so. Participation in the environmental impact assessment process is one likely medium for such activity. When the macroenvironmental stressors are not preventable—for example, regional economic change—the major role of the community mental health professional is to mitigate their effects. Techniques such as anticipatory guidance and attribution therapy, carried out individually and through the media, may be of value [p. 23].[3]

McLean and Tarnopolsky (1977) have reviewed the published work on how noise affects humans and animals from the standpoint of mental health. They have concluded that although under certain circumstances noise can be a stressor, the level of annoyance associated with various noise levels varies enormously, and very little reliable evidence exists connecting noise to subsequent mental illness. Since noise level and annoyance are largely independent of each other, these authors suggest that it is important to study the relation of annoyance with noise to mental health.

In a subsequent study of aircraft noise, Tarnopolsky, Barker, Wiggins, and McLean (1978) found that level of annoyance was clearly related to psychiatric measures. In particular, hypersensitivity to noise was associated with a high frequency of psychiatric symptoms (see also Graeven, 1974).

The federal government has become sufficiently concerned with the effects of the environment on health so that the Committee on Vital and Health Statistics of the National Center for Health Statistics convened a technical-consultant panel to advise the committee on statistical data that should be

---

[3]From "Task Force Report: The Macro-Environment and Community Mental Health," by J. Monahan and A. Vaux. In *Community Mental Health Journal*, 1980, 16, 14–26. Copyright 1980 by Human Sciences Press. Reprinted by permission.

collected that would help increase understanding of the health effects of the environment. The consultants concluded that preventing those environmental conditions that affect human health is a cost-effective strategy for preventing disease and impairment. In particular, they concluded that a large but hard-to-estimate proportion of the burden of such diseases as cancer and heart disease can be attributed to environmental exposures. The consultant panel recommended a series of studies that would help clarify the effects of environmental characteristics on health, such as the establishment of a national death index to permit determination of whether members of a group of persons of known environmental exposure have died and, if so, where and when the death occurred (U.S. Department of Health, Education and Welfare, 1977b).

Assessment of environments

In the history of efforts to understand human behavior, the most fundamental generally shared belief has been that human behavior is a consequence of the interactions of personal and environmental characteristics. Yet, until quite recently research has concentrated almost exclusively on attempts to understand behavior solely as a function of personal characteristics. There has been growing evidence, however, that much of the variability of human behavior can be accounted for by situational and environmental variables. Furthermore, it now seems recognized that there is an upper limit on the ability to predict human behavior solely on the basis of personal characteristics. What is perhaps of greatest concern, this upper limit is thought to be relatively low, leaving perhaps three-quarters of the variations in human behavior unexplained (Arthur, 1971; Barker, 1968; Barker & Gump, 1964; Ekehammar, 1974; Endler & Hunt, 1968; Moos, 1976; Proshansky, 1976; Wandersman & Moos, 1981). These ideas help explain the growth of interest in assessment of situational and environmental characteristics.

In review of the methods that have been used to conceptualize human environments, Moos (1973) has identified six interrelated practices. First, environments have been characterized by their *ecological dimensions,* such as geography, meteorology, or architecture, and the relations between these dimensions and human behavior—for example, the relation between climate and productivity or between environmental noise and social interaction—have been assessed. Second, largely through the work of Barker and his colleagues, certain environments have been identified as *behavior settings*—stable units external to the individual that have a powerful influence on the behavior that occurs within them (Wicker, 1979). A complex methodology has been developed for identifying and categorizing behavior settings (Barker, 1968). Third, organizational environments have been described in terms of their *size, staffing patterns,* and *supervisory structures,* and these characteristics have been shown to be related to organization members' behavior and attitudes. Other commonly studied aspects of organizational environments include *turnover rate* and *population density.* Fourth, environments have been described by the predominant *characteristics of their inhabitants,* and the behavior of newcomers—for example, college freshmen—has been shown to be related to characteristics of persons already in the environment. Fifth, behavior has been related to perceived *organizational climate,* which involves such factors as mutual involvement and support of members and likelihood of personal growth. Finally, environments have been viewed in terms of their *reinforcement practices*—that is, in terms of what behaviors are encouraged or discouraged.

There are two reasons to assess environmental characteristics and their impact on human behavior. First, since disordered human functioning may be rooted, to some extent, in the social system within which the functioning takes place, modifying environments may promote more effective behaviors. Virtually all social institutions—families, prisons, hospitals, business organizations, to mention but a few—are interested in creating environments that will have particular consequences for their members. Second, this type of assessment allows *environmental placement,* which means matching up a set of objectives with regard to a particular prospective college student or foster child, for example, with a university or family environment that will facilitate the attainment of those objectives.

Obviously, not all environments have been identified, much less studied. Environments that have received considerable attention thus far include junior and senior high school classrooms, correctional institutions, community-oriented psychiatric treatment programs, psychiatric wards, college campuses, and families. The psychological climate of psychiatric wards has been studied. The Ward Atmosphere Scale (Moos, 1974), which can be completed by patients or by staff, has been developed for this purpose (see Table 9–1). Public school classrooms are being studied by Moos and Trickett, who have developed a parallel scale for assessing classroom environments (Moos & Trickett, 1974; Trickett & Moos, 1973).

In a recent examination of alternative ways to assess classroom climate, Kaye, Trickett, and Quinlan (1976) contrasted three measures of teacher support and teacher control—two of the nine dimensions assessed by the Classroom Environment Scale—in a sample of 16 classrooms taught by 16 different teachers. The first measure was of perceived environment. (Measuring perceived environment is the method most commonly used for environmental assessment.) Certain items on the Classroom Environment Scale served this purpose. Second, global ratings of these two dimensions were made by outside observers. Third, analyses of specific aspects of teacher/student interactions were made by judges listening to tape recordings of classroom sessions. The authors found that the two dimensions under study (teacher support and teacher control) were not independent but, in fact, were strongly negatively correlated. They also found that the three measures of each dimension were in far higher agreement for teacher control than for teacher support, and on the basis of their findings they encouraged the use of multiple methods of environmental assessment. This conclusion is often reached by researchers in the field of personality assessment.

TABLE 9–1. Examples of items on the Ward Atmosphere Scale.
R denotes items scored in reverse.

Involvement
   1. Patients put a lot of energy into what they do around here.
   2. The patients are proud of this ward.
Support
   1. Doctors have very little time to encourage patients. *(R)*
   2. Staff are interested in following up patients once they leave the hospital.
Spontaneity
   1. Patients tend to hide their feelings from one another. *(R)*
   2. Patients say anything they want to the doctors.
Autonomy
   1. Patients are expected to take leadership on the ward.
   2. Patients here are encouraged to be independent.
Practical orientation
   1. New treatment approaches are often tried on this ward.
   2. Patients are encouraged to plan for the future.
Personal problem orientation
   1. Patients tell each other about their personal problems.
   2. Patients hardly ever discuss their sexual lives. *(R)*
Anger and aggression
   1. Patients often criticize or joke about the ward staff.
   2. Staff sometimes argue with each other.
Order and organization
   1. Patients' activities are carefully planned.
   2. The staff make sure that the ward is always neat.
Program clarity
   1. The patients know when doctors will be on the ward.
   2. If a patient's medicine is changed, a nurse or doctor always tells him why.
Staff control
   1. The staff very rarely punish patients by restricting them. *(R)*
   2. If a patient argues with another patient, he will get into trouble with the
      staff. *(R)*

From *Evaluating Treatment Environments: A Social Ecological Approach,* by R. H. Moos.
Copyright 1974 by John Wiley & Sons, Inc. Reprinted by permission.

In reviewing recent efforts to describe various environmental settings,
Insel and Moos (1974) have concluded that three environmental dimensions
are measured in all these efforts. The first they call the *relationship* dimension—
that is, the nature and intensity of personal relationships within the environment, including, for example, staff support, peer cohesion, and affiliation.
The second dimension is *personal development*—the opportunity offered to individuals in the environment for personal growth and the development of self-
esteem. The third dimension, *system maintenance and change,* has to do with
the extent to which the environment is orderly and clear in its expectations,
maintains control, and is responsive to change. You can see that the items of
the Ward Atmosphere Scale shown in Table 9–1 are designed to measure these
three dimensions.

   Kohn, Jeger, and Koretzky (1979) have challenged Moos's three-factor
theory of stable characteristics of environments. Kohn et al. believe the data

are better explained on the basis of only two somewhat differently described factors. They obtained data from a sample of patients and staff at a residential treatment center for emotionally disturbed and delinquent boys and girls. The patients completed an environmental assessment scale for both the classroom environment where they went to school and the cottages where they lived.

In contrast to Moos's view that most environments can be characterized by the three factors of relationship, personal development, and system maintenance, Kohn et al. found only the first and third factors in their data. On the basis of their analysis, they renamed the two factors (1) support-involvement versus disinterest and (2) order-organization versus disorder-disorganization. Trickett and Quinlan (1979), however, found support for the Moos three-factor theory of environments in their analysis of data they had collected regarding classroom environments.

Trickett and Wilkinson (1979) examined the question of level of analysis of environmental descriptions. Their rationale for this examination was rooted in both conceptual and methodological distinctions between individual and group data. They noted that "if one analyzes perceived environment data using individuals as the unit, one finds, strictly speaking, individual differences in how environments are perceived, not differences in environments per se. Methodologically, if the intent is to describe environments rather than individuals, statistical analyses should be based on group, not individual, data" (p. 498).

Basing their analysis on data obtained from nearly 3500 students in more than 200 classrooms who completed a scale describing classroom environments, Trickett and Wilkinson found that the pattern of intercorrelations of the various scales with each other was virtually identical whether individual-student or classroom scores were examined. Thus, although the difference between using individuals and classrooms as the unit of analysis is conceptually important, the two methods yield very similar results for purposes of understanding the perceived environment.

Family assessment

During most of our lives, no environment is more central to us than our family. Most of us grow up in a family, and when we become adults we start our own family. Consequently, it is hardly surprising that considerable attention is being devoted to conceptualizing and describing families and to studying how family characteristics determine individual behavior (see, for example, Framo, 1972; Kantor & Lehr, 1977; Levy & Munroe, 1938; Lewis, Beavers, Gossett, & Phillips, 1976; Winter & Ferreira, 1969).

The independent variables in these studies are family characteristics. Some techniques for assessing family characteristics are based on observation or on laboratory experiments (see, for example, Mishler & Waxler, 1968; Reiss, 1971; Strodtbeck, 1951), but most are based on self-report measures. The Family Agreement Measure, for example (Bodin, 1968), determines behavioral differences among family members. This questionnaire consists of 12 five-item clusters that tap such areas as family-group strengths, family-group problems, family leadership, communication problems, and family discipline. The Family Concept Test (Vander Veen, 1965) was designed for the purpose of understanding the importance of the family for the individual. Moos and Moos's (1976) Family Environment Scale was patterned after other environmental-assessment scales created by this group. Their 90-item scale assesses relationship, personal-growth, and family-system-maintenance dimensions. Scales in the relationship dimension measure cohesion, expressiveness, and conflict. Scales in the personal-growth dimension measure such variables as independence and achievement orientation. Scales in the system-maintenance dimension measure organization and control. Olson, Sprenkle, and Russell (1979) have developed the Family Adaptability and Cohesion Evaluation Scales, which are based on a complex two-dimensional conceptualization of families in terms of four levels of cohesion and four levels of adaptability.

Each of these scales is based on a particular conceptual orientation to family functioning. Table 9–2 shows examples of items from the Moos Family Environment Scale. These items are similar to those on most self-report measures of family functioning.

TABLE 9–2. Examples of items on the Moos Family Environment Scale: R denotes items scored in reverse.

Relationship dimension	
Cohesion	Family members really help and support one another.
Expressiveness	Family members often keep their feelings to themselves. (R)
Conflict	We fight a lot in our family.
Personal-Growth dimension	
Independence	We don't do things on our own very often in our family. (R)
Achievement Orientation	We feel it is important to be the best at whatever you do.
Intellectual-Cultural Orientation	We often talk about political and social problems.
Active-Recreational Orientation	We spend most weekends and evenings at home. (R)
Moral-Religious Emphasis	Family members attend church, synagogue, or Sunday school fairly often.
System-Maintenance dimension	
Organization	Activities in our family are pretty carefully planned.
Control	Family members are rarely ordered around. (R)

Adapted from "A Typology of Family Social Environments," by R. H. Moos and B. S. Moos. In *Family Process*, 1976, 15, 357–371. Reprinted by permission.

Person/environment interactions

Not all persons are affected in the same way by a particular environmental setting. A growing body of literature indicates that "substantial interactions exist between the type of person inhabiting a particular kind of setting and the characteristics of the setting itself" (Price, 1974, p. 296). What is needed, therefore, is a way of describing persons, a way of describing settings, and a way of describing the nature of the interaction between the two. Researchers in this last field of study—that is, how person characteristics interact with environmental characteristics—examine what is often called *person/environment fit*. They try to understand the person-in-the-environment—that is, how the community shapes and is shaped by the individual and how particular environments facilitate or hinder the growth and development of particular persons. This interactionist view constitutes a major theoretical orientation in psychology (Ekehammar, 1974; Jessor, 1956, 1958; Lewin, 1936, 1951; Murray, 1938, 1951).

Pervin (1968) has reviewed the literature on person/environment fit and has shown that both task performance and general satisfaction are enhanced when there is a good match between personal and environmental characteristics. Pervin has shown, for example, that dropping out of college is most often the result of a lack of congruence between personal needs and environmental characteristics, and he has suggested that educational objectives may very well be achieved in different ways for different types of students.

In a very different area of investigation, Sims and Baumann (1972), noting that tornado-caused deaths are far more frequent in the South than in the rest of the country, created a tornado death index—a measure of the agreement between the number of actual and the number of potential tornado casualties—and showed that the South had disproportionately high casualty rates, unexplainable on any meteorological or topological basis. These authors conclude that "man's confrontation with his physical environment is influenced not only by the facts of that environment, but by his ideas and feelings about it, and that these, in turn, are influenced by his personality and culture" (p. 1388).

To test this general hypothesis in one specific case, Sims and Baumann examined a small number of women in Illinois and Alabama. They showed that the Alabama subjects were significantly more fatalistic, passive, and distrustful of the organized systems for tornado warning than those in Illinois and, in general, believed more than the Illinois sample in an external rather than internal locus of control over their own behavior. The authors do not argue that this personality difference is the sole or even the primary determinant of tornado death rate but rather that their data constitute a suggestive illustration of how "man's personality is active in determining the quality of his interaction with nature" (p. 1391).

The difficulties in coming to confident conclusions about person/environment interactions can be seen in the work of Kelly and his colleagues (Edwards

& Kelly, 1980; Kelly, 1979). This group has undertaken a longitudinal study of coping and adaptation of adolescent males in two high schools that differed in turnover rate—that is, the proportions of students and teachers entering or leaving the system each year. Students were selected on the basis of their exploration preferences—high, medium, and low—with students at all levels of exploration preference in both schools. The principal hypothesis Kelly and his colleagues examined was that "students with high exploration preferences would have optimal adaptations in the high turnover environment and good but poorer adaptations in the low turnover environment. Conversely, the students with low preferences for exploration were expected to have better adaptations in the low turnover environment and the poorest adaptations in the high turnover school" (Edwards & Kelly, 1980, p. 204).

Neither the early cross-sectional studies nor the later longitudinal studies provided unequivocal support for the joint role of exploration preferences and varied environments in determining adaptations, although "interesting person, school, maturational, and interaction effects were found on measures of adolescent adaptation" (Edwards & Kelly, 1980, p. 205). Significant main effects were found, however, for school environment. Specifically, students in the high-turnover school desired "more physical change, perceived more opportunity, saw the principal as more positive and their school as being more excellent than students in the low turnover environment" (p. 210). In addition, high-turnover students participated in more extracurricular activities and felt more identified and more satisfied with school.

Significant main effects were also found for exploration preferences. High explorers had more active styles of adaptation and reported significantly higher self-esteem, higher need for social approval, more initiative, and less depression than either the medium or low explorers. High explorers also reported fewer social problems and higher levels of social performance, reported feeling more involved in their classes, participated more in extracurricular activities, and felt more a part of the school than the other exploration groups.

Edwards and Kelly note, in their summary statement, that "this study clearly reveals the need for further theoretical development of the person-environment transaction theory. This is especially true for the development of strong predictive hypotheses about similar environments such as high schools. We hope that the presentation of these findings, while offering only minimal support for the person-environment transaction theory, will encourage other investigators to continue to investigate this important area" (p. 214).

The interactionist approach has received considerable support in other studies, however (see Ekehammar, 1974, pp. 1036–1041; see also Endler & Hunt, 1966, 1968; Magnusson, 1974; Moos, 1973; Raush, Dittmann, & Taylor, 1959). In general, these studies suggest that certain psychological phenomena (anxiety, honesty, or particular forms of behavior, for example) can be significantly better accounted for by knowing characteristics of the person *and* the setting than by knowing about either the person *or* the setting.

Environmental change

The analysis of environments, or behavior settings, is important not only in its own right but also because the setting can have enormous impact on individual functioning, including physiological functioning (see Kiritz & Moos, 1974), because knowledge of the relations between individual behavior and the environmental setting can help guide environmental design, and because knowledge derived from such an analysis can facilitate the development of a new kind of competence—namely, the ability to change and to control the environment within which one functions.

To test this last possibility—that environmental assessment techniques can play a role in facilitating environmental change—Moos (1974) developed an approach to environmental change consisting of four basic components. First, a *systematic analysis* must be made of how the environment is perceived by all members and what they consider an ideal social system. Second, *individualized feedback* must be provided to allow identification of similarities and differences in perceived environment among groups of persons within the environment (for example, patients and staff, or workers and management), and to allow identification of differences between the perceived and ideal environment. Third, *practical planning* for environmental change must take place, with the help of an expert in social-system change. And, fourth, *reassessment and revision* must be carried out if necessary. In a subsequent study, Moos (1975) was able to show that, by using this four-step strategy, it was possible to change the treatment environments in three different psychiatric programs.

A number of other reports have recently appeared describing efforts to modify environments. Here are two examples. Holahan (1979) has described his experiences in redesigning an admissions ward in a large municipal psychiatric hospital. He studied the consequences of that renovation for patient behavior by contrasting patient behavior on the redesigned ward with that of patients in an unrenovated admissions ward in the same hospital. Because patients were randomly assigned to the two wards, the hospital provided an excellent setting to examine the impact of environmental change on human behavior.

Holahan and his associates hoped that their design changes in the admissions ward would result in increased social interactions among patients. They tried to make the ward more attractive and to provide more alternatives for patient activities. In general, their hypotheses were supported; that is, they found that patients on the remodeled ward engaged in more social behavior and were less passive and withdrawn than patients on the other ward.

Holahan was aware of the limitations of environmental change in affecting the lives of psychiatric patients, however, and noted that "the physical design changes failed to improve noticeably the character of staff attitudes toward patients" (p. 256). In addition, he recognized that "the physical-design changes within the hospital context left totally unaltered the patients' life prospects after discharge" (p. 257).

Knapp and McClure (1978) described their efforts to increase quality of life in a Columbia, South Carolina, public housing unit. The program, requested by the housing authority, sought to increase quality of life by a combination of tutorial assistance, values-clarification workshops, psychological counseling, referral services, and constructive activities for people age 18 and younger, and monthly community meetings, referral services, and counseling services for adults. The program operated for five months.

Three separate but neighboring housing units were studied. Two units with a combined population of 900 persons served as the site for the experimental program; a single unit with a population of 1300 served as the control.

Four dependent measures were selected to assess the effectiveness of the program: locus-of-control scores, use of community health and social agencies, vandalism, and alcohol- and other drug-related arrests. It was hypothesized that the residents of the units in which the program was implemented would show increased internal locus of control, increased use of community agencies, and fewer drug-related arrests and that there would be less vandalism in the experimental housing units. Initial interviewing took place in December 1975, and postprogram interviews were conducted in April 1976.

Results of the experiment were generally quite positive. A significant change took place in locus of control, although the changes were not the same in children and adults. In children, significant increases in *external* locus of control took place in the control group, while insignificant changes took place in the experimental group. In adults, significant increases in *internal* locus of control took place in the experimental group, while the control group remained unchanged.

The hypothesis about community-agency use was confirmed; that is, whereas preexperimental level of use of community agencies was similar in the control and experimental groups, postexperimental use was significantly greater in the experimental than in the control group. There was some suggestion in the results that drug-related arrests decreased more in the experimental group than in the control group, but the experiment did not last long enough to provide enough data on which to base a clear decision. The authors believed, however, that the program was probably more effective in reducing drug-related arrests among adults than among children.

POPULATION RESEARCH

During the past 15 years, the scientific study of population growth has shown an accelerating rate of development, in large measure as a response to the growth of population itself. The scientific task is primarily to learn how varying population distributions affect human behavior. Underlying the increasing interest in this question are such crucial concerns as family planning, environmental protection, and the effects of famine, crime and violence, and crowding on the quality of life. The effects of high population density for animals as well as for human beings have been examined in the field and in the laboratory, by biologists, demographers, and other scientists. Public concern with the issue of uncontrolled population growth grew after the publication, in 1968, of *The Population Bomb*, by Paul R. Ehrlich, and many communities in the United States have engaged in heated debates about the possible consequences of changes in population or population density for community life.

At current birthrates and death rates, populations in developing countries are doubling at the rate of once every 25 to 30 years, while in most developed countries the rate is once every 40 to 60 years. Contrast these figures with earlier average doubling rates—1000 years in 1650, 200 years in 1850, and 80 years in 1930—and the acceleration of the growth rate of the world population becomes clear. But even if the birthrate were to be reduced to simple population replacement, the age structure of the population would ensure that total population would continue to grow for another 20 to 60 years, depending on the proportion of the population that is in the childbearing years. It has been estimated, for example, that if the birthrate were to be reduced to the level of simple population replacement in the next decade in the United States, a stationary population would not be achieved until the year 2030, at which time the population would be 271,000,000—a 20% increase over the 1980 population of 226,500,000. Compare this estimate with a similarly calculated one for India. There a stationary population would be achieved in the year 2040, but the population at that time would be 1,210,800,000—an increase of 77% over the 1980 population of 684,000,000. As for the People's Republic of China, if the birthrate were to be reduced to simple population replacement during the next decade, the population would not become stationary until 2050, at which time that total population would be 1,427,400,000—an increase of 45% over the 1980 population of 983,000,000 (Darroch, 1973). Thus, there seems little doubt that population and population density are destined to increase dramatically during the next generation and to bring with them major world crises.

Population density and animal behavior

Perhaps the classic series of studies of the consequences of unlimited population growth on animal behavior was the one reported by Calhoun (1962). In his earliest work, he confined a population of wild Norway rats in a quarter-acre enclosure and observed their population changes and behavior for more than two years.

> With an abundance of food and places to live and with predation and disease eliminated or minimized, only the animals' behavior with respect to one another remained as a factor that might affect the increase in their number. There could be no escape from the behavioral consequences of rising population density. By the end of 27 months the population had become stabilized at 150 adults. Yet adult mortality was so low that 5,000 adults might have been expected from the observed reproductive rate. The reason this larger population did not materialize

was that infant mortality was extremely high. Even with only 150 adults in the enclosure, stress from social interaction led to such disruption of maternal behavior that few young survived [p. 139].[4]

He then did a series of experiments with domesticated strains of the Norway rat under more controlled laboratory conditions. Population was permitted to increase to approximately twice the number that could comfortably occupy the available space.

> The consequences of the behavioral pathology we observed were most apparent among the females. Many were unable to carry pregnancy to full term or to survive delivery of their litters if they did. An even greater number, after successfully giving birth, fell short in their maternal functions. Among the males the behavior disturbances ranged from sexual deviation to cannibalism and from frenetic over-activity to a pathological withdrawal from which individuals would emerge to eat, drink and move about only when other members of the community were asleep [Calhoun, 1962, p. 139].

Freedman (1975) reviewed the research literature then in existence on the effects of crowding on animals and summarized that literature as follows:

> 1. At a certain point the population declines sharply; 2. There is greatly increased infant mortality caused primarily by inadequate nest building and care of the young by the females; 3. There is increased aggressiveness and a breakdown in normal social behavior; 4. Some animals become recluses and no longer engage in any social behavior; 5. The strongest animals survive and are able to breed, raise young, and in general live a normal life; 6. Adrenal activity is increased and male gonadal activity somewhat decreased by exposure to larger numbers of other animals, but density is relatively unimportant; 7. Emotionality and susceptibility to disease are not generally negatively affected [p. 23].[5]

More recent animal research has suggested, however, that the role of density on behavior is far more complex than originally thought. Freedman 1979 has concluded that

> psychologists have given too much weight to a few dramatic studies and have failed to keep up with new research. Now, most biologists and animal behaviorists agree that density has no simple, negative effect on nonhuman animals. Indeed, the effect on other animals is identical in form to that on humans. Density plays an important role in the regulation of population and has many physical and social effects, but all of these effects are complex and depend on other factors in the situation. . . . The available research on nonhuman animals indicates that density per se does not generally have harmful effects and that the effects it does have are determined mainly by other factors that psychologists had for believing

[4]From "Population Density and Social Pathology," by J. B. Calhoun, *Scientific American,* 1962, *206,* 139–148. This and all other quotations from this source are reprinted by permission.

[5]From *Crowding and Behavior,* by J. L. Freedman. Copyright 1975 by W. H. Freeman and Company. This and all other quotations from this source are reprinted by permission.

that high density would probably also be harmful to people. It is time to abandon that preconception and rely instead on the research findings regarding humans [pp. 81, 85].

Population density and human behavior

Studies relating population density to human behavior have produced far more equivocal findings. As we saw, studies on the effects of population density on animal behavior have defined density in terms of the number of animals per unit area. In human studies there are two other ways of defining population density. It can be defined, as in animal studies, as the number of persons per square mile or acre. There are, however, a host of difficulties in comparing areas (see Day & Day, 1973). A related but not identical concept of population density is the concept of *crowding,* generally measured in terms of the amount of dwelling-unit space per person (see Schmidt & Keating, 1979). A neighborhood of closely spaced, small single-family homes or a neighborhood of high-rise, large luxury apartments may be characterized as high in density but low in crowding; a lower-middle-class, suburban high-rise apartment building may be high in crowding but, if located in the countryside, low in density. The concept of crowding is also a psychological one— a feeling, or subjective experience, of being crowded. This feeling may be quite independent of the externally quantified concepts of density and crowding. It is even possible to feel crowded when totally alone.

An illustration of the complexity in this field of investigation can be seen in Schmitt's work in Hawaii. In his first study (1966) Schmitt found that crowding in Honolulu was unrelated to various measures of health and social disorganization but that density was significantly related to seven of the nine measures he used. These measures, including death rate, psychiatric-hospital admission rate, and rate of juvenile delinquency, remained significantly related to density even when crowding, education, and income were held constant. But a later study (Schmitt, Zane, & Nishi, 1978) did not successfully replicate the 1966 findings. None of the density measures revealed a consistently strong relationship with the dependent social-disequilibrium variables. Schmitt and his colleagues concluded that the relationships between crowding, density, and social disequilibrium are more complex and less direct than seemed likely in their earlier study.

Levy and Herzog (1974), as part of a research program in social ecology, investigated the relationship of population density and crowding to scores on a variety of indicators of social pathology, including psychopathology, using as units of investigation the 125 geographic areas in the Netherlands, one of the most densely populated countries in the world. They hypothesized that density and crowding would be significantly associated with the measures of social pathology even when social class and religion were controlled for. They found, as Schmitt had, that density was far more closely and significantly related to their dependent variables than crowding was.

In a recent review of the research literature on crowding and human behavior, Lawrence (1974) has indicated that studies linking population density (variously defined) with measures of sociopathic behavior often show significant results, only to have these findings vanish when corrections are made for social class or ethnicity. Even when the relationships remain significant, it is impossible to determine what factor was causal. Finally, studies of the relationship of population density to infectious disease and to suicide rate have yielded positive results in one community but not in others. Lawrence has concluded that

> the field is confused—by definitions, by conflicting data, and . . . by popular conjecture. The animal data are most easily interpreted and possibly of least use to man. The urban findings are inconclusive, demonstrating no unequivocal relationship between population density and social ills. Finally, clinical and experimental models are at odds, and the results of experiments are again inconclusive. Perhaps the only certain conclusion that can be drawn at this time is that there is no clear demonstrable linear relationship between high density and aberrant human behaviors, or between the social crowding of the individual and aggression. It is impossible to do more than speculate further [1974, pp. 717–718].

More recent studies have equally ambiguous results. Giel and Ormel (1977) examined the relationship between crowding and subjective reports of health in a sample of adults in the Netherlands. They found, on the basis of an interview survey with more than 1000 persons aged 25 and above, a negligible relationship between dwelling-unit density and a number of self-reported measures of health and illness. These authors proposed two possible explanations for their negative findings: perhaps crowding in the Netherlands does not reach a stressful level, or perhaps the relatively high standard of living in the Netherlands compensates for high dwelling-unit density.

Schweitzer and Su (1977) examined the relation of population density to rates of psychiatric hospitalization in Brooklyn, New York, and on the basis of their analysis they felt that population density might be a significant intervening variable in the development of mental illness. They state: "The results of this study do not absolutely implicate population density in the production of mental illness. They do however suggest that if density is pathogenic it is likely that its effect will be routed through family contact. Further study of density should therefore pay attention to the presence or absence of family social supports as well as measures of family stress" (p. 1171).

Thus, for human beings, the relationship of population density or crowding to various forms of social disequilibrium is far from clear. Moos (1979) has reviewed the literature linking population density and crowding to measures of health and has concluded that although crowded conditions can adversely affect health, the social climate (for example, how space is used, interpersonal proximity, friendship patterns, and level of cohesion) as well as architectural and physical design (for example, presence of gardens and open space, balconies, quiet rather than noisy surroundings, or sunlight) can have mediating effects on that relationship.

We can also illustrate the complexity of these relationships using crime rate, a matter of enormous importance throughout the world. Crime rate is far higher in cities than in rural areas—five times as high, on the average. Major crimes are largely high-population phenomena. But it does not necessarily follow that the crime rate is highest in areas of high population density or crowding. Freedman, Heshka, and Levy (see Freedman, 1975, pp. 55–69, 137–142) correlated measures of population, population density, income, and ethnic composition with overall crime rate and with the crime rate for six specific crimes (murder, rape, assault, robbery, burglary, and car theft) across 97 Standard Metropolitan Statistical Areas (see Chapter 8) and found that, regardless of which crime rate was examined, population density was never the most highly correlated variable. The variable most highly correlated with overall crime rate and with three specific crime rates was population. For the other three specific crime rates, ethnic composition (percentage non-white) was the most highly correlated variable. When statistical corrections were introduced for the variations in socioeconomic affluence, the relationship between crime rate and population density, small to begin with, disappeared.

Furthermore, if one were to argue that high population density results in feelings of anger and aggression, one would have to show population density to be more closely related to crimes of violence than to crimes against property. The opposite has been found; that is, the lowest correlations between population density and crime rate are found for crimes of violence. Similar studies (Pressman & Carol, 1971; Galle, Gove, & McPherson, 1972; Galle, McCarthy, & Gove, 1974) found no stable significant relationships between density or crowding and any measure of social pathology (for example, alcoholism) or crime. Thus, there seems to be very little evidence that population density is a factor leading to crime. In fact, examinations of areas characterized by relatively low per-capita income have shown population density to be negatively correlated with crime rate (see Freedman, 1975). Freedman has concluded that,

> in general, this research provides no evidence to support the notion that high density is bad for people. . . . There is no relationship between how crowded a city or neighborhood is and how much crime it has. . . . Poor neighborhoods have more crime than rich ones. Poor people tend to commit more crimes than people with money. . . . There are a great many reasons why people commit crimes, many factors in modern, complex society that cause crime, but there is no evidence that crowding is one of them [pp. 68–69].

No one who is aware of the major concerns of U.S. citizens can fail to realize that our cities are sources of special anguish. To the community mental health professional, the issue is how one can maintain the strengths and excitement of the city and still have it be a fit place for human habitation. Are cities doomed to be the domain of the ill and destitute, or will ways be found to preserve cities' economic and social heterogeneity and viability? In comparison with many U.S. cities, European cities seem safe, strong, and alive. Mass transit works well, and the high population density serves to enhance the special city charm—an outdoor cafe on nearly every street corner, people walking on the street night and day, shopping within easy reach without an automobile. This is not to suggest that European cities are without their problems but only that a greater understanding of how they function may help the social scientist who is committed to improving the quality of U.S. city life achieve that objective.

Population control and family planning

It would be most appropriate, in discussing general issues in population research of interest to the community mental health professional, to comment on the status of family-planning programs both worldwide and in the United States. As with numerous other problems, biological knowledge here far exceeds our psychological and sociological knowledge.

Remarkable developments have been made in contraceptive technology—developments that have brought about those extraordinary changes in human sexual behavior often called the "sexual revolution." Primary responsibility for contraception has been transferred from the man to the woman, and women now have far more freedom in the sexual arena. New procedures are currently being developed for the hormonal suppression of ovulation and for hormonal contraception without ovulation suppression, as well as for suppression of sperm production and for reduction of the fertilizing capacity of sperm. And the time may not be too distant when common contraceptive methods will include once-a-month anti-ovulant pills and tablets to alter the biochemical constitution of seminal fluid or to inhibit spermatogenesis.

Yet, the first systematic worldwide survey of fertility-control practices found that, as of 1971, 70% of an estimated 500 million women at risk of having an unwanted pregnancy were using no contraceptive method at all (Robbins, 1973). Of the 150 million women practicing some form of contraception, about half were using the most effective methods—the pill, the IUD, sterilization, or abortion. The other half were using the less effective, more traditional methods—the condom, the diaphragm, the rhythm method (more recently called the symptothermal method or natural family planning), spermicides, or withdrawal. The survey showed that the most common birth-control method worldwide was abortion. In 1971 there were an estimated 55 million induced abortions—four abortions for every ten live births. The projected world population figures presented earlier in this chapter, ominous as they are, are conservative estimates, based on the assumption that family-planning efforts will successfully achieve zero population gain within the next decade. As the results of the 1971 survey suggest, there is very little hope that these efforts will be successful that quickly.

Although the concept of family planning includes helping couples have wanted children as well as helping them avoid having unwanted children, there is no doubt that the latter activity is, in practice, given more attention.

In a reminiscence, C. P. Blacker (1973) describes the early days of the family-planning movement, according special credit to two courageous women—Margaret Sanger and Marie Stopes, "eloquent and persuasive speakers possessed of the fervour of missionaries" (p. 494). He wrote:

> I retain some vivid memories of the adverse tide of that time. When, for example, in 1927 I entered for some reason the amiable presence of the Treasurer of the Royal College of Physicians, he asked me if I was the secretary of a committee formed to investigate birth control. I replied that I was, at the same time wondering if his friendly features would show signs of distaste or pleasure. In fact, an expression of dire distress crossed his face. "I have no doubt," he said, "that what you are doing is timely. It is a pity that the subject is so sordid." This view was then widely held, not least strongly by gynaecologists [p. 495].

The family-planning movement had its start in the early 1920s, but it was not until after World War II that the movement began to develop its current vigor. The development of antibiotic drugs and insecticides was driving death rates down, and the world was becoming aware of the population explosion. The pill and the IUD were introduced, and techniques for voluntary sterilization were perfected and later legalized. Attitudes toward birth control are still very mixed, though increasingly favorable, and attitudes toward death control are just beginning to be examined. The topic of voluntary death is increasingly finding itself on the front pages, and courts of law are being asked to decide under what circumstances, if any, one may choose death for oneself or for someone for whom one has legal and moral responsibility. The issues of birth and death control have ethical, moral, religious, and political implications (see Smith, 1972). Under these circumstances, the community mental health professional can make a significant contribution simply by reviewing and summarizing what appear to be the scientific facts and by examining the awareness of and attitudes toward these facts in the community he or she serves. This kind of contribution embodies one of the principles of professional functioning that will be outlined later in this chapter.

Sexual experience among the unmarried is increasingly common. Kantner and Zelnik (1972, 1973) reported that 46% of unmarried women aged 15–19 had had intercourse. In a more recent survey (Zelnik & Kantner, 1980) that proportion had increased to 50%. Among never-married males aged 17–21 living in metropolitan areas, 69% reported having had intercourse. The proportion of the population with coital experience at any age was inversely related to socioeconomic status and was higher among persons raised by one parent than by two. The level of knowledge concerning the period of greatest likelihood of conception during the menstrual cycle was found to be low—one-third of 19-year-old white females whose mothers had had a college education could not identify the period of greatest risk.

With regard to contraceptive use, in 1973 more than half of 15–19-year-old sexually active females reported that they had failed to use any kind of contraceptive in their most recent intercourse, and fewer than 20% reported that they used contraceptives consistently By 1979, 34% of sexually active women aged 15–19 reported that they consistently used contraceptives. Many females reported that they did not use contraceptives because they did not believe they would become pregnant. Yet, as of 1973, among sexually experienced young women, the reported incidence of pregnancy was substantial— 10% among whites and 40% among blacks. By 1979, the risk of premarital pregnancy had increased among sexually active women aged 15–19. Among women who reported always using contraceptives, 13% became pregnant. Among inconsistent contraceptive users, the risk of pregnancy increased to 30%, and among nonusers, the risk exceeded 60%. Except for consistent contraceptive users, pregnancy risk continued to be higher for blacks than for whites. The high risk of pregnancy among contraceptive users appears to be due, in part, to the fact that less effective methods tend to be used. Attitudes toward abortion paralleled attitudes toward contraception. Those females who were most favorable to abortion were also those most likely to be using contraceptives.

In a related study, Blake (1973) found that more than 70% of a sample of men and women aged 18 and older favored birth-control education at the high school level. About half the survey respondents approved providing birth-control services to teenage girls who request them. Yet, Blake found no evidence of a correspondingly permissive attitude toward premarital sexual relations. These attitudes were age-related—the older respondents tended to be less permissive. Among younger respondents (Hunt, 1974), premarital sexual relations were considered acceptable for an emotionally involved couple by more than 70% of women and 80% of men.

Family planning in the United States

In 1979 more than 8.6 million women in the United States visited family-planning clinics, a 16% increase over the previous year (National Center for Health Statistics, 1981b). Not included in this number were women who visited private physicians' offices or group medical practices. Nearly all the women visiting such clinics were under age 30, and one-third of the visits were made by teenagers. Nearly 40% of the visits were made by women with less than a high school education, and 14% were made by women living in families receiving public assistance. Almost half the visits were made by women who had never been pregnant.

Nearly all the visits to a family-planning clinic resulted in the adoption or continued use of some contraceptive method. The overwhelming choice was oral contraception. The pill was the choice of about two-thirds of all women, but its use decreased with age, ranging from 77% among teenagers to 45% among women over 30, because of the increasing appeal of sterilization among older women.

There are excess health risks associated with the use of oral contraceptives among women over age 35. Those risks have been documented by Hoover,

Bain, Cole, and MacMahon (1978) on the basis of a two-stage questionnaire survey of more than 65,000 married women in the greater Boston area in 1970 and in 1973. The questionnaire requested information on lifetime oral-contraceptive use, reproductive history, education, and hospitalization experience during the previous year. Oral-contraceptive use was associated with increased risk of hospitalization for thromboembolic disease, mental illness, hyperthyroidism, hypertension, and cancer of the cervix. In addition, oral-contraceptive users were hospitalized for many non-life-threatening conditions 20 to 40% more frequently than nonusers. There is some evidence, however, that use of the newer lower-dose oral contraceptives decreases the risk of upper-genital-tract infection, menstrual cramps and anemia due to menstrual bleeding, and fibrocystic breast disease (Hatcher, Stewart, Stewart, Guest, Josephs, & Dale, 1982).

Among currently married women in 1976, according to a study by the National Center for Health Statistics (1978b), about 30% of couples were sterile (nearly always as a consequence of surgical sterilization), nearly 50% were using contraceptives, 13% were either pregnant, postpartum, or seeking pregnancy, and the remaining 7% were other nonusers of contraceptives. Between 1965 and 1975 there was a continued increase in the proportion of married couples currently using contraception and a continued decline in the proportion that had never used contraception (National Center for Health Statistics, 1979). Although the pill continues to be the most popular method of family planning among couples married less than ten years, among couples married ten years or longer, the most commonly used method is surgical sterilization.

About half the women in this study reported using a different contraceptive method in 1975 than they had used in 1970. For most the change was to surgical sterilization from some other method, particularly among older women who already had as many children as they wished.

With the exception of sterilization (tubal ligation or vasectomy), every contraceptive method has a significant failure rate. A study of contraception failure conducted by the National Center for Health Statistics of the U.S. Public Health Service (1978a), based on a national sample of 9800 ever-married women aged 15–44, found that the failure rate ranged from 2.0% for the pill to 19.1% for the rhythm method. Condoms, foams, and the diaphragm had failure rates ranging from 10% to 15%.

The National Center for Health Statistics (1981a) recently completed a study of induced terminations of pregnancy in an eight-state area. During 1978 there were approximately three induced terminations for every ten live births (not appreciably lower than the worldwide average), but this ratio varied as a function of a number of demographic characteristics. Induced abortions were highest among the youngest and oldest groups of women, averaging between six and seven per ten live births among women under 20 and about eight per ten live births among women 40 and above. The abortion-to-live-birth ratio was slightly higher among black than among white women. More than one-quarter of induced abortions occurred among married women. More than half the women had had no previous live births, and three-quarters had had no prior abortions.

In a study of more than 1500 women who were obtaining abortions in a free-standing abortion clinic in New York state, Howe, Kaplan, and English (1979) contrasted the women who were having their first abortions (83% of the sample) with those having repeat abortions (17%). Repeaters were more likely to be using contraceptives than first-timers but were also more active sexually. Noncontracepting repeaters listed medical contraindications or lack of supplies as the major reasons for not contracepting and indicated that they had tried one or more methods of contraception since their first abortions. Both first-timers and repeaters overwhelmingly rejected the premise that abortion is a primary or even a secondary birth-control method. "The essential difficulty for repeaters appears to be that they are victims of technological, organizational, and logistical inadequacies as well as statistical probabilities rather than motivationally deficient or indifferent to the dangers of unprotected sexual intercourse" (p. 1242).

Research literature has generally confirmed the common wisdom that unplanned children are at unusually high risk of a variety of developmental difficulties (Blake, 1981; Matejcek, Dytrych, & Schuller, 1978; Rader, Bekker, Brown, & Richardt, 1978). Yet, unwanted pregnancies are far from rare, even in the United States. Between 1973 and 1976 there was a slight decrease in the proportion of births that were described as wanted. In 1976 more than 13% of births were unwanted (National Center for Health Statistics, 1980). The proportion of unwanted births was lowest among mothers aged 20–29 and was higher among those both younger and older. The proportion of wanted births tended to decrease with increasing numbers of children already born to the couple and was substantially lower among black mothers than among white mothers. The highest proportion of wanted births was among women with the highest level of education.

The report on unwanted births concludes by stating that, in general,

> the groups experiencing the greatest numbers of unintended pregnancies (unwanted and undetermined combined) . . . are the very young mothers and the oldest, the mothers who have the largest number of children, those with the least education and income, and the mothers who are without husbands or who have experienced marital disruption. The large differences between white and black mothers in the proportions of wanted and unwanted births probably reflect substantial differences in these social and economic conditions [p. 7].

The especially high birthrate among adolescent women has been of considerable concern to social scientists and physicians, mainly because of the severe psychosocial and economic complications that so often follow (Furstenberg, 1976). Schinke, Gilchrist, and Small have noted:

> Each year over 600,000 women in the United States become mothers before they become adults. In 1975, children born to women less than 19 years old constituted 19% of all births; 13,000 births that year were to women under 15. These children—

born to mothers hardly more than children themselves—show heightened risks of infant mortality, prematurity, and congenital neurological impairments, including blindness, deafness, and mental retardation. For young parents, adolescent pregnancy interrupts or terminates education; the result often is reduced earning power and dependence on public assistance and the social welfare system. Teenage parents encounter additional stresses of ill-considered marriages and increased likelihood of marital problems and divorce [1979, p. 81].

If pregnant adolescent women receive early and comprehensive prenatal care, however, the risks of infant mortality or low birth weight are no higher than for babies born to women over age 20 (Granadio, 1981; Perkins, Nakashima, Mullin, Dubansky, & Chin, 1978).

Shelton (1977) has examined the factors that appear to be associated with the recent fall in birthrate among women under age 15 in Georgia—a fall that is of recent origin and has followed a generally rising birthrate in this group. In Georgia a 1972 law that allowed minors to obtain contraceptive services without parental consent did not appear to result in a reduced birthrate. In 1974, however, the rate began to fall, and according to Shelton this fall can be understood as a likely consequence of the 1973 U.S. Supreme Court decision allowing increased access to induced abortion.

Shelton found that the decline in births occurred first in those communities where abortion utilization was the highest and occurred in those subgroups of women whose abortion utilization is the highest. Although the availability of abortion appears to have had the greatest impact in lowering the birthrate, Shelton believes that efforts toward providing contraceptives should be continued. These efforts will not easily succeed, however. Shelton notes that

> the reasons for low utilization of contraception by teenagers are multiple and complex. All of the asserted reasons—ignorance, misinformation, lack of motivation, restrictive societal and physician attitudes, legal constraints, financial constraints, reluctance to admit one's sexuality, fear of the physical examination, lack of futuristic thinking—are without a doubt increased for the very young adolescent. When faced with the reality of an unwanted pregnancy, however, it appears that many very young teenagers will eventually take the definite action of having an abortion—if the abortion is readily accessible [p. 620].

Ebaugh and Haney (1980) have examined shifts in attitudes toward abortion in the United States between 1972 and 1978 and have contrasted these shifts with similar attitudes assessed during the 1960s. They summarize their findings as follows:

> Attitudes toward legalized abortion have changed significantly among the American public over the past 15 years. While there has been an increasing liberalization of attitudes during the 1960s and early 1970s, by 1975 the trend began to change and attitudes became slightly more conservative. By 1978, that trend was pronounced. A comparison of respondents by age, sex, and educational characteristics shows important differences between the 1960 and 1970 data. In the 1960s it was male, better educated, older people who were most liberal in their abortion

attitudes. In the 1970s, male-female differences are not so consistent and vary by year. The age trend reversed itself with younger people being more liberal in their attitudes than older people. While a positive relationship between education and liberal attitudes persists in the 1970s, the college educated remained relatively constant in their attitudes while respondents with only a high school education became more favorable toward abortion over the decade [p. 499].[6]

In a subsequent analysis of 1980 survey data, Ebaugh and Haney (1982) found that the conservative trend in attitudes toward legalized abortion that had begun in 1975 had not continued. Rather, attitudes toward abortion were found to be more liberal than in 1978, and in some cases even more so than in the two or three previous years. In the 1978 survey, 6% of respondents firmly disapproved of abortion while 30% firmly approved of abortion. In the 1980 survey, 6% of respondents again firmly disapproved of abortion while 37% firmly approved of abortion. The change between 1978 and 1980 was particularly noticeable among respondents with less than a college degree and among those who were weekly churchgoers.

A substantial body of literature is accumulating testifying to the safety (both physical and psychological) of legal abortion (see, for example, Ewing & Rouse, 1973; Osofsky & Osofsky, 1972; Smith, 1973), even for women with histories of psychiatric disability. Yet, attitudes toward legalized abortion, like attitudes toward other forms of contraception and premarital sexual behavior, vary tremendously. Identifying community attitudes toward family planning and the implications of these attitudes for human behavior are complex but perhaps necessary tasks for the community mental health professional.

By way of summary, sexual behavior has changed dramatically in most communities during the past two decades, largely as a consequence of the availability of more effective contraceptives. In spite of the rapid increase in availability of family-planning programs, there are a large number of unwanted pregnancies among married as well as unmarried women, and in the United States as well as the rest of the world, there are a very large number of abortions. Fortunately, legal abortions appear to present virtually no risk to women's physical well-being.

Birth-control methods are not invariably successful. All forms of contraception except sterilization have a nontrivial failure rate, and those with the lowest failure rates often have the most dangerous side effects. These facts may help account for the dramatic increase in voluntary sterilizations during the past decade as well as the continuing high demand for abortions.

Public attitudes toward premarital sexual relations are not uniformly favorable by any means, and abortion as a method of birth control is even more controversial (Blake & Del Pinal, 1981). Yet, few women who seek abortion view abortion as their preferred method of birth control, and few seek

[6]From "Shifts in Abortion Attitudes: 1972–1978," by H. R. F. Ebaugh and C. A. Haney. In *Journal of Marriage and the Family*, 1980, 42, 491–499. Copyrighted 1980 by the National Council on Family Relations. Reprinted by permission.

abortions as a consequence of thoughtless disregard of what they know to be the risks associated with sexual intercourse. Rather, abortion is, for most women, the family-planning method of last resort.

It seems reasonably clear that the number of pregnancies and births, particularly among adolescents, can be reduced by a combination of improved sex education and increased availability of birth-control services, including prompt abortions. Lindemann and Scott have concluded that there are two paths to pregnancy in early adolescence—one path taken by women who want to become pregnant and the other by women who do not. They suggest three distinct intervention strategies:

> The first strategy is directed toward preventing unwanted pregnancies. A central feature of these efforts . . . consists of disseminating information about reproductive physiology and the effective use of birth control. It also may entail the delivery of contraceptive services to adolescents. . . . The second category of intervention strategies involves attempts to convert those who "want" to get pregnant to the position that it is preferable to avoid pregnancy when very young. . . . This conversion is not necessarily affected by exposure to increasing information concerning sex and reproduction. Intervention strategies in these cases face the task of introducing those females not yet pregnant, but who have a predisposition toward early pregnancy, to ways of fulfilling their psychological and social needs without having a baby. . . . Converting those who want to get pregnant to the position that it is preferable to avoid pregnancy at very young ages requires intervention strategies directed at the social structure and values of society. . . . Finally, the third intervention strategy is directed to those early adolescents who already are pregnant. For this group, intervention requires counseling about abortion, keeping the baby or giving it up for adoption, acquiring health care, making the transition to the role of mother, and minimizing the negative social and economic effects of early pregnancy [1981, pp. 191–192].[7]

Surveys reveal an astonishing lack of accurate information about human reproduction throughout the population, and there is some evidence that, regardless of people's attitudes toward sexual behavior among the unmarried, there is general support for educating the young in the "facts of life," though less agreement on whether public schools should play any role in that education.

SOME PRINCIPLES OF COMMUNITY INTERVENTION

No community is free of problems. A child is murdered by a psychiatric outpatient being treated for sexual deviation, and the community demands that all outpatients be committed to the public psychiatric hospital. A rash of robberies by juvenile delinquents arouses the interest of the community in taking some action. There is a growing problem of illicit drug use and drug abuse, or a string of tragic suicides, or concern with air or water pollution, or

---

[7]From "Wanted and Unwanted Pregnancy in Early Adolescence: Evidence from a Clinic Population," by C. Lindemann and W. J. Scott. In *Journal of Early Adolescence*, 1981, *1*, 185–193. Reprinted by permission.

the growing realization that many elderly people in the community cannot find adequate, affordable housing. If the community mental health center sees itself as able to allocate some resources to deal with these kinds of problems— problems only very indirectly related to the problems traditionally handled by the mental health service delivery system—or if other agencies have staff members who can turn their attention to these kinds of issues, how are they to proceed? What qualities must they have? How can they take what Kelly (1971) called the ecological perspective?

Kelly suggested that the premise of the ecological perspective is that intervention "should contribute to the development of the community" (1971, p. 897). Adopting the ecological perspective means

> shifting the focus in our communities away from our personal aspirations, our sponsoring institutions, and even the visible persons or institutions in town, and, instead, making the local conditions and the local events the forum for our work. . . . It means grasping the intricacies of the total community so as to identify talents and resources that are hidden yet present. It means locating the persons who care about their town. . . . Viewing a community ecologically means seeing how persons, roles, and organizations, as well as events, are interrelated [pp. 897–898].

Kelly has proposed that the mental health professional and the social scientist must work in the midst of the community in order to help resolve community concerns and that the mental health professional must have certain special qualities. First, every community mental health professional must have a small set of competencies—skills that are needed by the community and tailored to the setting in which he or she works. He or she must build on these competencies, continually work toward developing new ones, and share them with the host community. Second, community-based mental health professionals must identify and become involved with the total community and must care about the community and move freely throughout it, paying particular attention to those aspects that do not seem naturally and automatically congenial to them. Third, the mental health professional must not just tolerate but, rather, sincerely value diversity. He or she must appreciate and grow to understand the significance of differences among people and among groups within the community and how this variation can enhance the problem-solving process. Fourth, the community worker must be empathetic, interpersonally effective, and able to work with the diverse elements of the community. Among these diverse elements will be found the resources that need to be linked together to solve community problems. Fifth, the community mental health worker must be prepared to take prudent risks, to be the advocate of a worthwhile, though unpopular, cause, and to help the community progress. Risk taking means supporting the marginal person or enterprise and putting aside the need to bet only on winners. Sixth, working in the community requires a mixture of patience and zeal—an ability to see the long-term, slowly achieved goal in terms of a series of more easily attainable, short-term goals, an ability to know when to push and when to hold back. And, finally, work in the community demands a willingness to have success accrue to the community rather than to oneself, a willingness to enjoy quietly the fruits of one's labor, without demanding credit, recognition, and public applause, and an eagerness to face the challenge of a new and still more difficult task.

Modification of community characteristics requires a compassionate empirical analysis of the community—how its characteristics impinge on the lives of the persons who live in it, why apparently undesirable characteristics persist, how the power of growth-inducing community forces can be enhanced, and how life-styles that seem to be associated with social disequilibrium can be discouraged. Writing about modification of the environment as it applies to youth, Keniston has said "One reason the unrest of youth eludes psychological categories may be psychiatry's stress on the inner world and on those modes of adaptation that Heinz Hartmann has called autoplastic—efforts at self-change, at insight, at adaptation to the environment. Too little attention has been given to the positive value of alloplastic adaptations, which try to make the world a more livable place, to create new life styles, to change others" (1970, p. 1767).

During its initial years, the community mental health center program worked toward improving and expanding direct clinical services. Implicit in this early view of community mental health center objectives were certain assumptions about community structure. First, it was assumed that community residents could be sorted into those who were disadvantaged and those who were not. Second, it was assumed that some members of the community were caretakers and others were clients of caretakers. Third, it was assumed that the repository of wisdom about community mental health needs was the mental health professional and professionals in other social agencies.

This set of assumptions has become increasingly untenable. This is because, first, emphasis on the prevention of mental disorder has increased. It has become clear that although some sources of psychopathology are inside the skin, other sources are within the social systems in which we live, and prevention will therefore require more active involvement with the community. Second, it has become clear that if changes are to be made in these social systems to prevent or limit the disability associated with psychopathology, some forms of social or political action are required. Third, the legitimate area of concern of the mental health professional has been extended to include not just individual problems but also problems affecting the entire community and not just treatment of disorders but also improvement of the quality of life. Fourth, with a growing interest in socially generated psychopathology, the concepts of self-esteem and power have become very important. Fifth, even with respect to the provision of direct clinical services, it has become increasingly obvious that improvements have to be made in the organization and delivery of these services, in their financing, and in the control of their quality. These improvements may not be made without pressure from recipients or potential recipients of the services and thus may require social or political action. Finally, a much more compassionate view of the strengths and weaknesses of the community is appearing. In this view, a community is seen not as consisting of givers and takers but as a group of interdependent people, *all* of whom have needs that can be met by others and who have contributions to make to others (see Blackman & Goldstein, 1968). In this view, furthermore, *all* members of the community are seen as potentially disadvantaged by poverty and by poor health, to be sure, but also by loss of parents, by job dissatisfaction, by unhappy marriage, and by the lack of a meaningful social role. Jane Howard, in her book *A Different Woman,* describes this interdependence beautifully. In the beginning of this passage, she is writing about her mother.

> She was always doing people, who in turn did her, preferably when her feet were under their tables, or theirs under hers. . . . "Do" . . . means to take under one's wing, to shelter, succor, nurture, concentrate on, listen to, cause to feel central. It is not easy to do people in absentia, which was what my cousin Mary Louise was implying when she said to my mother over the phone, "Oh, Eleanor, I just wish you'd come over to Oak Park and put your feet under my table." The practice of doing continues. "Hey, go do Dr. Covington, she's standing all alone over there," Ann or I might whisper to each other at a party. We all do and in turn are done by our friends, who are all, from time to time, our caseloads, just as we are theirs. Everyone, according to an as yet unpublished monograph on the Caseload Theory of Interpersonal Relationships, is entitled now and then to be a caseload [pp. 20–21].[8]

Yolles wrote "There will be no effective national progress in community mental health unless psychiatrists and other core mental health professionals . . . accept their responsibilities as professionals to practice as community leaders and activists as well as clinicians" (1969, p. 3). Thus, a new relationship is required between the mental health professional and the community within which he or she lives and works. All members of the community, including those members who provide mental health services, must be seen as interdependent.

Efforts to prevent mental disorder by reducing the stresses under which people live have not been very common, nor, when undertaken, have they invariably been successful. But the literature increasingly calls for such programs. Although everyone functions in the face of counterproductive stresses, the poverty-stricken populations in our communities are clearly victims of greater stresses than the more affluent populations, and most of the theory and programming regarding stress reduction has concerned itself with poor neighborhoods. Clausen noted that

> it has been widely recognized that improvement of the quality of housing and education is a health-relevant goal. [Community health] centers can provide a

[8]From *A Different Woman,* by J. Howard. Copyright © 1973 by Jane Howard. Reprinted by permission of the publishers, E. P. Dutton & Co., Inc., and The Sterling Lord Agency, Inc.

base for organizing to deal with nagging urban problems and thereby become a means of overcoming feelings of powerlessness and of being exploited. Such centers would seem far more appropriate than the more specialized community mental health centers for dealing with problems of living deriving from lack of preparation for participation in the larger society and from other sources of frustration to which the poor are subject [1970, p. 8].

Another view of the potential of the community health center for reducing stresses under which the poor function can be seen in this statement by Scherl and English.

Involvement in meaningful decision making on issues intimately affecting one's own life seems to provide one response to a reality-based sense of hopelessness, helplessness, and anger. Through a Neighborhood Health Center, the poor can gain a measure of mobility of action and independence and add a measure of power to their voices. . . . The Neighborhood Health Center does not offer a panacea for poverty. But it is conceptualized in such a way that its effect may cover a wider area than the usual one to which health programs are limited. The centers have the opportunity to play some part in helping to alter outer (e.g., deficient education, jobs) and inner (e.g., attitudes) factors that impede the poor from rising out of poverty. Meaningful participation may turn out to be as important as providing treatment for the mentally ill [1969, pp. 1672–1673].

As you can see from this discussion, attempts to reduce stress typically involve soliciting community participation and rather quickly become highly political in character. Mental health professionals are rarely skilled politicians and are often too naive or uneasy about the potential conflict and stress to deal with communitywide programs. Perhaps because of the political character of programs attempting to reduce stress, only a handful of community mental health program directors have ventured into this arena. Yet, in spite of the risks associated with such activities, identifying and attempting to reduce environmental stresses may be the only way to achieve what President Kennedy proposed—namely, "general strengthening of our fundamental community, social welfare, and educational programs which can do much to eliminate or correct the harsh environmental conditions which often are associated with mental retardation and mental illness" (1963, p. 2).

One particularly interesting example of a possible favorable consequence of efforts to influence the distribution of power can be found in a paper by Solomon, Walker, O'Connor, and Fishman (1965). The authors present data that tend to document "the existence of an association between well-organized direct action for civil rights and a substantial reduction in crimes of violence committed by Negroes" (p. 227). Although Solomon et al. cautioned that their findings were by no means conclusive, they hypothesized that "Negroes release long dammed-up resentment of segregation by asserting themselves (directly or vicariously) in direct action for civil rights. Such emotional expression, when it occurs in a framework of community organization, may reduce the need for aggressive outbursts of a violent sort, thus reducing the incidence of such crimes" (p. 236).

From the discussion presented in this section, several principles can be derived to guide the development of programs to reduce stresses (see Bloom, 1971a). In order to illustrate how these principles might be employed, some of their implications for the field of family planning are provided.

Principle 1: Regardless of where your paycheck comes from, think of yourself as working for the community. Mental health programs in the community should be determined by a process of negotiation open to all members of the community. The ultimate power to decide the nature of the community-based mental health program should rest with the community, and mental health professionals should work in the community only as long as they feel a sufficient sense of congruence between the program the community wants and their own personal and professional value systems.

Work in the mental health field is a heavily value-laden enterprise, and values do not change easily. It is therefore particularly important in controversial issues, such as family planning, that the full spectrum of community opinion be solicited so that it can play a role in determining the character of social programs.

Principle 2: If you want to know about a community's mental health needs, ask the community. It is important that, in determining community mental health needs, planners not limit themselves to asking the opinions of human-service-agency personnel or extrapolating from present mental-health-service statistics. There are at least three other ways to identify community needs. First, public hearings can be held in which members of the community who have something to say about mental health needs—their own or those of their family, their friends, or the entire community—can be heard. Second, systematic household surveys can be undertaken in which a sample of persons are interviewed about their impressions of mental health needs in the community. Third, psychiatric patients themselves can be an invaluable source of information about community mental health needs. When patients are ready to be discharged from psychiatric care, for example, an opportunity presents itself to turn to them for help in exchange for the help they received. Ex-patients can be asked what they feel are the needs for mental-health-related services in the community. One question that would be particularly useful to ask former psychiatric patients is how the community (the neighborhood or the larger community) would have had to be structured in order for them not to have developed the disorganized or disturbing behaviors that resulted in their seeking psychiatric care. A related question would be what would have had to happen differently in their own lives in order for them not to have required care.

The training of community psychologists lends itself to a leadership role in community-need assessment. If family planning is an issue in the community, if family-planning services are lacking, if illegitimate births are increasing, little is served by having an incomplete understanding of the magnitude or dimensions of the problem. Need-assessment procedures can identify the problem and begin to illuminate its origins and persistence. Which groups appear to be at special risk? How has the problem changed in recent years? Is the problem more acute in some sections of the city? Answers to these questions can help enrich understanding of the problem and ultimately facilitate its solution.

Principle 3: As you learn about community mental-health-related needs, you have the responsibility to tell the community what you are learning. This principle puts the mental health professional in the role of community educator. The mental health professional is in an excellent position to learn about conditions in the community that need to be corrected and should bring to the community's attention these unmet mental health needs and the proposals for action designed to meet them.

The competent community knows itself. Need assessment is the beginning of a process that educates, that increases the community's wisdom. A skillfully undertaken inquiry into community values and community needs, skillfully reported in the media, can inaugurate debate that has the potential for problem resolution, for it often becomes clear that people share many areas of agreement where few were thought possible. In the area of family planning, for example, most people might agree that unwanted babies are at a special disadvantage and that they weaken the family and the community.

Principle 4: Help the community establish its own priorities. When community mental health needs have been identified, it is reasonable to expect that the resources available to the community will not be sufficient to meet all of them. Representatives of the community should play a major role in deciding which needs will be met first and how the limited resources will be divided among the various needs. It is possible, of course, for needs to conflict with each other; that is, in the very act of meeting one need, a program can exacerbate the situation with respect to another need. When such conflicts are identified, programs can emerge that come closer to satisfying the entire community.

Problems associated with family-planning services will vary in intensity in different communities and should have different priorities. Community debate can help establish appropriate priorities, and the community psychologist can help inaugurate and maintain constructive priority setting.

Principle 5: You can help the community decide among various courses of action in its efforts to solve its own problems. This is a special and perhaps unique role for community psychologists, who are acquainted not only with needs and with strategies for meeting them used by other communities but also with empirical research results. This knowledge can help them advise the community when it tries to decide among various courses of action. The mental health professional can identify high-risk groups in the community and discuss alternative ways of dealing with the problems of these groups.

Regarding family planning, for example, how serious is the problem locally? How have other communities dealt with the issue? Are some communities more successful than others, and if so, how can this community profit from knowing how other communities have dealt with the problem? What appear to be the consequences of ignoring the problem? This kind of information can make it easier for policy-making groups to come to decisions about social-program planning.

Principle 6: In the event that the community being served is so disorganized that representatives of various facets of the community cannot be found, you have the responsibility to help find such representatives. It is crucial for mental health professionals to be in good communication with the entire community and its representatives, not merely with selected members of an entrenched power group. For example, mental health professionals should be certain that the members of the policy-making board of the mental health center represent all sociocultural groups and socioeconomic levels within the community.

This is the principle underlying the field of community organization. The potential cast of characters in the family-planning debate is generally well known, and the community psychologist can help ensure that each has an appropriate voice in community debate and social-policy formulation.

Principle 7: You should work toward the equitable distribution of power in the community. Although it is difficult to make generalizations about optimal distribution of power, the most equitable way of distributing power appears to be in direct proportion to the size of the various identifiable ethnic, linguistic, and economic subgroups within the community. Equitable power distribution in the family-planning debate is also difficult to specify, but inequitable power distribution can be identified. Power is inequitable when births of unwanted children to teenagers are increasing while schools are not permitted to provide sex education, or when pregnant unmarried young women find that the community provides no feasible alternatives other than to complete their pregnancies, or when prevailing community attitudes toward such women are fundamentally hostile or punitive.

To the extent that these principles are followed, the community becomes involved in its own mental health and emotional vitality. Its members increase their power over their own lives, which leads to an increase in their competence and self-esteem, which in turn leads to increased emotional robustness and improved mental health.

CONCLUSIONS AND OVERVIEW

This chapter has attempted to provide an introduction to the field of community psychology, that field that looks outside the individual to find the sources of stress and the keys to prevention and remediation. We have examined how mental health professionals go about conceptualizing and assessing the community or the more narrowly defined environment or setting. We have examined selected aspects of population-focused issues and research and have identified and illustrated a set of principles that most community psychologists keep in mind as they attempt to institute community change. These principles are designed to provide community members with an optimal sense of control over their lives and over their community. The assumption governing the community psychology enterprise is that increased control over one's life results in increased self-esteem, which in turn results in increased psychological well-being.

Emotional disorders will not be eradicated, however, just because members of the community have developed increased self-esteem and increased power over their own lives. Not all psychopathology can be traced to powerlessness or lack of competence or to defects in social systems. Yet, it seems crucial to test the limits of these theories of psychopathology and this dynamic view of the community as a system of interdependent human beings.

Programs under the sponsorship of community mental health centers appear to be returning to more traditional direct clinical services. Thus, to move beyond community mental health may require moving beyond the community mental health center. How successful these moves will be—out of the mental health center and into schools, city government, social institutions, the general health service delivery system, the workplace, and the community at large—may be the critical question of the coming decade.

REFERENCES

Aakster, C. W. Psycho-social stress and health disturbances. *Social Science and Medicine*, 1974, *8*, 77–90.

Aanes, D., Klaessy, D., & Wills, J. The impact of a community hospital's psychiatric unit on a regional state hospital. *Hospital & Community Psychiatry*, 1975, *26*, 596–598.

Abernathy, W. B. The microcomputer as a community mental health public information tool. *Community Mental Health Journal*, 1979, *15*, 192–202.

Abrahams, R. B. Mutual help for the widowed. *Social Work*, 1972, *17*, 54–61.

Abrahams, R. B., & Patterson, R. D. Psychological distress among the community elderly: Prevalence, characteristics and implications for service. *International Journal of Aging and Human Development*, 1978–1979, *9*, 1–18.

Abramson, L. Y., Seligman, M. E. P., & Teasdale, J. D. Learned helplessness in humans: Critique and reformulation. *Journal of Abnormal Psychology*, 1978, *87*, 49–74.

Achterberg, J., Simonton, O. C., & Matthews-Simonton, S. *Stress, psychological factors, and cancer*. Fort Worth, Tex.: New Medicine Press, 1976.

Adam, C. T. A descriptive definition of primary prevention. *Journal of Primary Prevention*, 1981, *2*, 67–79.

Adelson, D., & Lurie, L. Mental health education: Research and practice. In S. E. Golann & C. Eisdorfer (Eds.), *Handbook of community mental health*. New York: Appleton-Century-Crofts, 1972.

Adler, L. M. The relationship of marital status to incidence of and recovery from mental illness. *Social Forces*, 1953, *32*, 185–194.

Adler, P. T. The community as a mental health system. *MH (Mental Hygiene)*, 1972, *56*, 28–32.

Adler, P. T. The community mental health center in the community: Another look. *Journal of Community Psychology*, 1977, *5*, 116–123.

Aguilera, D. C., & Messick, J. M. *Crisis intervention: Theory and methodology* (2nd ed.). St. Louis, MO.: Mosby, 1974.

Aiello, T. J. Short-term group therapy of the hospitalized psychotic. In H. Grayson (Ed.), *Short-term approaches to psychotherapy*. New York: Human Sciences Press, 1979.

Albee, G. W. Models, myths, and manpower. *Mental Hygiene*, 1968, *52*, 168–180.

Albee, G. W. Primary prevention. *Canada's Mental Health*, 1979, *27*, 5–9.

Albee, G. W. The fourth mental health revolution. *Journal of Prevention*, 1980, *1*, 67–70.

Albee, G. W. Politics, power, prevention, and social change. In J. M. Joffe & G. W. Albee (Eds.), *Prevention through political action and social change*. Hanover, N.H.: University Press of New England, 1981.

Aldrich, C. K. Brief psychotherapy: A reappraisal of some theoretical assumptions. *American Journal of Psychiatry*, 1968, *125*, 585–592.

Allen, G. F., Chinsky, J. M., Larcen, S. W., Lochman, J. E., & Selinger, H. E. *Community psychology and the schools: A behaviorally oriented multilevel preventive approach*. Hillsdale, N.J.: Erlbaum, 1976.

Altrocchi, J. Mental health consultation. In S. E. Golann & C. Eisdorfer (Eds.), *Handbook of community mental health*. New York: Appleton-Century-Crofts, 1972.

Altrocchi, J., Spielberger, C. D., & Eisdorfer, C. Mental health consultation with groups. *Community Mental Health Journal*, 1965, *1*, 127–134.

American Psychological Association. Federal court upholds right to treatment. *APA Monitor*, 1972, *3* (5), 1.

433

American Public Health Association. *Mental disorders: A guide to control methods.* New York: Author, 1962.

Anderson, L. S., Cooper, S., Hassol, L., Klein, D. C., Rosenblum, G., & Bennett, C. C. *Community psychology: A report of the Boston Conference on the Education of Psychologists for Community Mental Health.* Boston: Boston University, 1966.

Andrews, F. M. Social indicators of perceived life quality. *Social Indicators Research,* 1974, *1,* 279–299.

Andrews, F. M., & Withey, S. B. Developing measures of perceived life quality: Results from several national surveys. *Social Indicators Research,* 1974, *1,* 1–26.

Andrews, F. M., & Withey, S. B. *Social indicators of well-being: Americans' perceptions of life quality.* New York: Plenum Press, 1976.

Andrews, G., Tennant, C., Hewson, D. M., & Vaillant, G. E. Life event stress, social support, coping style, and risk of psychological impairment. *Journal of Nervous and Mental Disease,* 1978, *166,* 307–316.

Andriola, J., & Cata, G. The oldest mental hospital in the world. *Hospital & Community Psychiatry,* 1969, *20,* 42–43.

Antonovsky, A. *Health, stress, and coping: New perspectives on mental and physical wellbeing.* San Francisco, Calif.: Jossey-Bass, 1979.

Applebaum, S. A. Parkinson's law in psychotherapy. *International Journal of Psychoanalytic Psychotherapy,* 1975, *4,* 426–436.

Apsler, R., & Hodas, M. B. Evaluating hotlines with simulated calls. *Crisis Intervention,* 1975, *6,* 14–21.

Argyle, M., Bryant, B., & Trower, P. Social skills training and psychotherapy: A comparative study. *Psychological Medicine,* 1974, *4,* 435–443.

Argyle, M., Trower, P., & Bryant, B. Explorations in the treatment of personality disorders and neuroses by social skills training. *British Journal of Medical Psychology,* 1974, *47,* 63–72.

Aring, C. D. The Gheel experience: Eternal spirit of the chainless mind! *Journal of the American Medical Association,* 1974, *230,* 998–1001.

Arnhoff, F. N. Social consequences of policy toward mental illness. *Science,* 1975, *188,* 1277–1281.

Arthur, R. J. Success is predictable. *Military Medicine,* 1971, *136,* 539–545.

Askenasy, A. R., Dohrenwend, B. P., & Dohrenwend, B. S. Some effects of social class and ethnic group membership on judgments of the magnitude of stressful life events: A research note. *Journal of Health and Social Behavior,* 1977, *18,* 432–439.

Auerbach, S. M., & Kilmann, P. R. Crisis intervention: A review of outcome research. *Psychological Bulletin,* 1977, *84,* 1189–1217.

Avnet, H. H. How effective is short-term therapy? In L. R. Wolberg (Ed.), *Short-term psychotherapy.* New York: Grune & Stratton, 1965. (a)

Avnet, H. H. Short-term treatment under auspices of a medical insurance plan. *American Journal of Psychiatry,* 1965, *122,* 147–151. (b)

Bachrach, L. L. *Marital status of discharges from psychiatric inpatient units of general hospitals, United States, 1970–1971: I. Analysis by age, color and sex.* NIMH Statistical Note 82. Washington, D.C.: U.S. Government Printing Office, 1973.

Bachrach, L. L. *Marital status and mental disorder: An analytical review.* DHEW Pub. No. (ADM) 75–217. Washington, D.C.: U.S. Government Printing Office, 1975.

Bachrach, L. L. *Deinstitutionalization: An analytical review and sociological perspective.* DHEW Pub. No. (ADM) 76–351. Washington, D.C.: U.S. Government Printing Office, 1976.

Baizerman, M., & Hall, W. T. Consultation as a political process. *Community Mental Health Journal,* 1977, *13,* 142–149.

Baker, F., Schulberg, H. C., & O'Brien, G. M. The changing mental hospital—its perceived image and contact with the community. *Mental Hygiene,* 1969, *53,* 237–244.

Baldwin, B. A. Crisis intervention: An overview of theory and practice. *Counseling Psychologist,* 1979, *8,* 43–52.

Bandura, A. Self-efficacy: Toward a unifying theory of behavioral change. *Psychological Review*, 1977, 84, 191–215.

Bane, M. J. Marital disruption and the lives of children. In G. Levinger & O. Moles (Eds.), *Divorce and separation: Context, causes and consequences*. New York: Basic Books, 1979.

Bard, M. *Training police as specialists in family crisis intervention*. Washington, D.C.: U.S. Government Printing Office, 1970.

Bard, M., & Berkowitz, B. Training police as specialists in family crisis intervention: A community psychology action program. *Community Mental Health Journal*, 1967, 3, 315–317.

Bard, M., & Berkowitz, B. A community psychology consultation program in police family crisis intervention: Preliminary impressions. *International Journal of Social Psychiatry*, 1969, 15, 209–215.

Barker, R. *Ecological psychology*. Stanford, Calif.: Stanford University Press, 1968.

Barker, R., & Gump, P. *Big school, small school*. Stanford, Calif.: Stanford University Press, 1964.

Barrett, J. E. The relationship of life events to the onset of neurotic disorders. In J. E. Barrett, R. M. Rose, & G. L. Klerman (Eds.), *Stress and mental disorder*. New York: Raven Press, 1979.

Bartemeier, L. *Hearings before the Subcommittee on Health, the Committee on Labor and Public Welfare, U.S. Senate, March 5, 6, 7, 1963*. Washington, D.C.: U.S. Government Printing Office, 1963.

Barthell, C. N., & Holmes, D. S. High school yearbooks: A nonreactive measure of social isolation in graduates who later became schizophrenic. *Journal of Abnormal Psychology*, 1968, 73, 313–316.

Bass, R. D. *Consultation and education services: Federally funded community mental health centers, 1973*. NIMH Statistical Note 108, DHEW Pub. No. (ADM) 75–108. Washington, D.C: U.S. Government Printing Office, 1974.

Bassuk, E. L., & Gerson, S. Deinstitutionalization and mental health services. *Scientific American*, 1978, 238, 46–53.

Bates, J. E. The concept of difficult temperament. *Merrill-Palmer Quarterly*, 1980, 26, 11–22.

Bauer, R. (Ed.). *Social indicators*. Cambridge, Mass.: M.I.T. Press, 1966.

Baum, A., Singer, J. E., & Baum, C. S. Stress and the environment. *Journal of Social Issues*, 1981, 37, 4–35.

Baumrind, D. The contributions of the family to the development of competence in children. *Schizophrenia Bulletin*, 1975, Issue No. 14, 12–37.

Beaver, W., Buck, F. M., & McWilliams, S. A. Issues in replicating the trauma-stren conversion. *American Journal of Community Psychology*, 1979, 7, 129–136.

Beisser, A. R., & Green, R. *Mental health consultation and education*. Palo Alto, Calif.: National Press Books, 1972.

Belfer, M. L., Mulliken, J. B., & Cochran, T. C. Cosmetic surgery as an antecedent of life change. *American Journal of Psychiatry*, 1979, 136, 199–201.

Bell, B. D. The limitations of crisis theory as an explanatory mechanism in social gerontology. *International Journal of Aging and Human Development*, 1975, 6, 153–168.

Bell, D. (Ed.). *Toward the year 2000: Work in progress*. Boston, Mass.: Beacon Press, 1967.

Bell, R., Sundel, M., Aponte, J. F., Murrell, S. A., & Lin, E. (Eds.). *Assessing health and human service needs: Concepts, methods and applications*. New York: Human Sciences Press, 1982.

Bellak, L., & Small, L. *Emergency psychotherapy and brief psychotherapy*. New York: Grune & Stratton, 1965.

Bellak, L., & Small, L. *Emergency psychotherapy and brief psychotherapy* (2nd ed.). New York: Grune & Stratton, 1978.

Bene-Kociemba, A., Cotton, P. G., & Frank, A. Predictors of community tenure of discharged state hospital patients. *American Journal of Psychiatry*, 1979, 136, 1556–1561.

Bennett, D. Deinstitutionalization in two cultures. *Milbank Memorial Fund Quarterly*, 1979, *57*, 516–531.

Bergin, A. E., & Garfield, S. L. (Eds.). *Handbook of psychotherapy and behavior change: An empirical analysis.* New York: Wiley, 1971.

Bergler, E. *The basic neurosis, oral regression and psychic masochism.* New York: Grune & Stratton, 1949.

Berkman, L. F., & Syme, S. L. Social networks, host resistance, and mortality: A nine-year follow up study of Alameda County residents. *American Journal of Epidemiology*, 1979, *109*, 186–204.

Berlin, I. Resistance to mental health consultation directed at change in public institutions. *Community Mental Health Journal*, 1979, *15*, 119–128.

Bernard, J. *The sociology of community.* Glenview, Ill.: Scott, Foresman, 1973.

Bernstein, R. Are we still stereotyping the unmarried mother? *Social Work*, 1960, *5*, 22–28.

Bethel, H. *Provisional patient movement and administrative data: State and county mental hospital inpatient services, July 1, 1971–June 30, 1972.* NIMH Statistical Note 77. Washington, D.C.: U.S. Government Printing Office, 1973.

Bethel, H. *Provisional patient movement and administrative data: State and county mental hospital inpatient services, July 1, 1972–June 30, 1973.* NIMH Statistical Note 106. Washington, D.C.: U.S. Government Printing Office, 1974.

Bethel, H., & Redick, R. W. *Provisional patient movement and administrative data: State and county mental hospital inpatient services, July 1, 1970–June 30, 1971.* NIMH Statistical Note 60. Washington, D.C.: U.S. Government Printing Office, 1972.

Bey, R. D., & Lange, J. Waiting wives: Women under stress. *American Journal of Psychiatry*, 1974, *131*, 283–286.

Bindman, A. J. Mental health consultation: Theory and practice. *Journal of Consulting Psychology*, 1959, *23*, 473–482.

Bindman, A. J. Problems associated with community mental health programs. *Community Mental Health Journal*, 1966, *2*, 333–338.

Blacker, C. P. The confluence of psychiatry and demography. *British Journal of Psychiatry*, 1973, *123*, 493–500.

Blackman, S., & Goldstein, K. M. Some aspects of a theory of community mental health. *Community Mental Health Journal*, 1968, *4*, 83–90.

Blake, J. The teenage birth control dilemma and public opinion. *Science*, 1973, *180*, 708–712.

Blake, J. Family size and the quality of children. *Demography*, 1981, *18*, 421–442.

Blake, J., & Del Pinal, J. H. Negativism, equivocation, and the wobbly assent: Public "support" for the prochoice platform on abortion. *Demography*, 1981, *18*, 309–320.

Blaufarb, H., & Levine, J. Crisis intervention in an earthquake. *Social Work*, 1972, *17*, 16–19.

Bleach, G., & Claiborn, W. L. Initial evaluation of hot-line telephone crisis centers. *Community Mental Health Journal*, 1974, *10*, 387–394.

Bloom, B. L. Definitional aspects of the crisis concept. *Journal of Consulting Psychology*, 1963, *27*, 498–502.

Bloom, B. L. A census tract analysis of socially deviant behaviors. *Multivariate Behavioral Research*, 1966, *1*, 307–320.

Bloom, B. L. Psychotherapy and the community mental health movement. In C. J. Frederick (Ed.), *The future of psychotherapy.* Boston, Mass.: Little, Brown, 1969.

Bloom, B. L. Strategies for the prevention of mental disorders. In Division 27, American Psychological Association, Task Force on Community Mental Health, *Issues in community psychology and preventive mental health.* New York: Behavioral Publications, 1971. (a)

Bloom, B. L. A university freshman preventive intervention program: Report of a pilot project. *Journal of Consulting and Clinical Psychology*, 1971, *37*, 235–242. (b)

Bloom, B. L. *Changing patterns of psychiatric care.* New York: Human Sciences Press, 1975.

Bloom, B. L. *Community mental health: A general introduction.* Monterey, Calif.: Brooks/ Cole, 1977. (a)

Bloom, B. L. Current issues in mental health continuing education. *American Journal of Community Psychology,* 1977, *5,* 121–130. (b)

Bloom, B. L. Social and community interventions. *Annual review of psychology,* 1980, *31,* 111–142.

Bloom, B. L. Focused single-session therapy: Initial development and evaluation. In S. E. Budman (Ed.), *Forms of brief therapy.* New York: Guilford Press, 1981. (a)

Bloom, B. L. The logic and urgency of primary prevention. *Hospital & Community Psychiatry,* 1981, *32,* 839–843. (b)

Bloom, B. L., & Asher, S. J. Patient rights and patient advocacy: A historical and conceptual appreciation. In B. L. Bloom & S. J. Asher (Eds.), *Psychiatric patient rights and patient advocacy: Issues and evidence.* New York: Human Sciences Press, 1982. (a)

Bloom, B. L., & Asher, S. J. (Eds.). *Psychiatric patient rights and patient advocacy: Issues and evidence.* New York: Human Sciences Press, 1982. (b)

Bloom, B. L., Asher, S. J., & White, S. W. Marital disruption as a stressor: A review and analysis. *Psychological Bulletin,* 1978, *85,* 867–894.

Bloom, B. L., & Caldwell, R. A. Sex differences in adjustment during the process of marital separation. *Journal of Marriage and the Family,* 1981, *43,* 693–701.

Bloom, B. L., Hodges, W. F., & Caldwell, R. A. A preventive intervention program for the newly separated: Initial evaluation. *American Journal of Community Psychology,* 1982, *10,* 251–264.

Bloom, B. L., Hodges, W. F., Caldwell, R. A., Systra, L., & Cedrone, A. R. Marital separation: A community survey. *Journal of Divorce,* 1977, *1,* 7–19.

Bloom, B. L., & Parad, H. J. Professional activity patterns in community mental health centers. In I. Iscoe, B. L. Bloom, & C. D. Spielberger (Eds.), *Community psychology in transition.* Washington, D.C.: Hemisphere, 1977.

Blum, R. H. Case identification in psychiatric epidemiology—methods and problems. *Milbank Memorial Fund Quarterly,* 1962, *40,* 253–288.

Blumenthal, M. D. Mental health among the divorced. *Archives of General Psychiatry,* 1967, *16,* 603–608.

Bockoven, J. S. *Moral treatment in American psychiatry.* New York: Springer, 1963.

Bockoven, J. S., & Solomon, H. C. Comparison of two five-year follow-up studies: 1947 to 1952 and 1967 to 1972. *American Journal of Psychiatry,* 1975, *132,* 796–801.

Bodin, A. The family agreement measure. In P. McReynolds (Ed.), *Advances in psychological measurement.* Palo Alto, Calif.: Science and Behavior Books, 1968.

Bolman, W. M. An outline of preventive psychiatric programs for children. *Archives of General Psychiatry,* 1967, *17,* 5–8.

Bolman, W. M., & Bolian, G. C. Crisis intervention as primary or secondary prevention. In J. D. Noshpitz (Ed.), *Basic handbook of child psychiatry* (Vol. 4). New York: Basic Books, 1979.

Bolman, W. M., Halleck, S. L., Rice, D. G., & Ryan, M. L. An unintended side effect in a community psychiatric program. *Archives of General Psychiatry,* 1969, *20,* 508–513.

Bolman, W. M., & Westman, J. C. Prevention of mental disorder: An overview of current programs. *American Journal of Psychiatry,* 1967, *123,* 1058–1068.

Bonn, E. M. The impact of redeployment of funds on a model state hospital. *Hospital & Community Psychiatry,* 1975, *26,* 584–586.

Bower, E. M. Slicing the mystique of prevention with Occam's razor. *American Journal of Public Health,* 1969, *59,* 478–484.

Bower, E. M. K.I.S.S. and kids: A mandate for prevention. *American Journal of Orthopsychiatry,* 1972, *42,* 556–565.

Bowlby, J. *Attachment and loss.* Vol. 1: *Attachment.* New York: Basic Books, 1969.

Bradley, J. P., Daniels, L. F., & Jones, T. C. *The international dictionary of thoughts.* Chicago, Ill.: Ferguson, 1969.

Brand, J. L. The United States: An historical perspective. In R. H. Williams & L. D. Ozarin (Eds.), *Community mental health: An international perspective*. San Francisco, Calif.: Jossey-Bass, 1968.

Brandwein, R. A., Brown, C. A., & Fox, E. M. Women and children last: The social situation of divorced mothers and their families. *Journal of Marriage and the Family*, 1974, *36*, 498–514.

Braun, P., Kochansky, G., Shapiro, R., Greenberg, S, Gudeman, J. E., Johnson, S., & Shore, M. F. Overview: Deinstitutionalization of psychiatric patients—a critical review of outcome studies. *American Journal of Psychiatry*, 1981, *138*, 736–749.

Brenner, M. H. *Mental illness and the economy*. Cambridge, Mass.: Harvard University Press, 1973.

Breslow, L., Fielding, J. E., & Lave, L. B. (Eds.). *Annual review of public health*. Palo Alto, Calif.: Annual Reviews, 1980.

Breuer, J., & Freud, S. *Studies on hysteria*. New York: Basic Books, 1957. (Originally published, 1895.)

Briscoe, C. W., Smith, J. B., Robins, E., Marten, S., & Gaskin, F. Divorce and psychiatric disease. *Archives of General Psychiatry*, 1973, *29*, 119–125.

Brockopp, G. W., & Oughterson, E. D. Legal and procedural aspects of telephone emergency services. *Crisis Intervention*, 1972, *4*, 15–25.

Brogan, D. R., & James, L. D. Physical environment correlates of psychosocial health among urban residents. *American Journal of Community Psychology*, 1980, *8*, 507–521.

Bromet, E. J., Parkinson, D. K., Schulberg, H. C., Dunn, C. O., & Gondek, P. C. Mental health of residents near the Three Mile Island reactor: a comparative study of selected groups. *Journal of Preventive Psychiatry*, 1982, *1*, 225–276.

Brown, B. S., & Cain, H. P. The many meanings of "comprehensive." *Journal of Orthopsychiatry*, 1964, *34*, 834–839.

Brown, G. W. Meaning, measurement, and stress of life events. In B. S. Dohrenwend & B. P. Dohrenwend (Eds.), *Stressful life events: Their nature and effects*. New York: Wiley, 1974.

Brown, G. W., & Birley, J. L. T. Crises and life changes and the onset of schizophrenia. *Journal of Health and Social Behavior*, 1968, *9*, 203–214.

Brown, G. W., Harris, T. O., & Peto, J. Life events and psychiatric disorders: II. Nature of the causal link. *Psychological Medicine*, 1973, *3*, 159–176.

Brown, G. W., Sklair, F., Harris, T. O., & Birley, J. L. T. Life events and psychiatric disorders: 1. Some methodological issues. *Psychological Medicine*, 1973, *3*, 74–87.

Brown, P. Social implications of deinstitutionalization. *Journal of Community Psychology*, 1980, *8*, 314–322.

Brown, S. D. Coping skills training: An evaluation of a psychoeducational program in a community mental health setting. *Journal of Counseling Psychology*, 1980, *27*, 340–345.

Bry, B. H. Reducing the incidence of adolescent problems through preventive intervention: One and five year follow-up. *American Journal of Community Psychology*, 1982, *10*, 265–276.

Budman, S. H., Bennett, M. J., & Wisneski, M. J. Short-term group psychotherapy: An adult developmental model. *International Journal of Group Psychotherapy*, 1980, *30*, 63–76.

Budman, S. H., Bennett, M. J., & Wisneski, M. J. An adult developmental model of short-term group psychotherapy. In S. H. Budman (Ed.), *Forms of brief therapy*. New York: Guilford Press, 1981.

Budman, S. H., & Clifford, M. Short-term group therapy for couples in a health maintenance organization. *Professional Psychology*, 1979, *10*, 419–429.

Budman, S., Demby, A., & Randall, M. Short-term group psychotherapy: Who succeeds, who fails? *Group*, 1980, *4*, 3–16.

Bunn, A. R. Ischaemic heart disease mortality and the business cycle in Australia. *American Journal of Public Health*, 1979, 69, 772–781.

Bunn, A. R. II. IHD mortality and the business cycle in Australia. *American Journal of Public Health*, 1980, 70, 409–411.

Bunn, T. A., & Clarke, A. M. Crisis intervention: An experimental study of the effects of a brief period of counselling on the anxiety of relatives of seriously injured or ill hospital patients. *British Journal of Medical Psychology*, 1979, 52, 191–195.

Bureau of the Census, U.S. Department of Commerce. *Marital status and living arrangements*. Current Population Reports, Series P–20, No. 271. Washington, D.C.: U.S. Government Printing Office, 1974.

Bureau of the Census, U.S. Department of Commerce. *A statistical portrait of women in the U.S.* Current Population Reports, Series P–23, No.58. Washington, D.C.: U.S. Government Printing Office, 1976.

Burke, F. *Urban growth models and methods of studying social areas.* CMHE Working Paper No. 56. Nashville, Tenn.: Center for Community Studies, George Peabody College, 1974.

Burke, J. D., White, H. S., & Havens, L. L. Which short-term therapy? *Archives of General Psychiatry*, 1979, 36, 177–186.

Burke, R. J., & Weir, T. Marital helping relationships: The moderators between stress and well-being. *Journal of Psychology*, 1977, 95, 121–130.

Butcher, J. N., & Koss, M. P. Research on brief and crisis-oriented therapies. In S. L. Garfield & A. E. Bergin (Eds.), *Handbook of psychotherapy and behavior change: An empirical analysis* (2nd ed.). New York: Wiley, 1978.

Butcher, J. N., & Maudal, G. R. Crisis intervention. In I. Weiner (Ed.), *Clinical methods in psychology.* New York: Wiley, 1976.

Byers, E. S., Cohen, S., & Harshbarger, D. D. Impact of aftercare services on recidivism of mental hospital patients. *Community Mental Health Journal*, 1978, 14, 26–34.

Caffey, E. M., Galbrecht, C. R., & Klett, C. J. Brief hospitalization and aftercare in the treatment of schizophrenia. *Archives of General Psychiatry*, 1971, 24, 81–86.

Calhoun, J. B. Population density and social pathology. *Scientific American*, 1962, 206, 139–148.

Campbell, A. *The sense of well-being in America: Recent patterns and trends.* New York: McGraw-Hill, 1981.

Cancer: A progress report. *Newsweek*, November 2, 1981.

Cannon, W. B. *Bodily changes in pain, hunger, fear and rage.* New York: D. Appleton, 1929.

Caplan, G. *An approach to community mental health.* New York: Grune & Stratton, 1961. (a)

Caplan, G. (Ed.). *Prevention of mental disorders in children: Initial explorations.* New York: Basic Books, 1961. (b)

Caplan, G. *Manual for psychiatrists participating in the Peace Corps program.* Washington, D.C.: Medical Program Division, Peace Corps, 1962.

Caplan, G. Types of mental health consultation. *American Journal of Orthopsychiatry*, 1963, 33, 470–481.

Caplan, G. *Principles of preventive psychiatry.* New York: Basic Books, 1964.

Caplan, G. *The theory and practice of mental health consultation.* New York: Basic Books, 1970.

Caplan, G. Mastery of stress: Psychological aspects. *American Journal of Psychiatry*, 1981, 138, 413–420.

Caplan, G., & Grunebaum, H. Perspectives on primary prevention: A review. *Archives of General Psychiatry*, 1967, 17, 331–346.

Carkhuff, R. R. *The art of helping.* Amherst, Mass.: Human Resources Press, 1973.

Carlson, B. E., & Davis, L. V. Prevention of domestic violence. In R. H. Price, R. F. Ketterer, B. C. Bader, & J. Monahan (Eds.), *Prevention in mental health: Research, policy, and practice.* Beverly Hills, Calif.: Sage Publications, 1980.

Carpenter, M. D. Residential placement for the chronic psychiatric patient: A review and evaluation of the literature. *Schizophrenia Bulletin*, 1978, 4, 384–398.

Carpenter, W. T., Tamarkin, N. R., & Raskin, D. E. Emergency psychiatric treatment during a mass rally: The march on Washington. *American Journal of Psychiatry*, 1971, 127, 1327–1332.

Cassel, J. Social science theory as a source of hypotheses in epidemiological research. *American Journal of Public Health*, 1964, 54, 1482–1488.

Cassel, J. The relation of the urban environment to health: Implications for prevention. *Mount Sinai Journal of Medicine*, 1973, 40, 539–550.

Cassel, J. An epidemiological perspective of psychosocial factors in disease etiology. *American Journal of Public Health*, 1974, 64, 1040–1043. (a)

Cassel, J. Psychosocial processes and "stress": Theoretical formulation. *International Journal of Health Services*, 1974, 4, 471–482. (b)

Cassel, J. The contribution of the social environment to host resistance. *American Journal of Epidemiology*, 1976, 104, 107–123.

Castelnuovo-Tedesco, P. The twenty-minute hour: An approach to the postgraduate teaching of psychiatry. *American Journal of Psychiatry*, 1967, 123, 786–791.

Castelnuovo-Tedesco, P. The "20–minute hour" revisited: A follow-up. *Comprehensive Psychiatry*, 1970, 11, 108–122.

Castelnuovo-Tedesco, P. Decreasing the length of psychotherapy: Theoretical and practical aspects of the problem. In S. Arieti (Ed.), *The world biennial of psychiatry and psychotherapy* (Vol. 1). New York: Basic Books, 1971.

Catalano, R., & Dooley, C. D. Economic predictors of depressed mood and stressful life events in a metropolitan community. *Journal of Health and Social Behavior*, 1977, 18, 292–307.

Catalano, R., & Dooley, D. Economic change in primary prevention. In R. H. Price, R. F. Ketterer, B. C. Bader, & J. Monahan (Eds.), *Prevention in mental health: Research, policy and practice*. Beverly Hills, Calif.: Sage Publications, 1980.

Cauffman, J. G., Wingert, W. A., Friedman, D. B., Warburton, E. A., & Hanes, B. Community health aides: How effective are they? *American Journal of Public Health*, 1970, 60, 1904–1909.

Chan, K. B. Individual differences in reactions to stress and their personality and situational determinants: Some implications for community mental health. *Social Science and Medicine*, 1977, 11, 89–103.

Cherniss, C. Creating new consultation programs in community mental health centers. *Community Mental Health Journal*, 1977, 13, 133–141.

Chiriboga, D. A., Coho, A., Stein, J. A., & Roberts, J. Divorce, stress and social supports: A study in helpseeking behavior. *Journal of Divorce*, 1979, 3, 121–135.

Chiriboga, D. A., & Cutler, L. Stress responses among divorcing men and women. *Journal of Divorce*, 1977, 1, 95–106.

Chiriboga, D. A., Roberts, J., & Stein, J. A. Psychological well-being during marital separation. *Journal of Divorce*, 1978, 2, 21–36.

Chu, F. D. The Nader report: One author's perspective. *American Journal of Psychiatry*, 1974, 131, 775–779.

Chu, F. D., & Trotter, S. *The madness establishment*. New York: Grossman, 1974.

Clark, C. C. Simulation gaming: A new teaching strategy in nursing education. *Nurse Education*, 1976, 1, 4–9.

Clarke, G. J. In defense of deinstitutionalization. *Milbank Memorial Fund Quarterly*, 1979, 57, 461–479.

Clausen, J. A. *Social psychiatry and mental health programs in the United States*. Paper presented at the 7th World Congress of Sociology, Varna, Bulgaria, September, 1970.

Clayton, P. J. The effect of living alone on bereavement symptoms. *American Journal of Psychiatry*, 1975, 132, 133–137.

Cleary, P. J. A checklist for life event research. *Journal of Psychometric Research*, 1980, 24, 199–207.

Cline, D. W., & Chosy, J. J. A prospective study of life changes and subsequent health changes. *Archives of General Psychiatry*, 1972, 27, 51–53.

Cobb, S. A model for life events and their consequences. In B. S. Dohrenwend & B. P. Dohrenwend (Eds.), *Stressful life events: Their nature and effects.* New York: Wiley, 1974.

Cobb, S. Social support as a moderator of life stress. *Psychosomatic Medicine*, 1976, 38, 300–314.

Cochran, R., & Robertson, A. The life events inventory: A measure of the relative severity of psycho-social stressors. *Journal of Psychosomatic Research*, 1973, 17, 135–139.

Cochrane, A. L. *Effectiveness and efficiency: Random reflections on health services.* London: Nuffield Provincial Hospitals Trust, 1972.

Coddington, R. D. The significance of life events as etiologic factors in the diseases of children: I. A survey of professional workers. *Journal of Psychosomatic Research*, 197, 16, 7–18. (a)

Coddington, R.D. The significance of life events as etiologic factors in the diseases of children: II. A study of a normal population. *Journal of Psychosomatic Research*, 1972, 16, 205–213. (b)

Cohen, A. *Teachings of Maimonides.* London: Routledge, 1927.

Cohen, F. Personality, stress, and the development of physical illness. In G. C. Stone, F. Cohen, & N. E. Adler (Eds.), *Health psychology—a handbook.* San Francisco, Calif.: Jossey-Bass, 1979.

Cohen, F., & Lazarus, R. S. Coping with the stresses of illness. In G. C. Stone, F. Cohen, & N. E. Adler (Eds.), *Health psychology—a handbook.* San Francisco, Calif.: Jossey-Bass, 1979.

Cohen, L. D. Consultation as a method of mental health intervention. In B. Brower & L. E. Abt (Eds.), *Progress in clinical psychology.* New York: Grune & Stratton, 1966.

Cohen, W. J. Education and learning. *Annals of the American Academy of Political and Social Science*, 1967, 373, 79–101.

Cole, J. O. Comment. *American Journal of Psychiatry*, 1974, 131, 781–782.

Cole, J. O., & Gerard, R. W. (Eds.). *Psychopharmacology: Problems in evaluation.* Publication 583. Washington, D.C.: National Academy of Sciences, 1959.

Committee on Interstate and Foreign Commerce, Subcommittee on Public Health and Safety. *Committee report, August 21, 1963* (No. HR694). Washington, D.C.: U.S. Government Printing Office, 1963.

Conger, J. C., & Keane, S. P. Social skills intervention in the treatment of isolated or withdrawn children. *Psychological Bulletin*, 1981, 90, 478–495.

Conger, W. D., Shepard, M., & Szot, T. *Social report: 1977. Human Resources Department, City of Boulder.* Boulder, Colo.: City of Boulder, 1978.

Connery, R. H., Backstrom, C. H., Friedman, J. R., Marden, R. H., Meekison, P., Deener, D. R., Kroll, M., McCleskey, C., & Morgan, J. A., Jr. *Politics of mental health: Organizing community mental health in metropolitan areas.* New York: Columbia University Press, 1968.

Conoley, J. C. (Ed.). *Consultation in schools: Theory, research, procedures.* New York: Academic Press, 1981.

Cooke, D. J., & Greene, J. G. Types of life events in relation to symptoms at the climacterium. *Journal of Psychosomatic Research*, 1981, 25, 5–11.

Cooper, B., & Sylph, J. Life events and the onset of neurotic illness: An investigation in general practice. *Psychological Medicine*, 1973, 3, 421–435.

Cooper, J. E., Kendell, R. E., Gurland, B. J., Sartorius, N., & Farkas, T. Cross-national study of diagnosis of the mental disorders: Some results from the first comparative investigation. *American Journal of Psychiatry*, 1969, 125 (No. 10 Suppl.), 21–29.

Cooper, S., & Hodges, W. F. (Eds.). *The field of mental health consultation.* New York: Human Sciences Press, 1983.

Cope, Z. *Florence Nightingale and the doctors.* New York: Lippincott, 1958.

Cowen, E. L. Emergent directions in school mental health. *American Scientist*, 1971, *59*, 723–733.

Cowen, E. L., Dorr, D., Izzo, L. D., Madonia, A., & Trost, M. A. The Primary Mental Health Project: A new way of conceptualizing and delivering school mental health services. *Psychology in the Schools*, 1971, *8*, 216–225.

Cowen, E. L., Gesten, E. L., Boike, M., Norton, P., Wilson, A. B., & DeStefano, M. A. Hairdressers as caregivers: I. A descriptive profile of interpersonal help-giving involvements. *American Journal of Community Psychology*, 1979, *7*, 633–648.

Cowen, E. L., Gesten, E. L., Davidson, E., & Wilson, A. B. Hairdressers as caregivers: II. Relationships between helper characteristics and helping behaviors and feelings. *Journal of Prevention*, 1981, *1*, 225–239.

Cowen, E. L., Gesten, E. L., & Wilson, A. B. The Primary Mental Health Project (PMHP): Evaluation of current program effectiveness. *American Journal of Community Psychology*, 1979, *7*, 292–303.

Cowen, E. L., Izzo, L. D., Miles, H., Telschow, E. F., Trost, M. A., & Zax, M. A mental health program in the school setting: Description and evaluation. *Journal of Psychology*, 1963, *56*, 307–356.

Cowen, E. L., Pederson, A., Babigian, H., Izzo, L. D., & Trost, M. A. Long-term follow-up of early detected vulnerable children. *Journal of Consulting and Clinical Psychology*, 1973, *41*, 438–446.

Cowen, E. L., Zax, M., Izzo, L. D., & Trost, M. A. The prevention of emotional disorders in the school setting: A further investigation. *Journal of Consulting Psychology*, 1966, *30*, 381–387.

Crago, M. A. Psychopathology in married couples. *Psychological Bulletin*, 1972, *77*, 114–128.

Craig, T. J., & Lin, S. P. Death and deinstitutionalization. *American Journal of Psychiatry*, 1981, *138*, 224–227.

Crandall, J. E., & Lehman, R. E. Relationship of stressful life events to social interest, locus of control, and psychological adjustment. *Journal of Consulting and Clinical Psychology*, 1977, *45*, 1208.

Crandell, D. L., & Dohrenwend, B. P. Some relations among psychiatric symptoms, organic illness, and social class. *American Journal of Psychiatry*, 1967, *123*, 1527–1538.

Cresswell, D. L., Corre, B. H., & Zautra, A. A needs assessment of perceived life quality and life stressors among medical hospital employees. *Journal of Community Psychology*, 1981, *9*, 153–161.

Crook, T., & Eliot, J. Parental death during childhood and adult depression: A critical review of the literature. *Psychological Bulletin*, 1980, *87*, 252–259.

Cumming, E., & Cumming, J. *Closed ranks: An experiment in mental health education.* Cambridge, Mass.: Harvard University Press, 1957.

Cumming, E., & Cumming, J. Some questions on community care. *Canada's Mental Health*, 1965, *13*, 7–12.

Cummings, N. A. The anatomy of psychotherapy under national health insurance. *American Psychologist*, 1977, *32*, 711–718. (a)

Cummings, N. A. Prolonged (ideal) versus short-term (realistic) psychotherapy. *Professional Psychology*, 1977, *8*, 491–501. (b)

Cummings, N. A., & Follette, W. T. Psychiatric services and medical utilization in a prepaid health plan setting: Part II. *Medical Care*, 1968, *6*, 31–41.

Cypress, B. K. *Office-visits for preventive care, National Ambulatory Medical Care Survey: United States, 1977–1978.* National Center for Health Statistics. No. 69. April 1981. DHHS Pub. No. (PHS) 81–1250. Washington, D.C.: U.S. Government Printing Office, 1981.

Dain, N. *Concepts of insanity in the United States, 1789–1865.* Rutgers, N.J.: Rutgers University Press, 1964.

Daley, B. S., & Koppenaal, G. S. The treatment of women in short-term women's groups. In S. H. Budman (Ed.), *Forms of brief therapy.* New York: Guilford Press, 1981.

Dalzell-Ward, A. J. The new frontier of preventive medicine. *Public Health London,* 1976, *90,* 101–109.

Daniels, R. S. Community psychiatry—a new profession, a developing subspecialty, or effective clinical psychiatry? *Community Mental Health Journal,* 1966, *2,* 47–54.

Danish, S. J., D'Augelli, A. R., & Brock, G. W. An evaluation of helping skills training: Effects on helpers' verbal responses. *Journal of Counseling Psychology,* 1976, *23,* 259–266.

Danish, S. J., & Hauer, A. L. *Helping skills: A basic training program.* New York: Behavioral Publications, 1973. (a)

Danish, S. J., & Hauer, A. L. *Helping skills: A basic training program—leader's manual.* New York: Behavioral Publications, 1973. (b)

Darbonne, A. R. Crisis: A review of theory, practice, and research. *Psychotherapy: Theory, research and practice,* 1967, *4,* 49–56.

Darroch, R. K. Psychologists and population research: A need for discipline planning? *American Psychologist,* 1973, *28,* 683–693.

Datan, N., & Ginsberg, L. H. (Eds.). *Life-span developmental psychology: Normative life crises.* New York: Academic Press, 1975.

D'Augelli, A. R., Handis, M. H., Brumbaugh, L., Illig, V., Searer, R., Turner, D. W., & D'Augelli, J. F. The verbal helping behavior of experienced and novice telephone counselors. *Journal of Community Psychology,* 1978, *6,* 222–228.

D'Augelli, A. R., & Levy, M. The verbal helping skills of trained and untrained human service paraprofessionals. *American Journal of Community Psychology,* 1978, *6,* 23–30.

Davis, J. A. *Education for positive mental health.* Chicago, Ill.: Aldine, 1965.

Day, A. T., & Day, L. H. Cross-national comparison of population density. *Science,* 1973, *181,* 1016–1023.

Dean, A., & Lin, N. The stress-buffering role of social support: Problems and prospects for systematic investigation. *Journal of Nervous and Mental Disease,* 1977, *165,* 403–417.

Deibert, A. N. Community mental health: In? For? By? *Professional Psychology,* 1971, *2,* 394–400.

Delaney, J., Seidman, E., & Willis, G. Crisis intervention and the prevention of institutionalization: An interrupted time series analysis. *American Journal of Community Psychology,* 1978, *6,* 33–45.

Delbecq, A. *Group techniques for program planning: A guide to nominal group and Delphi processes.* Glenview, Ill.: Scott, Foresman, 1975.

DeLeon, P. H. Commentary on Brown's "Social implications of deinstitutionalization." *Journal of Community Psychology,* 1982, *10,* 84–87.

Department of Hospitals. *The State Psychiatric Hospital, Center for Family Care, Geel.* Geel, Belgium: Ministry of Public Health and the Family, n. d.

Depue, R. A., & Monroe, S. M. Learned helplessness in the perspective of the depressive disorders: Conceptual and definitional issues. *Journal of Abnormal Psychology,* 1978, *87,* 3–20.

Deutsch, A. *The mentally ill in America* (2nd ed.). New York: Columbia University Press, 1949.

DeVol, T. I. Does level of professional training make a difference in crisis intervention counseling? *Journal of Community Health,* 1976, *2,* 31–35.

DeWild, D. W. Toward a clarification of primary prevention. *Community Mental Health Journal,* 1981, *16,* 306–316.

Dibner, S. S. Newspaper advice columns as a mental health resource. *Community Mental Health Journal,* 1974, *10,* 147–155.

Dickens, C. *American notes for general circulation* (Vol. 1). London: Chapman & Hall, 1842.

Dohrenwend, B. P. Social status, stress, and psychological symptoms. *Milbank Memorial Fund Quarterly,* 1969, *47,* 137–150.

Dohrenwend, B. P. Psychiatric disorder in general populations: Problem of the untreated "case." *American Journal of Public Health,* 1970, *60,* 1052–1064.

Dohrenwend, B. P. Stressful life events and psychopathology: Some issues of theory and method. In J. E. Barrett, R. M. Rose, & G. L. Klerman (Eds.), *Stress and mental disorder.* New York: Raven Press, 1979.

Dohrenwend, B. P., & Chin-Shong, E. Social status and attitude toward psychological disorder: The problem of tolerance of deviance. *American Sociological Review,* 1967, *32,* 417–433.

Dohrenwend, B. P., & Dohrenwend, B. S. The problem of validity in field studies of psychological disorder. *Journal of Abnormal Psychology,* 1965, *70,* 52–69.

Dohrenwend, B. P., & Dohrenwend, B. S. *Social status and psychological disorder: A causal inquiry.* New York: Wiley-Interscience, 1969.

Dohrenwend, B. P., & Dohrenwend, B. S. Social and cultural influences on psychopathology. *Annual Review of Psychology,* 1974, *25,* 417–452.

Dohrenwend, B. P., Egri, G., & Mendelsohn, F. S. Psychiatric disorder in general populations: A study of the problem of clinical judgment. *American Journal of Psychiatry,* 1971, *127,* 1304–1312.

Dohrenwend, B. P., Shrout, P. E., Egri, G., & Mendelsohn, F. S. Nonspecific psychological distress and other dimensions of psychopathology: Measures for use in the general population. *Archives of General Psychiatry,* 1980, *37,* 1229–1236.

Dohrenwend, B. S. Life events as stressors: A methodological inquiry. *Journal of Health and Social Behavior,* 1973, *14,* 167–175. (a)

Dohrenwend, B. S. Social status and stressful life events. *Journal of Personality and Social Psychology,* 1973, *28,* 225–235. (b)

Dohrenwend, B. S. Social stress and community psychology. *American Journal of Community Psychology,* 1978, *6,* 1–14.

Dohrenwend, B. S., & Dohrenwend, B. P. *Stressful life events: Their nature and effects.* New York: Wiley, 1974.

Dohrenwend, B. S., & Dohrenwend, B. P. Some issues in research on stressful life events. *Journal of Nervous and Mental Disease,* 1978, *166,* 7–15.

Dohrenwend, B. S., & Dohrenwend, B. P. Life stress and psychopathology. In D. A. Regier & G. Allen (Eds.), *Risk factor research in the major mental disorders.* DHHS Pub. No. (ADM) 81–1068. Washington, D.C.: U.S. Government Printing Office, 1981. (a)

Dohrenwend, B. S., & Dohrenwend, B. P. (Eds.). *Stressful life events and their contexts.* New York: Prodist, 1981. (b)

Dohrenwend, B. S., Krasnoff, L., Askenasy, A. R., & Dohrenwend, B. P. Exemplification of a method of scaling life events: The PERI life events scale. *Journal of Health and Social Behavior,* 1978, *19,* 205–229.

Donner, J., & Gamson, A. Experience with multifamily, time-limited, outpatient groups at a community psychiatric clinic. *Psychiatry,* 1968, *31,* 126–137.

Donovan, J. M., Bennett, M. J., & McElroy, C. M. The crisis group—an outcome study. *American Journal of Psychiatry,* 1979, *136,* 906–910.

Dooley, D., & Catalano, R. Economic, life, and disorder changes: Time-series analyses. *American Journal of Community Psychology,* 1979, *7,* 381–396.

Dooley, D., & Catalano, R. Economic change as a cause of behavioral disorder. *Psychological Bulletin,* 1980, *87,* 450–468.

Douglas, D. F., Westley, B. H., & Chaffee, S. H. An information campaign that changed community attitudes. *Journalism Quarterly,* 1970, *47,* 479–492.

Doyle, W. W., Jr., Foreman, M. E., & Wales, E. Effects of supervision in the training of nonprofessional crisis-intervention counselors. *Journal of Counseling Psychology,* 1977, *24,* 72–78.

Dreiblatt, I. S., & Weatherley, D. An evaluation of the efficacy of brief-contact therapy with hospitalized psychiatric patients. *Journal of Consulting and Clinical Psychology,* 1965, *29,* 513–519.

Drewnowski, J., & Wolfe, S. *The level of living index.* Report No. 4. Geneva: United Nations Research Institute for Social Development, 1966.

Driscoll, J. M., Meyer, R. G., & Schanie, C. F. Training police in family crisis intervention. *Journal of Applied Behavioral Science,* 1973, *9,* 62–82.

Dubos, R. *Mirage of health: Utopias, progress, and biological change.* New York: Harper & Row, 1959.

Dubos, R. *Man adapting.* New Haven, Conn.: Yale University Press, 1965.

Duhl, L. J., & Leopold, R. L. (Eds.). *Mental health and urban social policy: A casebook of community action.* San Francisco, Calif.: Jossey-Bass, 1968.

Duncan, D. F. Mental health and health education: An emerging partnership. *Urban Health,* 1979, *10,* 12–13.

Dunham, H. W. Community psychiatry: The newest therapeutic bandwagon. *Archives of General Psychiatry,* 1965, *12,* 303–313.

Dunham, H. W. Discussion. In E. H. Hare & J. K. Wing (Eds.), *Psychiatric epidemiology.* London: Oxford University Press, 1970.

Dunner, D. L., Patrick, V., & Fieve, R. R. Life events at the onset of bipolar affective illness. *American Journal of Psychiatry,* 1979, *136,* 508–511.

Durlak, J. A. Comparative effectiveness of paraprofessional and professional helpers. *Psychological Bulletin,* 1979, *86,* 80–92.

Durlak, J. A. Evaluating comparative studies of paraprofessional and professional helpers: A reply to Nietzel and Fisher. *Psychological Bulletin,* 1981, *89,* 566–569.

Dworkin, A. L., & Dworkin, E. P. A conceptual overview of selected consultation models. *American Journal of Community Psychology,* 1975, *3,* 151–159.

Dynes, R. R., & Quarantelli, E. L. Group behavior under stress: A required convergence of organizational and collective behavior perspectives. *Sociology and Social Research,* 1968, *52,* 416–429.

Eastwood, M. R. *The relation between physical and mental illness.* Toronto: University of Toronto Press, 1975.

Eaton, W. W. Life events, social supports, and psychiatric symptoms: A re-analysis of the New Haven data. *Journal of Health and Social Behavior,* 1978, *19,* 230–234.

Ebaugh, H. R. F., & Haney, C. A. Shifts in abortion attitudes: 1972–1978. *Journal of Marriage and the Family,* 1980, *42,* 491–499.

Edwards, D. W., & Kelly, J. G. Coping and adaptation: A longitudinal study. *American Journal of Community Psychology,* 1980, *8,* 203–215.

Edwards, G., Orford, J., Egert, S., Guthrie, S., Hawker, A., Hensman, C., Mitcheson, M., Oppenheimer, E., & Taylor, C. Alcoholism: A controlled trial of "treatment" and "advice." *Journal of Studies on Alcohol,* 1977, *38,* 1004–1031.

Ehrlich, P. R. *The population bomb.* New York: Ballantine Books, 1968.

Ehrlich, R. P. Prevention, health promotion and the mass media: "Peace yourself together." *American Psychological Association Division of Community Psychology Newsletter,* 1981, *15,* 10–11.

Ehrlich, R. P., D'Augelli, A. R., & Danish, S. J. Comparative effectiveness of six counselor verbal responses. *Journal of Counseling Psychology,* 1979, *26,* 390–398.

Eisenberg, L. If not now, when? *American Journal of Orthopsychiatry,* 1962, *32,* 781–793.

Eisenberg, L. A research framework for evaluating the promotion of mental health and prevention of mental illness. *Public Health Reports,* 1981, *96,* 3–19.

Eisler, R. M., & Frederiksen, L. W. *Perfecting social skills: A guide to interpersonal behavior development.* New York: Plenum Press, 1980.

Ekehammar, B. Interactionism in personality from a historical perspective. *Psychological Bulletin,* 1974, *81,* 1026–1048.

Elias, M. J. Helping emotionally disturbed children through prosocial television. *Exceptional Children,* 1979, *46,* 217–218.

Endicott, J., Herz, M. L., & Gibbon, M. Brief versus standard hospitalization: The differential costs. *American Journal of Psychiatry*, 1978, *135*, 707–712.

Endler, N. S., & Hunt, J. McV. Sources of behavioral variance as measured by the S-R Inventory of Anxiousness. *Psychological Bulletin*, 1966, *65*, 338–346.

Endler, N. S., & Hunt, J. McV. S-R Inventories of hostility and comparisons of the proportion of variance from persons, responses, and situations for hostility and anxiousness. *Journal of Personality and Social Psychology*, 1968, *9*, 309–315.

Engel, G. L. The need for a new medical model: A challenge for biomedicine. *Science*, 1977, *196*, 129–136.

Engel, G. L. The clinical application of the biopsychosocial model. *American Journal of Psychiatry*, 1980, *137*, 535–544.

Engs, R. C., & Kirk, R. H. The characteristics of volunteers in crisis intervention centers. *Public Health Reports*, 1974, *89*, 459–464.

Erickson, M. T. *Child psychopathology* (2nd ed.). Englewood Cliffs, N.J.: Prentice-Hall, 1982.

Erikson, K. T. *Everything in its path: Destruction of community in the Buffalo Creek flood.* New York: Simon and Schuster, 1976. (a)

Erikson, K. T. Loss of communality at Buffalo Creek. *American Journal of Psychiatry*, 1976, *133*, 302–305. (b)

Essen-Moller, E. Individual traits and morbidity in a Swedish rural population. *Acta Psychiatrica et Neurologica Scandinavica*, 1956, Suppl. No. 100.

Ewalt, J. R., & Ewalt, P. L. History of the community psychiatry movement. *American Journal of Psychiatry*, 1969, *126*, 43–52.

Ewing, C. P. *Crisis intervention as psychotherapy.* New York: Oxford University Press, 1978.

Ewing, J. A., & Rouse, B. A. Therapeutic abortion and a prior psychiatric history. *American Journal of Psychiatry*, 1973, *130*, 37–40.

Faden, V. B., & Taube, C. A. *Length of stay of discharges from non-federal general hospital psychiatric inpatient units, United States, 1975.* NIMH Statistical Note 133. Washington, D.C.: U.S. Government Printing Office, 1977.

Farberow, N. L., & Shneidman, E. S. *The cry for help.* New York: McGraw-Hill, 1961.

Faris, R. E. L., & Dunham, H. W. *Mental disorders in urban areas.* Chicago, Ill.: University of Chicago Press, 1939.

Farnsworth, D. L. Comment. *American Journal of Psychiatry*, 1974, *131*, 779.

Farrelly, F., & Brandsma, J. *Provocative therapy.* Cupertino, Calif.: Meta Publications, 1974.

Feldman, S. Ideas and issues in community mental health. *Hospital & Community Psychiatry*, 1971, *22*, 325–329.

Felner, R. D., Ginter, M., & Primavera, J. Primary prevention during school transitions: Social support and environmental structure. *American Journal of Community Psychology*, 1982, *10*, 227–290.

Fenton, F. R., Tessier, L., & Struening, E. L. A comparative trial of home and hospital psychiatric care: One year follow-up. *Archives of General Psychiatry*, 1979, *36*, 1073–1079.

Ferri, E. Characteristics of motherless families. *British Journal of Social Work*, 1973, *3*, 91–100.

Fiester, A. R., & Rudestam, K. E. A multivariate analysis of the early drop-out process. *Journal of Consulting and Clinical Psychology*, 1975, *43*, 528–535.

Figley, C. R. (Ed.). *Stress disorders among Vietnam veterans: Theory, research and treatment.* New York: Brunner/Mazel, 1978.

Filipczak, J., Archer, M., & Friedman, R. M. In-school social skills training: Use with disruptive adolescents. *Behavior Modification*, 1980, *4*, 43–263.

Finkel, N. J. Strens, traumas, and trauma resolution. *American Journal of Community Psychology*, 1975, *3*, 173–178.

Fisher, B. *When your relationship ends: The divorce process rebuilding blocks.* Boulder, Colo.: Family Relationships Learning Center, 1978.

Flanagan, J. C. Evaluation and validation of research data in primary prevention. *American Journal of Orthopsychiatry,* 1971, *41,* 117–123.

Flanagan, J. C. A research approach to improving our quality of life. *American Psychologist,* 1978, *33,* 138–147.

Flay, B. R., DiTecco, D., & Schlegel, R. P. Mass media in health promotion: An analysis using an extended information-processing model. *Health Education Quarterly,* 1980, *7,* 127–147.

Follette, W., & Cummings, N. A. Psychiatric services and medical utilization in a prepaid health plan setting. *Medical Care,* 1967, *5,* 25–35.

Framo, J. L. (Ed.). *Family interaction: A dialogue between family researchers and family therapists.* New York: Springer, 1972.

Frances, A., & Clarkin, J. F. No treatment as the prescription of choice. *Archives of General Psychiatry,* 1981, *38,* 542–545.

Frank, E., & Rowe, D. A. Primary prevention: Parent education, mother-infant groups in a general hospital setting. *Journal of Preventive Psychiatry,* 1981, *1,* 169–178.

Frank, J. D. *Persuasion and healing.* Baltimore: Johns Hopkins Press, 1973.

Fraser, J. R. P., & Froelich, J. E. Crisis intervention in the court room: The case of the night prosecutor. *Community Mental Health Journal,* 1979, *15,* 237–247.

Freedman, A. M. Historical and political roots of the Community Mental Health Centers Act. *American Journal of Orthopsychiatry,* 1967, *37,* 487–494.

Freedman, J. L. *Crowding and behavior.* San Francisco, Calif.: W. H. Freeman, 1975.

Freedman, J. L. Reconciling apparent differences between the responses of humans and other animals to crowding. *Psychological Review,* 1979, *86,* 80–85.

Freeman, H. Mental health and the environment. *British Journal of Psychiatry,* 1978, *132,* 113–124.

Fried, M. Social problems and psychopathology. In L. J. Duhl (Ed.), *Urban America and the planning of mental health services.* New York: Group for the Advancement of Psychiatry, 1964.

Fried, M., & Lindemann, E. Socio-cultural factors in mental health and illness. *American Journal of Orthopsychiatry,* 1961, *31,* 87–101.

Friedman, M., & Rosenman, R. H. *Type A behavior and your heart.* New York: Knopf, 1974.

Frings, J. What about brief services?—a report of a study of short-term cases. *Social Casework,* 1951, *32,* 236–241.

Furstenberg, F. F., Jr. The social consequences of teenage parenthood. *Family Planning Perspectives,* 1976, *8,* 148–164.

Galle, O. R., Gove, W. R., & McPherson, J. M. Population density and pathology: What are the relations for man? *Science,* 1972, *176,* 23–30.

Galle, O. R., McCarthy, J. D., & Gove, W. Population density and pathology. Paper presented at the annual meeting of the Population Association of America, New York, April 1974.

Gallin, R. S. Life difficulties, coping, and the use of medical services. *Culture, Medicine, and Psychiatry,* 1980, *4,* 249–269.

Garmezy, N. The current status of research with children at risk for schizophrenia and other forms of psychopathology. In D. A. Regier & G. Allen (Eds.), *Risk factor research in the major mental disorders.* DHHS Pub. No. (ADM) 81–1068. Washington, D.C.: U.S. Government Printing Office, 1981.

Gatz, M., Barbarin, O. A., Tyler, F. B., Mitchell, R. B., Moran, J. A., Wirzbicki, P. J., Crawford, J., & Engleman, A. Enhancement of individual and community competence: The older adult as community worker. *American Journal of Community Psychology,* 1982, *10,* 291–303.

Gerson, S., & Bassuk, E. Psychiatric emergencies: An overview. *American Journal of Psychiatry,* 1980, *137,* 1–11.

Gersten, J. C., Langner, T. S., Eisenberg, J. G., & Orzek, L. Child behavior and life events: Undesirable change or change per se. In B. S. Dohrenwend & B. P. Dohrenwend (Eds.), *Stressful life events: Their nature and effects.* New York: Wiley, 1974.

Gersten, J. C., Langner, T. S., Eisenberg, J. C., & Simcha-Fagan, O. An evaluation of the etiologic role of stressful life-change events in psychological disorder. *Journal of Health and Social Behavior,* 1977, *18,* 228–244.

Getz, W. L., Fujita, B. N., & Allen, D. The use of paraprofessionals in crisis intervention: Evaluation of an innovative program. *American Journal of Community Psychology,* 1975, *3,* 135–144.

Gibbs, M., Lachemeyer, J., & Sigal, J. *Community psychology: Theoretical and empirical approaches.* New York: Gardner Press, 1980.

Giel, R., & Ormel, J. Crowding and subjective health in the Netherlands. *Social Psychiatry,* 1977, *12,* 37–42.

Gildea, M. C.-L., Glidewell, J. C., & Kantor, M. B. The St. Louis school mental health project: History and evaluation. In E. L. Cowen, E. A. Gardner, & M. Zax (Eds.), *Emergent approaches to mental health problems.* New York: Appleton-Century-Crofts, 1967.

Gillis, A. R. High-rise housing and psychological strain. *Journal of Health and Social Behavior,* 1977, *18,* 418–431.

Gillman, R. D. Brief psychotherapy: A psychoanalytic view. *American Journal of Psychiatry,* 1965, *122,* 601–611.

Gist, R., & Stolz, S. B. Mental Health promotion and the media: community response to the Kansas City hotel disaster. *American Psychologist,* 1982, *37,* 1136–1139.

Glass, A. J. The future of large public mental hospitals. *Mental Hospitals,* 1965, *16,* 9–22.

Glasscote, R. M., & Gudeman, J. E. *The staff of the mental health center: A field study.* Washington, D.C.: American Psychiatric Association Joint Information Service, 1969.

Glick, I. D., Hargreaves, W. A., & Goldfield, M. D. Short vs. long hospitalization: A prospective controlled study: I. The preliminary results of a one-year follow-up of schizophrenics. *Archives of General Psychiatry,* 1974, *30,* 363–369.

Glick, I. D., Hargreaves, W. A., Raskin, M., & Kutner, S. J. Short versus long hospitalization: A prospective controlled study: II. Results for schizophrenic inpatients. *American Journal of Psychiatry,* 1975, *132,* 385–390.

Glidewell, J. C. A design for an experimental program. In R. H. Williams & L. D. Ozarin (Eds.), *Community mental health: An international perspective.* San Francisco, Calif.: Jossey-Bass, 1968.

Glidewell, J. C. Priorities for psychologists in community mental health. In Division 27, American Psychological Association, Task Force on Community Mental Health, *Issues in community psychology and preventive mental health.* New York: Behavioral Publications, 1971.

Glidewell, J. C., Gildea, M. C.-L., & Kaufman, M. K. The preventive and therapeutic effects of two school mental health programs. *American Journal of Community Psychology,* 1973, *1,* 295–329.

Glidewell, J. C., & Swallow, C. S. *The prevalence of maladjustment in elementary schools: A report prepared for the Joint Commission on the Mental Health of Children.* Chicago, Ill.: University of Chicago Press, 1969.

Goffman, E. *Asylums: Essays on the social situation of mental patients and other inmates.* Chicago, Ill.: Aldine, 1961.

Golan, N. *Treatment in crisis situations.* New York: Free Press, 1978.

Goldberg, D. P. *The detection of psychiatric illness by questionnaire.* London: Oxford University Press, 1972.

Goldberg, E. L., & Comstock, G. W. Life events and subsequent illness. *American Journal of Epidemiology,* 1976, *104,* 146–158.

Goldberg, I. D., Krantz, G., & Locke, B. Z. Effect of a short-term outpatient psychiatric therapy benefit on the utilization of medical services in a prepaid group practice medical program. *Medical Care*, 1970, *8*, 419-428.

Goldsmith, S. B. The status of health status indicators. *Health Services Reports*, 1972, *87*, 212-220.

Goldstein, A. P. *Structured learning therapy: Toward a psychotherapy for the poor.* New York: Academic Press, 1973.

Goldston, S. E. (Ed.). *Concepts of community psychiatry: A framework for training.* DHEW Pub. No. 1319. Washington, D.C.: U.S. Government Printing Office, 1965.

Goldston, S. E. Mental health education in a community mental health center. *American Journal of Public Health*, 1968, *58*, 693-699.

Goldston, S. E. An overview of primary prevention programming. In D. C. Klein & S. E. Goldston (Eds.), *Primary prevention: An idea whose time has come.* Washington, D.C.: U.S. Government Printing Office, 1977.

Gomes-Schwartz, B. The modification of schizophrenic behavior. *Behavior Modification*, 1979, *3*, 439-468.

Gonzales, L. R., Hays, R. B., Bond, M. A., & Kelly, J. G. Community mental health. In M. Herson, A. E. Kazdin, & A. S. Bellack (Eds.), *The clinical psychology handbook.* New York: Pergamon Press, in press.

Goode, W. J. Problems in post-divorce adjustment. *American Sociological Review*, 1949, *14*, 394-401.

Goode, W. J. *After divorce.* New York: Free Press, 1956.

Goodstein, L. D. *Consulting with human service systems.* Reading, Mass.: Addison-Wesley, 1978.

Goodstein, L. D., & Sandler, I. Using psychology to promote human welfare: A conceptual analysis of the role of community psychology. *American Psychologist*, 1978, *33*, 882-892.

Goodwin, R. H. The family life educator as change agent: A participant in problems and solutions. *Family Coordinator*, 1972, *21*, 303-312.

Goplerud, E. N. Unexpected consequences of deinstitutionalization of the mentally disabled elderly. *American Journal of Community Psychology*, 1979, *7*, 315-328.

Gordon, R. H. Efficacy of a group crisis-counseling program for men who accompany women seeking abortions. *American Journal of Community Psychology*, 1978, *6*, 239-246.

Gordon, R. H., & Kilpatrick, C. A. A program of group counseling for men who accompany women seeking legal abortions. *Community Mental Health Journal*, 1977, *13*, 291-295.

Gordon, S. B., Lerner, L. L., & Keefe, F. J. Responsive parenting: An approach to training parents of problem children. *American Journal of Community Psychology*, 1979, *7*, 45-56.

Gordon, T. *Parent Effectiveness Training.* New York: Wyden, 1977.

Gore, S. The effect of social support in moderating the health consequences of unemployment. *Journal of Health and Social Behavior*, 1978, *19*, 157-165.

Gorwitz, K. *Mental hygiene statistics newsletter: Length of hospitalization.* Dec. 10, 1969. Annapolis: Maryland Department of Health and Mental Hygiene, 1969.

Goshen, C. E. *Documentary history of psychiatry: A source book on historical principles.* New York: Philosophical Library, 1967.

Gottlieb, B. H. Re-examining the preventive potential of mental health consultation. *Canada's Mental Health*, 1974, *22*, 4-6.

Gottschalk, L. A., Fox, R. A., & Bates, D. E. A study of prediction and outcome in a mental health crisis clinic. *American Journal of Psychiatry*, 1973, *130*, 1107-1111.

Gottschalk, L. A., Mayerson, P., & Gottlieb, A. A. Prediction and evaluation of outcome in an emergency brief psychotherapy clinic. *Journal of Nervous and Mental Disease*, 1967, *144*, 77-96.

Gove, W. R. Societal reaction as an explanation of mental illness: An evaluation. *American Sociological Review*, 1970, *35*, 873-884. (a)

Gove, W. R. Who is hospitalized: A critical review of some sociological studies of mental illness. *Journal of Health and Social Behavior*, 1970, *11*, 294–303. (b)

Grad, J., & Sainsbury, P. Evaluating the community psychiatric service in Chichester: Results: *Milbank Memorial Fund Quarterly*, 1966, *44*, 246–278.

Grady, M. A., Gibson, M. J. S., & Trickett, E. J. (Eds.). *Mental health consultation theory, practice, and research: 1973–1978*. Washington, D.C.: U.S. Government Printing Office, 1981.

Graeven, D. B. The effects of airplane noise on health: An examination of three hypotheses. *Journal of Health and Social Behavior*, 1974, *15*, 336–343.

Granadio, F. Young pregnant teenagers: The impact of comprehensive care. *Journal of Adolescent Health*, 1981, *1*, 193–197.

Grant, I., Gerst, M., & Yager, J. Scaling of life events by psychiatric patients and normals. *Journal of Psychosomatic Research*, 1976, *20*, 141–149.

Granvold, D. K., Pedler, L. M., & Schellie, S. G. A study of sex-role expectancy and female post-divorce adjustment. *Journal of Divorce*, 1979, *2*, 383–393.

Graves, E., & Lovato, C. Utilization of short-stay hospitals in the treatment of mental disorders: 1974–1978. *Vital and Health Statistics of the National Center for Health Statistics*. No. 70. May 22, 1981. Washington, D.C.: U.S. Government Printing Office, 1981.

Greenberg, B. G., Harris, M. E., MacKinnon, C. F., & Chipman, S. S. A method for evaluating the effectiveness of health education literature. *American Journal of Public Health and the Nation's Health*, 1953, *45*, 1147–1155.

Greenblatt, M. Historical forces affecting the closing of mental hospitals. In S. C. Plog (Ed.), *Where is my home? Proceedings of a conference on the closing of state mental hospitals*. Menlo Park, Calif.: Stanford Research Institute, 1974.

Greenley, J. R., Gillespie, D. P., & Lindenthal, J. J. A race riot's effect on psychological symptoms. *Archives of General Psychiatry*, 1975, *32*, 1189–1195.

Greer, F. L. The application of crisis theory: A review of the research. *Crisis Intervention*, 1979, *10*, 43–87.

Grob, G. N. *State and the mentally ill: A history of Worcester State Hospital in Massachusetts, 1830–1920*. Chapel Hill, N.C.: University of North Carolina Press, 1966.

Groddeck, G. *The unknown self*. New York: Funk & Wagnalls, 1951.

Group for the Advancement of Psychiatry. *Crisis in psychiatric hospitalization*. No. 72. New York: Author, 1969.

Gruenberg, E. M. Benefits of short-term hospitalization. In R. Cancro, N. Fox, & L. E. Shapiro (Eds.), *Strategic intervention in schizophrenia: Current developments in treatment*. New York: Behavioral Publications, 1974.

Gruenberg, E. M. The failures of success. *Milbank Memorial Fund Quarterly*, 1977, *55*, 3–24.

Gruenberg, E. M. Mental disorders. In J. M. Last (Ed.), *Maxcy-Rosenau public health and preventive medicine* (11th ed.). New York: Appleton-Century-Crofts, 1980.

Gruenberg, E. M. Risk factor research methods. In D. A. Regier & G. Allen (Eds.), *Risk factor research in the major mental disorders*. DHHS Pub. No. (ADM) 81–1068. Washington, D.C.: U.S. Government Printing Office, 1981.

Gurin, G., Veroff, J., & Feld, S. *Americans view their mental health*. New York: Basic Books, 1960.

Hagedorn, H. J., Beck, K. J., Neubert, S. F., & Werlin, S. H. *A working manual of simple program evaluation techniques for community mental health centers*. DHEW Pub. No. (ADM) 76–404. Washington, D.C.: U.S. Government Printing Office, 1976.

Hagnell, O. *A prospective study of the incidence of mental disorder*. Stockholm: Svenska Bokforlaget Norstedts-Bonniers, 1966.

Haley, J. *Strategies of psychotherapy*. New York: Grune & Stratton, 1963.

Haley, J. *Uncommon therapy: The psychiatric techniques of Milton H. Erickson, M.D.* New York: W. W. Norton, 1973.

Hall, A. D., & Fagan, R. E. Definition of system. *General Systems*, 1956, *1*, 18–28.

Hallowitz, E. The role of a neighborhood service center in community mental health. *American Journal of Orthopsychiatry,* 1968, *38,* 705–714.

Hallowitz, E., & Riessman, F. The role of the indigenous nonprofessional in a community mental health neighborhood service center program. *American Journal of Orthopsychiatry,* 1967, *37,* 766–778.

Halpern, H. A. Crisis theory: A definitional study. *Community Mental Health Journal,* 1973, *9,* 342–349.

Halpern, W. I. The community mental health aide. *Mental Hygiene,* 1969, *53,* 78–83.

Handal, P. J., Barling, P. W., & Morrissy, E. Development of perceived and preferred measures of physical and social characteristics of the residential environment and their relationship to satisfaction. *Journal of Community Psychology,* 1981, *9,* 118–124.

Hargreaves, W. A., Attkisson, C. C., Siegal, L. M., & McIntyre, M. H. (Eds.). *Resource materials for community mental health program evaluation.* Part II: *Needs assessment and planning.* San Francisco, Calif.: National Institute of Mental Health, 1974.

Hargreaves, W. A., Attkisson, C. C., & Sorensen, J. E. *Resource materials for community mental health program evaluation.* DHEW Pub. No. (ADM) 79–328. Washington, D.C.: U.S. Government Printing Office, 1977.

Hargreaves, W. A., Glick, I. D., Drues, J., Shaustack, J. A., & Feigenbaum, E. Short vs. long hospitalization: A prospective controlled study: VI. Two-year follow-up results for schizophrenics. *Archives of General Psychiatry,* 1977, *34,* 305–311.

Harris, R. *Sacred trust.* New York: Penguin, 1969.

Hartman, L. M. The preventive reduction of psychological risk in asymptomatic adolescents. *American Journal of Orthopsychiatry,* 1979, *49,* 121–135. (a)

Hartman, L. M. The primary prevention of behavior pathology: An empirical investigation. *Psychiatric Journal,* 1979, *4,* 260–267. (b)

Hatcher, R. A., Stewart, G. K., Stewart, F., Guest, F., Josephs, N., & Dale, J. *Contraceptive technology* (11th rev. ed.). New York: Irvington, 1982.

Havik, O. E. Psychological intervention in physical illness: A review concerning patient information and education. In B. Christiansen (Ed.), *Does psychology return its costs? Research in Clinical Psychology,* Report No. 2. Oslo: Norwegian Council for the Sciences and Humanities, 1981.

Haynes, L. A., & Avery, A. W. Training adolescents in self-disclosure and empathy skills. *Journal of Counseling Psychology,* 1979, *26,* 526–530.

Hefferin, E. A. Life-cycle stressors: An overview of research. *Family and Community Mental Health,* 1980, *2,* 71–101.

Heffron, E. F. Project outreach: Crisis intervention following natural disaster. *Journal of Community Psychology,* 1977, *5,* 103–11.

Heisel, J. S., Ream, S., Raitz, R., Rappaport, M., & Coddington, R. D. The significance of life events as contributing factors in the diseases of children. *Behavioral Pediatrics,* 1973, *83,* 119–123.

Heller, K., & Monahan, J. *Psychology and community change.* Homewood, Ill. Dorsey Press, 1977.

Heller, K., & Monahan, J. Individual process consultation. In S. Cooper & W. F. Hodges (Eds.), *The field of mental health consultation.* New York: Human Sciences Press, 1983.

Heller, K., Price, R. H., & Sher, K. J. Research and evaluation in primary prevention: Issues and guidelines. In R. H. Price, R. F. Ketterer, B. C. Bader, & J. Monahan (Eds.), *Prevention in mental health: Research, policy, and practice.* Beverly Hills, Calif.: Sage Publications, 1980.

Hennon, C. B., & Peterson, B. H. An evaluation of a family life education delivery system for young families. *Family Relations,* 1981, *30,* 387–394.

Henry, J. The future hustle. *New Republic,* February 4, 1978, pp. 16–18, 20.

Hereford, C. F. *Changing parental attitude through group discussion.* Austin, Tex.: University of Texas Press, 1963.

Herman, S. J. Women, divorce and suicide. *Journal of Divorce,* 1977, *1,* 107–117.

Hersch, C. The discontent explosion in mental health. *American Psychologist,* 1968, *23,* 497–506.

Herz, M. I., Endicott, J., & Spitzer, R. L. Brief hospitalization of patients with families: Initial results. *American Journal of Psychiatry*, 1975, *132*, 413–418.

Herz, M. I., Endicott, J., & Spitzer, R. L. Brief versus standard hospitalization: The families. *American Journal of Psychiatry*, 1976, *133*, 795–801.

Hetherington, E. M., Cox, M., & Cox, R. Divorced fathers. *Family Coordinator*, 1976, *25*, 417–428.

Hetherington, E. M., Cox, M., & Cox, R. The aftermath of divorce. In J. H. Stevens, Jr., & M. Matthews (Eds.), *Mother-child, father-child relations*. Washington, D.C.: National Association for the Education of Young Children, 1977.

Hinkle, L. E., Jr. The effect of exposure to cultural change, social change, and changes in interpersonal relationships on health. In B. S. Dohrenwend & B. P. Dohrenwend (Eds.), *Stressful life events: Their nature and effects*. New York: Wiley, 1974.

Hirschfeld, R. M. A., & Cross, C. K. Psychosocial risk factors for depression. In D. A. Regier & G. Allen (Eds.), *Risk factor research in the major mental disorders*. DHHS Pub. No. (ADM) 81–1068. Washington, D.C.: U.S. Government Printing Office, 1981.

Hirschowitz, R. G. An attempt to delineate the field of community psychiatry. *Hospital & Community Psychiatry*, 1970, *21*, 209–212.

Hirschowitz, R. G. Mental health consultation: The state of the art. *Psychiatric Quarterly*, 1973, *47*, 1–14.

Hoch, P. H. Short-term versus long-term therapy. In L. W. Wolberg (Ed.), *Short-term psychotherapy*. New York: Grune & Stratton, 1965.

Hoffman, D. L., & Remmel, M. L. Uncovering the precipitant in crisis intervention. *Social Casework*, 1975, *56*, 259–267.

Hoke, B. Promotive medicine and the phenomenon of health. *Archives of Environmental Health*, 1968, *16*, 269–278.

Holahan, C. J. Redesigning physical environments to enhance social interactions. In R. F. Muñoz, L. R. Snowden, & J. G. Kelly (Eds.), *Social and psychological research in community settings*. San Francisco, Calif.: Jossey-Bass, 1979.

Holahan, C. J., & Moos, R. H. Social support and psychological distress: A longitudinal analysis. *Journal of Abnormal Psychology*, 1981, *90*, 365–370.

Hollingshead, A. B., & Redlich, F. C. *Social class and mental illness: A community study*. New York: Wiley, 1958.

Hollister, W. G. The concept of strens in education: A challenge to curriculum development. In E. M. Bower & W. G. Hollister (Eds.), *Behavioral science frontiers in education*. New York: Wiley, 1967.

Holloway, W. H. Short-term contractual group treatment and working through. In H. Grayson (Ed.), *Short-term approaches to psychotherapy*. New York: Human Sciences Press, 1979.

Holmes, T. H. Development and application of a quantitative measure of life change magnitude. In J. E. Barrett, R. M. Rose, & G. L. Klerman (Eds.), *Stress and mental disorder*. New York: Raven Press, 1979.

Holmes, T. H., & Masuda, M. Life change and illness susceptibility. In B. S. Dohrenwend & B. P. Dohrenwend (Eds.), *Stressful life events: Their nature and effects*. New York: Wiley, 1974.

Holmes, T. H., & Rahe, R. H. The Social Readjustment Rating Scale. *Journal of Psychosomatic Research*, 1967, *11*, 213–218.

Hoover, R., Bain, C., Cole, P., & MacMahon, B. Oral contraceptive use: Association with frequency of hospitalization and chronic disease risk factors. *American Journal of Public Health*, 1978, *68*, 335–341.

Hoppe, E. W. Treatment dropouts in hindsight: A follow-up study. *Community Mental Health Journal*, 1977, *13*, 307–313.

Horowitz, M. J., & Solomon, G. F. Delayed stress response syndromes in Vietnam veterans. In C. R. Figley (Ed.), *Stress disorders among Vietnam veterans*. New York: Brunner/Mazel, 1978.

Horowitz, M. J., Wilner, N., & Alvarez, W. Impact of Event Scale: A measure of subjective stress. *Psychosomatic Medicine*, 1979, 51, 209–218.

Howard, J. *A different woman*. New York: Dutton, 1973.

Howe, B., Kaplan, H. R., & English, C. Repeat abortions: Blaming the victims. *American Journal of Public Health*, 1979, 69, 1242–1246.

Hudgens, R. W., Robins, E., & Delong, W. B. The reporting of recent stress in the lives of psychiatric patients. *British Journal of Psychiatry*, 1970, 117, 635–643.

Hughes, C. C., Trembly, M. A., Rapoport, R. N., & Leighton, A. H. *People of cove and woodlot*. New York: Basic Books, 1960.

Hunt, M. *Sexual behavior in the seventies*. Chicago: Playboy Press, 1974.

Ilgenfritz, M. P. Mothers on their own—widows and divorcees. *Marriage and Family Living*, 1961, 23, 38–41.

Insel, P. M. Task force report: The social climate of mental health. *Community Mental Health Journal*, 1980, 16, 62–78.

Insel, P. M., & Moos, R. H. Psychological environments: Expanding the scope of human ecology. *American Psychologist*, 1974, 29, 179–188.

Irvine, E. E. Children at risk. *Case Conference*, 1964, 10, 293–296.

Iscoe, I. Community psychology and the competent community. *American Psychologist*, 1974, 29, 607–613.

Iscoe, I., Bloom, B. L., & Spielberger, C. D. (Eds.). *Community psychology in transition: Proceedings of the National Conference on Training in Community Psychology*. New York: Hemisphere, 1977.

Ivey, A. E. *Microcounseling: Innovations in interview training*. Springfield, Ill.: Charles C Thomas, 1971.

Jacobs, D., Charles, E., Jacobs, T., Weinstein, H., & Mann, D. Preparation for treatment of the disadvantaged patient: Effects on disposition and outcome. *American Journal of Orthopsychiatry*, 1972, 43, 666–674.

Jacobs, S. C., Prusoff, B. A., & Paykel, E. S. Recent life events in schizophrenia and depression. *Psychological Medicine*, 1974, 4, 444–453.

Jaffe, P. G., Thompson, J. K., & Paquin, M. J. Immediate family crisis intervention as preventive mental health: The family consultant service. *Professional Psychology*, 1978, 9, 551–560.

Jameson, J., Shuman, L. J., & Young, W. W. The effects of outpatient psychiatric utilization on the costs of providing third-party coverage. *Medical Care*, 1978, 16, 383–399.

Jenkins, C. D. Psychosocial modifiers of response to stress. In J. E. Barrett, R. M. Rose, & G. L. Klerman (Eds.), *Stress and mental disorder*. New York: Raven Press, 1979.

Jenkins, C. D., Tuthill, R. W., Tannenbaum, S. I., & Kirby, C. Social stressors and excess mortality from hypertensive diseases. *Journal of Human Stress*, 1979, 5, 29–40.

Jessor, R. Phenomenological personality theories and the data language of psychology. *Psychological Review*, 1956, 63, 173–180.

Jessor, R. The problem of reductionism in psychology. *Psychological Review*, 1958, 65, 170–178.

Johnson, D. L., & Breckenridge, J. N. The Houston Parent-Child Development Center and the primary prevention of behavior problems in young children. *American Journal of Community Psychology*, 1982, 10, 305–316.

Johnson, J. H., & Sarason, I. G. Life stress, depression and anxiety: Internal-external control as a moderator variable. *Journal of Psychosomatic Research*, 1978, 22, 205–208.

Johnson, J. H., & Sarason, I. G. Moderator variables in life stress research. In I. G. Sarason & C. D. Spielberger (Eds.), *Stress and anxiety* (Vol. 6). Washington, D.C.: Halstead, 1979.

Joint Commission on Mental Health of Children. *Crisis in child mental health: Challenge for the 1970's*. New York: Harper & Row, 1969.

REFERENCES

Joint Commission on Mental Illness and Health. *Action for mental health.* New York: Basic Books, 1961.

Jones, E. *The life and work of Sigmund Freud.* New York: Basic Books, 1955.

Jones, K. Revolution and reform in the mental health services. *Medical Care,* 1963, *1,* 155–160.

Jones, K. R., & Vischi, T. R. Impact of alcohol, drug abuse and mental health treatment on medical care utilization: A review of the research literature. *Medical Care,* 1979, *17* (Suppl.), 1–82.

Jones, M. *Social psychiatry in practice: The idea of a therapeutic community.* New York: Penguin, 1968.

Joslyn-Scherer, M. S. Communication in the human services: A guide to therapeutic journalism. In A. Lauffer (Ed.), *Sage Human Service Guides.* Beverly Hills, Calif.: Sage Publications, 1980.

Kaffman, M. Short term family therapy. *Family Process,* 1963, *2,* 216–234.

Kahn, A. J. *Theory and practice of social planning.* New York: Russell Sage Foundation, 1969.

Kahn, E. J., Jr. The sporting scene. *New Yorker,* March 10, 1980, pp. 53–68.

Kalafat, J., Boroto, D. R., & France, K. Relationships among experience level and value orientation and the performance of paraprofessional telephone counselors. *American Journal of Community Psychology,* 1979, *7,* 167–179.

Kantner, J. F., & Zelnik, M. Sexual experience of young unmarried women in the United States. *Family Planning Perspectives,* 1972, *4,* 9–18.

Kantner, J. F., & Zelnik, M. Contraception and pregnancy: Experience of young unmarried women in the United States. *Family Planning Perspectives,* 1973, *5,* 21–35.

Kantor, D., & Lehr, W. *Inside the family: Toward a theory of family process.* San Francisco, Calif.: Jossey-Bass, 1975.

Kantor, M. B., Gildea, M. C.-L., & Glidewell, J. C. Preventive and therapeutic effects of maternal attitude change in the school setting. *American Journal of Public Health,* 1969, *59,* 490–502.

Kaplan, D. M., & Mason, E. A. Maternal reactions to premature birth viewed as an acute emotional disorder. *American Journal of Orthopsychiatry,* 1960, *30,* 539–552.

Kaseman, C. M., & Anderson, R. G. Clergy consultation as a community mental health program. *Community Mental Health Journal,* 1977, *13,* 84–91.

Kasl, S. V. Mortality and the business cycle: Some questions about research strategies when utilizing macro-social and ecological data. *American Journal of Public Health,* 1979, *69,* 784–788.

Kasl, S. V. Problems in the analysis and interpretation of ecological data. *American Journal of Public Health,* 1980, *70,* 413–414.

Kasl, S. V., & Harburg, E. Mental health and the urban environment: Some doubts and second thoughts. *Journal of Health and Social Behavior,* 1975, *16,* 268–282.

Kaswan, J. Comment on Brown's "Social implications of deinstitutionalization." *Journal of Community Psychology,* 1982, *10,* 88–89.

Kaye, S., Tricket, E. J., & Quinlan, D. M. Alternative methods for environmental assessment: An example. *American Journal of Community Psychology,* 1976, *4,* 367–377.

Kazanjian, V., Stein, S., & Weinberg, W. L. *An introduction to mental health consultation.* Public Health Monograph No. 69. Washington, D.C.: U.S. Government Printing Office, 1962.

Keilson, M. V., Dworkin, F. H., & Gelso, C. J. The effectiveness of time-limited psychotherapy in a university counseling center. *Journal of Clinical Psychology,* 1979, *35,* 631–636.

Kellam, S. G., Branch, J. D., Agrawal, K. C., & Ensminger, M. E. *Mental health and going to school: The Woodlawn program of assessment, early intervention, and evaluation.* Chicago: University of Chicago Press, 1975.

Kellam, S. G., Branch, J. D., Agrawal, K. C., & Grabill, M. E. Woodlawn Mental Health Center: An evolving strategy for planning in community mental health. In S. E. Golann & C. Eisdorfer (Eds.), *Handbook of community mental health*. New York: Appleton-Century-Crofts, 1972.

Kellam, S. G., & Schiff, S. K. Adaptation and mental illness in the first-grade classrooms of an urban community. In M. Greenblatt, P. E. Emery, & B. C. Glueck, Jr. (Eds.), *Poverty and mental health*. Psychiatric Research Report No. 21. Washington, D.C.: American Psychiatric Association, 1967.

Keller, H. R. Behavioral consultation. In J. C. Conoley (Ed.), *Consultation in schools: Theory, research, procedures*. New York: Academic Press, 1981.

Kelly, J. Divorce: The adult perspective. In B. Wolman & G. Stricker (Eds.), *Handbook of developmental psychology*. New York: Prentice-Hall, 1982.

Kelly, J. G. Antidotes for arrogance. *American Psychologist*, 1970, *25*, 524–531.

Kelly, J. G. Qualities for the community psychologist. *American Psychologist*, 1971, *26*, 897–903.

Kelly, J. G. *The high school: Students and social contexts in two Midwestern communities*. Hillsdale, N.J.: Erlbaum, 1979.

Keniston, K. We have much to learn from youth. *American Journal of Psychiatry*, 1970, *126*, 1767–1768.

Kennedy, J. F. *Message from the president of the United States relative to mental illness and mental retardation*. (88th Congress, First Session, U.S. House of Representatives Document No. 58). Washington, D.C.: U.S. Government Printing Office, 1963.

Kentsmith, D. K., Menninger, W. W., & Coyne, L. A survey of state hospital admissions from an area served by a mental health center. *Hospital & Community Psychiatry*, 1975, *26*, 593–596.

Kessler, M., & Albee, G. W. Primary prevention. *Annual review of psychology*, 1975, *26*, 557–591.

Kessler, R. C. A strategy for studying differential vulnerability to the psychological consequences of stress. *Journal of Health and Social Behavior*, 1979, *20*, 100–108. (a)

Kessler, R. C. Stress, social status, and psychological distress. *Journal of Health and Social Behavior*, 1979, *20*, 259–272. (b)

Ketterer, R. F. *Consultation and education in mental health: Problems and prospects*. Beverly Hills, Calif.: Sage Publications, 1981.

Kety, S. S., & Kinney, D. K. Biological risk factors in schizophrenia. In D. A. Regier & G. Allen (Eds.), *Risk factor research in the major mental disorders*. DHHS No. (ADM) 81–1068. Washington, D.C.: U.S. Government Printing Office, 1981.

Kiesler, D. J. Some myths of psychotherapy research and the search for a paradigm. *Psychological Bulletin*, 1966, *65*, 110–136.

King, G. D. An evaluation of the effectiveness of a telephone counseling center. *American Journal of Community Psychology*, 1977, *5*, 75–83.

Kinney, J. M., Madsen, B., Fleming, T., & Haapala, D. A. Homebuilders: Keeping families together. *Journal of Consulting and Clinical Psychology*, 1977, *45*, 667–673.

Kinston, W., & Rosser, R. Disaster: Effects on mental and physical state. *Journal of Psychosomatic Research*, 1974, *18*, 437–456.

Kiritz, S., & Moos, R. H. Physiological effects of social environments. *Psychosomatic Medicine*, 1974, *36*, 96–114.

Kirk, S. A., & Therrien, M. E. Community mental health myths and the fate of former hospitalized patients. *Psychiatry*, 1975, *38*, 209–217.

Kirschenbaum, D. S., DeVoge, J. B., Marsh, M. E., & Steffen, J. J. Multimodal evaluation of therapy versus consultation components in a large inner-city early intervention program. *American Journal of Community Psychology*, 1980, *8*, 587–601.

Kitson, G. C., Lopata, H. Z., Holmes, W. M., & Meyering, S. W. Divorcees and widows: Similarities and differences. *American Journal of Orthopsychiatry*, 1980, *50*, 291–301.

Kitson, G. C., & Sussman, M. B. The impact of divorce on adults. *Conciliation Courts Review*, 1977, *15*, 20–24.

Klassen, D., Roth, A., & Hornstra, R. K. Perception of life events as gains or losses in a community survey. *Journal of Community Psychology*, 1974, *2*, 330–336.

Klee, G. D., Spiro, E., Bahn, A. K., & Gorwitz, K. An ecological analysis of diagnosed mental illness in Baltimore. In R. R. Monroe, G. D. Klee, & E. B. Brody (Eds.), *Psychiatric epidemiology and mental health planning* (Research Report No. 22). Washington, D.C.: American Psychiatric Association, 1967.

Klein, D. C., & Lindemann, E. Approaches to pre-school screening. *Journal of School Health*, 1964, *34*, 365–373.

Klein, D. C., & Ross, A. Kindergarten entry: A study of role transition. In M. Krugman (Ed.), *Orthopsychiatry and the school*. New York: American Orthopsychiatric Association, 1958.

Klerman, G. L. Better but not well: Social and ethical issues in the deinstitutionalization of the mentally ill. *Schizophrenia Bulletin*, 1977, *3*, 617–631.

Klos, D. M., & Rosenstock, I. M. Some lessons from the North Karelia project. *American Journal of Public Health*, 1982, *72*, 53–54.

Knapp, F., & McClure, L. F. Quasi-experimental evaluation of a quality of life intervention. *Journal of Community Psychology*, 1978, *6*, 280–290.

Kobasa, S. C. Personality and resistance to illness. *American Journal of Community Psychology*, 1979, *7*, 413–423.

Koegler, R. R. Brief therapy with children. In G. W. Wayne & R. R. Koegler (Eds.), *Emergency psychiatry and brief therapy*. Boston, Mass.: Little, Brown, 1966.

Kogan, L. S. The short-term case in a family agency: Part I. The study plan. *Social Casework*, 1957, *38*, 231–238. (a)

Kogan, L. S. The short-term case in a family agency: Part II. Results of study. *Social Casework*, 1957, *38*, 296–302. (b)

Kogan, L. S. The short-term case in a family agency: Part III. Further results and conclusion. *Social Casework*, 1957, *38*, 366–374. (c)

Kohn, M., Jeger, A. M., & Koretzky, M. B. Social-ecological assessment of environments: Toward a two-factor model. *American Journal of Community Psychology*, 1979, *7*, 481–495.

Kohn, M. L. Social class and schizophrenia: A critical review. In D. Rosenthal & S. S. Kety (Eds.), *The transmission of schizophrenia*. Oxford: Pergamon Press, 1968.

Kolb, L. C. Community mental health centers: Some issues in their transition from concept to reality. *Hospital & Community Psychiatry*, 1968, *19*, 335–340. (a)

Kolb, L. C. *Noye's modern clinical psychiatry*. Philadelphia, Pa.: Saunders, 1968. (b)

Korchin, S. J. *Modern clinical psychology: Principles of intervention in the clinic and community*. New York: Basic Books, 1976.

Kornberg, M. S., & Caplan, G. Risk factors and preventive intervention in child psychotherapy. *Journal of Prevention*, 1980, *1*, 71–133.

Kramer, M. Cross-national study of diagnosis of the mental disorders: Origin of the problem. *American Journal of Psychiatry*, 1969, *125*, Suppl. No. 10, 1–11.

Kubie, L. S. Pitfalls of community psychiatry. *Archives of General Psychiatry*, 1968, *18*, 257–266.

Kuehnel, T., & Kuehnel, J. Mental health consultation: An educative approach. In. S. Cooper & W. F. Hodges (Eds.), *The field of mental health consultation*. New York: Human Sciences Press, 1983.

Lalonde, M. *A new perspective on the health of Canadians*. Ottawa: Canadian Government Printing Office, 1974.

Lamb, H. R., & Zusman, J. Primary prevention in perspective. *American Journal of Psychiatry*, 1979, *136*, 12–17.

Langner, T. S. A twenty-two item screening score of psychiatric symptoms indicating impairment. *Journal of Health and Human Behavior*, 1962, *3*, 269–276.

Langner, T. S., & Michael, S. T. *Life stress and mental health*. New York: Macmillan, 1963.

Lawrence, J. E. S. Science and sentiment: Overview of research on crowding and human behavior. *Psychological Bulletin*, 1974, *81*, 712–720.

Lawton, M. P., Lipton, M. B., Fulcomer, M. C., & Kleban, M. H. Planning for a mental hospital phasedown. *American Journal of Psychiatry,* 1977, *134,* 1386–1390.

Lazare, A., Cohen, F., Jacobson, A. M., Williams, M. W., Mignone, R. J., & Zisook, S. The walk-in patient as a "customer": A key dimension in evaluation and treatment. *American Journal of Orthopsychiatry,* 1972, *42,* 872–883.

Lazarus, R. S. *Psychological stress and the coping process.* New York: McGraw-Hill, 1966.

Lazarus, R. S. *Patterns of adjustment* (3rd ed.). New York: McGraw-Hill, 1976.

Leff, M. J., Roatch, J. F., & Bunney, W. E. Environmental factors preceding the onset of severe depression. *American Journal of Psychiatry,* 1970, *33,* 293–311.

Leighton, A. H. *My name is legion.* New York: Basic Books, 1959.

Leighton, D. C., Harding, J. S., Macklin, D. B., MacMillan, A. M., & Leighton, A. H. *The character of danger.* New York: Basic Books, 1963.

Lemkau, P. V. Assessing a community's need for mental health services. *Hospital & Community Psychiatry,* 1967, *18,* 65–70.

Levenson, R. W., & Gottman, J. M. Toward the assessment of social competence. *Journal of Consulting and Clinical Psychology,* 1978, *46,* 453–462.

Leventhal, H., Safer, M. A., Cleary, P. D., & Gutmann, M. Cardiovascular risk modification by community-based programs for life-style change: Comments on the Stanford study. *Journal of Consulting and Clinical Psychology,* 1980, *48,* 150–158.

Levine, D. S., & Willner, S. G. *The cost of mental illness, 1974.* NIMH Statistical Note 125. Washington, D.C.: U.S. Government Printing Office, 1976.

Levine, M. *The history and politics of community mental health.* New York: Oxford University Press, 1981.

Levine, M., & Brocking, M. Mental health consultation with senior nursing students. *American Journal of Community Psychology,* 1974, *2,* 229–242.

Levy, J., & Munroe, R. *The happy family.* New York: Knopf, 1938.

Levy, L. The state mental hospital in transition: A review of principles. *Community Mental Health Journal,* 1965, *1,* 353–356.

Levy, L., & Herzog, A. N. Effects of population density and crowding on health and social adaptation in the Netherlands. *Journal of Health and Social Behavior,* 1974, *15,* 228–240.

Levy, L., & Rowitz, L. *Ecology of mental disorders.* New York: Behavioral Publications, 1972.

Levy, S. R., Iverson, B. K., & Walberg, H. J. Nutrition-education research: An interdisciplinary evaluation and review. *Health Education Quarterly,* 1980, *7,* 107–127.

Lew, E. A. Mortality and the business cycle: How far can we push the association? *American Journal of Public Health,* 1979, *69,* 782–783.

Lew, E. A. Heart disease mortality: Changing terminology, diagnostic fashions, and capabilities. *American Journal of Public Health,* 1980, *70,* 411–412.

Lewin, K. *Principles of topological psychology.* New York: McGraw-Hill, 1936.

Lewin, K. *Field theory in social science: Selected theoretical papers.* New York: Harper, 1951.

Lewin, K. K. *Brief encounters: Brief psychotherapy.* St. Louis, Mo.: Warren H. Green, 1970.

Lewis, J. M., Beavers, W. R., Gossett, J. T., & Phillips, V. A. *No single thread: Psychological health in family systems.* New York: Brunner/Mazel, 1976.

Lewis, M. S., Gottesman, D., & Gutstein, S. The course and duration of crisis. *Journal of Consulting and Clinical Psychology,* 1979, *47,* 128–134.

Libo, L. M., & Griffith, C. R. Developing mental health programs in areas lacking professional facilities: The community consultation approach in New Mexico. *Community Mental Health Journal,* 1966, *2,* 163–169.

Lieberman, M. A., & Borman, L. D. The impact of self-help groups on widows' mental health. *National Reporter,* 1981, *4,* 2–6.

Lifton, R. J. Statement on the Buffalo Creek disaster. In H. J. Parad, H. L. P. Resnik, & L. G. Parad (Eds.), *Emergency and disaster management: A mental health sourcebook.* Bowie, Md.: Charles Press, 1976.

Lifton, R. J., & Olson, E. The human meaning of total disaster: The Buffalo Creek experience. *Psychiatry*, 1976, *39*, 1–18.

Lin, N., Simeone, R. S., Ensel, W. M., & Kuo, W. Social support, stressful life events, and illness: A model and an empirical test. *Journal of Health and Social Behavior*, 1979, *20*, 108–119.

Lindemann, C., & Scott, W. J. Wanted and unwanted pregnancy in early adolescence: Evidence from a clinic population. *Journal of Early Adolescence*, 1981, *1*, 185–193.

Lindemann, E. Symptomatology and management of acute grief. *American Journal of Psychiatry*, 1944, *101*, 141–148.

Lindsay, W. R., Symons, R. S., & Sweet, T. A program for teaching social skills to socially inept adolescents: Description and evaluation. *Journal of Adolescence*, 1979, *2*, 215–228.

Litman, R. E., & Farberow, N. L. Emergency evaluation of self destructive potentiality. In N. L. Farberow & E. S. Shneidman (Eds.), *The cry for help*. New York: McGraw-Hill, 1961.

Littlepage, G. E., Kosloski, K. D., Schnelle, J. F., McNees, M. P., & Gendrich, J. C. The problems of early outpatient terminations from community mental health centers: A problem for whom? *Journal of Community Psychology*, 1976, *4*, 164–167.

Locke, H. J. *Predicting adjustment in marriage*. New York: Holt, 1951.

Lombana, J. H. Counseling the elderly: Remediation plus prevention. *Personnel and Guidance Journal*, 1976, *55*, 143–144.

Lowenthal, M. F., & Haven, C. Interaction and adaptation: Intimacy as a critical variable. *American Sociological Review*, 1968, *33*, 20–30.

Lowy, F. H., Wintrob, R. M., & Dhindsa, B. Man and his anxiety: Psychiatric emergencies at Expo '67. *Laval Medical*, 1969, *40*, 966–970.

Lukton, R. C. Crisis theory: Review and critique. *Social Service Review*, 1974, *48*, 384–402.

Lynch, J. J. *The broken heart*. New York: Basic Books, 1977.

Maccoby, N., & Alexander, J. Reducing heart disease risk using the mass media: Comparing the effects on three communities. *Social and psychological research in community settings*. San Francisco, Calif.: Jossey-Bass, 1979.

Maccoby, N., & Farquhar, J. W. Communication for health: Unselling heart disease. *Journal of Communication*, 1975, *25*, 114–126.

Maccoby, N., Farquhar, J. W., Wood, P. D., & Alexander, J. Reducing the risk of cardiovascular disease: Effects of a community based campaign on knowledge and behavior. *Journal of Community Health*, 1977, *3*, 100–114.

MacLennan, B. W., Montgomery, S. L., & Stern, E. G. *The analysis and evaluation of the consultation component in a community mental health center*. Laboratory Paper No. 36, Mental Health Study Center. Adelphi, Md.: National Institute of Mental Health, 1970.

MacMahon, B., & Pugh, T. F. Suicide in the widowed. *American Journal of Epidemiology*, 1965, *81*, 23–31.

MacMahon, B., & Pugh, T. F. *Epidemiology: Principles and methods*. Boston, Mass.: Little, Brown, 1970.

MacMahon, B., Pugh, T. F., & Hutchison, G. B. Principles in the evaluation of community mental health programs. *American Journal of Public Health*, 1961, *51*, 963–968.

MacMahon, B., Pugh, T. F., & Ipsen, J. *Epidemiologic methods*. Boston, Mass.: Little, Brown, 1960.

Magnusson, D. The individual in the situation: Some studies on individuals' perception of situations. *Studia Psychologica*, 1974, *16*, 124–132.

Maier, S. F., & Seligman, M. E. P. Learned helplessness: Theory and evidence. *Journal of Experimental Psychology: General*, 1976, *105*, 3–46.

Malan, D. H. *A study of brief psychotherapy*. London: Tavistock, 1963.

Malan, D. H. *The frontier of brief psychotherapy: An example of the convergence of research and clinical practice*. New York: Plenum, 1976.

Malan, D. H., Heath, E. S., Bacal, H. A., & Balfour, F. H. G. Psychodynamic changes in untreated neurotic patients: II. Apparently genuine improvements. *Archives of General Psychiatry*, 1975, 32, 110–126.

Malzberg, B. Marital status and mental disease among Negroes in New York State. *Journal of Nervous and Mental Disease*, 1956, 123, 457–465.

Malzberg, B. Marital status and the incidence of mental disease. *International Journal of Social Psychiatry*, 1964, 10, 19–26.

Mandell, A. J. The fifteen minute hour. *Diseases of the Nervous System*, 1961, 22, 559–562.

Manis, J. G., Brewer, M. J., Hunt, C. L., & Kerchner, L. C. Estimating the prevalence of mental illness. *American Sociological Review*, 1964, 29, 84–89.

Mann, J. *Time-limited psychotherapy*. Cambridge, Mass.: Harvard University Press, 1973.

Mann, P. A. *Community psychology: Concepts and applications*. New York: Free Press, 1978.

Mannino, F. V. Empirical perspectives in mental health consultation. *Journal of Prevention*, 1981, 1, 147–155.

Mannino, F. V., & MacLennan, B. W. *Monitoring and evaluating mental health consultation and education services*. DHEW Pub. No. (ADM) 77–550. Washington, D.C.: U.S. Government Printing Office, 1978.

Mannino, F. V., MacLennan, B. W., & Shore, M. F. (Eds.). *The practice of mental health consultation*. DHEW Pub. No. (ADM) 74–12. Washington, D.C.: U.S. Government Printing Office, 1975.

Mannino, F. V., & Shore, M. F. *Consultation research in mental health and related fields*. Public Health Monograph No. 79. Washington, D.C.: U.S. Government Printing Office, 1971.

Mannino, F. V., & Shore, M. F. The effects of consultation: A review of empirical studies. *American Journal of Community Psychology*, 1975, 3, 1–21.

Marchant, W. C. Counseling and/or consultation: A test of the education model in the elementary school. *Elementary School Guidance and Counseling*, 1972, 7, 4–8.

Marks, I. Risk factors in anxiety disorders. In D. A. Regier & G. Allen (Eds.), *Risk factor research in the major mental disorders*. DHHS Pub. No. (ADM) 81–1068. Washington, D.C.: U.S. Government Printing Office, 1981.

Marmor, J. (Ed.). *Modern psychoanalysis*. New York: Basic Books, 1968.

Marmor, J. Comment. *American Journal of Psychiatry*, 1974, 131, 780.

Marmor, J. The relationship between systems theory and community psychiatry. *Hospital & Community Psychiatry*, 1975, 26, 807–811.

Marmor, J. Short-term dynamic psychotherapy. *American Journal of Psychiatry*, 1979, 136, 149–155.

Marshall, C. L. *Toward an educated health consumer: Mass communication and quality in medical care*. U.S. Public Health Service Pub. No. (NIH) 77–881. Washington, D.C.: U.S. Government Printing Office, 1977.

Martin, R. L., & Guze, S. B. Risk factors and personality disorders. In D. A. Regier & G. Allen (Eds.), *Risk factor research in the major mental disorders*. DHHS Pub. No. (ADM) 81–1068. Washington, D.C.: U.S. Government Printing Office, 1981.

Marvald, M. M. An indictment of the Community Mental Health Centers Acts—caveat emptor. *Hospital & Community Psychiatry*, 1971, 22, 79–83.

Masterpasqua, F. Toward a synergism of developmental and community psychology. *American Psychologist*, 1981, 36, 782–786.

Matejcek, Z., Dytrych, Z., & Schuller, V. Children from unwanted pregnancies. *Acta Psychiatrica Scandinavica*, 1978, 57, 67–90.

Mattes, J. A., Rosen, B., & Klein, D. F. Comparison of the clinical effectiveness of "short" versus "long" stay psychiatric hospitalization: II. Results of a 3-year posthospital follow-up. *Journal of Nervous and Mental Disease*, 1977, 165, 387–394.

Mattes, J. A., Rosen, B., Klein, D. F., & Millan, D. Comparison of the clinical effectiveness of "short" versus "long" stay psychiatric hospitalization: III. Further results of a 3-year posthospital follow-up. *Journal of Nervous and Mental Disease*, 1977, 165, 395–402.

Mazade, N. A. Consultation and education practice and organizational structure in ten community mental health centers. *Hospital & Community Psychiatry*, 1974, 25, 673–675.

McAlister, A., Puska, P., Salonen, J. T., Tuomilehto, J., & Koskela, K. Theory and action for health promotion: Illustrations from the North Karelia project. *American Journal of Public Health*, 1982, 72, 43–50.

McClure, L., Cannon, D., Belton, E., D'Ascoli, C., Sullivan, B., Allen, S., Connor, P., Stone, P., & McClure, G. Community psychology concepts and research base: Promise and product. *American Psychologist*, 1980, 35, 1000–1011.

McCord, J. B., & Packwood, W. T. Crisis centers and hotlines: A survey. *Personnel and Guidance Journal*, 1973, 51, 723–728.

McGee, R. K. *Crisis intervention in the community.* Baltimore, MD.: University Park Press, 1974.

McGrath, J. E. (Ed.). *Social and psychological factors in stress.* New York: Holt, Rinehart & Winston, 1970.

McLean, E. K., & Tarnopolsky, A. Noise, discomfort and mental health: A review of the socio-medical implications of disturbance by noise. *Psychological Medicine*, 1977, 7, 19–62.

McMillen, R., & Williams, R. T. (Eds.). *Ideas: Newsletter of the National Committee for Mental Health Education.* Special issue, March 1977. Available from R. T. Williams, University of Wisconsin Extension, Madison, Wis.

McMurray, L. Emotional stress and driving performance: The effect of divorce. *Behavioral Research in Highway Safety*, 1970, 1, 100–114.

McNees, M. P., Hannah, J. T., Schnelle, J. F., & Bratton, K. M. The effects of aftercare programs on institutional recidivism. *Journal of Community Psychology*, 1977, 5, 128–133.

McPheeters, H. L. Primary prevention and health promotion in mental health. *Preventive Medicine*, 1976, 5, 187–198.

Measuring the quality of life. *New Human Services Newsletter*, 1971, 1(4).

Mechanic, D. *Mental health and social policy.* Englewood Cliffs, N.J.: Prentice-Hall, 1969.

Mechanic, D. Social class and schizophrenia: Some requirements for a plausible theory of social influence. *Social Forces*, 1972, 50, 305–309.

Medalie, J. H., & Goldbourt, U. Angina pectoris among 10,000 men. *American Journal of Medicine*, 1976, 60, 910–921.

Meltzoff, J., & Kornreich, M. *Research in psychotherapy.* New York: Atherton, 1970.

Mendel, W. M. Brief hospitalization techniques. In J. Masserman (Ed.), *Current psychiatric therapies: 1966* (Vol. 6). New York: Grune & Stratton, 1967.

Menninger, K. *The vital balance.* New York: Viking Press, 1963.

Meyer, A. The life chart and the obligation of specifying positive data in psychopathological diagnosis. In E. E. Winters (Ed.), *The collected papers of Adolf Meyer* (Vol. 3): *Medical Teaching.* Baltimore, Md.: Johns Hopkins Press, 1951.

Meyer, A. J., Nash, J. D., McAlister, A. L., Maccoby, N., & Farquhar, J. W. Skills training in a cardiovascular health education campaign. *Journal of Consulting and Clinical Psychology*, 1980, 48, 129–142.

Meyer, N. G. *Provisional patient movement and administrative data: State and county mental hospital inpatient services, July 1, 1973–June 30, 1974.* NIMH Statistical Note 114. Washington, D.C.: U.S. Government Printing Office, 1975.

Meyer, N. G., & Taube, C. A. *Length of stay of admissions to state and county mental hospitals, United States, 1971.* NIMH Statistical Note 74. Washington, D.C.: U.S. Government Printing Office, 1973.

Meyers, J. Mental health consultation. In J. C. Conoley (Ed.), *Consultation in schools: Theory, research, procedures.* New York: Academic Press, 1981.

Mico, P. R., & Ross, H. S. *Health education and behavioral science.* Oakland, Calif.: Third Party Associates, 1975.

Miller, J. G. The nature of living systems. *Behavioral Science*, 1971, 16, 277–301.

Miller, T. W., Wilson, G. C., & Dumas, M. A. Development and evaluation of social skills training for schizophrenic patients in remission. *Journal of Psychiatric Nursing and Mental Health*, 1979, *17*, 42–46.

Miller, W. B. Psychiatric consultation: Part 1. A general systems approach. *Psychiatry in Medicine*, 1973, *4*, 135–145.

Mills, C. W. *The sociological imagination.* Oxford: Oxford University Press, 1959.

Mishara, B. L., & Patterson, R. D. *Consumer's guide to mental health.* New York: New York Times Books, 1977.

Mishler, E. G., & Waxler, N. E. *Interaction in families: An experimental study of family processes and schizophrenia.* New York: Wiley, 1968.

Mitchell, R. E., & Trickett, E. J. Task force report: Social networks as mediators of social support—an analysis of the effects and determinants of social networks. *Community Mental Health Journal*, 1980, *16*, 27–44.

Moed, G., & Muhich, D. E. Some problems and parameters of mental health consultation. *Community Mental Health Journal*, 1972, *8*, 232–239.

Monahan, J., & Vaux, A. Task force report: The macro-environment and community mental health. *Community Mental Health Journal*, 1980, *16*, 14–26.

Monti, P. M., Curran, J. P., Corriveau, D. P., DeLancey, A. L., & Hagerman, S. M. Effects of social skills training groups and sensitivity training groups with psychiatric patients. *Journal of Consulting and Clinical Psychology*, 1980, *48*, 241–248.

Moore, H. E. *And the winds blew.* Austin, Tex.: Hogg Foundation for Mental Health, 1964.

Moos, R. H. Conceptualizations of human environments. *American Psychologist*, 1973, *28*, 652–665.

Moos, R. H. *Evaluating treatment environments: A social ecological approach.* New York: Wiley, 1974.

Moos, R. H. *Evaluating correctional and community settings.* New York: Wiley, 1975.

Moos, R. H. Evaluating and changing community settings. *American Journal of Community Psychology*, 1976, *4*, 313–326.

Moos, R. H. Social-ecological perspectives on health. In G. C. Stone, F. Cohen, & N. E. Adler (Eds.), *Health psychology—a handbook.* San Francisco, Calif.: Jossey-Bass, 1979.

Moos, R. H., & Moos, B. S. A typology of family social environments. *Family Process*, 1976, *15*, 357–371.

Moos, R. H., & Trickett, E. J. *Classroom environment scale manual.* Palo Alto, Calif.: Consulting Psychologists Press, 1974.

Morrice, J. K. W. *Crisis intervention: Studies in community care.* New York: Pergamon Press, 1976.

Morrison, J. K., & Libow, J. A. The effect of newspaper publicity on a mental health center's community visibility. *Community Mental Health Journal*, 1977, *13*, 58–62.

Morrissy, E., & Handal, P. J. Characteristics of the residential environment scale: Reliability and differential relationship to neighborhood satisfaction in divergent neighborhoods. *Journal of Community Psychology*, 1981, *9*, 125–132.

Mueller, D. P., Edwards, D. W., & Yarvis, R. M. Stressful life events and psychiatric symptomatology: Change or undesirability. *Journal of Health and Social Behavior*, 1977, *18*, 307–317.

Mueller, D. P., Edwards, D. W., & Yarvis, R. M. Stressful life events and community mental health center patients. *Journal of Nervous and Mental Disease*, 1978, *166*, 16–24.

Muench, G. A. An investigation of the efficacy of time-limited psychotheraphy. *Journal of Counseling Psychology*, 1965, *12*, 294–299.

Mulford, H. A., & Wilson, D. W. *Identifying problem drinkers in a household health survey.* PHS Pub. No. 1000, Series 2, No. 16. Washington, D.C.: U.S. Government Printing Office, 1966.

Muller, A. Evaluation of the costs and benefits of motorcycle helmet laws. *American Journal of Public Health*, 1980, 70, 586–592.

Mulvey, E. P., & Reppucci, N. D. Police crisis intervention: An empirical investigation. *American Journal of Community Psychology*, 1981, 9, 527–547.

Mumford, E., Schlesinger, H. J., & Glass, G. V. The effects of psychological intervention on recovery from surgery and heart attacks: An analysis of the literature. *American Journal of Public Health*, 1982, 72, 141–151.

Muñoz, R. F., Glish, M., Soo-Hoo, T., & Robertson, J. The San Francisco mood-survey project: Preliminary work toward the prevention of depression. *American Journal of Community Psychology*, 1982, 10, 317–329.

Munõz, R. F., Snowden, L. R., & Kelly, J. G. (Eds.). *Social and psychological research in community settings*. San Francisco, Calif.: Jossey-Bass, 1979.

Murphy, J. G., & Datel, W. E. A cost-benefit analysis of community versus institutional living. *Hospital & Community Psychiatry*, 1976, 27, 165–170.

Murray, H. A. *Explorations in personality*. New York: Oxford University Press, 1938.

Murray, H. A. Toward a classification of interaction. In T. Parsons & E. A. Shils (Eds.), *Toward a general theory of action*. Cambridge, Mass.: Harvard University Press, 1951.

Myers, J. K., Lindenthal, J. J., & Pepper, M. P. Life events, social integration and psychiatric symptomatology. *Journal of Health and Social Behavior*, 1975, 16, 421–427.

Nagler, S., & Cook, P. E. Some ideological considerations underlying a mental health consultation program to the public schools. *Community Mental Health Journal*, 1973, 9, 244–252.

National Center for Health Statistics. *Mortality from selected causes by marital status*. Series 20, Nos. 8A & 8B. Washington, D.C.: U.S. Government Printing Office, 1970.

National Center for Health Statistics. *Summary report: Final divorce statistics, 1971*. Monthly Vital Statistics Report, Vol. 23, No. 8, Suppl. 3. Washington, D.C.: U.S. Government Printing Office, 1974.

National Center for Health Statistics. *Contraceptive efficacy among married women 15–44 years of age in the United States, 1970–1973*. No. 26, April 6, 1978. Washington, D.C.: U.S. Government Printing Office, 1978. (a)

National Center for Health Statistics. *Contraceptive utilization in the United States: 1973 and 1976*. No. 36, August 18, 1978. Washington, D.C.: U.S. Government Printing Office, 1978. (b)

National Center for Health Statistics. *Patterns of aggregate and individual changes in contraceptive practice: United States, 1965–1975*. DHEW Pub. No. (PHS) 79–1401. Washington, D.C.: U.S. Government Printing Office, 1979.

National Center for Health Statistics. *Wanted and unwanted births reported by mothers 15–44 years of age: United States, 1976*. No. 56, January 24, 1980. Washington, D.C.: U.S. Government Printing Office, 1980.

National Center for Health Statistics. Induced terminations of pregnancy: Reporting states, 1977 and 1978. *Monthly Vital Statistics Report*, 1981, 30 (Sept. 28), 1–27. (a)

National Center for Health Statistics. *Visits to family planning clinics: United States, 1979*. No. 74, September 4, 1981. Washington, D.C.: U.S. Government Printing Office, 1981. (b)

National Institute of Mental Health. *Consultation and education*. USPHS Pub. No. 1478. Washington, D.C.: U.S. Government Printing Office, 1966.

National Institute of Mental Health. *Special report: The first U.S. mission on mental health to the U.S.S.R.* PHS Pub. No. 1893. Washington, D.C.: U.S. Government Printing Office, 1969.

National Institute of Mental Health. *Staffing of mental health facilities, United States, 1972*. DHEW Pub. No. (ADM) 74–28. Washington, D.C.: U.S. Government Printing Office, 1974.

National Institute of Mental Health. *Mental health demographic profile system description: Purpose, contents and sampler of uses*. DHEW Pub. No. (ADM) 76–263. Washington, D.C.: U.S. Government Printing Office, 1975. (a)

National Institute of Mental Health. *A typological approach to doing social area analysis.* DHEW Pub. No. (ADM) 76–262. Washington, D.C.: U.S. Government Printing Office, 1975. (b)

New definitions: Report of the 1972–1973 Joint Committee on Health Education Terminology. *Journal of School Health,* 1974, *44,* 33–35.

Newman, C. J. Children of disaster: Clinical observations at Buffalo Creek. *American Journal of Psychiatry,* 1976, *133,* 306–312.

Newman, F. L., Chapman, J., Deegan, E., & Wescott, W. Decision versus policy in crisis intervention. *American Journal of Community Psychology,* 1979, *7,* 543–563.

A new racial poll. *Newsweek,* February 26, 1979.

Nietzel, M. T., & Fisher, S. G. Effectiveness of professional and paraprofessional helpers: A comment on Durlak. *Psychological Bulletin,* 1981, *89,* 555–565.

Norris, E. L., Larsen, J. K., Arutunian, C., Kroll, J., & Murphy, S. *Allocating resources: Priorities in mental health services delivery.* Palo Alto, Calif.: American Institutes for Research, 1975.

North Carolina Department of Public Instruction, Division of Health, Safety, and Physical Education. *Life skills for health: Focus on mental health* (4 vols.). Raleigh, N.C.: Department of Public Instruction, 1974.

Oborn, P. T. *Review of the literature on social indicators.* Denver, Colo.: Social Welfare Research Institute, University of Denver, 1972.

O'Donnell, J. M., & George, K. The use of volunteers in a community mental health center emergency and reception service: A comparative study of professional and lay telephone counseling. *Community Mental Health Journal,* 1977, *13,* 3–12.

Office of the White House Press Secretary. *Executive order: President's Commission on Mental Health.* Washington, D.C.: White House, 1977. (a)

Office of the White House Press Secretary. *Remarks of the president and Mrs. Carter and question and answer session upon announcing the President's Commission on Mental Health.* Washington, D.C.: White House, 1977. (b)

Oliver, J. M., & Pomicter, C. Depression in automotive assembly-line workers as a function of unemployment variables. *American Journal of Community Psychology,* 1981, *9,* 507–512.

Ollendick, D. G., & Hoffmann, S. M. Assessment of psychological reactions in disaster victims. *Journal of Community Psychology,* 1982, *10,* 157–167.

Olson, D. H., Sprenkle, D. H., & Russell, C. S. Circumplex model of marital and family systems: I. Cohesion and adaptability dimensions, family types, and clinical applications. *Family Process,* 1979, *18,* 3–28.

Osofsky, J. D., & Osofsky, H. J. The psychological reaction of patients to legalized abortion. *American Journal of Orthopsychiatry,* 1972, *42,* 48–60.

Ozarin, L. D., & Feldman, S. Implications for health service delivery: The Community Mental Health Centers Amendments of 1970. *American Journal of Public Health,* 1971, *61,* 1780–1784.

Ozarin, L. D., & Levinson, A. I. The future of the public mental hospital. *American Journal of Psychiatry,* 1969, *125,* 1647–1652.

Ozarin, L. D., & Sharfstein, S. S. The aftermaths of deinstitutionalization: Problems and solutions. *Psychiatric Quarterly,* 1978, *50,* 128–132.

Parad, H. J. (Ed.). *Crisis intervention: Selected readings.* New York: Family Service Association of America, 1965.

Parad, H. J., & Parad, L. G. A study of crisis-oriented planned short-term treatment: Part I. *Social Casework,* 1968, *49,* 346–355.

Parad, H. J., Resnik, H. L. P., & Parad, L. G. *Emergency and disaster management.* Bowie, Md.: Charles Press, 1976.

Parad, L. G. Short-term treatment: An overview of historical trends, issues, and potentials. *Smith College Studies in Social Work,* 1971, *41,* 119–146.

Parad, L. G., & Parad, H. J. A study of crisis-oriented planned short-term treatment: Part II. *Social Casework,* 1968, *49,* 418–426.

Parkes, C. M. Evaluation of a bereavement service. *Journal of Preventive Psychiatry*, 1981, *1*, 179–188.

Pasamanick, B. What is mental illness and how can we measure it? In S. B. Sells (Ed.), *The definition and measurement of mental health*. Washington, D.C.: U.S. Government Printing Office, 1968.

Pasamanick, B., Scarpitti, F. R., & Dinitz, S. *Schizophrenics in the community*. New York: Appleton-Century-Crofts, 1967.

Paykel, E. S. Contribution of life events to causation of psychiatric illness. *Psychological Medicine*, 1978, *8*, 245–253.

Paykel, E. S. Causal relationships between clinical depression and life events. In J. E. Barrett, R. M. Rose, & G. L. Klerman (Eds.), *Stress and mental disorder*. New York: Raven Press, 1979.

Paykel, E. S., Myers, J. K., Dienelt, M. N., Klerman, G. L., Lindenthal, J. J., & Pepper, M. P. Life events and depression. *Archives of General Psychiatry*, 1969, *21*, 753–760.

Pearlin, L. I., & Johnson, J. S. Marital status, life-strains and depression. *American Sociological Review*, 1977, *42*, 704–715.

Pearlin, L. I., & Schooler, C. The structure of coping. *Journal of Health and Social Behavior*, 1978, *19*, 2–21.

Penick, E. C., Powell, B. J., & Sieck, W. A. Mental health problems and natural disaster: Tornado victims. *Journal of Community Psychology*, 1976, *4*, 64–68.

Perez, R. Provision of mental health services during a disaster: The Cuban immigration of 1980. *Journal of Community Psychology*, 1982, *10*, 40–47.

Perkins, R., Nakashima, I., Mullin, M., Dubansky, L., & Chin, M. Intensive care in adolescent pregnancy. *Obstetrics and Gynecology*, 1978, *52*, 179–188.

Perlmutter, F. D. Consultation and education in rural community mental health centers. *Community Mental Health Journal*, 1979, *15*, 58–68.

Perlmutter, F. D., & Silverman, H. A. Conflict in consultation-education. *Community Mental Health Journal*, 1973, *9*, 116–122.

Perlmutter, F. D., & Vayda, A. M. Barriers to prevention programs in community mental health centers. *Administration in Mental Health*, 1978, *5*, 140–153.

Perlmutter, F. D., Vayda, A. M., & Woodburn, P. K. An instrument for differentiating programs in prevention—primary, secondary, and tertiary. *American Journal of Orthopsychiatry*, 1976, *46*, 533–541.

Pervin, L. A. Performance and satisfaction as a function of individual-environment fit. *Psychological Bulletin*, 1968, *69*, 56–68.

Phillips, D. L., & Clancy, K. J. Response bias in field studies of mental illness. *American Sociological Review*, 1970, *35*, 503–515.

Phillips, D. L., & Segal, B. E. Sexual status and psychiatric symptoms. *American Sociological Review*, 1969, *34*, 58–72.

Phillips, E. L., & Johnston, M. S. H. Theoretical and clinical aspects of short-term parent-child psychotherapy. *Psychiatry*, 1954, *17*, 267–275.

Phillips, E. L., & Wiener, D. N. *Short-term psychotherapy and structured behavior change*. New York: McGraw-Hill, 1966.

Pinel, P. A. A treatise on insanity. *History of Medicine Series*, 1962, *14*. (Originally published, 1806.)

Pipes, R. B. Consulting in organizations: The entry problem. In J. C. Conoley (Ed.), *Consultation in schools: Theory, research, procedures*. New York: Academic Press, 1981.

Poindexter, H. A. Meeting the needs of the older person. *Journal of the National Medical Association*, 1976, *68*, 131–134.

Polak, P. R., Deever, S., & Kirby, M. W. On treating the insane in sane places. *Journal of Community Psychology*, 1977, *5*, 380–387.

Polak, P. R., Egan, D., Vandenbergh, R., & Williams, W. V. Prevention in mental health: A controlled study. *American Journal of Psychiatry*, 1975, *132*, 146–149.

Polak, P. R., & Kirby, M. W. A model to replace psychiatric hospitals. *Journal of Nervous and Mental Disease*, 1975, *162*, 13–22.

Prange, A. J., Jr., & Loosen, P. T. Somatic findings in affective disorders: Their status as risk factors. In D. A. Regier & G. Allen (Eds.), *Risk factor research in the major mental disorders*. DHHS Pub. No. (ADM) 81–1068. Washington, D.C.: U.S. Government Printing Office, 1981.

President's Commission on Mental Health. *Report to the president* (Vol. 1). Washington, D.C.: U.S. Government Printing Office, 1978.

President's Committee on Health Education. *Report*. New York: Author, 1973.

Pressman, L., & Carol, A. Crime as a diseconomy of scale. *Review of Social Economy*, 1971, *29*, 227–236.

Price, R. H. Etiology, the social environment, and the prevention of psychological dysfunction. In P. M. Insel & R. H. Moos (Eds.), *Health and the social environment*. Lexington, Mass.: Heath, 1974.

Proshansky, H. M. Environmental psychology and the real world. *American Psychologist*, 1976, *31*, 303–310.

Puryear, D. A. *Helping people in crisis*. San Francisco, Calif.: Jossey-Bass, 1979.

Pyle, R. R. Mental health consultation: Helping teachers help themselves. *Professional Psychology*, 1977, *8*, 192–198.

Pyszka, R. H., & Hall, D. C. *A survey-based methodology for mental health needs assessment*. Menlo Park, Calif.: Stanford Research Institute, 1975.

Quarantelli, E. L. The behavior of panic participants. *Sociology and Social Research*, 1957, *41*, 187–194.

Quarantelli, E. L., & Dynes, R. R. Response to social crisis and disaster. *Annual review of sociology*, 1977, *3*, 23–49.

Rabiner, C. J., & Lurie, A. The case for psychiatric hospitalization. *American Journal of Psychiatry*, 1974, *131*, 761–764.

Rabkin, J. G. Stressful life events and schizophrenia: A review of the research literature. *Psychological Bulletin*, 1980, *87*, 408–425.

Rabkin, J. G., & Struening, E. L. Life events, stress, and illness. *Science*, 1976, *194*, 1013–1020.

Rabkin, R. *Strategic psychotherapy: Brief and symptomatic treatment*. New York: Basic Books, 1977.

Rader, G. E., Bekker, L. D., Brown, L., & Richardt, C. Psychological correlates of unwanted pregnancy. *Journal of Abnormal Psychology*, 1978, *87*, 373–376.

Radloff, L. Sex differences in depression: The effects of occupation and marital status. *Sex Roles*, 1975, *1*, 249–265.

Rahe, R. H. Life-change measurement as a predictor of illness. *Proceedings of the Royal Society of Medicine*, 1968, *61*, 44–46.

Rahe, R. H. The pathway between subjects' recent life changes and their near-future illness reports: Representative results and methodological issues. In B. S. Dohrenwend & B. P. Dohrenwend (Eds.), *Stressful life events: Their nature and effects*. New York: Wiley, 1974.

Rahe, R. H. Life change events and mental illness: An overview. *Journal of Human Stress*, 1979, *5*, 2–10.

Rahe, R. H., McKean, J. E., Jr., & Arthur, R. J. A longitudinal study of life-change and illness patterns. *Journal of Psychosomatic Research*, 1967, *10*, 355–366.

Rangell, L. Discussion of the Buffalo Creek disaster: The course of psychic trauma. *American Journal of Psychiatry*, 1976, *133*, 313–316.

Raphael, B. Preventive intervention with the recently bereaved. *Archives of General Psychiatry*, 1977, *34*, 1450–1454.

Rappaport, J. *Community psychology: Values, research, and action*. New York: Holt, Rinehart & Winston, 1977.

Rappoport, L., & Kren, G. What is a social issue? *American Psychologist*, 1975, *30*, 838–841.

Raschke, H. J. The role of social participation in post-separation and post-divorce adjustment. *Journal of Divorce*, 1977, 129–140.

Raush, H. L., Dittmann, A. T., & Taylor, T. J. Person, setting and change in social interaction. *Human Relations*, 1959, *12*, 361–378.

Redick, R. W., & Johnson, C. *Marital status, living arrangements and family characteristics of admissions to state and county mental hospitals and outpatient psychiatric clinics, United States 1970*. NIMH Statistical Note 100. Washington, D.C.: U.S. Government Printing Office, 1974.

Redlich, F. C., & Pepper, M. Are social psychiatry and community psychiatry subspecialties of psychiatry? *American Journal of Psychiatry*, 1968, *124*, 1343–1350.

Regier, D. A., & Allen, G. (Eds.). *Risk factor research in the major mental disorders*. DHHS Pub. No. (ADM) 81–1068. Washington, D.C.: U.S. Government Printing Office, 1981.

Regier, D. A., Goldberg, I. D., & Taube, C. A. The de facto U.S. mental health services system. *Archives of General Psychiatry*, 1978, *35*, 685–693.

Reid, D. D. Precipitating proximal factors in the occurrence of mental disorders: Epidemiological evidence. In E. M. Gruenberg & M. Huxley (Eds.), *Causes of mental disorders: A review of epidemiological knowledge, 1959*. New York: Milbank Memorial Fund, 1961.

Reid, W. J., & Shyne, A. *Brief and extended casework*. New York: Columbia University Press, 1969.

Reider, N. A type of psychotherapy based on psychoanalytic principles. *Bulletin of the Menninger Clinic*, 1955, *19*, 111–128.

Reiff, R. Social intervention and the problem of psychological analysis. *American Psychologist*, 1968, *23*, 524–531.

Reiff, R. Ya gotta believe. In I. Iscoe, B. L. Bloom, & C. D. Spielberger (Eds.), *Community psychology in transition*. Washington, D.C.: Hemisphere, 1977.

Reiss, D. Intimacy and problem solving: An automated procedure for testing a theory of consensual experience in families. *Archives of General Psychiatry*, 1971, *25*, 442–455.

Rheinstein, M. *Marriage stability, divorce and the law*. Chicago: University of Chicago Press, 1972.

Richard, W. C. Crisis intervention services following natural disaster: The Pennsylvania recovery project. *Journal of Community Psychology*, 1974, *2*, 211–219.

Ridenour, N. *Mental health education: Principles in the effective use of materials*. New York: Mental Health Materials Center, 1969.

Rieder, R. O. Hospitals, patients, and politics. *Schizophrenia Bulletin*, 1974, *11*, 9–15.

Riessman, C. K., Rabkin, J. G., & Struening, E. L. Brief versus standard psychiatric hospitalization: A critical review of the literature. *Community Mental Health Review*, 1977, *2*, 2–10.

Robbins, H. H. Commentary on Brown, "Social implications of deinstitutionalization." *Journal of Community Psychology*, 1982, *10*, 82–83.

Robbins, J. Unmet needs in family planning: A world survey. *Family Planning Perspectives*, 1973, *5*, 232–242.

Robbins, P. R., Spencer, E. C., & Frank, D. A. Some factors influencing the outcome of consultation. *American Journal of Public Health*, 1970, *60*, 524–534.

Roberts, C. A. *Primary prevention of psychiatric disorders*. Toronto: University of Toronto Press, 1968.

Robertson, N. C. The relationship between marital status and the risk of psychiatric referral. *British Journal of Psychiatry*, 1974, *124*, 191–202.

Robin, S. S., & Wagenfeld, M. O. *Paraprofessionals in the human services*. New York: Human Sciences Press, 1981.

Robins, L. N. Sturdy childhood predictors of adult outcomes: Replications from longitudinal studies. In J. E. Barrett, R. M. Rose, & G. L. Klerman (Eds.), *Stress and mental disorder*. New York: Raven Press, 1979.

Roen, S. R. Parameters of a community mental health approach. *Public Health Reports*, 1962, *77*, 755–762.

Roosens, E. *Mental patients in town life: Geel—Europe's first therapeutic community.* Beverly Hills, Calif.: Sage Publications, 1979.

Rose, R. M., Hurst, M. W., & Herd, A. J. Cardiovascular and endocrine responses to work and the risk for psychiatric symptomatology among air traffic controllers. In J. E. Barrett, R. M. Rose, & G. L. Klerman (Eds.), *Stress and mental disorder.* New York: Raven Press, 1979.

Rose, S. M. Deciphering deinstitutionalization: Complexities in policy and program analysis. *Milbank Memorial Fund Quarterly,* 1979, *57,* 429–460.

Rosen, B., Katzoff, A., Carrillo, C., & Klein, D. F. Clinical effectiveness of "short" vs. "long" psychiatric hospitalization: I. Inpatient results. *Archives of General Psychiatry,* 1976, *33,* 1316–1322.

Rosen, G. *A history of public health.* New York: MD Publications, 1958.

Rosen, J. C., & Wiens, A. N. Changes in medical problems and use of medical services following psychological intervention. *American Psychologist,* 1979, *34,* 420–431.

Rosenbaum, A., & Calhoun, J. F. The use of the telephone hotline in crisis intervention: A review. *Journal of Community Psychology,* 1977, *5,* 325–339.

Rosenbaum, C. P. Events of early therapy and brief therapy. *Archives of General Psychiatry,* 1964, *10,* 506–512.

Rosenbaum, C. P., & Beebe, J. E., III. *Psychiatric treatment: Crisis/clinic/consultation.* New York: McGraw-Hill, 1975.

Rosenblatt, S. M., Gross, M. M., Malenowski, B., Broman, M., & Lewis, E. Marital status and multiple psychiatric admissions for alcoholism: A cross-validation. *Quarterly Journal for the Study of Alcoholism,* 1971, *32,* 1092–1096.

Rosenhan, D. L. On being sane in insane places. *Science,* 1973, *179,* 250–258.

Rosenstein, M. J., & Milazzo-Sayre, L. J. *Characteristics of admissions to selected mental health facilities, 1975: An annotated book of charts and tables.* DHHS Pub. No. (ADM) 81–1005. Washington, D.C.: U.S. Government Printing Office, 1981.

Rosenthal, A. J., & Levine, S. V. Brief psychotherapy with children: A preliminary report. *American Journal of Psychiatry,* 1970, *127,* 646–651.

Rosenthal, A. J., & Levine, S. V. Brief psychotherapy with children: Process of therapy. *American Journal of Psychiatry,* 1971, *128,* 141–146.

Roskin, M. Coping with life changes—A preventive social work approach. *American Journal of Community Psychology,* 1982, *10,* 331–340.

Rossi, A. M. Some pre-World War II antecedents of community mental health theory and practice. *Mental Hygiene,* 1962, *46,* 78–94.

Rossi, P. M. Community social indicators. In A. Campbell & P. E. Converse (Eds.), *The human meaning of social change.* New York: Russell Sage Foundation, 1972.

Rossi, R. J., & Gilmartin, K. J. *Handbook of social indicators: Sources, characteristics, and analysis.* New York: Garland STPM Press, 1980.

Rotter, J. B. Generalized expectancies for internal versus external control of reinforcement. *Psychological Monographs: General and Applied,* 1966, *80,* 1–28.

Rowland, K. F. Environmental events predicting death for the elderly. *Psychological Bulletin,* 1977, *84,* 349–372.

Rowland, L. W. Personal communication, December 1, 1975.

Rubin, Z., & Mitchell, C. Couples research as couples counseling. *American Psychologist,* 1976, *36,* 17–25.

Ruch, L. O. A multidimensional analysis of the concept of life change. *Journal of Health and Social Behavior,* 1977, *18,* 71–83.

Ryan, W. Preventive services in the social context: Power, pathology, and prevention. In B. L. Bloom & D. P. Buck (Eds.), *Preventive services in mental health programs.* Boulder, Colo.: Western Interstate Commission for Higher Education, 1967.

Ryan, W. Community care in historical perspective. *Canada's Mental Health,* 1969, Suppl. No. 60.

Ryan, W. Emotional disorder as a social problem: Implications for mental health programs. *American Journal of Orthopsychiatry,* 1971, *41,* 638–645.

Sabin, J. E. Short-term group psychotherapy: Historical antecedents. In S. H. Budman (Ed.), *Forms of brief therapy.* New York: Guilford Press, 1981.

Sadock, B., Newman, L., & Normand, W. C. Short-term group psychotherapy in a psychiatric walk-in clinic. *American Journal of Orthopsychiatry,* 1968, *38,* 724–732.

Sallis, J., & Henggeler, S. W. Needs assessment: A critical review. *Administration in Mental Health,* 1980, *7,* 200–209.

Sameroff, A. J., & Chandler, M. J. Reproductive risk and the continuum of caretaking casualty. In F. D. Horowitz (Ed.), *Review of Child Development Research,* Vol. 4. 1975, 187–244.

Sanders, I. T. *The community: An introduction to a social system* (2nd ed.). New York: Ronald Press, 1966.

Sandler, I. N., & Block, M. Life stress and maladaptation of children. *American Journal of Community Psychology,* 1979, *7,* 425–440.

Sandler, I. N., & Ramsay, T. B. Dimensional analysis of children's stressful life events. *American Journal of Community Psychology,* 1980, *8,* 285–302.

Sanford, N. Is the concept of prevention necessary or useful? In S. E. Golann & C. Eisdorfer (Eds.), *Handbook of community mental health.* New York: Appleton-Century-Crofts, 1972.

Sank, L. Community disasters: Primary prevention and treatment in a health maintenance organization. *American Psychologist,* 1979, *34,* 334–338.

Sarason, I. G. Life stress, self-preoccupation and social supports. In I. G. Sarason & C. D. Spielberger (Eds.), *Stress and anxiety* (Vol. 7). Washington, D.C.: Halstead, 1980.

Sarason, I. G., Johnson, J. H., & Siegel, J. M. Assessing the impact of life changes: Development of the Life Experiences Survey. In I. G. Sarason & C. D. Spielberger (Eds.), *Stress and anxiety* (Vol. 6). New York: Hemisphere, 1979.

Sarason, S. B. *The psychological sense of community: Prospects for a community psychology.* San Francisco, Calif.: Jossey-Bass, 1974.

Sauber, R. S. *Preventive educational intervention for mental health.* Cambridge, Mass.: Ballinger, 1973.

Scheidlinger, S., Struening, E. L., & Rabkin, J. G. Evaluation of a mental health consultation service in a ghetto area. *American Journal of Psychotherapy,* 1970, *23,* 485–493.

Scherl, D. J., & English, J. T. Community mental health and comprehensive health service programs for the poor. *American Journal of Psychiatry,* 1969, *125,* 1666–1674.

Schiff, S. K. Free inquiry and the enduring commitment: The Woodlawn mental health center 1963–1970. In S. E. Golann & C. Eisdorfer (Eds.), *Handbook of community mental health.* New York: Appleton-Century-Crofts, 1972.

Schiff, S. K., & Kellam, S. G. A community-wide mental health program of prevention and early treatment in first grade. In M. Greenblatt, P. E. Emery, & B. C. Glueck, Jr. (Eds.), *Poverty and mental health.* Psychiatric Research Report No. 21. Washington, D.C.: American Psychiatric Association, 1967.

Schinke, S. P., Gilchrist, L. D., & Small, R. W. Preventing unwanted adolescent pregnancy: A cognitive-behavioral approach. *American Journal of Orthopsychiatry,* 1979, *49,* 81–88.

Schlesinger, B. The one-parent family in perspective. In B. Schlesinger (Ed.), *The one-parent family.* Toronto: University of Toronto Press, 1969.

Schless, A. P., Schwartz, L., Goetz, C., & Mendels, J. How depressives view the significance of life events. *British Journal of Psychiatry,* 1974, *125,* 406–410.

Schless, A. P., Teichman, A., Mendels, J., & DiGiacomo, J. N. The role of stress as a precipitating factor of psychiatric illness. *British Journal of Psychiatry,* 1977, *130,* 19–22.

Schmale, A. H. Depression as affect, character style, and symptom formation. *Psychoanalysis and Contemporary Science,* 1972, *1,* 327–351.

Schmale, A. H., & Iker, H. Hopelessness as a predictor of cervical cancer. *Social Science and Medicine,* 1971, *5,* 95–100.

Schmidt, D. E., & Keating, J. P. Human crowding and personal control: An integration of the research. *Psychological Bulletin*, 1979, *86*, 680–700.

Schmitt, R. C. Density, health and social disorganization. *Journal of the American Institute of Planners*, 1966, *32*, 38–40.

Schmitt, R. C., Zane, L. Y., & Nishi, S. Density, health, and social disorganization revisited. *Journal of the American Institute of Planners*, 1978, *44*, 209–211.

Schmuck, R. A. System-process mental health models. In S. Cooper & W. F. Hodges (Eds.), *The field of mental health consultation*. New York: Human Sciences Press, 1983.

Schwartz, A. C. Reflection on divorce and remarriage. *Social Casework*, 1968, *49*, 213–217.

Schwartz, A. N. An observation on self-esteem as the linchpin of quality of life for the aged: An essay. *Gerontologist*, 1975, *15*, 470–472.

Schwartz, M. D. Situation/transition groups: A conceptualization and review. *American Journal of Orthopsychiatry*, 1975, *45*, 744–755.

Schwartz, S., & Johnson, J. *Psychopathology of childhood: A clinical-experimental approach*. New York: Pergamon Press, 1981.

Schwartz, S. L. A review of crisis intervention programs. *Psychiatric Quarterly*, 1971, *45*, 498–508.

Schwebel, R. Youth—a view from Berkeley. In D. Adelson (Ed.), *Man as the measure*. New York: Behavioral Publications, 1972.

Schweitzer, L., & Su, W. H. Population density and the rate of mental illness. *American Journal of Public Health*, 1977, *67*, 1165–1172.

Scrignar, C. B. One-session cure of a case of speech anxiety with a 10 year follow-up. *Journal of Nervous and Mental Disease*, 1979, *167*, 315–316.

Seagull, A. A. Must the deeply disturbed have long-term treatment? *Psychotherapy: Theory, Research and Practice*, 1966, *3*, 36–42.

Segal, J. (Ed.). *Research in the service of mental health: Report of the Research Task Force of the National Institute of Mental Health*. DHEW Pub. No. (ADM) 75–236. Washington, D.C.: U.S. Government Printing Office, 1975.

Segal, S. J. Contraceptive technology: Current and prospective methods. *Milbank Memorial Fund Quarterly*, 1971, *49* (Part 2), 145–171.

Selye, H. The General Adaptation Syndrome and the diseases of adaptation. *Journal of Clinical Endocrinology*, 1946, *6*, 117–230.

Selye, H. *The stress of life*. New York: McGraw-Hill, 1956.

Selzer, M. L., & Vinokur, A. Life events, subjective stress and traffic accidents. *American Journal of Psychiatry*, 1974, *131*, 903–906.

Shachnow, J., & Matorin, S. Community psychiatry welcomes the nonprofessional. *Psychiatric Quarterly*, 1969, *43*, 492–511.

Shatan, C. Community psychiatry—stretcher bearer of the social order? *International Journal of Psychiatry*, 1969, *7*, 312–321.

Sheldon, E. B., & Freeman, H. E. Notes on social indicators: Promises and potential. *Policy Sciences*, 1970, *1*, 97–111.

Sheldon, E. B., & Parke, R. Social indicators. *Science*, 1975, *188*, 693–699.

Shelton, J. D. Very young adolescent women in Georgia: Has abortion or contraception lowered their fertility? *American Journal of Public Health*, 1977, *67*, 616–620.

Shevky, E., & Bell, W. *Social area analysis: Theory, illustrative application, and computational procedure*. Stanford, Calif.: Stanford University Press, 1955.

Shin, D. C. Subjective indicators and the comparative evaluation of the quality of community life. *American Journal of Community Psychology*, 1980, *8*, 523–535.

Shneidman, E. S., & Farberow, N. L. Statistical comparisons between attempted and committed suicides. In N. L. Farberow & E. S. Shneidman (Eds.), *The cry for help*. New York: McGraw-Hill, 1961.

Shore, M. F., & Shapiro, R. The effect of deinstitutionalization on the state hospital. *Hospital & Community Psychiatry*, 1979, *30*, 605–608.

Shoulberg, D. J. Psychoanalytically oriented brief psychotherapy and the community mental health clinician. *Journal of Social Welfare*, 1976, *3*, 65–74.

Shryock, R. H. In the 1840's. In I. Galdston (Ed.), *Social medicine: Its derivations and objectives*. New York: Commonwealth Fund, 1949.

Shure, M. B. Training children to solve interpersonal problems: A preventive mental health program. In R. F. Muñoz, L. R. Snowden, & J. G. Kelly (Eds.), *Social and psychological research in community settings*. San Francisco, Calif.: Jossey-Bass, 1979.

Shure, M. B., & Spivack, G. Interpersonal problem solving in young children: A cognitive approach to prevention. *American Journal of Community Psychology*, 1982, 10, 341–356.

Shyne, A. W. What research tells us about short-term cases in family agencies. *Social Casework*, 1957, 38, 223–231.

Siegel, L. M., Attkisson, C. C., & Cohn, A. H. Mental health needs assessments: Strategies and techniques. In W. A. Hargreaves, C. C. Attkisson, & J. E. Sorensen (Eds.), *Resource materials for community mental health program evaluation* (2nd ed.). Washington, D.C.: U.S. Government Printing Office, 1977.

Sifneos, P. E. Two different kinds of psychotherapy of short duration. *American Journal of Psychiatry*, 1967, 123, 1069–1074.

Sifneos, P. E. *Short-term psychotherapy and emotional crisis*. Cambridge, Mass.: Harvard University Press, 1972.

Sifneos, P. E. *Short-term dynamic psychotherapy: Evaluation and technique*. New York: Plenum Medical Book Co., 1979.

Signell, K. A., & Scott, P. A. Mental health consultation: An interaction model. *Community Mental Health Journal*, 1971, 7, 288–302.

Silverman, D. C. Sharing the crisis of rape: Counseling the mates and families of victims. *American Journal of Orthopsychiatry*, 1978, 48, 166–173.

Silverman, P. R. Services to the widowed: First steps in a program of preventive intervention. *Community Mental Health Journal*, 1967, 3, 37–44.

Silverman, P. R. Widowhood and preventive intervention. *Family Coordinator*, 1972, 21, 95–102.

Silverman, P. R., MacKenzie, D., Pettipas, M., & Wilson, E. *Helping each other in widowhood*. New York: Health Sciences, 1975.

Silverman, W. H., & Beech, R. P. Are dropouts, dropouts? *Journal of Community Psychology*, 1979, 7, 236–242.

Simonton, O. C., Matthews-Simonton, S., & Sparks, T. F. Psychological intervention in the treatment of cancer. *Psychosomatics*, 1980, 21, 226–233.

Simonton, O. C., & Simonton, S. S. Belief systems and management of the emotional aspects of malignancy. *Journal of Transpersonal Psychology*, 1975, 1, 29–47.

Sims, J. H., & Baumann, D. D. The tornado threat: Coping styles of the North and South. *Science*, 1972, 176, 1386–1392.

Sirbu, W., Cotler, S., & Jason, L. A. Primary prevention: Teaching parents behavioral child rearing skills. *Family Therapy*, 1978, 5, 163–170.

Sleet, D. A. The use of games and simulations in health instruction. *California School Health*, 1975, 9, 11–14.

Sleet, D. A., & Stadsklev, R. Annotated bibliography of simulations and games in health education. *Health Education Monographs*, 1977, 5, 74–91.

Sloane, R. B., Staples, F. R., Cristol, A. H., Yorkton, N. J., & Whipple, K. Short-term analytically oriented psychotherapy versus behavior therapy. *American Journal of Psychiatry*, 1975, 132, 373–377.

Small, L. *The briefer psychotherapies* (Rev. ed.). New York: Brunner/Mazel, 1979.

Smith, E. M. A follow-up study of women who request abortion. *American Journal of Orthopsychiatry*, 1973, 43, 574–585.

Smith, M. B. The revolution in mental health care—a "bold new approach"? *Trans/Action*, 1968, 5, 19–23.

Smith, M. B. Ethical implications of population policies: A psychologist's view. *American Psychologist*, 1972, 27, 11–15.

Smith, M. B., & Hobbs, N. The community and the community mental health center. *American Psychologist*, 1966, 21, 499–509.

Smith, M. L. & Glass, G. V. Meta-analysis of psychotherapy outcome studies. *American Psychologist,* 1977, *32,* 752–760.

Smith, W. G. Critical life-events and prevention strategies in mental health. *Archives of General Psychiatry,* 1971, *25,* 103–109.

Smith, W. G., & Hart, D. W. Community mental health: A noble failure? *Hospital & Community Psychiatry,* 1975, *26,* 581–583.

Solomon, F., Walker, W. L., O'Connor, G. J., & Fishman, J. R. Civil rights activity and the reduction of crime among Negroes. *Archives of General Psychiatry,* 1965, *12,* 227–236.

Somers, A. R. (Ed.). *Promoting health: Consumer education and national policy.* Germantown, Md.: Aspen, 1976.

Spanier, G. B., & Casto, R. F. Adjustment to separation and divorce: An analysis of 50 case studies. *Journal of Divorce,* 1979, *2,* 241–253.

Spaulding, R. C., Edwards, D., & Fichman, S. The effect of psychiatric hospitalization in crisis. *Comprehensive Psychiatry,* 1976, *17,* 457–460.

Speers, R. W. Brief psychotherapy with college women: Technique and criteria for selection. *American Journal of Orthopsychiatry,* 1962, *32,* 434–444.

Spencer, H. *The study of sociology.* New York: Appleton, 1882.

Spielberger, C. D. A mental health consultation program in a small community with limited professional mental health resources. In E. L. Cowen, E. A. Gardner, & M. Zax (Eds.), *Emergent approaches to mental health problems.* New York: Appleton-Century-Crofts, 1967.

Spivack, G., & Shure, M. B. *Social adjustment of young children: A cognitive approach to solving real-life problems.* San Francisco, Calif.: Jossey-Bass, 1973.

Spoon, D., & Southwick, J. Promoting mental health through family life education. *Family Coordinator,* 1972, *21,* 279–286.

Srole, L., Langner, T. S., Michael, S. T., Opler, M. K., & Rennie, T. A. C. *Mental health in the metropolis.* New York: McGraw-Hill, 1962.

Stein, R. L. The economic status of families headed by women. *Monthly Labor Review,* December, 1970, pp. 3–10.

Steinberg, H. R., & Durell, J. A stressful social situation as a precipitant of schizophrenic symptoms: An epidemiological study. *British Journal of Psychiatry,* 1968, *114,* 1097–1105.

Stern, G. M. *The Buffalo Creek disaster: The story of the survivors' unprecedented lawsuit.* New York: Random House, 1976. (a)

Stern, G. M. From chaos to responsibility. *American Journal of Psychiatry,* 1976, *133,* 300–301. (b)

Stewart, A., Lafave, H. G., Grunberg, F., & Herjanic, M. Problems in phasing out a large public psychiatric hospital. *American Journal of Psychiatry,* 1968, *125,* 82–88.

Stone, G. L., Hinds, W. C., & Schmidt, G. W. Teaching mental health behaviors to elementary school children. *Professional Psychology,* 1975, *6,* 34–40.

Straker, M. A review of short term psychotherapy. *Diseases of the Nervous System,* 1977, *38,* 813–816.

Strodtbeck, F. L. Husband-wife interaction over revealed differences. *American Sociological Review,* 1951, *16,* 468–473.

Stuart, M. R., & Mackey, K. J. Defining the differences between crisis intervention and short-term therapy. *Hospital & Community Psychiatry,* 1977, *28,* 527–529.

Strupp, H. H. *Psychotherapy: Clinical, research, and theoretical issues.* New York: Jason Aronson, 1973.

Strupp, H. H. Success and failure in time-limited psychotherapy. *Archives of General Psychiatry,* 1980, *37,* 595–603. (a)

Strupp, H. H. Success and failure in time-limited psychotherapy: A systematic comparison of two cases, comparison 2. *Archives of General Psychiatry,* 1980, *37,* 708–716. (b)

Strupp, H. H. Success and failure in time-limited psychotherapy with special reference

to the performance of a lay counselor. *Archives of General Psychiatry*, 1980, *37*, 831–841. (c)

Strupp, H. H. Success and failure in time-limited psychotherapy: Further evidence (comparison 4). *Archives of General Psychiatry*, 1980, *37*, 947–954. (d)

Strupp, H. H., & Hadley, S. W. Specific vs. nonspecific factors in psychotherapy. *Archives of General Psychiatry*, 1979, *36*, 1125–1136.

Sucato, V. The problem-solving process in short-term and long-term service. *Social Service Review*, 1978, *52*, 244–264.

Sue, S., & Zane, N. Learned helplessness theory and community psychology. In M. Gibbs, J. Lachemeyer, & J. Sigal (Eds.), *Community psychology: Theoretical and empirical approaches*. New York: Gardner Press, 1980.

Sundberg, N. D., Snowden, L. R., & Reynolds, W. M. Toward assessment of personal competence and incompetence in life situations. *Annual review of psychology*, 1978, *29*, 179–221.

Sundel, M., & Lawrence, H. A systematic approach to treatment planning in time-limited behavior groups. *Journal of Behavior Therapy and Experimental Psychiatry*, 1977, *8*, 395–399.

Sundel, M., Rhodes, G. B., & Ferguson, E. The impact of a psychiatric hospital crisis unit on admissions and the use of community resources. *Hospital & Community Psychiatry*, 1978, *9*, 569–570.

Sundel, M., & Schanie, C. F. Community mental health and mass media preventive education: The alternatives project. *Social Service Review*, 1978, *52*, 297–306.

Swartzburg, M., & Schwartz, A. A five-year study of brief hospitalization. *American Journal of Psychiatry*, 1976, *133*, 922–924.

Swisher, J. D. Mental health—the core of preventive health education. *Journal of School Health*, 1976, *46*, 386–391.

Syme, S. L. Behavioral factors associated with the etiology of physical disease: A social epidemiological approach. *American Journal of Public Health*, 1974, *64*, 1043–1045.

Syme, S. L., & Torfs, C. P. Epidemiologic research in hypertension: A critical appraisal. *Journal of Human Stress*, 1978, *4*, 43–48.

Tableman, B., Marciniak, D., Johnson, D., & Rodgers, R. Stress management training for women on public assistance. *American Journal of Community Psychology*, 1982, *10*, 357–367.

Talbott, J. A. Deinstitutionalization: Avoiding the disasters of the past. *Hospital & Community Psychiatry*, 1979, *30*, 621–624.

Tannenbaum, S. A. Three brief psychoanalyses. *American Journal of Urology and Sexology*, 1919, *15*, 145–151.

Taplin, J. R. Crisis theory: Critique and reformulation. *Community Mental Health Journal*, 1971, *7*, 13–23.

Tarnopolsky, A., Barker, S. M., Wiggins, R. D., & McLean, E. K. The effect of aircraft noise on the mental health of a community sample: A pilot study. *Psychological Medicine*, 1978, *8*, 219–233.

Tauss, W. A note on the prevalence of mental disturbance. *Australian Journal of Psychology*, 1967, *19*, 121–123.

Taylor, D. G., Aday, L. A., & Andersen, R. A. A social indicator of access to medical care. *Journal of Health and Social Behavior*, 1975, *16*, 39–49.

Tennant, C., & Andrews, G. A scale to measure the stress of life events. *Australian and New Zealand Journal of Psychiatry*, 1976, *10*, 27–32.

Tennant, C., & Andrews, G. The pathogenic quality of life event stress in neurotic impairment. *Archives of General Psychiatry*, 1978, *35*, 859–863.

Tennant, C., Smith, A., Bebbington, P., & Hurry, J. The contextual threat of life events: The concept and its reliability. *Psychological Medicine*, 1979, *9*, 525–528.

Tennant, C., Smith, A., Bebbington, P., & Hurry, J. Parental loss in childhood. *Archives of General Psychiatry*, 1981, *38*, 309–314.

Test, M. A., & Stein, L. I. Community treatment of the chronic patient: Research overview. *Schizophrenia Bulletin*, 1978, *4*, 350–364.

Theorell, T., & Rahe, R. H. Life changes in relation to the onset of myocardial infarction. In T. Theorell (Ed.), *Psychosocial factors in relation to the onset of myocardial infarction and to some metabolic variables—a pilot study.* Stockholm: Department of Medicine, Seraphimer Hospital, Karolinska Institute, 1970.

Thomas, D. S., & Locke, B. Z. Marital status, education and occupational differentials in mental disease. *Milbank Memorial Fund Quarterly,* 1963, *41,* 145–160.

Thomasson, E., Berkovitz, T., Minor, S., Cassle, G., McCord, D., & Milner, J. S. Evaluation of a family life education program for rural high-risk families: A research note. *Journal of Community Psychology,* 1981, *9,* 246–249.

Titchener, J. L., & Kapp, F. T. Family and character change at Buffalo Creek. *American Journal of Psychiatry,* 1976, *133,* 295–299.

Titchener, J. L., Kapp, F. T., & Winget, C. The Buffalo Creek syndrome: Symptoms and character change after a major disaster. In H. J. Parad, H. L. P. Resnik, & L. G. Parad (Eds.), *Emergency and disaster management: A mental health sourcebook.* Bowie, Md.: Charles Press, 1976.

Titmuss, R. M. Community care of the mentally ill: Some British observations. *Canada's Mental Health,* 1965, Suppl. No. 49.

Tobiessen, J., & Shai, A. A comparison of individual and group mental health consultation with teachers. *Community Mental Health Journal,* 1971, *7,* 218–226.

Totman, R. What makes life events stressful? A retrospective study of patients who have suffered a first myocardial infarction. *Journal of Psychosomatic Research,* 1979, *23,* 193–201.

Totman, R., Kiff, J., Reed, S. E., & Craig, J. W. Predicting experimental colds in volunteers from different measures of recent life stress. *Journal of Psychosomatic Research,* 1980, *24,* 155–163.

Trickett, E. J., & Moos, R. H. Social environment of junior high and high school classrooms. *Journal of Educational Psychology,* 1973, *65,* 93–102.

Trickett, E. J., & Quinlan, D. M. Three domains of classroom environment: Factor analysis of the Classroom Environment Scale. *American Journal of Community Psychology,* 1979, *7,* 279–291.

Trickett, E. J., & Wilkinson, L. Using individual or group scores on perceived environment scale: Classroom Environment Scale as example. *American Journal of Community Psychology,* 1979, *7,* 497–502.

Tryon, R. C., & Bailey, D. E. *Cluster analysis.* New York: McGraw-Hill, 1970.

Tunley, R. *The American health scandal.* New York: Harper & Row, 1966.

Tuomilehto, J., Koskela, K., Puska, P., Björkqvist, S., & Salonen, J. A community anti-smoking programme: Interim evaluation of the North Karelia project. *International Journal of Health Education,* 1978, *21,* 3–15.

Turner, R. J. The epidemiological study of schizophrenia: A current appraisal. *Journal of Health and Social Behavior,* 1972, *13,* 360–369.

Twentyman, C. T., & Zimering, R. T. Behavioral training of social skills: A critical review. *Progress in Behavior Modification,* 1979, *3,* 319–400.

Udell, B., & Hornstra, R. K. Hospitalization and presenting problems. *Comprehensive Psychiatry,* 1975, *16,* 573–580.

Ulmer, R. A., & Kupferman, S. C. An empirical study of the process and outcome of psychiatric consultation. *Journal of Clinical Psychology,* 1970, *26,* 323–326.

Ulrici, D., L'Abate, L., & Wagner, V. The E-R-A model: A heuristic framework for classification of skill training programs for couples and families. *Family Relations,* 1981, *30,* 307–315.

United Nations. *Internation definition and measurement of standards and levels of living.* New York: Author, 1954.

Ursano, R. J. The Viet Nam era prisoner of war: Precaptivity personality and the development of psychiatric illness. *American Journal of Psychiatry,* 1981, *138,* 315–318.

Ursano, R. J., Boydstun, J. A., & Wheatley, R. D. Psychiatric illness in U. S. Air Force

Viet Nam prisoners of war: A five-year follow-up. *American Journal of Psychiatry*, 1981, *138*, 310–314.

Ursano, R. J., & Dressler, D. M. Brief versus long-term psychotherapy: Clinician attitudes and organizational design. *Comprehensive Psychiatry*, 1977, *18*, 55–60.

U.S. Congress. *P.L. 79-487—the National Mental Health Act*. Washington, D.C.: U.S. Government Printing Office, 1946.

U.S. Congress. *P.L. 84-182—the Mental Health Study Act of 1955*. Washington, D.C.: U.S. Government Printing Office, 1955.

U.S. Congress. *P.L. 88-164—Mental Retardation Facilities and Community Mental Health Centers Construction Act of 1963*. Washington, D.C.: U.S. Government Printing Office, 1963.

U.S. Congress. *P.L. 89-105—Mental Retardation Facilities and Community Mental Health Centers Construction Act Amendments of 1965*. Washington, D.C.: U.S. Government Printing Office, 1965.

U.S. Congress. *P.L. 90-31—Mental Health Amendments of 1967*. Washington, D.C.: U.S. Government Printing Office, 1967.

U.S. Congress. *P.L. 90-574—Public Health Service Act, Amendment*. Washington, D.C.: U.S. Government Printing Office, 1968.

U.S. Congress. *P.L. 91-211—Community Mental Health Centers Amendments of 1970*. Washington, D.C.: U.S. Government Printing Office, 1970. (a)

U.S. Congress. *P.L. 91-513—Comprehensive Drug Abuse Prevention and Control Act of 1970*. Washington, D.C.: U.S. Government Printing Office, 1970. (b)

U.S. Congress. *P.L. 93-45—Health Programs Extension Act of 1973*. Washington, D.C.: U.S. Government Printing Office, 1973.

U.S. Congress. *P.L. 93-344—Congressional Budget and Impoundment Control Act of 1974*. Washington, D.C.: U.S. Government Printing Office, 1974.

U.S. Congress. *P.L. 94-63—Public Health Service Act, Amendments*. Washington, D.C.: U.S. Government Printing Office, 1975.

U.S. Congress. *P.L. 95-622—Community Mental Health Centers Act*. Washington, D.C.: U.S. Government Printing Office, 1978.

U.S. Congress. *P.L. 96-398—Mental Health Systems Act*. Washington, D.C.: U.S. Government Printing Office, 1980.

U.S. Department of Health, Education and Welfare. *Planning of facilities for mental health services: Goals, principles, action*. PHS Pub. No. 808. Washington, D.C.: U.S. Government Printing Office, 1961.

U.S. Department of Health, Education and Welfare. *Mental health activities and the development of comprehensive health programs in the community*. PHS Pub. No. 995. Washington, D.C.: U.S. Government Printing Office, 1963.

U.S. Department of Health, Education and Welfare. Regulations, Title 2, P.L. 88–164. *Federal Register*, May 6, 1964, pp. 5951–5956.

U.S. Department of Health, Education and Welfare. *Toward a social report*. Washington, D.C.: U.S. Government Printing Office, 1969.

U.S. Department of Health, Education and Welfare. *An annotated bibliography: Violence at home*. DHEW Pub. No. (ADM) 75–136. Washington, D.C.: U.S. Government Printing Office, 1974.

U.S. Department of Health, Education and Welfare. Births, marriages, divorces, and deaths for 1975. *Monthly Vital Statistics Report*, 1976, 24(10).

U.S. Department of Health, Education and Welfare. *Guide to mental health education materials*. USPHS Pub. No. (ADM) 77–35. Washington, D.C.: U.S. Government Printing Office, 1977. (a)

U.S. Department of Health, Education and Welfare. *Statistics needed for determining the effects of the environment on health*. DHEW Pub. No. (HRA) 77–1457. Washington, D.C.: U.S. Government Printing Office, 1977. (b)

U.S. Department of Health, Education and Welfare. *Field manual for human service work-*

ers in major disasters. DHEW Pub. No. (ADM) 78–537. Washington, D.C.: U.S. Government Printing Office, 1978. (a)

U.S. Department of Health, Education and Welfare. *Health: United States, 1978.* DHEW Pub. No. (PHS) 78–1232. Washington, D.C.: U.S. Government Printing Office, 1978. (b)

U.S. Department of Health, Education and Welfare. *Crisis intervention programs for disaster victims in smaller communities.* DHEW Pub. No. (ADM) 79–675. Washington, D.C.: U.S. Government Printing Office, 1979. (a)

U.S. Department of Health, Education and Welfare. *Healthy people: The Surgeon General's report on health promotion and disease prevention.* Washington, D.C.: U.S. Government Printing Office, 1979. (b)

U.S. Department of Health, Education and Welfare. *Smoking and health: A report of the surgeon general.* DHEW Pub. No. (PHS) 79–50066. Washington, D.C.: U.S. Government Printing Office, 1979. (c)

U.S. Department of Health and Human Services. *Annual summary for the United States, 1979: Births, deaths, marriages, and divorces.* DHHS Pub. No. (PHS) 81–1120. Washington, D.C.: U.S. Government Printing Office, 1980. (a)

U.S. Department of Health and Human Services. *Promoting health/preventing disease: Objectives for the nation.* Washington, D.C.: U.S. Government Printing Office, 1980. (b)

U.S. Department of Health and Human Services. *Aircraft accidents: Emergency mental health problems.* DHHS Pub. No. (ADM) 81–956. Washington, D.C.: U.S. Government Printing Office, 1981. (a)

U.S. Department of Health and Human Services. *Manual for child health workers in major disasters.* DHHS Pub. No. (ADM) 81–1070. Washington, D.C.: U.S. Government Printing Office, 1981. (b)

U.S. Office of Management and Budget. *Social indicators.* Washington, D.C.: U.S. Government Printing Office, 1973.

U.S. Senate Committee on Labor and Public Welfare. *Full Opportunity Act: Hearings on Senate Bill 5, 91st Congress, 1st and 2nd sessions.* Washington, D.C.: U.S. Government Printing Office, 1970.

U.S. Senate Committee on Labor and Public Welfare. *Community Mental Health Centers Act: History of the program and current problems and issues.* Washington, D.C.: U.S. Government Printing Office, 1973.

Vacher, C. D., & Stratas, N. E. *Consultation-education: Development and evaluation.* New York: Human Sciences Press, 1976.

Vachon, M. L. S., Lyall, W. A. L., Rogers, J., Freedman-Letofsky, K., & Freeman, S. J. J. A controlled study of self-help intervention for widows. *American Journal of Psychiatry, 1980, 137,* 1380–1384.

Vander Veen, F. The parent's concept of the family unit and child adjustment. *Journal of Counseling Psychology, 1965, 12,* 196–200.

van Rooijen, L. Widows' bereavement: Stress and depression after 1½ years. In I. G. Sarason & C. D. Spielberger (Eds.), *Stress and anxiety* (Vol. 6). Washington, D.C.: Hemisphere, 1979.

Vidaver, R. M. The mental health technician: Maryland's design for a new health career. *American Journal of Psychiatry, 1969, 125,* 1013–1023.

Viney, L. L. The concept of crisis: A tool for clinical psychologists. *Bulletin of the British Psychological Society, 1976, 29,* 387–395.

Vinokur, A., & Selzer, M. L. Life events, stress and mental disorders. *Proceedings, 81st Annual Convention, American Psychological Association,* 1973, 329–330.

Vinokur, A., & Selzer, M. L. Desirable versus undesirable life events: Their relationship to stress and mental distress. *Journal of Personality and Social Psychology, 1975, 32,* 329–337.

Wagner, E. H. The North Karelia project: What it tells us about the prevention of cardiovascular disease. *American Journal of Public Health, 1982, 73,* 51–53.

Walker, K. N., MacBride, A., & Vachon, M. L. S. Social support networks and the crisis of bereavement. *Social Science and Medicine,* 1977, *11,* 35–41.

Wallace, C. J., Nelson, C. J., Liberman, R. P., Aitchison, R. A., Lukoff, D., Elder, J. P., & Ferris, C. A review and critique of social skills training with schizophrenic patients. *Schizophrenia Bulletin,* 1980, *6,* 42–63.

Wallerstein, J. S., & Kelly, J. B. Effects of divorce on the visiting father-child relationship. *American Journal of Psychiatry,* 1980, *137,* 1534–1539.

Walton, E. G., & Russell, R. D. Affective mental health education with sight and sound experiences. *Journal of School Health,* 1978, *48,* 661–666.

Wandersman, A., & Moos, R. H. Assessing and evaluating residential environments: A sheltered living environments example. *Environment and Behavior,* 1981, *13,* 481–508.

Warheit, G. J. Life events, coping, stress, and depressive symptomatology. *American Journal of Psychiatry,* 1979, *136,* 502–507.

Warheit, G. J., Bell, R. A., & Schwab, J. J. *Needs assessment approaches: Concepts and methods.* DHEW Pub. No. (ADM) 79–492. Washington, D.C.: U.S. Government Printing Office, 1977.

Warren, R. L. *Studying your community.* New York: Free Press, 1965.

Warren, R. L. *The community in America* (2nd ed.). Chicago, Ill.: Rand McNally, 1972.

Watson, G. S., Zador, P. L., & Wilks, A. The repeal of helmet use laws and increased motorcyclist mortality in the United States, 1975–1978. *American Journal of Public Health,* 1980, *70,* 579–585.

Watson, G. S., Zador, P. L., & Wilks, A. Helmet use, helmet use laws, and motorcyclist fatalities. *American Journal of Public Health,* 1981, *71,* 297–300.

Watzlawick, P. *The language of change: Elements of therapeutic communication.* New York: Basic Books, 1978.

Watzlawick, P., Weakland, J., & Fisch, R. *Change: Principles of problem formation and problem resolution.* New York: W. W. Norton, 1974.

Wechsler, H., & Pugh, T. F. Fit of individual and community characteristics and rates of psychiatric hospitalization. *American Journal of Sociology,* 1967, *73,* 331–338.

Wechsler, H., Thum, D., Demone, H. W., Jr., & Dwinnell, J. Social characteristics and blood alcohol level. *Quarterly Journal for the Study of Alcoholism,* 1972, *33,* 132–147.

Weiss, R. S. The emotional impact of marital separation. *Journal of Social Issues,* 1976, *32,* 135–145.

Weiss, R. S. *Going it alone.* New York: Basic Books, 1979.

Weissman, M. M., & Klerman, G. L. Epidemiology of mental disorders: Emerging trends in the United States. *Archives of General Psychiatry,* 1978, *35,* 705–712.

Wellner, A. M., & Simon, R. A survey of associate-degree programs for mental health technicians. *Hospital & Community Psychiatry,* 1969, *20,* 166–169.

Wells, K. C., Hersen, M., Bellack, A. S., & Himmelhoch, J. Social skills training in unipolar nonpsychotic depression. *American Journal of Psychiatry,* 1979, *136,* 1331–1332.

White, R. W. Motivation reconsidered: The concept of competence. *Psychological Review,* 1959, *66,* 297–333.

Whiteside, T. A. A countervailing force. *New Yorker,* October 8, 1973, pp. 50ff.

Whittington, H. G. The third psychiatric revolution—really? *Community Mental Health Journal,* 1965, *1,* 73–80.

Wicker, A. W. Ecological psychology: Some recent and prospective developments. *American Psychologist,* 1979, *34,* 755–765.

Wilcox, L. D., Brooks, R. M., Beal, G. M., & Klonglan, G. E. *Social indicators and societal monitoring: An annotated bibliography.* San Francisco, Calif.: Jossey-Bass, 1972.

Wildman, R. C., & Johnson, D. R. Life change and Langner's 22-item mental health index: A study and partial replication. *Journal of Health and Social Behavior,* 1977, *18,* 179–188.

Williams, R. T. Mental health education: The untapped resource. Unpublished paper, University of Wisconsin Extension, 1979.

Williams, T. *Post-traumatic stress disorders of the Vietnam veteran: Observations and recommendations for the psychological treatment of the veteran and his family.* Cincinnati, Ohio: Disabled American Veterans, 1980.

Williams, W. V., & Polak, P. R. Follow-up research in primary prevention: A model of adjustment in acute grief. *Journal of Clinical Psychology,* 1979, *35,* 35–45.

Williamson, G. S. & Pearse, I. H. *Science, synthesis and sanity.* Chicago, Ill.: Henry Regnery, 1966.

Wilson, G. T. Behavior therapy as a short-term therapeutic approach. In S. H. Budman (Ed.), *Forms of brief therapy.* New York: Guilford Press, 1981.

Winslow, C. E. A. *The evolution and significance of the modern public health campaign.* New Haven, Conn.: Yale University Press, 1923.

Winter, W. D., & Ferreira, A. J. (Eds.). *Research in family interaction: Readings and commentary.* Palo Alto, Calif.: Science and Behavior Books, 1969.

Witkin, M. J. *Provisional patient movement and selective administrative data, state and county mental hospitals, inpatient services by state: United States 1976.* Statistical Note 153. Washington, D.C.: U.S. Government Printing Office, 1979.

Witkin, M. J. *Provisional patient movement and selective administrative data, state and county mental hospitals, by state: United States, 1977.* Statistical Note 156. Washington, D.C.: U.S. Government Printing Office, 1981.

Wolberg, L. R. Methodology in short-term therapy. *American Journal of Psychiatry,* 1965, *122,* 135–140. (a)

Wolberg, L. R. *Short-term psychotherapy.* New York: Grune & Stratton, 1965. (b)

Wolberg, L. R. The technic of short-term psychotherapy. In L. R. Wolberg (Ed.), *Short-term psychotherapy.* New York: Grune & Stratton, 1965. (c)

Wolberg, L. R. Short-term psychotherapy. In J. Marmor (Ed.), *Modern psychoanalysis.* New York: Basic Books, 1968.

Wolf, A. Short-term group psychotherapy. In L. R. Wolberg (Ed.), *Short-term psychotherapy.* New York: Grune & Stratton, 1965.

Wolfer, J. A., & Visintainer, M. A. Pediatric surgical patients' and parents' stress responses and adjustment. *Nursing Research,* 1975, *24,* 244–255.

Wolff, H. G. Life stress and bodily disease—a formulation. In H. G. Wolff, S. G. Wolf, Jr., & C. C. Hare (Eds.), *Life stress and bodily disease.* Baltimore, Md.: Williams & Wilkins, 1950.

Wolkon, G. H. Crisis theory, the application for treatment, and dependency. *Comprehensive Psychiatry,* 1972, *13,* 459–464.

Wolpert, J., & Wolpert, E. R. The relocation of released mental hospital patients into residential communities. *Policy Sciences,* 1976, *7,* 31–51.

Woody, R. H. Process and behavioral consultation. *American Journal of Community Psychology,* 1975, *3,* 277–285.

World Health Organization. *Epidemiology of mental disorders.* WHO Technical Report No. 185. Geneva: Author, 1960.

Yolles, S. F. Past, present and 1980: Trend projections. In L. Bellak & H. H. Barten (Eds.), *Progress in community mental health* (Vol. 1). New York: Grune & Stratton, 1969.

Young, C. E., True, J. E., & Packard, M. E. A national survey of associate degree mental health programs. *Community Mental Health Journal,* 1974, *10,* 466–474.

Zacker, J., Rutter, E., & Bard, M. Evaluation of attitudinal changes in a program of community consultation. *Community Mental Health Journal,* 1971, *7,* 236–241.

Zarle, T. H., Hartsough, D. M., & Ottinger, D. R. Tornado recovery: The development of a professional-paraprofessional response to a disaster. *Journal of Community Psychology,* 1974, *2,* 311–320.

Zautra, A., & Beier, E. The effects of life crisis on psychological adjustment. *American Journal of Community Psychology,* 1978, *6,* 125–135.

Zautra, A., Beier, E., & Cappel, L. The dimensions of life quality in a community. *American Journal of Community Psychology,* 1977, *5,* 85–97.

NAME INDEX

479

SUBJECT INDEX

Abortion, 419, 420–421,
422–424
crisis intervention and,
150–151
Accidents, traffic, *see* Traffic
accidents
Additive burden hypothesis,
251, 252
Admission rates, to
hospitals, 210–211, 212,
223–224, 262, 370
Adults, competency training
for, 344–346
Aftercare, 15–16, 41, 43, 45,
46, 47 (*see also*
Deinstitutionalization)
recidivism rates and, 45
Air traffic controllers, and
stress, 279
Alcoholics and alcoholism,
30, 32, 66, 95–96, 167,
222, 261
marital status and, 226, 227
provision of services to
prevent, 25–26, 50
social support and, 281
Alternatives Project, 329–331
Angina pectoris, and social
support, 284–285
Anxiety-provoking short-
term psychotherapy, of
Sifneos, 75–77
Appraisal, and reactions to
stressful life events, 250
Asian Americans, *see* Chinese
Americans
Assessment, *see* Evaluation;
Need assessment
Athletes, and crisis
intervention, 119–120
Attitudes:
toward abortion, 422–424
toward blacks, 318
toward health, 319–320
toward length of therapy,
60, 101–102

Attitudes (*continued*)
of mental health
professionals, 60,
101–102
toward mentally ill, 16
toward mental retardation,
332
toward psychopathology
and psychiatric patients,
42–43, 47
toward time, 76
Authority figures, erosion of
status of, 35
Automobile accidents, *see*
Traffic accidents

Behavior:
attitude, *see* Attitudes
crowding, 414–417
grief, 105–106, 145–146
human, 403
Behavior modification, 59
Benevolent profiteering, 40
Bereavement, and crisis
intervention, 145–146
Biopsychosocial medical
model, 37
Bipolar manic-depressive
disorder, 255
Birth control, *see*
Contraception; Family
planning
Blacks, 264, 291, 428
attitudes toward, 318
consultation programs for,
182
Brief confrontive therapy of
Lewin, 72–75
Brief contact therapy, 89–91
Brief strategic therapy of
Erickson, 83–85
Brief therapy, 57–102 (*see also*
Planned short-term
therapy)
Buffalo Creek disaster of
1972, 122–124, 131

Cancer:
lung, and rate of death,
211, 213
stressful life events and,
260–261
Cardiovascular disease, 318,
323
social support and,
284–285
Catchment area (health),
24–25, 36
definition of, 3
Census tracts, 359–360
analysis of, 360–370, 401
ranges, means, and
definitions of variables,
362–363
Central nervous system,
injuries to, 204
Change:
social, 237, 261
stress and, 277
Child, unwanted, and
developmental
difficulties, 421
Child abuse, programs to
reduce, 340–341
Childbirth, as stressful life
event, 255
Childhood disorders:
schizophrenia, 206–207
stressful life events and,
257–258, 288–290
Children, 13, 172, 242 (*see
also* Parents; Schools)
coping skills training for, 229
disorders in, and stressful
life events, 257–258,
288–290
elective surgery and, 324
mental health services for,
13, 16, 26, 30, 50, 92, 93,
162–163, 201, 229–230
prevention of
psychopathology in,
206–207

489